THE BLOOMSBURY HANDBOOK OF CARE ETHICS

Also available from Bloomsbury

The Bloomsbury Handbook of Ethics, edited by Christian Miller

The Bloomsbury Handbook of Plato, edited by Gerald A. Press and Mateo Duque

The Bloomsbury Handbook of 21st-Century Feminist Theory, edited by Robin Truth Goodman

The Bloomsbury Handbook to the Medical-Environmental Humanities, edited by Scott Slovic, Swarnalatha Rangarajan and Vidya Sarveswaran

The Bloomsbury Handbook of Existentialism, edited by Jack Reynolds, Ashley Woodward and Felicity Joseph

THE BLOOMSBURY HANDBOOK OF CARE ETHICS

Edited by Matilda Carter

BLOOMSBURY ACADEMIC
LONDON • NEW YORK • OXFORD • NEW DELHI • SYDNEY

BLOOMSBURY ACADEMIC
Bloomsbury Publishing Plc
50 Bedford Square, London, WC1B 3DP, UK
1385 Broadway, New York, NY 10018, USA
29 Earlsfort Terrace, Dublin 2, Ireland

BLOOMSBURY, BLOOMSBURY ACADEMIC and the Diana logo are
trademarks of Bloomsbury Publishing Plc

First published in Great Britain 2025

Cover design by Terry Woodley
Cover image: People holding hands and offering assistance to a person in need.
(© stellalevi / Getty Images)

A catalogue record for this book is available from the British Library.

A catalog record for this book is available from the Library of Congress.

ISBN: HB: 978-1-3504-2837-9
ePDF: 978-1-3504-2838-6
eBook: 978-1-3504-2839-3

Series: Bloomsbury Handbooks

Typeset by Integra Software Services Pvt. Ltd.

For product safety related questions contact productsafety@bloomsbury.com.

To find out more about our authors and books visit www.bloomsbury.com
and sign up for our newsletters.

CONTENTS

List of Figures vii
List of Tables viii
List of Contributors ix
Acknowledgements xiii

Introduction 1
Matilda Carter

Part 1 Understanding care ethics

1 Care ethics and Chinese philosophy 9
Michael Slote

2 Reconceptualizing care: mature care and asymmetric relationships 17
Tove Pettersen

3 Dependency as a core concept for care ethics: a chronology (and a plea) 41
Simon van der Weele

4 A metaethics of care? Revisiting the normative authority of care ethics 61
Mercer E. Gary

5 Care ethics and phenomenology 81
Carlo Leget

6 Necessary care, moral practices and the cultivation of competent carers 97
Matilda Carter

7 Freedom to care, for women of colour 113
Asha Leena Bhandary

8 Political perspectives on care: what can we learn from Nancy Fraser? 133
Christine Noël Lemaitre

9 Care, justice and equality 141
Costanza Porro

10 Care ethics and structural injustice 157
Stephanie Collins

11 Normative questions, empirical burdens and global justice: perspectives from care ethics 179
Fiona Robinson

12 The ethics of care as a transformation in moral philosophy 195
Sandra Laugier

Part 2 Applying care ethics

13 The importance of enduring and living complex care-ethical inquiry: a plea for intimacy and reciprocity in collaborative care-ethical research 215
Alistair Niemeijer and Gustaaf Bos

14 Inquiring into materialized care: hospital beds as living landscapes of care 231
Merel Visse and Alistair Niemeijer

15 Care ethics and care policies in South Korea 251
Hee-Kang Kim

16 Notes from a care network: lessons from the pandemic 267
Sunita George and Raymond Greene

17 Queer care and pleasure activism 281
Amy McKiernan

18 Imagining care ethics: disability, violence and caring spaces – Trudy's mothering story 299
Chrissie Rogers

19 Care in unexpected places: punishment and forensic detention 317
Helen Brown Coverdale

20 Care ethics and public administration: an overview of the field and a look forward 335
Petr Urban

21 Care ethics, maternity and reproductive justice 355
Inge van Nistelrooij and Rodante van der Waal

22 Care ethics and conflicts in needs: balancing disabled and feminist perspectives and experiences in personalized social care services 377
Kirstein Rummery

23 Cultivating moral epiphanies through care 395
Maurice Hamington

24 Feminist care ethics and temporality 409
Sophie Bourgault

INDEX 428

FIGURES

14.1 Scenery 1: Watercolour and ink on paper 240

14.2 Scenery 2: Watercolour, ink and charcoal on paper 240

14.3 Scenery 3: Unexpected scenery in a Dutch hospital 241

14.4 Scenery 4: Unexpected scenery in a US hospital 241

TABLES

21.1	Two models of morality	363
21.2	Maternal thinking and midwifery thinking	367
22.1	Universal provision: Denmark, Sweden and Iceland	382
22.2	Partnership-based provision: Germany and the Netherlands	382
22.3	France and the Netherlands: formal schemes	388
22.4	The UK and the United States: semi-formal schemes	389
22.5	Austria and Italy: informal schemes	389

CONTRIBUTORS

Asha Leena Bhandary is Associate Professor of Philosophy at the University of Iowa, USA. She has made substantial contributions to the field of care ethics, including examining its interactions with liberalism in her 2020 monograph *Freedom to Care: Liberalism, Dependency Care, and Culture*, and with issues of race and gender in her standalone journal article 'Caring for Whom? Racial Practices of Care and Liberal Constructivism' (*philosophies*, 2022).

Gustaaf Bos is Assistant Professor in Care Ethics at the University of Humanistic Studies, Utrecht, Netherlands. He has published extensively on issues related to care ethics in both English and Dutch. His notable works include 'The Value of Inequality' (*Social Inclusion*, 2016, co-authored with Doortje Kal) and 'Responding to Otherness: The Need for Experimental-Relational Spaces' (*Evaluation for a Caring Society* edited by Merel Visse and Tineke A. Abma, 2018, co-authored with Tineke Abma).

Sophie Bourgault is Professor of Political Studies at the University of Ottawa, Canada. Her notable publications include 'Prolegomena to a Caring Bureaucracy' (*European Journal of Women's Studies*, 2017) and 'Epistemic Injustice, Face-to-Face Encounters and Caring Institutions' (*International Journal of Care and Caring*, 2020).

Helen Brown Coverdale is a Lecturer in Political Theory at University College London, UK. She has published extensively on the ethics of care in the area of criminal justice, and has an emerging research interest in the ethical qualities of human relationships with technology. Her notable publications include 'Caring and the Prison in Philosophy, Policy and Practice: Under Lock and Key' (*Journal of Applied Philosophy,* 2021) and 'Social Connection, Interdependence and Being Sure of Ourselves' (*Analysis*, 2022).

Matilda Carter is a British Academy Postdoctoral Fellow in Philosophy, based at the University of Glasgow, UK. Her primary research arc concerns the interactions between relational egalitarianism and social care practices, with particular emphasis on the care of people living with dementia. She explores these issues at length in her monograph *Relating to People Living with Dementia as Equals* (2025).

Stephanie Collins is Associate Professor of Philosophy at Monash University, Australia, specializing in theories of collective agency and collective responsibility in moral, social and political philosophy. Her notable works include the monographs *The Core of Care Ethics* (2015) and *Group Duties: Their Existence and Their Implications for Individuals* (2019).

Mercer E. Gary is Assistant Professor of Philosophy at Drexel University, USA, and a Presidential Scholar at the Hastings Center, specializing in feminist ethics and bioethics.

Her notable publications include 'Care Robots, Crises of Capitalism, and the Limits of Human Caring' (*International Journal of Feminist Approach to Bioethics*, 2021), 'From Care Ethics to Pluralist Care Theory: The State of the Field' (*Philosophy Compass*, 2022) and 'Relational Approaches in Bioethics: A Guide to Their Differences' (*Bioethics*, 2023).

Sunita George is Professor of Geography at Western Illinois University, USA, with research expertise in population geography and public health.

Raymond Greene is a researcher with expertise in geography, who has previously collaborated with Sunita George in the book chapter 'Care Ethics in the Time of Covid-19: Are We Our Brother's Keepers? Some Insights from the Efforts of "Food for Chennai", India' (*Systemic Inequality, Sustainability and Covid-19*, edited by Seela Aladuwaka and Barbara Wejnert, 2022).

Maurice Hamington is Professor of Philosophy at Portland State University, USA. He has published extensively on feminist philosophy and the ethics of care, including the monographs *Embodied Care* (2004) and *Revolutionary Care: Commitment and Ethos* (2024).

Hee-Kang Kim is Professor in the Department of Public Administration at Korea University, South Korea. She has research expertise in care ethics, justice theory, feminist theory, and normative policy analysis, and her notable publications include: 'Marriage Migration between South Korea and Vietnam: A Gender Perspective' (*Asian Perspective*, 2012) and 'Should Feminism Transcend Nationalism? A Defense of Feminist Nationalism in South Korea' (*Women's Studies International Forum*, 2009).

Sandra Laugier is Professor of Philosophy at Université Paris 1 Panthéon Sorbonne, France, and a Senior Member of Institut Universitaire de France. She serves as the Director of the Sorbonne Centre for Contemporary Philosophy, and has published extensively on issues relevant to the ethics of care in both English and French. Her notable works include the books *Tous vulnérables? Le care, les animaux et l'environnement* (2012) and *Why We Need Ordinary Language Philosophy* (2013).

Carlo Leget is Professor of Care Ethics at the University of Humanistic Studies, Utrecht, Netherlands, serving as chair of the Care Ethics department and the director of research. He has published extensively on applied issues around the ethics of care, including in the article 'Analyzing Dignity: A Perspective from the Ethics of Care' (*Medicine, Health Care and Philosophy*, 2013) and in his book *Art of Living, Art of Dying: Spiritual Care for a Good Death* (2017).

Christine Noël Lemaitre is a philosopher based at Aix-Marseille University, France. She specializes in moral and political philosophy and in the application of philosophers such as Hannah Arendt and Simone Weil to contemporary social issues. Her notable works in English include 'Thinking about the Institutionalization of Care with Hannah Arendt: A Nonsense Filiation?' (*philosophies*, 2022, co-authored with Catherine Chaberty) and 'Learning from Greek Philosophers: The Foundational and Structural Conditions of Ethical Training in Business Schools' (*Journal of Business Ethics*, 2018, co-authored with

Sandrine Frémaux and Grant Michelson). She has also published notable work in French, including the 2019 book *Arendt Pas à Pas*.

Amy McKiernan is Associate Professor of Philosophy at Dickinson College, Pennsylvania, USA. Her notable publications include 'Blaming from Inside the Birdcage: Strawsonian Accounts of Blame and Feminist Care Ethics' (*Feminist Philosophy Quarterly*, 2022) and 'Do Metaphors Matter? Fibromyalgia and Women's Embodiment' (*International Journal of Feminist Approaches to Bioethics*, 2018).

Alistair Niemeijer is Assistant Professor in Care Ethics at the University of Humanistic Studies, Utrecht, Netherlands. His research focuses on precarious practices of care and the wellbeing of the vulnerable, and his notable works include 'Challenging Standard Concepts of "Humane" Care through Relational Auto-Ethnography' (*Social Inclusion*, 2016, co-authored with Merel Visse) and 'Be a Good Sport: A Care Ethical Inquiry into Sport Parenting' (*Sport, Ethics and Philosophy*, 2024, co-authored with Esther Schoots and Gustaaf Bos).

Inge van Nistelrooij is Assistant Professor of Care Ethics at the University of Humanistic Studies, Utrecht, Netherlands. Her notable publications include 'Against Dichotomies: On Mature Care and Self-Sacrifice in Ethics' (*Nursing Ethics*, 2016, co-authored with Carlo Leget) and 'Beyond Demarcation: Care Ethics as an Interdisciplinary Field of Inquiry' (*Nursing Ethics*, 2019, co-authored with Carlo Leget and Merel Visse).

Tove Pettersen is Professor of Philosophy at the University of Oslo, Norway, specializing in feminist philosophy and the ethics of care. She has published extensively in these fields, with notable contributions including the journal articles 'The Ethics of Care: Normative Structures and Empirical Implications' (*Care Analysis*, 2011) and 'Conceptions of Care: Altruism, Feminism and Mature Care' (*Hypatia*, 2012), alongside her 2008 monograph *Comprehending Care: Problems and Possibilities in the Ethics of Care*.

Costanza Porro is a Lecturer in Political Philosophy at the University of Lancaster, UK, specializing in relational equality and the ethics of care. Her notable works include 'Esteem, Social Norms, and Status Inequality' (*Ethical Theory and Moral Practice*, 2021) and 'Criminal Blame, Exclusion and Moral Dialogue' (*Criminal Law and Philosophy*, 2021).

Fiona Robinson is Professor of Political Science at Carleton University, Canada, specializing in International Relations and Political Theory. She has made substantial contributions to the field of care ethics, and her notable works include the monographs *The Ethics of Care: A Feminist Approach to Human Security* (2011) and *Globalizing Care: Ethics, Feminist Theory and International Relations* (1999).

Chrissie Rogers is Professor of Sociology at the University of Kent, UK. She has published extensively on intellectual disability, mothering, and the ethics of care, including the books *Parenting and Inclusive Education: Discovering Difference, Experiencing Difficulty* (2007) and *Intellectual Disability and Being Human: A Care Ethics Model* (2016).

Kirstein Rummery is Professor in Sociology, Social Policy and Criminology at the University of Stirling, UK. She has research expertise in comparative care policy and gender equality, disability support, women's politicization and partnership working between health and social care. Her notable outputs include the monograph *Disability, Citizenship and Community Care: A Case for Welfare Rights?* (2002) and the journal article 'Partnerships and Collaborative Governance in Welfare: The Citizenship Challenge' (*Social Policy and Society*, 2006).

Michael Slote is Professor of Ethics at the University of Miami, USA. A longstanding and influential contributor to the field of care ethics, his notable publications include the books *Goods and Virtues* (1983), *The Ethics of Care and Empathy* (2007) and *Moral Sentimentalism* (2010).

Petr Urban is Senior Researcher at the Institute of Philosophy, Czech Academy of Sciences, where he serves as Deputy Head of the Department of Applied Philosophy and Ethics and Vice Chair of the Board of the Institute of Philosophy. He has expertise in political theory, applied ethics and phenomenology and his notable publications include 'Toward an Expansion of an Enactive Ethics with the Help of Care Ethics' (*Frontiers in Psychology*, 2014) and 'Enactivism and Care Ethics: Merging Perspectives' (*Filozofia*, 2015).

Merel Visse is Associate Professor at the University of Humanistic Studies, Utrecht, Netherlands. Her research centres on the relations between care, morality and creativity, involving the development of both scholarly publications and artistic works. Her notable publications include the book *Evaluation for a Caring Society* (2018) (co-edited with Tineke Abma) and the book chapter 'Your Thoughts Don't Have Words Everyday: Aesthetic Quality in the Health Professions' (*Wonder, Silence and Spaces for Human Flourishing: Towards a Humanization of the Professions of Health & Care, Welfare and Education*, edited by Finn Hansen, Solveig Eide and Carlo Leget, 2023).

Rodante van der Waal is a PhD candidate in Care Ethics at the University of Humanistic Studies, Utrecht, Netherlands. They are also an independent midwife in Amsterdam and a member of the Critical Midwifery Studies Collective. Their notable publications include 'Specter(s) of Care: A Symposium on Midwifery, Relationality, and Reproductive Justice To Come' (*Frontiers*, 2023) and 'The "Dead Baby Card" and the Early Modern Accusation of Infanticide: Situating Obstetric Violence in the Bio- and Necropolitics of Reproduction' (*Feminist Theory*, 2024).

Simon van der Weele is a philosopher and qualitative researcher based at the University of Humanistic Studies, Utrecht, Netherlands. He conducts interdisciplinary research at the intersection of ethics and anthropology, and his published works include 'Shadowing as a Qualitative Method for Intellectual Disability: Opportunities and Challenges' (*Journal of Intellectual Development and Disability*, 2021, co-authored with Femmianne H. Bredewold) and '"Doing" Normativity in Disability Studies: Soft Suggestions Towards an Empirical Ethics of Disability' (*Disability & Society*, 2024).

ACKNOWLEDGEMENTS

This collection was collated and edited while Matilda Carter was in receipt of a British Academy Postdoctoral Fellowship.

Introduction

MATILDA CARTER

Psychologist and feminist theorist Carol Gilligan was not the first to notice gendered differences in psychological tests of moral reasoning, nor the first to speculate as to their origins. Her seminal 1982 text *In a Different Voice: Psychological Theory and Women's Development* broke new ground, however, by placing these differences on an equal footing. Rejecting Lawrence Kohlberg's theory of moral development, Gilligan argued that the interpersonal forms of moral reasoning that prior studies had found more often used by women and girls were not indicators of moral immaturity, but representative of a distinct ethical perspective, no less valuable or developed than the focus on abstract and impersonal principles and rights that was more typically associated with men and boys.[1]

Insofar as it is rightly understood as a branch of feminist philosophy, care ethics (or the ethics of care) has its origins in interpretations of Gilligan's work. Nel Noddings, for example, draws on the proposed gendered distinction in moral perspectives to ground the approach to ethics she develops in her influential 1984 text *Caring: A Feminine Approach to Ethics and Moral Education*.[2] In a more critical vein, Joan Tronto identifies limitations in Gilligan's work in her 1993 book *Moral Boundaries: A Political Argument for an Ethic of Care*, emphasizing the need to place the care perspective within its political context in order to develop a theory that can 'fulfil the promise of transforming the place in our society of women and others who care'.[3]

Today, care ethics has developed into a flourishing field whose adherents include ethicists, social and political philosophers, and social scientists. Sharing the key starting points of inevitable dependence, human interdependence, and the non-voluntary, partial nature of obligations in human relationships, scholars working within this field have generated new insights by bringing these elements to bear on pressing moral and empirical issues. Much of this work continues in the feminist tradition sparked by Gilligan's work, but as the field has grown it has come to encompass scholars who understand its intellectual heritage as older and geographically wider.

Michael Slote, for example, has suggested that care ethics falls within the broader movement of moral sentimentalism, placing his empathy-based account in dialogue with Scottish Enlightenment thinkers like David Hume and Adam Smith.[4] Tove Pettersen has identified a separate, practice-oriented strain within the tradition whose intellectual origins lie in Christian ethics and the ethics of proximity.[5] And Maurice Hamington has drawn connections between care ethics and the tradition of American pragmatism, emphasizing in particular the work of Jane Addams.[6]

Efforts have also been made to situate the work of care ethicists in a global context of similar intellectual traditions. Amanda Gouws and Mikki van Zyl, for instance, have identified common themes between what they call 'Northern' care ethics and the South

African communitarian worldview of Ubuntu, and have made a case for synthesizing the two.[7] Similarly, in a 1994 article Chenyang Li made connections between care ethics and Confucian *ren* ethics, sparking a debate about the compatibility of the two traditions that persists in contemporary scholarship.[8]

With the field becoming increasingly rich and diverse, it is unsurprising that areas of internal disagreement have begun to emerge. Contemporary care ethicists certainly share a common set of assumptions, but the theory's conceptual underpinnings admit of a great deal of disagreement. Indeed, theorists can often struggle even to come to an agreement on how its central concept, 'care', ought to be defined. Speaking to this concern, Virginia Held has noted that much care ethics literature has proceeded without defining the term precisely, sometimes with 'the tacit understanding that of course to a considerable extent we know what we are talking about when we speak of taking care of a child or providing care for the ill'.[9]

Further fractures become apparent when theorists expound on the relationship between care and other central moral concepts like justice. Honouring Gilligan's initial interpretation of gendered differences in moral psychology, some care ethicists see the ethic of care and the ethic of justice as distinct, often contradictory frameworks. Defending this sort of view, Held has sought to provide answers to the question of how their demands ought to be balanced, arguing that both are relevant to most spheres of life, but that there are areas in which one ought to be prioritized over the other.[10]

Others have sought to situate care ethics within the broader scholarship concerned with the nature of justice, seeking to reformulate the latter concept with insights from the former. For example, Eva Feder Kittay has offered a modification of John Rawls's influential framework that takes explicit account of inevitable human dependence and the necessity of dependency workers.[11] More recently, Daniel Engster has argued for a theory of justice that places care at its heart, tracing our duties to one another back to the claims to be cared for that we have made on others and have assumed to be legitimate.[12]

There is also a lack of clarity about how the insights of care ethicists interact with concepts like equality and freedom. Kittay's work is explicitly egalitarian, building into her 1999 monograph *Love's Labor: Essays on Women, Equality, and Dependency* a 'connection-based' equality on the fact of our inevitable dependence – that we are all 'some mother's child'.[13] Marilyn Friedman has offered a similar reformulation of the neo-republican conception of freedom as non-domination, arguing that its identification of domination with the mere capacity to interfere arbitrarily in another's choices renders a vast swathe of dependents in receipt of care unavoidably unfree.[14] For those that separate the ethics of care from the ethics of justice, however, reformulations of such concepts are not typically taken to be necessary. Held, for example, has suggested that concepts like equality and freedom, though important, belong to the impartial ethics of justice, while the ethics of care deals with attentiveness to particular needs in actual circumstances.[15]

One final area of contention worth drawing attention to concerns the approach to and implied view of gender within care ethics. Despite starting life, at least to some extent, as a branch of feminist ethics, significant concerns have been raised by other feminist theorists about the extent to which it incorporates essentialist or otherwise repressive attitudes towards gender. Michele Moody-Adams, for instance, has raised the worry that care ethics generalizes about women's experiences, disregarding those women for whom caring does not take moral priority over impartial rules and rights.[16] In a similar vein, Claudia Card has criticized care ethics for making a virtue out of the attitudes and behaviours shaped by the conditions of women's oppression.[17] These are critiques that are in one sense external, but how care ethicists ought to respond to the concerns raised are a matter of internal debate.

On the one hand, there are theorists who have sought to address feminist suspicion of care ethics directly and bolster its feminist credentials. Tronto's work, in the sense that she reframes care ethics as a moral theory that 'includes the values traditionally associated with women', rather than a distinctive 'women's morality', can be understood in this way.[18] More recently, Fiona Robinson has argued that the theory continues to resonate in spite of feminist concern 'because it speaks to a widespread sense of unease that somehow our priorities are wrong – that what really matters to us, in a deeply moral sense, has somehow been left behind'. Far from valorizing the conditions of women's oppression or placing them outside of the scope of evaluation, care ethics in her view provides us with a critical lens that exposes the social processes that sustain the power relations that determine the priority given to care and the expectations about how it is to be provided.[19]

On the other hand, there are theorists who have sought to deflate concerns about the approach to gender in care ethics by embracing (qualified and caveated versions of) gender essentialism. For example, Slote has noted that there is a significant amount of evidence that suggests that women tend to be more empathetic than men, some of which has been linked to biological differences in hormone levels. Rather than treating this is a reason to be suspicious, however, he has questioned why we ought to be uncomfortable with a theory that implies a natural moral superiority of women over men, especially if that difference is not so great as to prevent it from functioning as an appropriate moral standard for all genders.[20]

It is in this context of increasing intellectual maturity and diversity that this handbook brings together a series of chapters from both established scholars and rising stars at the forefront of care ethics research today. This is a collection that is wide-ranging: drawing on care ethics as it has been developed in multiple philosophical subdisciplines, including political philosophy and aesthetics, alongside work in the social sciences. It is also work that is global in scope, featuring contributions from scholars across the international research community. Nevertheless, it is also a collection that has limits in its content and international reach. While the collection does feature work that deals with care ethics in practical contexts, it is regrettable that we have been unable to include a piece on the relationship between care ethics and nursing ethics. Likewise, while the collection reaches beyond Western scholarship into South Korean and Indian contexts, its contributions are primarily focused on and written by scholars situated in the Global North.

Naturally, a collection of this size could not encompass all the topics, internal distinctions, and applications that fall under the banner of care ethics. Nevertheless, this is a handbook of rigorous, thematically diverse and intellectually accessible scholarship, serving both as an invaluable introductory resource for those new to the field and as a vehicle for making progress in exploring the theory's central themes while generating new insights through novel applications.

THE STRUCTURE OF THE HANDBOOK

This handbook is divided into two sections. In the first, contributors explore the contours of care ethics: its history, its connections with other intellectual traditions, its relationships with nearby concepts and the shape of its internal debates. In the second, contributors apply the theory, exploring issues in applied philosophy and presenting social scientific research findings.

We begin with a contribution from eminent care ethicist Michael Slote, in which he explores connections between care ethics and concepts in Chinese philosophy, using his experience as a longstanding scholar in the field to intervene in an emerging and exciting set of discussions about the relationship between Western and non-Western intellectual traditions. Slote also provides us with his own take on the development of care ethics as a theory, examining its thematic links with the work of the eighteenth-century moral sentimentalists.

This is then followed by two contributions examining central concepts in care ethics. Tove Pettersen discusses the concept of care, making a series of arguments for differentiating what she calls *mature care* from its *altruistic* counterpart and using the former, rather than the latter, as a grounding for care ethics. Drawing on similar themes, Simon van der Weele explores the role of the concept of dependency in care ethics, offering a robust defence of its centrality for the theory in the light of attempts to move away from it. Mercer Gary's contribution complements these chapters by digging deeper into the conceptual underpinnings of care ethics by examining its relationship with normative authority. Carlo Leget then moves away from normative questions towards examining the relationship between care and phenomenology.

The next set of chapters in the first section examines care ethics as a theory within political philosophy. In my chapter, I introduce the concept of *necessary care*, arguing that this is a vital concept for building the care ethicist's case against liberal individualism and fleshing out the content of its moral prescriptions. I then make a case for a thick conception of necessary care, including within it the practices necessary to rear minimally competent carers. This is followed by a piece by Asha Bhandary, who offers a summary of her work on the concept of liberal dependency care and an analysis of the interactions of care ethics and race.

Continuing in this vein, Christine Noël Lemaitre offers an analysis of the work of Nancy Fraser, teasing out its implications for care ethics in the arena of political philosophy. Costanza Porro then engages in a close examination of the concepts of care, justice and equality, identifying some new avenues of inquiry that must be addressed to develop an integrated approach to the three concepts. Drawing on similar themes, Stephanie Collins then offers an analysis of the relationship between care ethics and the concept of structural justice, followed by a discussion from Fiona Robinson on care ethics and global justice. Sandra Laugier closes the first half of the handbook by discussing the impact of care ethics on moral philosophy, arguing that it represents a transformation in this field.

The second section of the handbook begins with two methodological contributions. Alistair Niemeijer and Gustaaf Bos discuss in their chapter the role of intimacy and reciprocity in research, drawing on their own experiences of conducting empirical care ethics studies. Merel Visse, also writing with Niemeijer, then offers a model of inquiry that can be used to conduct care ethics studies that involve a material dimension, using the example of hospital beds.

We then move to some applications of the care approach in specific contexts. Hee-Kang Kim offers an exploration of public policy in South Korea from a care ethics perspective. Sunita George and Raymond Greene's chapter reports on and analyses a concrete example of a care network in Chennai, India. Amy McKiernan examines the connections between care ethics, queer theory and pleasure activism. Then Chrissie Rogers offers a report on the experiences of a mother caring for an adult child with complex care needs.

The next three chapters engage in an analysis of care in underexplored and unusual contexts. Helen Brown Coverdale discusses the roles of care in the criminal justice system and in cases of forensic detention. Petr Urban explores care in the context of public administration. This is followed by two chapters that reflect on public policy questions using the resources of care ethics. The first, from Inge van Nistelrooij and Rodante van der Waal, explores questions of maternity care and reproductive justice. The second, from Kirstein Rummery, explores feminist and disabled perspectives on social services.

The final pair of chapters close out the collection by exploring broader applied questions about care ethics, offering a chance for readers to reflect on the content of the handbook when taken as a whole. Maurice Hamington explores the concept of moral epiphanies and the role care ethics can play in sparking them. Sophie Bourgault then closes by reflecting on care ethics and temporality.

This handbook, in sum, is a collection of timely and novel contributions to the field of care ethics that both consolidates the key literature that has come before it and takes it in new and valuable directions.

NOTES

1. Carol Gilligan, *In a Different Voice: Psychological Theory and Women's Development* (Cambridge: Harvard University Press, 1982),16–23.
2. Nel Noddings, *Caring: A Feminine Approach to Ethics & Moral Education* (Berkeley and Los Angeles: University of California Press, 1984), 75–103.
3. Joan C. Tronto, *Moral Boundaries: A Political Argument for an Ethic of Care* (London: Psychology Press, 1993), 96.
4. Michael Slote, *The Ethics of Care and Empathy* (London: Routledge, 2007), 3–4.
5. Tove Pettersen, 'Conceptions of Care: Altruism, Feminism, and Mature Care', *Hypatia* 27, no. 2 (2012): 367–9.
6. Maurice Hamington, *Embodied Care: Jane Addams, Maurice Merleau-Ponty, and Feminist Ethics* (Champaign: University of Illinois Press, 2010), 89–121.
7. Amanda Gouws and Mikki van Zyl, 'Towards a Feminist Ethics of Ubuntu: Bridging Rights and Ubuntu', in *Care Ethics and Political Theory*, ed. Daniel Engster and Maurice Hamington (New York: Oxford University Press, 2015), 164–86.
8. Chenyang Li, 'The Confucian *Ren* and Care Debate: Reassessment, Development, and Future Directions', *Philosophy Compass* 17, no. 9 (2022): e12868.
9. Virginia Held, *The Ethics of Care: Personal, Political, and Global* (New York: Oxford University Press, 2005), 29.
10. Virginia Held, 'Care and Justice, Still', in *Care Ethics and Political Theory*, ed. Daniel Engster and Maurice Hamington (New York: Oxford University Press, 2015), 18–36.
11. Eva F. Kittay, *Love's Labor: Essays on Women, Equality, and Dependency* (London: Psychology Press, 1999), 82–113.
12. Daniel Engster, *The Heart of Justice: Care Ethics and Political Theory* (Oxford: Oxford University Press on Demand, 2007), 21–65.
13. Kittay, *Love's Labor,* 66–71.
14. Marilyn Friedman, 'Pettit's Civic Republicanism and Male Domination', in *Republicanism and Political Theory*, ed. Cécile Laborde and John Maynor (Malden: Blackwell Publishing, 2008), 254–65.
15. Held, 'Care and Justice, Still', 21–3.
16. Michele M. Moody-Adams, 'Gender and the Complexity of Moral Voices', in *Feminist Ethics*, ed. Claudia Card (Lawrence: University of Kansas Press, 1991), 196–201.

17. Claudia Card, *The Unnatural Lottery: Character and Moral Luck* (Philadelphia: Temple University Press, 1996), 7–8.
18. Tronto, *Moral Boundaries,* 2–3.
19. Fiona Robinson, 'Care Ethics, Political Theory, and the Future of Feminism', in *Care Ethics and Political Theory*, ed. Daniel Engster and Maurice Hamington (New York: Oxford University Press, 2015), 305–6.
20. Slote, *The Ethics of Care and Empathy*, 67–74.

BIBLIOGRAPHY

Card, Claudia. *The Unnatural Lottery: Character and Moral Luck*. Philadelphia: Temple University Press, 1996.

Engster, Daniel. *The Heart of Justice: Care Ethics and Political Theory*. Oxford: Oxford University Press on Demand, 2007.

Friedman, Marilyn. 'Pettit's Civic Republicanism and Male Domination', in *Republicanism and Political Theory*, edited by Cécile Laborde and John Maynor, 246–68. Malden: Blackwell, 2008.

Gilligan, Carol. *In a Different Voice: Psychological Theory and Women's Development*. Cambridge: Harvard University Press, 1982.

Gouws, Amanda, and Mikki Van Zyl. 'Towards a Feminist Ethics of Ubuntu: Bridging Rights and Ubuntu', in *Care Ethics and Political Theory*, edited by Daniel Engster and Maurice Hamington, 164–86. New York: Oxford University Press, 2015.

Hamington, Maurice. *Embodied Care: Jane Addams, Maurice Merleau-Ponty, and Feminist Ethics*. Champaign: University of Illinois Press, 2010.

Held, Virginia. *The Ethics of Care: Personal, Political, and Global*. New York: Oxford University Press, 2005.

Held, Virginia. 'Care and Justice, Still', in *Care Ethics and Political Theory*, edited by Daniel Engster and Maurice Hamington, 18–36. New York: Oxford University Press, 2015.

Kittay, Eva F. *Love's Labor: Essays on Women, Equality, and Dependency*. London: Psychology Press, 1999.

Li, Chenyang. 'The Confucian *Ren* and Care Debate: Reassessment, Development, and Future Directions', *Philosophy Compass* 17, no. 9 (2022), e12868.

Moody-Adams, Michele M. 'Gender and the Complexity of Moral Voices', in *Feminist Ethics*, edited by Claudia Card, 195–212. Lawrence: University of Kansas Press, 1991.

Nath, Rekha. 'Relational Egalitarianism', *Philosophy Compass* 15, no. 7 (2020), e12686.

Noddings, Nel. *Caring: A Feminine Approach to Ethics and Moral Education*. Berkeley and Los Angeles: University of California Press, 1984.

Pettersen, Tove. 'Conceptions of Care: Altruism, Feminism, and Mature Care', *Hypatia* 27, no. 2 (2012), 366–89.

Robinson, Fiona. 'Care Ethics, Political Theory, and the Future of Feminism', in *Care Ethics and Political Theory*, edited by Daniel Engster and Maurice Hamington, 293–311. New York: Oxford University Press, 2015.

Slote, Michael. *The Ethics of Care and Empathy*. London: Routledge, 2007.

Tronto, Joan C. *Moral Boundaries: A Political Argument for an Ethic of Care*. London: Psychology Press, 1993.

PART ONE

Understanding care ethics

CHAPTER ONE

Care ethics and Chinese philosophy

MICHAEL SLOTE

INTRODUCTION

Care ethics has developed in many ways since Carol Gilligan introduced the idea of such an ethics in her classic 1982 book *In a Different Voice: Psychological Theory and Women's Development*.[1] Its reach has been extended, for example, to issues of overall social justice and to many other more specific political/legal issues. And its relation to non-Western ethical thinking has also been noted and discussed. In this chapter, I would like to take that relationship to a deeper and more integrating level, but before I do that, I would like to briefly offer some anecdotage (*sic*) about the history of care ethics, something that the editorship of this volume has asked me to do and that my decades-long history with care ethics puts me perhaps in a good position to do.

1

Let me begin by making a historical conjecture that will be familiar to at least some of you. I believe that all the talk today about caring can be traced back to Gilligan's 1982 book. Before that time, I don't remember anyone talking about caring the way we now do, and that cultural influence is so deeply realized (in one sense but not the other) that people who speak emphatically of caring have no idea where such talk originated.

Here's another point, one that hasn't at all been recognized. Care ethics from its inception put an emphasis on what we now call empathy, and discussions of empathy (sometimes using other language) can be traced all the way back to the eighteenth-century moral sentimentalist David Hume. But care ethics has also placed an unprecedented emphasis on relationships, and the influence of Martin Buber can be seen within that aspect of care ethics. But there is an earlier anticipation of care ethics that has never been pointed out in print, the work of (the Third Earl of) Shaftesbury that inaugurated the movement called moral sentimentalism.

Gilligan teaches us that connection with others is the cornerstone of the caring attitude and of any ethics of caring, but at the time she wrote, she didn't realize that something very similar had been said by Shaftesbury almost three centuries earlier. Strongly disagreeing with his tutor John Locke (yes, really!), Shaftesbury argues that human beings are not originally or ever isolated atomic units, but are actuated by sympathy in a way that connects them deeply with one another. This philosophical anticipation is worth noting, I think, in any history of the care ethics movement.

Let me now mention another more recent historical fact that may help to give us insight into the history of care ethics, and, again, the point is best made in relation to Gilligan. When she introduced the idea of care ethics in her book, she avoided speaking of reason or rationality, and I believe I know why she did (or didn't do) that. The book contrasts the emphasis on connection in care ethics with the emphasis on separateness or autonomy that can be attributed to philosophically familiar 'justice ethics', and it also contrasts the latter's emphasis on following rules or principles with the former's preference for direct action towards and on behalf of individuals. But the relation of care ethics or justice ethics to reason and/or rationality is left entirely out of the picture, and I think Gilligan had good (intellectual/moral) reason to do that.

If she had brought in rationality, it would have to have been on the side of justice ethics, and then care ethics would have in a most obvious way been saddled with the opposing notion of emotion or emotionality. This would immediately have been to the disadvantage of care ethics because it seems at least initially preferable to base moral law and moral principle on reason rather than on sheer emotion. So a focus on rationality would have risked nipping care ethics immediately in the bud. Gilligan presumably didn't want to allow that to happen, and it wasn't till a lecture given in 2015 that Gilligan began to talk seriously about rationality. (We needn't go into what she said, and nowadays there are other attempts to theorize rationality in a way consistent with care ethics.)

Finally, let me mention another aspect of the significance of care ethics that I believe is only now beginning to emerge. In the days since John Rawls and Elizabeth Anscombe, the field of normative ethics has been seen as divided among three influential and competing schools of thought: consequentialism, Kantian ethics and virtue ethics. But Gilligan's contrast between care ethics and justice ethics suggests another way of viewing our options in normative ethical theory. Justice ethics embodies or corresponds roughly to ethical rationalism; care ethics is pretty clearly a form of moral sentimentalism. And the stark contrast Gilligan drew between justice ethics and care ethics and her idea that these two moral 'orientations' have their roots in differences in the way boys and girls are raised can easily lead us to believe (as I myself now believe) that the main issue in normative ethics is between rationalism and sentimentalism rather than holding among the three more familiar opposing moral-theoretic isms. Gilligan's work and subsequent work in care ethics may persuade some of us that the history of ethics and the main issue or issues in ethics should be read very differently from the way that has in recent decades been standard among moral philosophers. Let me now proceed to my main business in this essay.

2

From its inception the relevance of empathy to care ethics has been noted in various ways. Gilligan makes only fleeting reference to empathy, but two years after Gilligan's book appeared, another book was published in which empathy played a crucial role. In her book *Caring: A Feminine Approach to Ethics and Moral Education*, Nel Noddings emphasized the importance of what we nowadays call empathy and she called 'engrossment' to caring motivation and actions.[2] But Noddings never went the further philosophical mile to offer us an overall account of moral right and wrong in terms of empathy/engrossment. She indicated that empathic caring, as with mothers and their children, is highly to be praised, but she never says what, in general, makes an act wrong (or not wrong and therefore in some sense right). Let me offer you my own view of this moral-theoretically central issue: an act is wrong if and only if it shows its agent to be lacking in empathic concern for others (or, more briefly, as lacking in empathy). I am not going to try to defend this general moral-sentimentalist criterion of morally wrong and morally right/permissible action. I have done that at length in other work, most notably my 2010 book *Moral Sentimentalism*.[3] Instead, I propose to show you how Chinese thought can help provide us with further and deeper understanding of why such a criterion is valid. Confucian philosophy has always emphasized benevolence as a virtue, but it has never clearly articulated the notion of empathy that plays such a crucial and foundational role in care ethics. However, Chinese ideas about benevolence and virtue more generally will not be the entry point of what I want to say by way of undergirding present-day care ethics with Chinese categories. The categories I believe can serve us in this way are yin and yang.

Perhaps the most familiar way of understanding yin and yang and their relationship treats them as opposed or contrary physical properties: yin as dark, wet and cold, and yang as bright, dry and warm. These contrary properties are then supposed to alternate with one another with each one driving out the other. Thus as things become darker, brightness eventually causes the darkness to vanish, and brightness is then driven out by darkness in due course. This sort of alternation was or has been supposed to explain why day follows night and night day, but such thinking is incompatible, of course, with modern-day scientific explanations of why day and night alternate (wherever they do). For that reason the oppositional view of yin and yang and of yin/yang as the relationship between them has long been rejected for philosophical use by Chinese thinkers.

Another major tradition of yin/yang thinking sees yin and yang as complementary rather than as contraries, and this is the tradition I shall be drawing on here. Chinese thought, for example, saw Earth as yin and Heaven as yang but saw them as potentially working together rather than as in any way opposites or contraries. To do philosophical and ethical work for us, the complementarian tradition of yin and yang has to be philosophically refined and made in a sense more abstract so that it no longer involves any supposition that yin and yang are the best way to explain the occurrence of natural phenomena. One way to do that is to think of yin as receptivity and of yang as directed active purpose. But for these factors or concepts to function respectively as yin and yang, they have to be shown to depend on one another in a 'friendly' non-oppositional way, something that I believe can be comfortably accomplished.

We can find an example the interpenetration or necessary mutual dependence of yin receptivity and yang directed purpose in the phenomenon of curiosity. The curious person wants to take in facts about some part or all of the world, and that amounts to cognitive receptivity. But by the same token the curious person focuses or pays attention to some part of their environment, and although this is usually non-self-conscious, such focusing or paying of attention involves the directed purpose of knowing. Focusing is a mental *action*, and the two aspects of curiosity, if you think about it, are absolutely inseparable. Let us turn now to ethics and our notions of moral virtue because something similar turns out to be true in that realm.

I first saw the relevance of yin and yang to ethics through theorizing about the nature of compassion. I assume you will grant that the compassionate person acts out of empathy with the distress or suffering of another person (or animal), and that means there are two psychological elements in compassion: empathy with another and motivation to help them. Now a person who wants to help might be killed or injured before they are actually able to help, but at the very least compassion involves an altruistic helping *motive*. Psychologists tend to assume these two elements are only contingently related, but there is, I think, reason to believe otherwise.

Consider a father who is empathically infected (as we say) by his daughter's enthusiasm for stamp collecting. This involves more than just some undifferentiated positive feeling of enthusiasm on the part of the father but ipso facto involves him in feeling enthusiastic *about stamp collecting*. Full-bodied empathy involves taking in positive or negative feeling *as directed towards some object of that feeling*. By the same token, then, if someone is distressed at or by the sharp pain they have in their arm, empathy with their suffering involves being distressed *at or by that very pain, their pain*. But think what this means. To be distressed by something is to wish it diminished or eliminated altogether, and the person distressed by pain in their arm by definition wants that pain to lessen or go away. So, if the empathic observer feels distress at the same pain, they too want to see it lessen or go away; and that represents motivation, altruistic motivation, to help relieve the other person's distress by doing away with or lessening the pain they feel in their arm. Therefore, the two components of compassion are not contingently related, as is so widely supposed, but, rather, the first empathic component necessarily and on purely conceptual grounds entails the altruistic motivation that is the hallmark of compassion.

But not just that. If we consider the altruism involved in compassion, we see that it and the compassion are unthinkable in the absence of any empathy with the sufferer: unthinkable as based on, say, a pure sense of duty. So, the two components of compassion are in a tight two-way connection, and this should remind you of what I said above about yin and yang because the empathy component embodies yin as receptivity and the necessarily related yang altruistic component embodies yang as directed active purpose. Compassion can be thought of, then, as a yin/yang phenomenon, and once we are aware of the categories of yin and yang as conceptualized, as we are conceptualizing them here, we can find a host of other mental or psychological phenomena that fall under those concepts. Let me offer you one more example.

Imagine a man who is sitting in his house and reading when he smells smoke. On investigating, he finds that his house is on fire and that the fire is fast approaching the room he is in. Recognizing the danger this represents to him, he flees out of the house via the only door available for that purpose. If he doesn't flee, that can only be because he doesn't really or fully recognize the danger he faces of a highly painful death, and that means that if he is fully yin receptive to what is happening and its implications for himself, he will be yang purposefully motivated to leave his house via the only available door. Similarly, the fearful yang motive of fleeing can only occur if there is a yin understanding of the dangers of his situation, so the case involves yin and yang in mutual necessitation. Now we think that a compassionate person or action is morally virtuous, but what the man facing a fire exhibits is not moral virtue so much as practical rationality or reasonableness.

Further, and this is important, the applicability of yin and yang to virtuous compassion and fire-fleeing practical rationality helps explain what is valuable about them. Receptivity (as opposed to sheer passivity) is a trait or disposition we think well of, and directed purpose is surely of greater value than purely random, disorderly or chaotic behaviour. If the two cannot be separated, then they constitute a unity of good things, and we think any unity of valuable things/factors has a value independently of – or above and beyond – the value that can be attributed to those factors/things when they are considered separately. We can say, then, that yin and yang and yin/yang may represent the source of the moral value we attribute to compassion (and related qualities of character) and the rational value we attribute to self-protective or prudent action. There is a difference here in the kind of value attributed in these two kinds of cases because we think of morally valuable traits as ones that tend to help others, whereas practical reason or rationality is mainly (though far from exclusively) a matter of traits helpful to oneself. But in either case we can say that yin and yang can be thought of as underlying and helping to explain the moral virtue(s) that care ethics describes and advocates and the rational values that care ethics has in fact had much less to say about.

But why should we want or need to bring in yin and yang as I just have? Why can't the care ethicist rest on or with more familiar categories and factors without appealing to these foreign concepts. It is no accident that there is no standard translation of 'yin' and 'yang' into English. These notions characterize Far Eastern thought insofar as it derives from the Chinese, but India and the West lack them altogether, and it still may not be clear to the reader why I am treating them as so philosophically helpful. In a nutshell, I believe that the basis and justification for bringing in these Chinese concepts is that in addition to relating and applying to familiar ethical ideas about what it is to be moral, they help us clarify and explain a whole host of philosophical issues that *surround* the questions moral philosophy and care ethics pursue on their own.

We have already seen one example of such an issue, the question, basically, of what makes it rational to act in one way or another. Care ethics, as I have said, ignores this question, but our above discussion indicates that both moral caring and individual practical rationality can be brought together under the aegis of yin/yang and the value we place on it. In general, theories seek to explain more and more, and bringing in yin, yang, and yin/yang allows care ethics to usefully and desirably extend its explanatory reach beyond sheer issues of moral right, moral wrong and moral goodness. But we can say more and, in the same vein, again making use of Chinese ideas. Chinese thought and, in particular, the concepts of yin and yang can help us to a better understanding of the human mind in general.

Philosophers seek to understand morality and rationality, and that is very important to many or most of them. But most philosophers have philosophical interests that lie beyond ethics narrowly or conventionally conceived, and philosophy itself, of course, contains disciplinary areas outside ethics proper. Philosophers are interested in the nature and process of knowing things about the world, and this area is called epistemology or theory of knowledge. They are interested in the nature of mathematical and logical truth and how these differ from ordinary knowledge of the world around us. They are interested in understanding aesthetic beauty or excellence in both art and nature. They are interested in exploring the nature of scientific thought and the reasons for its success. And, finally for present purposes, they are interested in the nature of the mind and of psychological functioning.

The last of these is of especial interest to most ethicists because right and wrong actions are anchored in human psychology, and there are issues about human psychology that philosophers (more than psychologists) find perplexing and/or worth studying. Anyone who believes in and wants to explore right and wrong will have to have some sort of view about whether human beings have enough freedom of will to be responsible for doing bad, or good, things. They will typically suppose that humans are capable of altruism and conscientiousness and are thus not totally self-centred selfish beings, but the philosopher wants to know how altruism and the like get a foothold, educationally or congenitally, in the human mind. And I could go on at greater length. The point is that issues in ethics touch on and are affected by what philosophers want to or should say about a whole host of related questions, and, most importantly, that means that if a given ethical view doesn't sit well with what philosophers think we need to say on philosophical or psychological issues outside ethics – especially, issues about knowledge and the nature of the mind – it becomes at least somewhat questionable.

By the same token, however, if plausible surrounding philosophical ideas fit well with some ethical view, that gives us reason, further reason, to be happy with that view. So if I can show you that yin and yang help illuminate issues about knowledge and the nature of the mind, that will support our use of them within ethics. Although care ethics is perfectly capable of proceeding without considering philosophical issues outside of ethics, it can be further supported if those outside issues or considerations fit well with what one wants to say in care ethics. There is reason or more reason to accept our previous explanation of moral and practically rational values in yin/yang terms if we can show that such ethical yin/yang is part of a larger picture in which yin and yang help us to better understanding of human knowledge and the human mind. That is what I would like to try to do in what follows.

3

The Chinese have never sharply distinguished between reason/cognition and emotion/feeling in the way that is typical in Western philosophical thinking. Here I have in mind not only what Chinese philosophers have held but also what is detectable in ordinary Chinese uses of language. The very widely used Chinese term *xin* is ordinarily translated as 'heart-mind' rather than as 'mind' because of the latter term's connotations or meaning in English – and similarly for equivalent terms in other Indo-European languages. In our languages such terms are thought to refer to thinking, reasoning and cognition independently of any emotions/feelings the mind may also contain. But the Chinese don't believe in this sort of thing, and that is why their term *xin* is better translated as heart-mind. The Chinese think all thinking involves emotion or feeling, and other societies of the Far East share this assumption. The Japanese term *kokoro* and the Korean *maum* are also standardly translated as heart-mind rather than mind.

Now someone might say that this just means that the Far East makes use of different concepts from ours and leave it at that. But I think that would be a mistake. Our own Western terms for cognition, belief, thinking and reasoning can apply only if there is feeling present, so it is a mistake to claim that our ways of thinking about the mind are perfectly in order in their own right. I want to claim that the difference between ourselves and the Chinese on the subject of the mind is not a matter of different concepts, but of the Chinese getting things right and our getting them wrong. But how to prove this?

In the West, beliefs about the world around us are generally thought to be independent of all feeling and emotion. We can believe something and also feel emotion *about* the belief or about other things, but it is held that the belief can stand on its own in the mind independently of any such emotion or feeling. All processes and states of a functioning mind involve believing something: reasoning, recognizing what falls under a certain category, planning for the future, criticizing some idea or view – all these demonstrably involve us in believing something or other.

But consider then what it is to believe some proposition p. It is to favour that proposition over competing or incompatible ideas, and favouring is an emotion – in this case a cognitive one. More significantly perhaps, many dictionaries define confidence as strong belief, and every philosopher grants that confidence that p involves a cognitively directed feeling. After all, we say that we *feel* confident that something is the case. But the dictionary definition puts belief *on the same scale* as confidence, understands it as involving a slightly or somewhat lesser degree of positive cognitive feeling towards some fact or proposition. In which case, belief, like confidence, is inseparable from cognitive or, as philosophers say, epistemic feeling, and to complete the scale one can also point out that certitude represents an even more positive epistemic evaluation of some fact or proposition than is entailed by confidence, much less belief.

What follows is that all mental or psychological functioning involves feeling, and that suggests, or more than suggests, that even we in the West have heart-minds rather than minds – contrary to the standard Western view of the matter. This can lead us towards yin/yang if we bring in some relevant further considerations. Take belief in a given sensory proposition about the world. To the extent we are being perceptually receptive to what is around us that belief can be characterized as yin. But where, then, is the yang?

Well, consider what it is to believe, say, that one is seeing a black swan for the first time. One has previously believed and heard that all swans are white, but here one is perceptually encountering an exception. But despite the exception one continues to believe all swans are white while at the same time recognizing that one is now confronting a black swan. Is such a thing possible? Arguably not, and that is because to believe a proposition is automatically to be disposed to make relevant inferences on the basis of that belief. But everyone agrees that inferring is an act of the mind – though as with focusing one is not usually aware that one is doing so. And in this case the inferring goes in a particular direction, towards the view that one or everyone has been mistaken to think all swans are white. Such directed active inferring clearly, then, exemplifies yang, and so all belief turns out to involve not only emotion/feeling but also yin/yang.

In the case where one's yin receptively takes in the surprising fact that there are black swans, one's belief is cognitively or epistemically rational or reasonable; and the cognitive disposition to yang make use of what one believes to correct a previous assumption is also rational. So, ordinary perceptual learning about the world around one is typically rational, and we can conceptualize that epistemic rationality in terms of yin and yang. In the case of the man faced with an oncoming fire, the yin/yang entails or amounts to a kind of practical rationality, rationality in overt actions. In the case of the person encountering a black swan, the yin/yang amounts to a kind of epistemic rationality, and the value or yin and yang can explain and justify the value we place on both epistemic and practical rationality. We are thus well beyond the area of morality. Empathically-based care ethics offers us an account of moral virtue and moral rightness and wrongness, but if we undergird them with yin/yang considerations, we are doing so in a way that makes deep contact with other areas of our values: with the cognitively and with the practically rational. So yin/yang theorizing can give us a broader picture of our values than care ethics can formulate on its own, and the picture is also a philosophically deeper one because the yin/yang explains the value we place on moral virtues like compassion or benevolence that lie at the heart of care-ethical thinking. But we can go somewhat further.

Belief within a functioning mind or heart-mind involves both yin and yang, and the rationality of such belief can be explained accordingly. But what about cases where the mind isn't functional, isn't functioning well? What can we say about them? Well, imagine that someone is so upset that they cannot think straight. They are not really receptive, then, to the facts of their situation and are also too disturbed to act in any kind of concerted fashion. Clearly, they are neither epistemically nor practically rational, but these conclusions can be explained by the fact that neither desirable yin receptivity nor desirable yang directedness of purpose is present in their thinking. So irrationality can be explained in terms of the absence of value when neither yin nor yang is present, and more particularly for moral cases the moral criticizability of indifference to the plight of others can also be criticized in yin/yang terms. If a person lacks empathy for others, they will be indifferent to their fate, but they also lack an important form of human cognitive yin receptivity in a way that we considerable morally undesirable. Their lack of interest in helping those who need help will then count as morally undesirable because of the absence of directed yang motivation that indifference amounts to.

I believe that every aspect of the functioning mind or heart-mind involves yin/yang and that every aspect of a dysfunctional mind shows an absence of both yin and yang. For example, a state of blind panic or of utter mental depression involves neither receptivity nor directed active purposiveness, and a general yin/yang account can explain why these states are dysfunctional and also irrational. Again, but in larger terms, yin/yang allows us to place morality in a wider and deeper philosophically explanatory and justificatory context, so, finally, I want to suggest that care ethicists take yin and yang on board in the way they deploy and develop their approach to normative morality. Moral philosophy takes in a wide variety of issues and subject matters, but it is only one part of philosophy, and all of us ethicists need to remember that.

NOTES

1. Carol Gilligan, *In a Different Voice: Psychological Theory and Women's Development* (Cambridge, MA: Harvard University Press, 1982).
2. Nel Noddings, *Caring: A Feminine Approach to Ethics and Moral Education* (Oakland: University of California Press, 1984).
3. Michael Slote, *Moral Sentimentalism* (New York: Oxford University Press, 2010).

BIBLIOGRAPHY

Gilligan, Carol. *In a Different Voice: Psychological Theory and Women's Development*. Cambridge, MA: Harvard University Press, 1982.

Noddings, Nel. *Caring: A Feminine Approach to Ethics and Moral Education*. Oakland: University of California Press, 1984.

Slote, Michael. *Moral Sentimentalism*. New York: Oxford University Press, 2010.

CHAPTER TWO

Reconceptualizing care

Mature care and asymmetric relationships

TOVE PETTERSEN

INTRODUCTION

Over the last four decades care ethics has developed into a broad field, and many care ethicists have great faith in this theory's potential for creating positive changes. Proponents of care ethics argue that many of our current social problems are due to inadequate care structures and the unwillingness to recognize the importance of care.[1] Global injustice and instability are, from the perspective of care ethics, viewed as largely due to neglect of the provisioning of care as well as the unjust allocation of care work and care resources.[2] If care became recognized as a central normative value for how to live and act, not in only our private lives but also in work life, in social policymaking and in global politics, it would change education, childcare, healthcare, the running of media, the production of culture, art and more. The needs of children, older adults, people with disabilities, and those experiencing poverty would then be at the very centre of our political attention, not at the margins.[3] If care was prioritized globally and domestically it would reduce violence and conflicts,[4] and lead us to take environmental and ecological concerns seriously.[5] As a normative theory, care ethics gives recommendations on how we ought to act and live. The recommendations are applicable to a variety of issues, from reproduction, abortion and childcare to professional care work, poverty, international relations, conflicts and peacekeeping, as well as environmental questions.[6,7] However, in order to act and live in accordance with care ethics, we need to know what it means to care.

In this chapter I want to direct attention to the core concept of an ethics of care – that of care itself. I take as my point of departure that even if a completely accepted and exhaustive definition of care probably never can be given, the normative core concept of any ethical theory should be elucidated. In order to have an operational theory and to avoid misunderstandings, we need to clarify our understanding of the theory's core concept. This holds true whether the central concept is justice, virtue, utility, freedom or, indeed, care. The overall concern here is whether the concepts of care we apply enable us to understand the phenomenon of care adequately, and consequently practise it in accordance with our normative goals.[8]

For many people the word 'care' intuitively has positive connotations; care is understood as doing something good for others; it is done in the best interest of others, often as a selfless, spontaneous and compassionate act. However, 'care' is not a neutral concept. It has a long history where the way we understand and handle care is closely linked to economic structures, colonial history, religion, to class and race, and to conceptions of gender and degree of able-bodiedness. Not only do these features influence our understanding of care, but indeed also people's possibilities for giving as well as receiving care. I will argue that in order to grasp care in a way that avoids holding us captive in bygone metaphysics or present-day prejudices, we carefully need to reconceptualize the concept of care. We need to understand care as referring to a relational activity, as explicitly pertaining to mutual interaction rather than something one party actively performs on a passive receiver. We need to scrutinize the distribution of power and resources in caring relations as well as our preconception of who and why somebody is in the 'giving' while others in the 'receiving' end of care. Such is the concept I have termed mature care, which will be elaborated on throughout the chapter.

In the first part of the chapter, I will shed light on two different understandings of care, an altruistic and a feminist understanding. Both traditions have some blind spots, and I therefore present three arguments to explain why I find it necessary to expound 'care' as 'mature care'. The *genealogy argument* is related to the necessity of getting rid of the adverse historical and cultural connotations that have accreted around the idea of 'care'. The *normative argument* aims at showing that, in accordance with the goals of care, we must have a notion of care that also gives room for caring for the carer. The ontological argument demonstrates that the relational ontology on which the ethics of care is founded also must be taken into account and applied to the new concept of care. In the second part of the chapter, I discuss some challenges with the traditional terminology. In the final section, I demonstrate how reconceptualizing 'care' into 'mature care' can shed light on a particular ethical and philosophical challenge, namely asymmetric caring, which constitutes a significant proportion of caring relationships.

2.1 TWO TRADITIONS AND THE NEED FOR REVISION

Roughly speaking, there are currently two dominant branches within the ethics of care, each one with a different set of conceptions of care.[9] Speaking in generalities, one branch centres primarily on the challenges associated with the caring professions such as nursing, psychiatry, elderly care and social work. Philosophically, it often relies on Martin Heidegger, Knud Løgstrup, Martin Buber and Emmanuel Levinas and its method is primarily phenomenological.[10] With regard to the different fields within philosophical ethics, it seems to focus more on applied ethics than on metaethics. Care ethicists in this branch often locate the historical roots of the ethics of care in the tradition of medicine and nursing, in diaconal practice and in Catholic and Christian ethics.[11] Moreover, care is often understood as altruistic caregiving, and neither gender, race, nor class have been prominent issues in this tradition.[12] Geographically, this version of care ethics appears to be the dominant stance in Europe.

The other main arena, still speaking in generalities, is feminist care ethics. Although feminist care ethics has a long history, the contemporary version is often viewed as having originated in the United States in the 1980s, and to have been deeply influenced by the women's movements of the 1960s and 1970s in Western Europe and the United States. It was the publication of Gilligan's *In a Different Voice*, Nel Noddings's *Caring: A Feminine Approach to Ethics and Moral Education* and Sara Ruddick's *Maternal Thinking: Towards a Politics of Peace* that sparked its development. In these groundbreaking works, gender differences related to care were a major concern. The empirical basis for contemporary feminist care ethics has mainly been the experience of women with unpaid care traditionally considered as *women's work*, such as caring for intimate others in the private sphere, not predominantly with professional caring.[13] Philosophically it is closely linked to feminist philosophy, feminist ethics and moral philosophy. Metaethics – in terms of remodelling and challenging the core concepts, the epistemology and ontology as well as the metaphysic of traditional ethics – is a main concern. This branch of care ethics aims at contributing to the theoretical development of care ethics as well as to the advancement of feminist ethics per se, and indeed to expand the ethics of care into the social as well as the global arena.[14] It has, as all feminist ethics, an explicit normative goal: to end the oppression of women and any other groups. Geographically, its chief location seems to be the United States.

Certainly, the two branches of care ethics that roughly can be characterized as an altruistic-oriented and a feminist-oriented ethics of care have much in common, the most obvious one being their focus on care, and the efforts to make care a central concern in normative thinking as well as practice. They also share taking practice and experience as important points of departure. Furthermore, both strands are critical of traditional moral philosophy and dominant ethical theories, such as deontology and utilitarianism. This critical approach is one reason why the altruistic care ethics tends to espouse phenomenologists such as Heidegger and Løgstrup; they represent alternatives to traditional moral. Within feminist care ethics, the criticism of traditional moral philosophy and ethics, has inspired the development of a new field within moral philosophy: feminist ethics. Clearly, more could be said about differences and similarities regarding these two schools of thought, but this sketch is hopefully sufficient to indicate why there are differences in the way the *concept of care* is used within these two branches of care ethics.

2.1.1 The genealogy argument

There are several indications that an altruistic care ethics is quite widespread.[15] 'Altruistic care', as I have explained elsewhere, expresses an ideal type; it refers to a cluster of culturally characteristic elements commonly used to comprehend care and to evaluate the practice of caring. Care is, in its altruistic version, understood as a *selfless* act that is performed *compassionately*, *spontaneously* and *unconditionally* to benefit a particular needy human being, an act during which the immediate interests and needs of the *particular other* take precedence over those of the carer.[16] The biblical parable of the Good Samaritan embodies altruistic care.[17] Such altruistic understanding of care can further be described as unidirectional, as opposed to bi- or multidirectional: one party in the relation performs the act of caring, another party receives it.[18]

Altruistic care might be what Anita Silvers targets when she claims that 'substituting the ethics of caring for the ethics of equality threatens an even more oppressive paternalism'.[19] When care was institutionalized, 'care-givers' were, according to Silvers, 'persons whose profession it became to channel charity by administering it properly to damaged individuals'. The group of disabled, Silvers continues, 'also became the means of production for members of another group, professional care-givers'.[20] Silvers also targets feminist care ethics: women with disabilities are rarely 'care-givers', they are 'care-receivers'. Moreover, being on the receiving end of care is not always voluntary. On the contrary, it is associated with a confinement of people with disabilities. Care, from the perspective of disability is not necessarily enabling, nor a social relationship to be valorized as it locates power with the carer while the cared-for is understood as a burden. Caring relationships are often asymmetric, and the cared-for is frequently conceptualized as a passive object under the control and power of the carer. The cared-for is viewed as being a dependent recipient of the commendable efforts of the carer[21] who 'is portrayed as a hero'.[22] In *Lesbian Ethics*, Sara Hoagland characterizes altruism as a slave virtue and sees it as an element of a 'phallocratic ethics', i.e. an ethics based on a master/slave dichotomy, whose function 'has been to insulate those on top to facilitate their access to the resources of those under them'.[23] Audre Lorde reflects in *A Burst of Light* on why so many Black women are *not* on the receiving end of care. Black women commonly care for others and shoulder the burdens of others at the expense of their own wellbeing.[24] Consequently, self-care as opposed to altruism can be an act of political warfare because when directing care towards oneself, one is also redirecting care away from what in a racist society is considered worthy of care. Silvers, Hoagland and Lorde's perspectives on care demonstrate, in my opinion, the need to ensure that care ethicists pay close attention to how care is understood and from what perspective.

Given that altruistic care ethics is historically linked to nursing and diaconal practice, which involve caring for the sick and the poor, it should come as no surprise that the main concern of this tradition is the 'needs of others'. Moreover, as altruistic care ethics is kin with Christian and Catholic ethics, which enjoin us to care compassionately for all God's children, to put the needs of the poor and vulnerable first, and where the stories of the Good Samaritan and of Jesus washing the feet of his disciples are taken to be paradigmatic examples of how to respond to the needs of others, it might explain why care is conceived as an unselfish gift to the other. And since we are instructed to take care of *all* God's children equally, it easily follows that little attention is paid to gender, race or other differences in this care tradition. Moreover, as each needy person's uniqueness, and the alleviation of the concrete individual suffering are at the forefront of the altruistic carer's attention, the political and cultural macrostructures that shape each individual's situation are easily moved to the background.

This emphasis on altruism is not prominent in the conception of care in the feminist care tradition even if some critics appear to think so.[25] Gilligan warned care ethicists against the problems associated with self-sacrifice and altruism. Since the feminist branch of care ethics originated precisely from feminist perspectives on women's traditional work, it also focuses on the well-being and rights of the carer (who is often a woman) while questioning the expectation to act altruistically. In *In a Different Voice* Gilligan actually quotes Elisabeth Cady Stanton who in *The Woman's Bible* claims that 'self-development is a higher duty than self-sacrifice'.[26] Furthermore, since the feminist focus on care work is historically linked also to other liberation movements including the anti-slavery movement, the image of washing the feet of others carries very different connotations for adherents of altruistic and feminist care ethics. This and similar images signify exploitation, structures of power, and the instrumentalization and naturalization of certain groups' work rather than genuine care. Since women have been, and many still are, forced into the role of being the carer, and expected to relinquish their own interests for the sake of caring for the needs of others, it is hard to envisage care as a voluntary gift of charity. The majority of working-class women, single mothers, women of colour and women from the Global South do not need to construct 'a class of dependents' in order to fulfil an altruistic calling, or in order to be moral, as Silvers suggests, as they have no other choice but to provide care.[27]

In the two traditions, as I roughly have described them, the concept of care carries very different connotations, and most likely there are several other ways of understanding it.

This in itself makes it all the more urgent to make explicit what is meant by care in order to avoid misunderstandings, and indeed also to get a more accurate understanding of what the normative core concept of this theory means. It is also essential for care ethicists to shatter any images of 'care' in which certain groups of people – women, people of colour, working-class people – are systematically expected to tend to the needs of others at the expense of their own. This conceptualization of care serves as an objectification of certain groups and a concealment of unjust social structures, and is exactly what a feminist ethics of care must distance itself from. The notion of 'mature care' is meant to explicitly surpass the traditional altruistic conception of care.

2.1.2 The normative argument

The second argument for a conception of care as mature care is related to the goals of care; it would be inconsistent as well as unethical not to let the goals of care apply to everyone – including the carer. The normative core value of an ethics of care is, as I see it, twofold: there is the universal condemnation of exploit and hurt, and there is the universal commitment to human flourishing. The first commitment bears certain similarities to the principle of non-maleficence; the second to the principle of beneficence.[28] There are, nevertheless, some important differences between the notion of care I am advocating here, and these two classical normative principles.

Commonly, the principle of non-maleficence is understood as *refraining* from inflicting harm on others. Although not inflicting harm is a core value of care, the normative ideal of an ethics of care involves more than passively refraining from harming – care usually means *active* intervention. Hence the principle of non-maleficence must be expanded to include active intervention to prevent, remove and even repair harm. If the principle of non-maleficence is restricted to refraining from inflicting harm, it is likely to permit passivity when the carer is confronted with the misfortune of others; the abuse next door, or the war abroad will in such a narrow ethical perspective not be part of your moral concern. Also, 'harm' must comprise more than physical harm; psychological, relational, emotional, sexual, economical as well as social and political harm must be included. What is more, the scope of the principle of non-maleficence must be specified not only to focus on harm done to others, but explicitly also to equally condemn and oppose harm to and exploitation of the carer. In an ethics of care the condemnation of harm and exploitation is universal, and a feminist ethics of care must clearly point out that the prevention of harm as well as the possibility to flourish are not restricted to others only. That would be an altruistic version of care.[29]

When the carer is an affluent do-gooder who views their acts of care as the donation of gifts, as charity, the carer will hardly have any reasons to highlight their own situation. As a matter of fact, when the social status between the carer and the cared-for is asymmetric in the sense that the carer is disproportionately well off, the carer might want to avoid drawing attention to their own prosperous situation. The one-sided altruistic focus on the other's care needs might be a convenient way of masking social and political issues, such as an illegitimate structure of power, or an unfair distribution of benefits and burdens. Uma Narayan reminds us that care has been used as an excuse to control others: in the colonial discourse, care was used to legitimate dominance and oppression. The colonizing projects were morally justified by a rhetoric that emphasized that the colonialist cared for and took responsibility for the colonized. This rhetoric was intended to convince the enslaved that it was both right and necessary that they were dominated, and to morally justify the oppression for the colonist themselves. Or in Narayan's own words: 'the colonising project was seen as being *in the interests of, for the good of*, and as *promoting the welfare of* the colonized and to morally justify the oppression for the colonists themselves'.[30]

However, there are many situations in which the carer has not chosen to play that role of her own volition, where her resources are scarce and caring for others increases her destitution.[31] If only the cared-for is entitled to be protected from harm and allowed to flourish, or if people are only expected or permitted to focus on doing good for others, these principles would prevent an agent from resisting oppression and harm – such as when a battered woman prefers not to report abuse because it will harm her abusive partner if she does.

As with the principle of beneficence, i.e. doing good for the benefit of others, the traditional understanding of this principle presents a complication because, apparently, it places no restrictions or limitations on the extent of our obligation to produce good nor does it include care for oneself. This principle, in its unrestrained version, underlies the altruistic understanding of care. It is often necessary to control good deeds, because limitless benevolence could harm and prevent the flourishing of the carer, the cared-for as well as possible third parties in various ways.[32]

It is often difficult to separate the prevention of harm and the promotion of flourishing, as they commonly are interwoven. In a parent–child relationship, for instance, the parent seeks to prevent harm, as well as promote the child's flourishing. In other relationships and caring practices, one of the concerns might be more prominent. When an emergency medic deals with a suicidal patient, the primary aim of care is to prevent harm; later, the therapist aims at alleviating and repairing trauma to enable the patient to eventually flourish. Some professions specialize in certain aspects; care in acute nursing is different from care in a nursery school. As friends, partners or parents, we are concerned with all these aspects, but emphasize different features depending on the circumstances. Refraining from doing harm, the prevention, removal and reparation of harm, and the promotion of flourishing could be envisaged as a continuum.

To prevent harm and to promote flourishing, these aims of caring must hold true for *both* the carer and the cared-for in a caring relationship. The nurse, therapist, teacher and mother are all entitled not to be harmed and not to have caring relationships permanently impede their own flourishing. Feminist care ethicists, among them Eva Kittay, have drawn attention to the fact that the interests of the one caring must also be attended to.[33] This amplification is derived, as I see it, from the fact that the normative value of care is comprehensive – it includes not only the cared-for, but also the carer and other persons for whom they might have a caring responsibility. On a general level, this means that the avoidance of harm and freedom to flourish should count equally for all relevant parties. This particular comprehension of care is included in what I term the concept of mature care. The concept of mature care recognizes that, in principle, one should care as much for oneself as for others – and vice versa – and that to care is more than refraining from harming yourself or others, but also to enable thriving and growth. A feminist ethics of care needs to explicitly ensure that the goals of care hold for *all* parties in a caring relationship. The term mature care is meant to affirm this commitment, and we will return to why and how this also holds true for asymmetric relationships.

2.1.3 The Ontological Argument

The third argument for reconceptualizing care as mature care, is that the relational ontology of feminist care ethics must be conveyed into the concept of care, together with an explicit attentiveness to how the relationships were established. Starting from the premise that all humans by nature are relational beings and participants in a network of relationships, and that the traditional views on women and men's caring capacity are cultural constructions as opposed to inherent, provides us with a completely different normative outlook.[34] It is certainly possible to understand care as the prevention of harm and the encouragement of flourishing also on the basis of traditional individualistic ontology. However, this conventional ontological model overlooks several features of the situation. The relational aspects of care disappear. Care understood on the basis of an individualistic ontology tends to see it as a mono-directional activity, transferred or given from the carer to the cared-for, or alternatively as something the cared-for has a right to deplete from the carer. Relationships without reciprocity will often end up either as paternalistic relationships where the carer neglects, abuses and violates the cared-for, or tyrannical relationships where the carer becomes a slave to the needs of others.[35] It is difficult to adequately grasp the reciprocity in 'care' without the relational ontology.

Although the altruistic tradition has its philosophical basis in phenomenology, where human interconnection is given greater prominence than in many other philosophical schools, the altruistic conception of care still seems to escape the relational view. Altruistic care actually chimes with a conventional individualistic ontology. A selfless devotion to others might also be a way of avoiding the responsibility for creating one's own life and for one's own deeds, as well as accepting being – or allowing oneself to become – a mere means for others.[36]

Within the feminist tradition the focus on the relational ontology has been more prominent, much thanks to Gilligan's work. This, combined with the fact that its adherents have been concerned also about the carer, explains why it is more common to acknowledge the reciprocal base in conceptualizations of care within the feminist tradition. However, as mentioned above, the feminist tradition has been criticized for allegedly having a too one-sided perspective on caring by disability scholars, post-colonialists, Black feminists and others. It has been pointed out that the view of the carer is the dominant perspective within an ethics of care, that this view sustains an image of people with disabilities as passive and helpless 'care-receivers'.[37] Moreover, it has been argued that feminist care ethics does not pay sufficient attention to the power dynamics within dependency relationships,[38] nor that the relationships which care ethicists take as their point of departure might have been established through coercion and exploitation[39] in a society where racism[40] and heterosexualism[41] exist. Feminist care ethics has also been alleged to be 'conservative' because of the perception that it reinforces traditional middle-class conceptions of femininity,[42] and idealizes and romanticizes the voices and values imposed on women by a patriarchal culture.[43]

It appears that work is required in both traditions of care ethics to better integrate the relational ontology with the concept of care, an ontology that starts from the premise that humans are interconnected in a web of relationships where significant asymmetry in power and resources often exists. Mature care is meant to express this, and also that care is a reciprocal activity, where mutuality and consent are aimed at and paternalism and tyranny kept at bay. A reconceptualization of care in which the relational ontology informs the view of what it is, and how it is, also has epistemological implications. It prevents a one-sided view of care from the perspective of the carer only, a perspective in which the cared-for easily can be perceived as a passive receiver. One avoids the perspective of the carer becoming 'the point of view from nowhere' and promotes an understanding of care in terms of dialogue, reciprocity and consent, rather than monologue, unilateralism and paternalism. Attentiveness towards the needs of others and oneself, as well as reflecting and assessing how caring is received and affects your own situation, is an important part of caring.[44] The concept of mature care aims at encompassing the idea of such a balance.

2.2 CARING ABOUT TERMINOLOGY

2.2.1 Why 'mature' care?

As pointed out, the normative goals of mature care are comprehensive: which means that the interests of the carer should *also* be taken into account. From a feminist perspective, this needs highlighting because the conceptual frameworks of many of our cultures (still) equate women with care in a way that envisages women as more naturally inclined than men to care for others. Consequently, many women are also expected to sacrifice their own interests for the sake of others. Without underscoring the assumption informing the ethics of care that the ability to care is a *human capacity*, and that caring is *work* someone must assume responsibility for and act on, one risks sustaining traditional gender roles.

This issue has been discussed within the contemporary feminist branch of care ethics (at least) since Gilligan published *In a Different Voice* in 1982, and most feminist care ethicists have explicitly rejected an essentialist view on women and caring, among them Gilligan herself, as well as Ruddick, Held, Tronto and Kittay. They all emphasize how empirical gender differences – also with regard to care – are engendered by socialization. But not everyone is this explicit. Nel Noddings has refused to reject essentialism when it comes to women and caring, though she prefers to explain gender differences by evolutionary biology rather than essentialism: 'evidence currently available suggests that women are more empathic than men, and this should not surprise us, given the thousands of years of female caregiving experience which evolution has had to work on'.[45] Within the altruistic tradition little attention is paid to the matter, and as a traditional concept of care carries a gendered metaphysic that upholds traditional structures, coining a feminist concept of care is required. Mature care is meant to be without any gendered connotation.

But why term a feminist reconceptualization of care 'mature' care? One inspiration comes from one of Gilligan's informants who in *In a Different Voice* described herself as 'mature' when she was able to weigh and mediate the interests of both self and others.[46] Another inspiration is Simone de Beauvoir's *Ethics of Ambiguity* and her concept of moral freedom where being able to recognize the interest of both self and other is the essence of ethics.[47] Understanding care in this reciprocal way, and having that understanding integrated in our terminology by terming it 'mature care', reveals that care does not espouse asceticism and self-denial, or a pure altruistic approach to the needs of others. It would be misconceived and evidence of a misunderstanding of what it means to care were we to equate care with self-sacrifice or self-denial, on the one hand, or with narrowly particularistic and self-centred concerns, on the other. Both perspectives would be one-sided, without reciprocity or mutual recognition. Care, understood as mature care, seeks a path between caring too little and caring too much, both for oneself and for others.

Neither my own interest, nor the interests of others, should serve as a general directive – but rather a template for acknowledging the interests of all affected.

'Mature', used in relation to care in this way, also denotes an affinity to Aristotle – more precisely, to his theory of the golden mean. The moral agent searches for a middle way between too little and too much care for themselves and others. Both selfishness and selflessness in their extreme forms are vices, as are pure egoism and altruism. This affinity with Aristotelian virtue ethics is not meant as an encouragement to understand care as yet another virtue, or care ethics as a type of virtue ethics, but rather to transcend the effect of dichotomies such as egoism and altruism, selflessness and selfishness. The focus on a middle way also infuses our conception of care with the anti-dichotomizing thinking that has figured as an important methodological approach for many feminist philosophers and feminist care theorists.[48] The benefit of leaning slightly towards Aristotle is that both excesses related to care, in either direction, are considered *vices*; neither of them are morally praiseworthy.[49]

'Mature' also, as I see it, suggests that the required state – mature care – comes about as a result of a developmental process, and is not an innate or gendered trait. The term connotes that this type of caring, a state of mutual recognition and equal consideration, is the result of a certain manner of growth. Maturity is obviously the obverse of immaturity, and I hold that only being capable of seeing the interests of oneself, or only the interests of the other, is a sign of immaturity. Contrary to Aristotle and other traditional views, the concept of mature care is intended to explicitly counter the cultural conception of women's development as completed when they manage to put the interests of others ahead of their own, and men as mature when they become capable of articulating and pursuing their own interests at the expense of others.

By incorporating both terms, i.e. maturity and immaturity, in the sense just explained, I also mean to make another epistemological point. The idea of maturity and immaturity challenges the sharp distinction between reason and emotion, or rather those mature enough to manage the balance between reason and emotion, and those who accentuate emotion or reason at the expense of the other.[50] Mature care demonstrates that the required cognitive capacities needed are acquired through growth, that neither reason nor emotions ought to be excluded, but can be present in various degrees. In addition to the ontological and epistemological consequences, conceptualizing care as mature care has further implications. One is how we apply other key concepts in an ethics of care, such as how we name the parties involved in a caring relationship. Let us inspect some of the care terminology more closely in light of the discussion above.

2.2.2 The problems with 'giving' and 'receiving' care

Terms such as 'care-giver' and 'care-receiver,' 'care-giving' and 'care-receiving,' as well as 'the object of care' and 'the recipient of care,' are frequently used in care literature by authors from both altruistic and feminist traditions.[51] I will refer to this terminology as 'traditional'.

The first problem with this vocabulary is that it conceals the *reciprocal interaction* in caring relationships, exactly what I have attempted to highlight and emphasize by the idea of mature care. Traditional terminology portrays one of the parties as a passive receiver, the other as an active giver. A feminist reconceptualization of care must avoid a terminology depicting care as a one-sided, unconditional gift of charity transferred from one individual to another. Also, a terminology based on the idea that one party gives and the other receives gainsays the relational ontology on which a feminist ethics of care is founded, while sustaining a traditional individualistic ontology.

Moreover, as disability scholars and others rightfully have suggested, people in need of support may be led to believe by traditional vocabulary that care ethicists might apply the perspective of *the dominator*, the one in control.[52] This is a hierarchical language that might reveal a perspective in which the one in need of care is perceived to be of lesser (moral) worth. Furthermore, objectifying terms like 'receiver' and 'giver' might disregard and disrespect both the autonomy and response of either party in the relationship. Although most users of these terms do not intend to evoke these connotations, they nevertheless follow from the traditional care vocabulary that evolved around the dichotomized concept of 'giving' and 'receiving'.

It is, however, difficult to find an alternative terminology capable of transcending these problems. What is required is a terminology that transcends the dichotomized conceptions used to address the parties in a relationship, and connote instead the relational aspect and mutual exchange in a (mature) caring relationship. An ideal terminology should not be objectifying, hierarchal or dominating. At the same time, we do not want a terminology that conceals the fact that one party is sometimes more dependent and has substantially less concrete freedom than the other. It is a fact that humans are vulnerable to different degrees, unequally situated and diverse with regard to support and help from others, and this should not be masked.

Within the existing literature, I find that Noddings's use of 'the one-caring' and 'the cared-for' avoids objectifying or pacifying one of the parties.[53] Now, one objection to Noddings's terminology is that caring also here is portrayed from the perspective of the carer. 'The cared-for', one could assert, might not experience or perceive the support as care, but rather as abusive, invasive, harmful or controlling. However, even if the expression 'the cared-for' is taken as seen from the perspective of the carer, 'the cared-for' does not imply anything with regard to whether and/or how the care is received, acknowledged and accepted. Nor does it say whether caring has reached its completion or not – as opposed to the expression 'care-receiver', which certainly carries these connotations. 'The cared-for' indicates only whom the carer has as their *intended addressee*; it says nothing about the result of their caring effort. As I see it, this terminology – 'the cared-for' – leaves (a conceptual) space where the cared-for can reject or consent to – partly as well as completely – the caring aimed at her. And when it is not presupposed that caring is accepted and completed, a more relational terminology encourages the carer to reflect over and inquire into the outcome of their caring, rather than simply assuming it has been successful. This cannot (at least not easily) be the case when the individualistic ontology and the altruistic comprehension of care are at work, under which caring is perceived as a gift from a benefactor to a beneficiary. Reciprocity, not one-sidedness, is one of the most prominent features of a caring relationship, even if this reciprocity manifests itself differently depending on the type of relationship.

2.3 MATURE CARE AND ASYMMETRIC RELATIONSHIPS

One might assert that although the concept of mature care may be applicable to symmetric relations – such as between partners, friends, colleagues – it appears to be inapt for asymmetric relationships – such as between parent and child, teacher and student, nurse and patient. Since, one might also assert, the main focus in asymmetric caring relationships ought to be on *the other's* best interests, and since resources and power are unequally balanced, requiring reciprocity seems to be impossible and perhaps even unethical. The performance of care in asymmetric relationships is an important part of care work and this objection is pertinent. We therefore need an account of how mature care can function as a normative guide for care provision also in asymmetric relationships.

The reply to the objection about not expecting a return from the cared-for is, in short, that if the relational aspect of the caring activity and the autonomy of the cared-for are to be taken seriously, mutuality should indeed not only be expected in the majority of asymmetrical relationships, but actually required and promoted. In order to support this view, I will start by identifying what I take to be some characteristic features of an asymmetric relationship, before proceeding to explain what reciprocity in asymmetric relationships means.

2.3.1 The asymmetric relationship

When we give an account of asymmetric relationships, such as between parent and child, teacher and student, nurse and patient, we commonly – and rightly – point out that that these relationships call for a different portrayal of moral agency than the model offered by traditional moral philosophy (such as deontology and utilitarianism).[54] An asymmetric caring relationship is not about promoting one's own interests in a group of equally rational, free and similarly situated agents, as is assumed by models based on contract theories. In asymmetric relationships, the agent gives priority to the interests of *others* – sometimes at the expense of her own interests. Very often, these relationships are not voluntary, they cannot easily (or by choice) be dissolved, and the parties are not equal in bargaining power or resources. Independence, strength, and freedom are *not* the most prominent features of an asymmetric relationship, but rather vulnerability, dependence and limitations.[55]

However, symmetric relationships can also have these characteristics. Symmetric relationships are not always completely balanced; exchanges are not without exception perfectly equal transactions based on the idea of me scratching your back, and you scratching mine. In a long-term relationship between, for instance, adult partners, one party may, for a certain period of time, need to be taken care of – in times of illness, crisis and distress. In the long run, however, partners alternate between taking care of each other. Vulnerability, attachment, dependency, giving attention and priority to the interests of the other, are not exclusive features of asymmetric relationships. They are indeed evident also in well-functioning symmetric relationships. The differences consist in how they manifest themselves. In symmetric relationships they do not *permanently* belong to *one* of the parties. Only *temporarily* is the one party more dependent than the other. If dependency becomes permanent, the relationship changes from symmetric to asymmetric. Even if features like those mentioned above are probably *more typical* of asymmetric relationships, they are still not sufficient conditions for terming the relationship asymmetric. So, what is the necessary condition for terming a relationship asymmetric?

The most significant feature of an asymmetric relationship is, in my view, the inability of the parties to *swap roles*. In equal relationships, this is indeed possible. In symmetric relationships the people involved take turns in being the carer and the cared-for. Actually, this is a constitutive feature of a symmetric relationship.[56] Not so in asymmetric relationships. A mother and child, a teacher and student, a nurse and patient *cannot* alternate between the roles of the carer and the cared-for. The inability to swap roles holds true whether the asymmetric relationship is personal or professional, and signifies the necessary condition for terming a relationship asymmetrical.

There are two obvious objections to using the inability to swap roles as the defining feature of the asymmetric relationship. First, if the roles cannot be swapped, where is the reciprocity previously advocated for in relation to mature care? Second, it might well be possible to swap roles in an asymmetric relationship too: children sometimes take care of their parents, for instance; patients care for their nurses, students for their teachers. The short answer to both objections is that an exchange of the caring responsibility cannot be done in a non-symmetric caring relationship without inflicting harm or impeding flourishing – the goals of care. 'Cannot' is a normative statement, not an empirical one. 'Cannot' means 'ought not'. When it comes to the responsibility for care, it ought not be swapped in an asymmetric relationship. However, other things related to the normative core of care, such as wishing each other well, respect, appreciation, trust, kindness, etc., can and indeed ought to be exchanged in unequal relationships as well. Asymmetric relationships are not without caring reciprocity, even if the roles as carer and the cared-for cannot be altered. Let me enlarge by way of an example.

Envisage ten-year-old Andy, who one morning makes breakfast for their mother. In a well-functioning asymmetric relationship, this breakfast arrangement does not indicate that Andy has become the carer, nor that the mother now is the cared-for. The reason is that the child is not responsible for promoting the mother's wellbeing, or for protecting her from harm. Andy's actions are approved and monitored by their carer (i.e. the mother): their actions are judged as not harmful, and probably as part of a learning process that in time will enable Andy to flourish and mature. The cared-for starts by modelling or copying others; later they will find their own way. As long as Andy is a child, however, they have no responsibility for taking care of their mother – or anybody else. True, they might have some duties within the family; maybe they are assigned the job of making breakfast on Saturday mornings, but the mother approves of this because she believes it to be in the cared-for's best interests to learn to take responsibility and acquire such skills and knowledge. There is indeed an exchange in the asymmetric relationship, but not of the same kind as in symmetric relationships.[57] There is an exchange of wishes for each other's wellbeing, for reciprocal learning, trust, attention, joy, disappointment, understanding, attentiveness, respect, etc. But there is not, i.e. ought not to be, an exchange of the *responsibility* for providing care. If Andy fails to make breakfast, others will make it without any harmful sanctioning of the ten-year-old.

However, if Andy were given and assumed total responsibility for their mother, which would be possible in a case where, for example, the mother is seriously ill without anybody else to take care of her, the situation is different. Andy's responsibility would conflict with the ideals of care, i.e. prevention or reparation of harm and promotion of flourishing. In an asymmetric relationship, the roles of carer and the one cared-for cannot be exchanged without violating the goals of care as explained above. In some circumstances, say when Andy turns fifteen, it might be difficult to determine whether it is harmful or not, or if it really prevents flourishing to take on the caring responsibility. This is nevertheless an empirical question.[58] Relationships can change; an asymmetric relationship can evolve into a symmetric one, and vice versa. Caring for one's ageing parent is an example of a relationship that has undergone such a change. Again, it's the normative goals of care, i.e., to prevent harm and promote flourishing, which authorize whether it is ethically acceptable or not to swap roles, and in an asymmetric relationship it is not. If it is, the relationship is symmetric, not asymmetric.

There are some differences between private and professional relationships, differences that cut across the distinction between symmetric and asymmetric relationships. In professional relationships the carer's attention to the cared-for will be more regulated, as well as focused on one or some *specific* and often predefined need(s) of the cared-for – such as their education or health. The professional relationship, as well as the provision of care, typically terminates when the pupil leaves the school, or the patient's health is restored. Emotional involvement is usually weaker and more regulated in professional caring relations, compared to many private relationships. In private relationships the concern for the other is not limited to certain attributes, nor confined to specific times or events. The care partners provide for one another, or parents for children, is usually broader and more prolonged than in a professional caring relationship. Many private relationships, such as family relationships and friendships, are commonly also longer lasting, some of them for life. Few professional relationships endure in the same way – though on occasion they can.

Also, the different degrees of asymmetry in uneven relationships should be mentioned, because some asymmetric relationships are 'dependency relationships'.[59] When one party depends on another person's care work to survive, their relationship is indeed asymmetric; it is a dependency relationship.[60] A teacher–student relationship is asymmetric, but it is not a 'dependency relationship' since the student can (relatively) easily replace one teacher with another or manage without. Professional ethics often proposes rules and guidelines exactly to prevent professional relationships from developing into relationships of dependency. A critically injured person, however, is asymmetrically dependent on people who can help. A child, in many respects, is dependent on their caretaker, as are people with disabilities in some circumstances. The one in need is considered dependent when her needs are basic, vital or critical.[61] The person in need is then in the custody of the carer, i.e. their health, welfare, safety, security and self-respect rest in the hands of the carer. The one in need cannot function without their efforts.

When the need for care in an asymmetrical relationship is basic, vital or critical, fulfilment of these needs is of course ethically defensible from the perspective of mature care. A requirement of ethical legitimacy is valid inasmuch as a failure to provide care, for example, by not caring for a newborn baby, helping a critically injured person or a person with dementia will inevitably cause harm and obstruct flourishing. From the perspective of mature care, behaviors that prevent flourishing are also harmful, such as exclusion from social life, education, the possibility to choose one's own partner, etc.

2.3.2 Asymmetry and ethical responsibility

According to the concept of mature care, the carer is also entitled to be protected from harm, to have their needs fulfilled and enjoy an opportunity to thrive. It nevertheless also follows from the discussion of asymmetric relationships that this cannot be done or reciprocated by the cared-for in an asymmetric relationship. The caring responsibility – the main responsibility not to inflict harm but to promote flourishing – cannot be exchanged in an asymmetric relationship; it falls upon the carer.[62] How, then, can the carer's interest be assured in an asymmetric relationship?

Eva Kittay has argued with her theory on nested obligations in *Love's Labor* that the carer's surroundings have obligations towards her when asymmetric care work takes its toll. An individual – as well as society – has, according to Kittay, an ethical obligation to the carer.[63] Still, I wish in what follows to scrutinize the view that even if some ethical responsibility rightly is handed over to a third party, the cared-for in (many) asymmetric relations still has ethical obligations. Only in certain types of asymmetric relationships will the cared-for have no ethical responsibilities, and these relationships do not constitute the majority. Let me elaborate on what kinds of reciprocated ethical obligation can be identified, also in most asymmetric relationships, from the perspective of mature care.

The ethically legitimate claim of the parties in many asymmetric relationships is dual. It is the normative core of care, to not inflict harm but to promote flourishing as explained above, which justifies both aspects of this claim. First there is the claim to have some particular needs satisfied in order not to be harmed and to be able to flourish. The cared-for's right to have their needs satisfied in an asymmetric relationship is ethically legitimate if not fulfilling them imposes harm or prevents flourishing. In asymmetrical relationships the cared-for can make this claim on the carer, but not so the other way round. The addressee for this part of the carer's claim must be a third party, as Kittay argues.[64] However, the parties' legitimate ethical claims in an asymmetric relationship extend *beyond* the satisfaction of vital needs. The second aspect of the ethically legitimate claim in an asymmetric caring relationship is to be protected against abuse or exploitation in the relationship. This aspect will generally apply to both parties – also in asymmetric caring relationships. The cared-for as well as the one caring must also request that their vulnerability and dependency are not exploited or abused. On the contrary, both have a rightful claim to have these factors taken into account.[65] Having vulnerability and dependency exploited is another way of harming and preventing flourishing.

The power wielded by the carer over the cared-for in consequence of their asymmetric relationship, and the ethical obligations resting on the former have been thoroughly examined in the literature, incorporated in legislation and addressed by professional codes of ethics. What has failed to attract as much attention is the opposite perspective in which the cared-for has the power to harm the carer, with the exceptions of Noddings and Kittay? Noddings has inquired into 'the ethics of being cared for',[66] and Kittay[67] into the situation of a particular asymmetric care worker whom she terms 'dependency-worker'. In what follows, I shall explore, like Kittay, the carer's situation in an asymmetric relationship where the cared-for is dependent. Unlike Kittay, however, I will focus mainly on the many asymmetric relationships in which the cared-for is autonomous. I will also, like Noddings, discuss what can ethically be expected from the cared-for, but put more emphasis on asymmetric reciprocity, which I will elucidate by using the concept of mature care.

My claim is that in a relationship – whether asymmetric or not – in which the cared-for is capable of deliberately violating the normative heart of care, the cared-for has ethical responsibilities and obligations as well. On this important ethical dimension of a caring relationship there is mutuality, and mature care can serve as an ideal. The cared-for is responsible for how they respond to the carer's attempts at caring. As long as the cared-for is not suffering from conditions that hamper their cognitive ability or emotional control, it would be a mistake of the carer not to expect or require the cared-for to assume responsibility for their conduct toward the carer. Treating the cared-for, even if they are dependent on others for some of their needs, as if they have no control over their behaviour shows them no respect. Expecting something from the cared-for is not to renounce responsibility. Rather, it might sustain and strengthen the relationship between the carer and the cared-for,[68] reduce harm, and promote development and flourishing. There will indeed be situations in which it is hard to determine exactly how and when one can expect moral responsiveness from the cared-for but these empirical difficulties do not alter the overall ethical point, that in many asymmetric relationships there also ought to be ethical reciprocity between the carer and the cared-for.

2.3.3 Intentionality and care

The focus on the cared-for's capacity to inflict harm consciously might help clarify how, when and why something can be required of the cared-for in an asymmetric relationship. Even if the cared-for cannot satisfy their own or their carer's needs, they might still be in a position to harm the carer. Only those who are *incapable of intentionally inflicting harm* cannot be held accountable for harm done, and have no moral obligations towards the carer. Hence, coma patients, the critically injured or a person with dementia are not expected to be ethically responsible. They are excused because they are incapable (if, say, they are unconscious) of deliberately harming, or the harm they are causing is unintentional (if they are critically ill or in shock, for example), or because they are not, given their current circumstances, completely autonomous and accountable (i.e., children and people with intellectual disabilities). If the cared-for is not capable of harming intentionally, they cannot act autonomously and they are therefore not a moral agent. This holds true whether we are talking about traditional or relational autonomy.[69] Ethics is per definition about our intentional conduct and attitudes. A coma patient or a neonate are not moral agents. Hence, their conduct is not addressed by ethics. These are situations where the cared-for is without moral responsibility, while the carer surely is responsible.

This brings us to an additional point – namely, how to use the term 'caring relationship'. Contrary to colloquial language, and in sync with Noddings, I hold that there is no 'caring relationship' between the carer and, say, a coma patient. Noddings puts it this way: 'To qualify as a caring encounter, the cared-for must contribute to the relation; the cared-for must show in some way that the caring has been received. This response completes the caring relation. Without it, we may acknowledge a carer's effort to care, but the encounter, episode, or relation cannot be said to be one of caring.'[70] However, Noddings's position needs to be refined by a small, but significant addition: the response also has to be intentional. The fact that a coma patient reacts (or not) to a particular treatment is indeed a response, but not an intentional one. In order for something to qualify as a caring relationship, it is not sufficient to determine whether caring is received or not, as Noddings suggests. In order to qualify as a 'caring relationship', there must be an intentional exchange that allows also the cared-for to acknowledge, challenge or reject the care provision. In other words, also in many asymmetric relations 'care' must be understood as a mutual interaction in accordance with mature care. Without this refinement we relapse from envisaging care as mature care, to figuring it as an altruistic gift that can be handed over to others without their consent. Without this additional aspect, we go back to perceiving our being in the world as separate, rather than connected, we encourage paternalism rather than relational autonomy. In a caring *relationship* there must be a 'circle of care' that allows the cared-for to respond and acknowledge – or challenge and reject – the care provision, and the one caring to receive feedback in order to continue, adjust or terminate their delivery of care.

How then, one may ask, can mature care accommodate caring for an unconscious being where no wilful response is present? If intentional reciprocity is impossible, nothing is expected from the cared-for. Consequently, it is intention, not asymmetry, that determines whether the cared-for also has ethical responsibility – for instance, not to exploit the carer. This situation by no means indicates that the carer is free of ethical obligations. Does this mean that the carer in these relationships must relapse from envisaging care as mature care to something one party actively does for or performs on a passive receiver, figuring it as an altruistic gift that can be handed over to the other without their consent? No. This would again imply that we go back to perceive our being in the world as separate, rather than connected, encouraging paternalism rather than relationality, and risking maltreatment rather than promoting flourishing. Even if there is no caring *relationship* with the unconscious, there is a causal connection between the way we tend to the needy and their wellbeing. We should, in sync with mature care, strive to understand their responses and adjust our treatment it accordingly. As mature carers, we are still embedded in a relational worldview, as well as committed to the dual core values of preventing harm and enabling flourishing. Consequently, we need to ponder how our acts affect the needy with regard to harm and flourishing. Additionally, a mature carer must also deem when nurturing others will inflict harm on herself, and when the assistance of a third party is required. Applying the altruistic concept of care may incline an excess of attention towards the helpless on the expenses of oneself and others, or a complacent involvement.

2.3 RECONCEPTUALIZING CARE

Reconceptualizing care as 'mature care' can, as I have argued in the first part of this chapter, help us eliminate the gendered connotations that have been attached to the idea of care (*the genealogy argument*). By doing so, we can include caring for the caregiver and infuse the concept of care with the relational ontology upon which the ethics of care is founded (*the normative argument*). Mature care is a conceptualization of care that recognizes the interconnectedness of individuals and emphasizes the importance of reciprocity, mutual consent and dialogue within caring relationships (*the ontological argument*). It avoids one-sided perspectives on care, which often arise from traditional non-feminist ethical frameworks, by considering the interests of both the carer and the cared-for, as well as the contextual structures in which caring takes place. Mature care seeks a balance between providing too little and too much care for oneself and others. It is not a gendered, racial or class-based conception. Instead, mature caring is viewed as the outcome of a developmental process involving both emotional and cognitive capacities. The normative foundation of mature care is universal: to prevent harm and enable flourishing for both those in need of care and those who provide care. When conceptualizing care as mature care, the care terminology must be non-hierarchal and not portray the cared-for as a passive receiver and the carer as an active giver as explained in above.

How can mature care, with its emphasis on mutual recognition and equal consideration, be applicable to asymmetric relationships where the carer must prioritize the interests of the cared-for, often at the expense of their own? I have addressed this concern in the last part of this chapter by examining the characteristics of asymmetric relationships and arguing that vulnerability, attachment, dependency, giving attention and priority to the interests of the other, are not exclusive features of asymmetric relationships. In times of illness and crises, these characteristics also manifest in symmetric relationships; they are constitutive features of a caring symmetric relationship. Being dependent on the care of others is a necessary but not sufficient condition for labelling a relationship 'asymmetric'. The most significant characteristic of an asymmetric relationship, I have argued, is the parties' inability to interchange roles between being the carer and the cared-for without causing harm and impeding the flourishing of the one in need of care, and thereby violating the normative goals of mature care. The responsibility not to inflict harm and to promote flourishing cannot be exchanged in an asymmetric relationship; it rests solely upon the carer.

Asymmetric care work can take a toll on the carer. From the perspective of mature care, caring for the carer is an ethical obligation of the relational network, be it friends, family or society. Moreover, if the cared-for is autonomous and capable of intentional action, they also have ethical obligations towards the carer. The cared-for is responsible for how they respond to the carer's attempts at care, for example, by not exploiting the carer's resources or causing harm.[71] Also, in many asymmetric relationships there can be an exchange of respect, acknowledgement, attentiveness, etc. In cases such as caring for a neonatal or a coma patient, where intentional exchange may be impossible, we cannot speak of a caring relationship. However, this does not mean we should revert to a unilateral, paternalistic and altruistic understanding of care that masks unfair distribution of benefits and burdens. Instead, in keeping with mature care, we should remain attentive to the needs of others and ourselves, as well as to the responsibilities of the third party. Reflecting on and assessing how care is received, how it affects one's own situation, and how it is allocated in the private and the public sphere are crucial aspects of the reconceptualized notion of care I have suggested: namely, mature care.

A reconceptualization is necessary because care ethicists aim at making the world a more caring place by placing care at the centre of our attention and prioritizations, and to ensure a just distribution of the benefits and burdens related to care. But as Virginia Held reminds us, no changes will take place unless we are able to imagine something new.[72] In order to imagine something new, it is often necessary to start by changing or refining our basic concepts – or by articulating new ones. This is so because there is a connection between the conceptual tools at our disposal, on the one hand, and our cognition, theorizing and practising, on the other. Our conceptual schemes constitute our worldview, our presumptions of what *is* and *how* it is. In a culturally and economic diverse world, there will obviously be different conceptions on what it means to care. Consequently, we need to pay close attention to how care and other related concepts are used, in ordinary language as well as in our theories. As I have tried to show, the traditional concepts at our disposal are not always good at doing their job. They can blur and disguise certain phenomena, exclude or confine some experiences. They might be based on a discriminatory anthropology, bigoted ontology and parochial epistemology. Or they might carry the imprint of certain cultures, traditions or eras different from those we are targeting. Sometimes, adequate notions are out of reach. As for the concept of care, paternalism and ignorance represent the failure to attend to the interests of the cared-for, while self-sacrifice and exploitation represent the failure to take the interests of the carer into account. These are the Scylla and Charybdis of caring. A reconceptualizing of the traditional understanding of care into mature care might help us to steer clear of them when practising care, as well as to avoid a parlance holding us hostage to the traditional gendered, individualistic and alienating way of understanding care.

NOTES

1. See: The Care Collective et al., *The Care Manifesto: The Politics of Interdependence* (New York: Verso Books, 2020); Kathleen Lynch, *Care and Capitalism* (Hoboken: John Wiley & Sons, 2022); Eva F. Kittay, *Love's Labor: Essays on Women, Equality, and Dependency* (London: Psychology Press, 1999); Joan C. Tronto, *Moral Boundaries: A Political Argument for an Ethic of Care* (New York: Routledge, 1993).
2. Fiona Robinson, 'Global Care Ethics: Beyond Distribution, Beyond Justice', *Journal of Global Ethics* 9, no. 2 (2013): 131–43; Maurice Hamington and Michael A. Flower (eds.), *Care Ethics in the Age of Precarity* (Minneapolis, MN: University of Minnesota Press, 2021).
3. Virginia Held, *The Ethics of Care: Personal, Political, and Global* (New York: Oxford University Press, 2006), 120, 154–168.
4. See: Virginia Held, 'Can the Ethics of Care Handle Violence?', *Ethics and Social Welfare* 4, no. 2 (2010): 115–29; Tove Pettersen, 'Feminist Care Ethics: Contributions to Peace Theory', in *Routledge Handbook of Feminist Peace Research*, ed. Tarja Väyrynen et al. (London: Routledge, 2021), 28–39; Sara Ruddick, *Maternal Thinking: Toward a Politics of Peace* (Boston: Beacon Press, 1989).
5. See: Fiona Robinson, *The Ethics of Care: A Feminist Approach to Human Security* (Philadelphia: Temple University Press, 2011); Karen Warren, *Ecofeminist Philosophy: A Western Perspective on What It Is and Why It Matters* (Lanham: Rowman & Littlefield, 2000); T. Pettersen, 'Caring for More than Humans: Ecofeminism and Care Ethics,' in *Conversation, in Between Closeness and Evil*, ed. Odin Lysaker, (Scandinavian Academic Press, 2020, pp. 183–213).
6. However, when feminist care ethics was new, it was in many feminist as well as non-feminist academic circles understood as a description of how women with a particular background reflected on their personal issues in the private sphere (Kohlberg 1984: 231, fn 2). Consequently, it was dismissed as an ethical theory as its validity was considered very limited. However, thanks to the work of many care ethicists, feminist care ethics has during the last decades developed into a promising normative theory on a par with deontology, utilitarianism and theories of justice. Consequently, very few people today would argue that care and care ethics are merely private and marginal issues, or that they are limited to personal relations in a certain cultural context only.
7. One might of course ask why care ethics holds the possibility for positive changes on so many levels. As I see it, it is due to some characteristic features of this ethical theory. Among them are the fact that it is based on a relational ontology, an epistemological situatedness, the view on care as gender-neutral work, and the view that care is a normative value – on a par with justice, freedom and equality. For a more extensive discussion of these features, see, for example: Tove Pettersen, 'Caring for More than Humans: Ecofeminism and Care Ethics in Conversation', in *Between Closeness and Evil*, ed. Odin Lysaker (Oslo: Scandinavian Academic Press, 2020), 183–213; and Pettersen, 'Feminist Care Ethics'; Virginia Held, *The Ethics of Care. Personal, Political, and Global.* (New York, Oxford: University Press, 2006).
8. Sally Haslanger, 'Gender and Social Construction: Who? What? When? Where? How?', in *Theorizing Feminisms: A Reader*, ed. Elizabeth Hackett and Sally Haslanger (New York: Oxford University Press, 2006), 16–23.

9. See: Tove Pettersen, *Comprehending Care: Problems and Possibilities in the Ethics of Care* (Lanham, MD: Lexington Books, 2008); Tove Pettersen, 'Conceptions of Care: Altruism, Feminism, and Mature Care', *Hypatia* 27, no. 2 (2012): 366–89.
10. See: Chris Gastmans, interview by Webteam, https://ethicsofcare.org/chris-gastmans/, last modified 16 April 2011; Kari Martinsen, *Omsorg, sykepleie og medisin: historisk-filosofiske essays* (Oslo: Tano, 1989); Kari Martinsen, *Øyet og kallet* (Bergen: Fagbokforlaget, 2000); Kari Martinsen, *Fenomenologi og omsorg* (Oslo: Universitetsforlaget, 2003); Per Nortvedt, *Sensitive Judgment: Nursing, Moral Philosophy, and an Ethics of Care* (Oslo: Tano Aschehoug, 1996); Per Nortvedt, 'Levinas, Justice, and Health Care', *Medicine, Health Care, and Philosophy* 6 (2003): 25–34; Per Nortvedt, 'Den etiske fordring – omsorgens kjerne', in *Livtag med den etiske fordring*, ed. David Bugge and Peter A. Sørensen (Århus: Klim, 2007), 175–88.
11. See: Knud E. Løgstrup, *Den etiske fordring* (Oslo: Cappelen, 1999); Martinsen, *Øyet og kallet*; Kari Martinsen, 'Kallet i går, i dag og i morgen – kan vi være foruten et kall?', *Kristent forum for sykepleiere og sykepleierstudenter* 3 (2003), 20–27; Per Nortvedt, *Omtanke: en innføring i sykepleiens etikk* (Oslo: Gyldendal Akademiske, 2012), 17–60.
12. See: Pettersen, *Comprehending Care*; Pettersen, 'Conceptions of Care', 366–89; Tove Pettersen, 'The Ethics of Care: Normative Structures and Empirical Implications', *Health Care Analysis* 19, no. 1 (2011): 51–64.
13. See: Carol Gilligan, *In a Different Voice: Psychological Theory and Women's Development* (Cambridge, MA: Harvard University Press, 1982); Virginia Held, *Feminist Morality: Transforming Culture, Society, and Politics* (Chicago, IL: University of Chicago Press, 1993); Kittay, *Love's Labor*; Ruddick, *Maternal Thinking*.
14. See: The Care Collective et al., *The Care Manifesto: The Politics of Interdependence* (New York: Verso Books, 2020); Lisa A. Eckenwiler, *Long-term Care, Globalization, and Justice* (Baltimore, MD: Johns Hopkins University Press, 2012); Held, *The Ethics of Care*; Rianne Mahon and Fiona Robinson, *Feminist Ethics and Social Policy: Towards a New Global Political Economy of Care* (Vancouver: University of British Columbia Press, 2011); Nel Noddings, *Caring: A Feminine Approach to Ethics and Moral Education* (Berkeley: University of California Press, 1984); Robinson, *The Ethics of Care*; Tronto, *Moral Boundaries*.
15. See: Marit H. Hem, 'Mature Care? An Empirical Study of Interaction Between Psychotic Patients and Psychiatric Nurses' (PhD diss., Oslo, 2008), Unipub; Marit H. Hem and Tove Pettersen, 'Mature Care and Nursing in Psychiatry: Notions Regarding Reciprocity in Asymmetric Professional Relationships', *Health Care Analysis* 19, no. 1 (2011): 65–76; Pettersen, *Comprehending Care*; Tove Pettersen and Marit H. Hem, 'Mature Care and Reciprocity: Two Cases from Acute Psychiatry', *Nursing Ethics* 18, no. 2 (2011): 217–31.
16. Pettersen, 'Conceptions of Care', 366–89.
17. See: Øyvind Foss, *Omsorgsetikk: søkelys på omsorgens motivasjon* (Oslo: Cappelen Damm Akademisk, 2005); Kari Martinsen, *Omsorg, sykepleie og medisin: historisk-filosofiske essays* (Oslo: Tano, 1989); Anthony Tuckett, 'Nursing Practice: Compassionate Deception and the Good Samaritan', *Nursing Ethics* 6, no. 5 (1999): 383–9.
18. Pettersen, 'Conceptions of Care', 367–74.
19. Anita Silvers, 'Reconciling Equality to Difference: Caring (F)or Justice for People with Disabilities', *Hypatia* 10, no. 1 (1995): 40.
20. Ibid., 44.

21. Anita Silvers, 'Disability', in *A Companion to Feminist Philosophy*, ed. Alison M. Jagger and Iris M. Young (Malden, MA: Blackwell Publishing, 1998), 330–40.
22. To overthrow this image and acquire status as an active participant in the caring relationship, disability organizations have sought to substitute the term care with other terms, such as personal assistance or help; see: Nick Watson et al., '(Inter)Dependence, Needs and Care', *Sociology* 38, no. 2 (2004): 331–50.
23. Sarah L. Hoagland, *Lesbian Ethics: Toward New Value* (Palo Alto, CA: Institute of Lesbian Studies, 1988), 82.
24. Audre Lorde, *A Burst of Light: Essays* (Ithaca, NY: Firebrand Books, 1988).
25. See: Hoagland, *Lesbian Ethics*; Silvers, 'Reconciling Equality to Difference', 30–55.
26. Gilligan, *In a Different Voice*, 129.
27. Silvers, 'Reconciling Equality to Difference', 30–55.
28. See: Pettersen, *Comprehending Care*; Pettersen, 'Conceptions of Care', 366–89; Pettersen, 'The Ethics of Care', 51–64.
29. Pettersen, *The Ethics of Care*, 51–64.
30. Uma Narayan, 'Colonialism and Its Others: Considerations on Rights and Care Discourses', *Hypatia* 10, no. 2 (1995): 134.
31. Kittay, *Love's Labor*, 48–50.
32. I have elaborated on different types of harm caused by altruistic care in Pettersen, 'Conceptions of Care', 366–89. See also: Kittay, *Love's Labor*; Eva F. Kittay, 'The Moral Harm of Migrant Carework', *Philosophical Topics* 37, no. 2 (2009): 53–73; and Joan C. Tronto, 'The "Nanny" Question in Feminism', *Hypatia* 17, no. 2 (2002): 34–51, for an elaboration of the harm the performance of care can inflict on the carer in different contexts.
33. See: Gilligan, *In a Different Voice*; Kittay, *Love's Labor*; Pettersen, *Comprehending Care*; Pettersen, 'Conceptions of Care', 366–89; Pettersen, 'The Ethics of Care', 51–64.
34. Consequently, a relational revision of philosophical concepts is not unusual among feminist philosophers – for example, of 'autonomy' (see Marilyn Friedman, 'Feminism in Ethics: Conceptions of Autonomy,' in *The Cambridge Companion to Feminism in Philosophy*, ed. Miranda Fricker and Jennifer Hornsby (Cambridge: Cambridge University Press, 2000), 205–24, 'the moral agent' (see: Held, *Feminist Morality*), 'responsibility' (see: Gilligan, In a Different Voice), and 'freedom' (see: Simone de Beauvoir, The Ethics of Ambiguity (New York: Columbia University Press, 1976)) – often with the aim of removing the individualistic and gendered metaphysics of traditional philosophy.
35. Kittay, *Love's Labor*, 48–50.
36. See: Simone de Beauvoir, 'Pyrrhus and Cineas', in *Simone de Beauvoir: Philosophical Writings*, ed. Margaret A. Simons, Marybeth Timmerman and Mary B. Mader (Urbana: University of Illinois Press, 2004), 77–150; Tove Pettersen, 'Acting for Others: Moral Ontology in Beauvoir's "Pyrrhus and Cineas"', *Simone de Beauvoir Studies* 26, no. 1 (2009): 18–27.
37. See: Silvers, 'Reconciling Equality to Difference'; Silvers, 'Disability'.
38. Rosemarie Garland-Thomson, 'Integrating Disability, Transforming Feminist Theory', in *Feminist Disability Studies*, ed. Kim Q. Hall (Bloomington: Indiana University Press, 2011), 29.
39. Narayan, 'Colonialism and Its Others', 133–40.
40. Lorde, *A Burst of Light*.
41. Hoagland, *Lesbian Ethics*.

42. Claudia Card, 'The Feistiness of Feminism', in *Feminist Ethics*, ed. Claudia Card (Lawrence: University of Kansas, 1991), 22.
43. Seyla Benhabib, 'From Identity Politics to Social Feminism', in *Politics at the Turn of the Century*, ed. Arthur M. Melzer, Jerry Weinberger and Richard M. Zinman (Lanham, MD: Rowman & Littlefield, 2001), 27–8.
44. See: Noddings, *Caring*; Pettersen, *Comprehending Care*; Pettersen, 'Conceptions of Care', 366–89; Tronto, *Moral Boundaries*; Vrinda Dalmiya, "Why Should a Knower Care?," *Hypatia* 17, 1 (2002): 34–52.
45. Nel Noddings, *The Maternal Factor: Two Paths to Morality* (Oakland: University of California Press, 2010), 23–57.
46. Pettersen, *Comprehending Care*.
47. Pettersen, 'Conceptions of Care', 366–89.
48. See: de Beauvoir, *The Ethics of Ambiguity*; Genevieve Lloyd, *The Man of Reason: 'Male' and 'Female' in Western Philosophy* (London: Routledge, 1984); Val Plumwood, *Feminism and the Mastery of Nature* (London: Routledge, 1993).
49. Tove Pettersen, 'Comprehending Care. Problems and Possibilities in Carol Gilligan's Ethics of Care' (PhD diss., University of Oslo, 2004), Unipub (Acta Humaniora no. 206), 205–36.
50. Rosalind Hursthouse, *On Virtue Ethics* (Oxford: Oxford University Press, 1999).
51. Kittay, Eva Feder Kittay, 'Precarity, Precariousness, and Disability', Care Ethics in the Age of Precarity, ed. Maurice Hamington and Michael Flower (University of Minnesota Press, 2021), 19–47; S. Tønnessen, A. Scott and P. Nortvedt, 'Safe and competent nursing care: An argument for a minimum standard?' Nursing Ethics, 27(6), 2020: 1396–1407; J. Tronto, *Moral Boundaries. A Political Argument for an Ethics of care* (New York: Routledge, 1993); J. Tronto, *Caring Democracy* (New York and London: New York University Press, 2013).
52. See: Narayan, 'Colonialism and Its Others', 133–40; Robinson, 'Global Care Ethics'; Silvers, 'Disability'; Watson, '(Inter)Dependence, Needs and Care', 331–50.
53. Noddings, *Caring*.
54. Many caring relationships are asymmetric. Neither the ontology, nor the models of the moral agent in traditional moral philosophy, can adequately grasp the interaction in these relationships. Several feminist ethicists have therefore created alternative theoretical models of the moral agent in order to understand and articulate more precisely what asymmetric caring and interaction mean. These theoretical endeavours are nevertheless not divorced from lived experience; they are often based on the care work traditionally assigned to women, such as childcare. Indeed, the mother–child relationship has informed the efforts of several prominent care ethicists to develop an ethics of care – Virginia Held, Eva Feder Kittay, Nel Noddings, Sara Ruddick, to mention just a few prominent contributors.
55. See: Gilligan, *In a Different Voice*; Kittay, *Love's Labor*; Noddings, *Caring*; Ruddick, *Maternal Thinking*; Held, *Feminist Morality*.
56. Noddings, *The Maternal Factor*, 46, 170.
57. Pettersen, *Comprehending Care*, 131.
58. An answer to how to act in a particular case cannot always be established by normative theory, but sometimes only by empirical research and observation. The fact that no pre-established, well-defined boundary can be drawn between what is harmful and not in every single case, does not alter my claim that the caring responsibility in an asymmetric relationship in principle cannot be exchanged between the two parties without violating the normative goals of mature care.

59. Kittay, *Love's Labor*.
60. These relationships can be private, professional or social in nature.
61. Kittay, *Love's Labor*.
62. This, as argued above, is precisely what defines the relationship as asymmetric. People in symmetric relationships can, if they want, have their caring needs met within the relationship, while *only* the cared-for's (vital) needs can be fulfilled within an asymmetric relationship.
63. Kittay, *Love's Labor*, 28, 107.
64. Kittay, *Love's Labor*, 28.
65. Ibid., 31.
66. Noddings, *Caring*.
67. Kittay, *Love's Labor*.
68. Noddings, *Caring*, 60.
69. Friedman, 'Feminism in Ethics', 205–24.
70. Noddings, *Maternal Thinking*, 48–9.
71. Kittay's Love's Labour, p. 34.
72. Held, *Feminist Morality*, 3.

BIBLIOGRAPHY

de Beauvoir, Simone. *The Ethics of Ambiguity*. New York: Columbia University Press, 1976.

de Beauvoir, Simone. 'Pyrrhus and Cineas', in *Simone de Beauvoir: Philosophical Writings*, edited by Margaret A. Simons, Marybeth Timmerman and Mary B. Mader, 77–150. Urbana: University of Illinois Press, 2004.

Benhabib, Seyla. 'From Identity Politics to Social Feminism', in *Politics at the Turn of the Century*, edited by Arthur M. Melzer, Jerry Weinberger and Richard M. Zinman, 27–41. Lanham, MD: Rowman & Littlefield, 2001.

Card, Claudia. 'The Feistiness of Feminism', in *Feminist Ethics*, edited by Claudia Card, 3–34. Lawrence: University of Kansas, 1991.

The Care Collective, Andreas Chatzidakis, Jamie Hakim, Jo Litter and Catherine Rottenberg. *The Care Manifesto: The Politics of Interdependence*. New York: Verso Books, 2020.

Dalmiya, Vrinda. "Why Should a Knower Care?" *Hypatia* 17, 1 (2002), 34–52.

Eckenwiler, Lisa A. *Long-term Care, Globalization, and Justice*. Baltimore, MD: Johns Hopkins University Press, 2012.

Foss, Øyvind. *Omsorgsetikk: søkelys på omsorgens motivasjon*. Oslo: Cappelen Damm Akademisk, 2005.

Friedman, Marilyn. 'Feminism in Ethics: Conceptions of Autonomy', in *The Cambridge Companion to Feminism in Philosophy*, edited by Miranda Fricker and Jennifer Hornsby, 205–24. Cambridge: Cambridge University Press, 2000.

Garland-Thomson, Rosemarie. 'Integrating Disability, Transforming Feminist Theory', in *Feminist Disability Studies*, edited by Kim Q. Hall, 13–47. Bloomington: Indiana University Press, 2011.

Gastmans, Chris. Interview by Webteam. https://ethicsofcare.org/chris-gastmans/. Last modified 16 April 2011.

Gilligan, Carol. *In a Different Voice: Psychological Theory and Women's Development*. Cambridge, MA: Harvard University Press, 1982.

Haslanger, Sally. 'Gender and Social Construction: Who? What? When? Where? How?', in *Theorizing Feminisms: A Reader*, edited by Elizabeth Hackett and Sally Haslanger, 16–23. New York: Oxford University Press, 2006.
Held, Virginia. *Feminist Morality: Transforming Culture, Society, and Politics*. Chicago, IL: University of Chicago Press, 1993.
Held, Virginia. *The Ethics of Care: Personal, Political, and Global*. New York: Oxford University Press, 2006.
Held, Virginia. 'Can the Ethics of Care Handle Violence?' *Ethics and Social Welfare* 4, no. 2 (2010): 115–29.
Hem, Marit H. 'Mature Care? An Empirical Study of Interaction Between Psychotic Patients and Psychiatric Nurses', PhD diss., Oslo, 2008. Unipub.
Hem, Marit H., and Tove Pettersen. 'Mature Care and Nursing in Psychiatry: Notions Regarding Reciprocity in Asymmetric Professional Relationships', *Health Care Analysis* 19, no. 1 (2011): 65–76.
Hoagland, Sarah L. *Lesbian Ethics: Toward New Value*. Palo Alto, CA: Institute of Lesbian Studies, 1988.
Hursthouse, Rosalind. *On Virtue Ethics*. Oxford: Oxford University Press, 1999.
Kittay, Eva F. *Love's Labor: Essays on Women, Equality, and Dependency*. London: Psychology Press, 1999.
Kittay, Eva F. 'The Moral Harm of Migrant Carework', *Philosophical Topics* 37, no. 2 (2009): 53–73.
Kohlberg, Lawrence. *The Psychology of Moral Development: The Nature and Validity of Moral Stages*. San Francisco: Harper & Row, 1984.
Løgstrup, Knud E. *Den etiske fordring*. Oslo: Cappelen, 1999.
Lloyd, Genevieve. *The Man of Reason: 'Male' and 'Female' in Western Philosophy*. London: Routledge, 1984.
Lorde, Audre. *A Burst of Light: Essays*. Ithaca, NY: Firebrand Books, 1988.
Lynch, Kathleen. *Care and Capitalism*. Hoboken, NJ: John Wiley & Sons, 2022.
Mahon, Rianne, and Fiona Robinson. *Feminist Ethics and Social Policy: Towards a New Global Political Economy of Care*. Vancouver: University of British Columbia Press, 2011.
Martinsen, Kari. *Omsorg, sykepleie og medisin: historisk-filosofiske essays*. Oslo: Tano, 1989.
Martinsen, Kari. *Øyet og kallet*. Bergen: Fagbokforlaget, 2000.
Martinsen, Kari. *Fenomenologi og omsorg*. Oslo: Universitetsforlaget, 2003.
Martinsen, Kari. 'Kallet i går, i dag og i morgen – kan vi være foruten et kall?' *Kristent forum for sykepleiere og sykepleierstudenter* 3 (2003): 20–7.
Narayan, Uma. 'Colonialism and Its Others: Considerations on Rights and Care Discourses', *Hypatia* 10, no. 2 (1995): 133–40.
Noddings, Nel. *Caring: A Feminine Approach to Ethics and Moral Education*. Berkeley: University of California Press, 1984.
Noddings, Nel. *The Maternal Factor: Two Paths to Morality*. Oakland: University of California Press, 2010.
Nortvedt, Per. *Sensitive Judgment: Nursing, Moral Philosophy, and an Ethics of Care*. Oslo: Tano Aschehoug, 1996.
Nortvedt, Per. 'Levinas, Justice, and Health Care', *Medicine, Health Care, and Philosophy* 6 (2003): 25–34.
Nortvedt, Per. 'Den etiske fordring – omsorgens kjerne', in *Livtag med den etiske fordring*, edited by David Bugge and Peter A. Sørensen, 175–88. Århus: Klim, 2007.

Nortvedt, Per. *Omtanke: en innføring i sykepleiens etikk*. Oslo: Gyldendal Akademiske, 2012.
Pettersen, Tove. 'Comprehending Care. Problems and Possibilities in Carol Gilligan's Ethics of Care', PhD diss., University of Oslo, 2004. Unipub (Acta Humaniora no. 206).
Pettersen, Tove. *Comprehending Care: Problems and Possibilities in the Ethics of Care*. Lanham, MD: Lexington Books, 2008.
Pettersen, Tove. 'Acting for Others: Moral Ontology in Beauvoir's "Pyrrhus and Cineas"', *Simone de Beauvoir Studies* 26, no. 1 (2009): 18–27.
Pettersen, Tove. 'The Ethics of Care: Normative Structures and Empirical Implications', *Health Care Analysis* 19, no. 1 (2011): 51–64.
Pettersen, Tove. 'Conceptions of Care: Altruism, Feminism, and Mature Care', *Hypatia* 27, no. 2 (2012): 366–89.
Pettersen, Tove. 'Caring for More than Humans: Ecofeminism and Care Ethics in Conversation', in *Between Closeness and Evil*, edited by Odin Lysaker, 183–213. Oslo: Scandinavian Academic Press, 2020.
Pettersen, Tove. 'Feminist Care Ethics: Contributions to Peace Theory', in *Routledge Handbook of Feminist Peace Research*, edited by Tarja Väyrynen, Swati Parashar, Élise Féron and Catia C. Confortini, 28–39. London: Routledge, 2021.
Pettersen, Tove, and Marit H. Hem. 'Mature Care and Reciprocity: Two Cases from Acute Psychiatry', *Nursing Ethics* 18, no. 2 (2011): 217–31.
Plumwood, Val. *Feminism and the Mastery of Nature*. London: Routledge, 1993.
Robinson, Fiona. *The Ethics of Care: A Feminist Approach to Human Security*. Philadelphia, PA: Temple University Press, 2011.
Robinson, Fiona. 'Global Care Ethics: Beyond Distribution, Beyond Justice', *Journal of Global Ethics* 9, no. 2 (2013): 131–43.
Ruddick, Sara. *Maternal Thinking: Toward a Politics of Peace*. Boston, MA: Beacon Press, 1989.
Silvers, Anita. 'Reconciling Equality to Difference: Caring (F)or Justice For People With Disabilities', *Hypatia* 10, no. 1 (1995): 30–55.
Silvers, Anita. 'Disability', in *A Companion to Feminist Philosophy*, edited by Alison M. Jagger and Iris M. Young, 330–40. Malden, MA: Blackwell Publishing, 1998.
Tronto, Joan C. *Moral Boundaries: A Political Argument for an Ethic of Care*. New York: Routledge, 1993.
Tronto, Joan C. 'The "Nanny" Question in Feminism', *Hypatia*17, no. 2 (2002): 34–51.
Tronto, Joan C. *Caring Democracy: Markets, Equality, and Justice*. New York: New York University Press, 2013.
Tuckett, Anthony. 'Nursing Practice: Compassionate Deception and the Good Samaritan', *Nursing Ethics* 6, no. 5 (1999): 383–9.
Warren, Karen. *Ecofeminist Philosophy: A Western Perspective on What It Is and Why It Matters*. Lanham, MD: Rowman & Littlefield, 2000.
Watson, Nick, Linda McKie, Bill Hughes, Debra Hopkins and Sue Gregory. '(Inter) Dependence, Needs and Care', *Sociology* 38, no. 2 (2004): 331–50.

CHAPTER THREE

Dependency as a core concept for care ethics

A chronology (and a plea)

SIMON VAN DER WEELE

INTRODUCTION

Dependency has been a core concept for care ethicists since the inception of care ethics as an ethical theory and a domain of moral philosophy.[1] Although care ethicists continue to debate the precise nature and value of dependency,[2] most would agree that dependency at least denotes the reliance each of us has on others to fulfil particular needs. We are all dependent on others to care for us, albeit some of us more intensely so than others. It is thus our condition of dependency that throws us into relationships and renders us relational beings. In this way, dependency provides care ethicists both with an alternative moral subject – relational rather than independent – and with the main wellspring of care-ethical thinking: our relationships to others and the responsibilities these entail. For these reasons, Stephanie Collins rightly locates dependency at the core of care ethics.[3]

In recent years, however, care ethicists have begun to stray away from dependency as care ethics' heart. Such care ethicists do not doubt the relevance of dependency for care ethics as such. They doubt, rather, whether dependency can truly carry the philosophical weight that care ethicists have traditionally encumbered it with. This leads such care ethicists to introduce related but distinct concepts, most notably interdependence,[4] vulnerability[5] and precariousness or precarity.[6] To be sure, the attention paid to these concepts reflects broader trends in moral and political philosophy, which have observed a surge in thinking about these concepts and their implications – most significantly for vulnerability[7] and precariousness.[8] Yet the rethinking of care ethics in terms of vulnerability or precariousness is no mere fad. What motivates it are serious questions about the viability of dependency as the heart of care ethics.

This chapter has two purposes. The first purpose is to draw a chronology of dependency as a concept for care ethics. What I present here is a reception history of sorts, in which I outline the care-ethical writing on dependency from the inception of care ethics to the present. My intention is to demonstrate why and how (1) care ethicists began to draw attention to dependency, (2) critics (notably, disability theorists) have decisively shaped the care-ethical discourse on dependency, and (3) some care ethicists moved away from dependency to interdependence, vulnerability or precariousness. To show these broad trends, I will have to paint in broad strokes. I hope my readers will grant me the odd historical reduction for the sake of the argument I present.

The second purpose of the chapter is to make a plea for keeping dependency at the conceptual heart of care ethics. There are good reasons for expanding the care-ethical vocabulary to include concepts like vulnerability and precariousness, but I believe that dependency ought to remain at its core. To explain why, I return to the earliest care-ethical writers, who first pointed at the intrinsic connection between our dependency and the moral import of relationships. Insofar as attention for relationships makes up the foremost care-ethical contribution to moral philosophy, it is dependency that ought to remain at the heart of care-ethical thinking.

3.1 DEPENDENCY IN CARE ETHICS' FOUNDATIONS

Let us begin by exploring the role of dependency in care-ethical thinking. Dependency was part of the care-ethical vocabulary from the get-go. Pioneering care ethicists such as Nel Noddings,[9] Sara Ruddick[10] and Virginia Held[11] all placed dependency at the forefront of their thinking. More politically oriented 'second-generation' care ethicists[12] like Joan Tronto[13] and Eva Kittay[14] also gave prominent roles to dependency in their variations of an ethic of care. In the work of these authors, dependency is not just one link in a chain of care-ethical concepts, such as responsibility, kindness, responsivity, trust and, of course, care; dependency also serves as the normative anchor that provides care ethics with its ethical force. What these authors emphasized is that it is dependency that instigates and necessitates caring. And since dependency is inevitable and ubiquitous, care will be ethically vital for humans to survive and thrive. To understand the precise role dependency plays in this classic care-ethical work, I will now consider how the concept surfaces in the writing of these authors.

Let us first take a look at what these authors have to say about what dependency *is*.[15] Interestingly, the 'early' care ethicists do not always provide succinct definitions of dependency, in spite of the concept's import for their thinking. However, all of them would likely subscribe to Sarah Clark Miller's helpful definition of dependency as 'situations of significant reliance on others that all persons undergo during the course of their lives'.[16] Dependency is thus defined by *need*: a need the dependent cannot meet herself, causing her to rely on another for tending to it. In this way, this need also gives rise to a dependency *relationship*, formed by someone who has a need (variously called the 'charge', 'care-receiver', 'cared-for', etc.) and someone who is to meet that need (variously called the 'dependency worker', the 'caregiver', the 'one caring', etc.).

Two points follow from this definition that particularly stand out for care ethicists. The first is that relationships of dependency are decidedly *unequal*. Tronto calls this 'the fact of inequality in relations of care'.[17] Since the dependency relationship is formed by a caregiver tending to a vital need that a care recipient cannot meet herself, power will be distributed asymmetrically by definition. For this reason, 'inequality of power is endemic to dependency relations', as Kittay puts it.[18] Care ethicists were quick to note that this 'fact of inequality' brings moral trouble to any dependency relationship and bestows caregivers with serious responsibilities. As we will see, it is also this 'fact of inequality' that incited a flurry of criticism at the first formulations of care-ethical thinking, precisely because it highlights the sheer vulnerability of those who receive care.

The second point of interest for care ethicists that follows from this definition of dependency is that there is absolutely nothing exceptional about dependency as such. Dependency, in the care-ethical understanding, is an inevitability in human life: fundamentally, dependency is part of the human life course, starting with the total dependency that characterizes our infancy, and then returning periodically in many lives – for instance, during times of sickness or injury and as we encounter the increasing frailties that mark old age. Disability (whether physical or intellectual) is another predicament that can have people experience dependency.[19]

Additionally, dependency also marks our lives in less obvious but no more trivial ways, if we think of our relationships to partners, friends, colleagues, teachers and all kinds of professional workers as dependency relationships – a fact made palpable when newly dubbed 'essential workers', such as nurses, refuse collectors and grocery store workers, suddenly gained public recognition in the early stages of the Covid-19 pandemic in 2020. This universal quality of dependency brought care ethicists to interrogate what they often call 'liberal' political and ethical theories for relying on overly individualized (and masculinized) notions of the subject or the person. After all, if dependency (and thus inequality) is endemic to human life, the liberal picture of human life that assumes universal equality is at least flawed, if not outright mistaken. Such feminist dissatisfaction with 'liberal' theorizing was an important motivation for care ethicists to start developing their more relationally attuned ethic of care.

With this conception of dependency in mind, what do care ethicists say about what dependency *does* for care ethics? Kittay perhaps puts it most succinctly when she writes that '[d]ependents require care'.[20] In other words, people who are dependent have needs that others need to attend to – which, for Kittay, is both an empirical truth and a normative claim. It is in this sense that dependency necessitates care. And, for Kittay, dependency thus engenders particular moral responsibilities. She goes on: 'neither the utterly helpless newborn who must be cared for in all aspects of her life nor a frail, but functioning, elderly person who needs only assistance to carry on with her life, will survive or thrive without another who meets her basic needs'.[21] For dependent human beings to live – let alone live decent lives – they will need care provided by others. This is what marks the moral urgency of care. And since (as we have seen) dependency is an inherent and inevitable element of our human condition, the moral stakes are high. As Kittay points out herself, 'no culture that endures beyond one generation can be secure against the claims of human dependency'.[22] In Kittay's rendering, care is a defining human activity *because* we humans are dependent.

Kittay's logic is mirrored in the writing of foundational care-ethical thinkers, both in form and in content. That is, many of them believe that dependency requires the moral response of care, and they too frame this as both an empirical and ethical claim. Ruddick, for instance, points to dependency as a 'source of normativity' for care ethics, in the sense that 'memories of caring and being cared for inspire a sense of obligation'.[23] She thus seems to think that experiences of being dependent and tending to dependency form us as ethical subjects who feel obliged to respond to the dependency of others. Similarly, Noddings (in a more phenomenological vein) regarded care as both a natural and moral response to witnessing the neediness of those whom she calls the 'cared-for'. A feeling of 'I must' 'sweeps over us … in response to the plight of the other', she writes.[24] In these writings, dependency secures the moral responsibility for caring.

3.2 THE ADVENT OF A 'DEPENDENCY DEBATE'

The writings of the 'early' care ethicists sparked plenty of debate, both within feminist philosophy and outside of it. Much of the controversy centred on the ontology of dependency and its moral ramifications. The ensuing academic debate on dependency, which I have elsewhere referred to as the 'dependency debate',[25] dominated care-ethical discourse in the 1990s and early 2000s. Unease about dependency's central role in care ethics chiefly came from two directions: from feminist philosophers and from disability scholars. I now consider their objections in turn, before detailing some of the rejoinders proffered by care ethicists in response.

3.2.1 Feminist critiques

Disputes around the nature and value of dependency were first triggered by feminist philosophers wary of the care-ethical project. Some of these philosophers chose to dismiss the care-ethical project in its entirety, because they feared that focusing on the more 'feminine' values of care and dependency over allegedly 'masculine' values like autonomy would only relegate women once more to the role of housekeepers in the private sphere. In other words, the worry was that the care-ethical project would hinder women's emancipatory efforts.[26] Others worried that the moral focus on concrete dependency relationships rendered care ethics parochial, insufficiently concerned with the wellbeing of strangers outside of our inner circle, and without an adequate vocabulary to tackle issues of justice.[27] For these philosophers, it was not the particular *rendition* of dependency that troubled feminist theorists, but rather the choice to centre care and dependency in the first place.

It is more interesting, however, to look at the concerns raised by feminist philosophers who were sympathetic to an ethic of care, but still sceptical of how care ethicists theorized dependency and its normative link to care. For them, the simple fact that dependency is endemic to the human condition could tell us nothing about how to value it, nor about how to value the care that it seems to demand. As I just showed, early care ethicists tended to justify the normative link between care and dependency in terms of the image of a mother caring for her child, which for them was an archetypical example of 'natural' care. But feminist critics chastised this move, for two reasons: (1) because it naturalized and romanticized the bond between mother and child; and (2) because it brought asymmetry to the heart of morality. Let me briefly develop these complaints in turn.

The first complaint is that care ethicists relied on a romanticized and empirically inaccurate depiction of the mother–child relationship to make their arguments work. Feminist philosophers argued that the image of a mother 'naturally' wanting to care for an infant was perhaps rhetorically compelling, but also far from realistic, let alone universal; several commentators identified the care-ethical point of view as ethnocentric: an example of white, middle-class feminism.[28] To draw a normative link between dependency and care through the mother–child image, the thought went, thus required a naturalization and idealization of a bond that was in reality not only multifarious, but also messy and frequently uncomfortable, exploitative or even violent. More importantly, these philosophers claimed, the image also relied on tropes that were harmful to women, who were stereotypically depicted as 'natural' carers in a romanticized mother-role.[29] (Indeed, fathers were notably absent in much early care-ethical work.)

The second complaint is that making one-sided, skewed relations of dependency the heart of care ethics means that the care-ethical project insufficiently attends to the possibility – and importance – of reciprocity and equality in care relationships. This is both an empirical and an ethical concern. On the one hand, so the argument goes, care ethicists simply failed to capture the full picture of caring by focusing on full dependency. Sarah Lucia Hoagland, for instance, wrote that 'the very purpose of parenting, as well as teaching and theraping which are also part of the model, is to wean the cared-for of dependency. Consequently, an ethic of caring whose model is a dependency relationship that is ideally transitory provides at best for an incomplete analysis of caring.'[30] But, on the other hand, there are normative concerns here, too: without reciprocity at the heart of care, care can become oppressive, both of caregivers and care recipients alike. Care ethics therefore needed a more complex account of dependency so that it could more adequately address issues of inequality and power.

3.2.2 Disability critiques

These critical feminist voices were soon joined by disability theorists, who questioned not only how care ethicists valued dependency, but also even the ontological inevitability of dependency itself. Authors such as Anita Silvers,[31] Jenny Morris,[32] Mike Oliver[33] and Tom Shakespeare worried that these care-ethical approaches to dependency overlooked the social nature of dependency faced by many disabled people.[34] Often drawing on the social model of disability, they contended that it was the practice of care itself that rendered disabled people dependent – and this dependency needed to be resisted rather than recognized.

Dependency, in this conception, is neither inevitable nor endemic to the human condition; rather, dependency is what Shakespeare called 'a product of particular social relations', both caused by and exacerbating the oppression of disabled people.[35] In essence, then, these disability scholars fundamentally challenged the normative link between care and dependency that care ethicists attempted to draw. For them, dependency did not 'require' care at all, to invoke Kittay's formulation. Rather, care precipitated dependency – which to them meant oppression and marginalization. In this rendition, dependency becomes practically synonymous with the social model account of disability itself: a form of socially induced oppression only contingently related to particular qualities of one's actual body or mind.

I want to give a sense of the logic of this disability critique by looking in more detail at Silvers's rendition of it, which to my mind is most engaged philosophically with the work of the early care ethicists. Silvers's main objective was to denaturalize dependency: to show that care ethicists too readily take for granted the asymmetrical relations of dependency that tether their moral theory. Silvers was willing to concede that some dependencies were inevitable and did require care. However, she also warned that 'a dependent stance is advantageous only if genuine – that is, if the putative dependent is truly incompetent'.[36] But many who find themselves dependent, not in the least disabled people, are not incompetent at all. For them, dependency is not 'genuine' but merely the 'pretence of helplessness'.[37]

Why would disabled people 'profess incompetence' in this way?[38] The answer lies in Silvers's specific understanding of care. If care is a celebrated moral disposition, she believed, then moral agents will need opportunities to display their moral competence through caring and helping. Disabled people are expected to provide such opportunities due to stereotypes about their supposed incompetence. And since disabled people do need support sometimes, they have no choice but to indulge these caregivers. In other words, the only way for disabled people to keep themselves intelligible as moral subjects worthy of help and support is to let themselves be cared for – which for Silvers meant acquiescing to asymmetrical relationships that enable exploitation and marginalization. In this way, disabled people are 'obligated to let ourselves be harmed simply to afford others opportunities to be virtuous', wrote Silvers.[39] Silvers thus problematized both the ontological ubiquity of dependency and the notion that an 'acceptable morality, feminist or otherwise, can flourish on dependence'.[40]

The comments of disability theorists such as Silvers may sound philosophically crude to some. Silvers, for instance, does not quite address the seeming inconsistency in her argument between her insistence that disabled people are 'consigned' to dependency and her more tacit acknowledgement that disabled people do need care, at least sometimes. It is important, therefore, to understand these arguments in their historical time and place. Authors such as Silvers were writing in a context in which disability activism was largely directed at achieving a greater degree of autonomy and self-determination for people with disabilities, moving away from residential-style care towards the personal assistance model, including cash-for-care and independent living schemes. The care-ethical emphasis on dependency and care was clearly at odds with the political rhetoric of this activism, which centred on the ideal of *in*dependence.[41] As we will see, as care ethicists began to articulate the political ramifications of their project more systematically, disability theorists soon began to find more common ground with them.

3.2.3 Care ethicists respond

The complaint against early care-ethical conceptualizations of dependency was thus twofold: feminists and disability theorists variously troubled the assumption that dependency is endemic to the human condition as well as the moral ramifications care ethicists drew from this assumption. From these objections arose a debate on the ontology and moral value of dependency. Should dependency be thought of as necessary or as imposed? As universal or as contingent? As temporary or as permanent? As helplessness or oppression? Depending on how one answered these questions, one's estimation of dependency – and of care itself – would shift dramatically. In this way, as I have written elsewhere, 'the concept of dependency became a Rorschach test of sorts for care theorists': what they saw in dependency revealed what they saw in care, too.[42]

How did care ethicists respond to these objections? I should note, first, that some of the strongest criticisms were not entirely fair to the sophisticated analyses presented by authors like Noddings and Ruddick. The concern that care ethicists do not adequately attend to reciprocity in dependency relationships, for instance, was in fact partially pre-empted by Noddings, who believed care (as an ideal) was only 'completed' when the cared-for accepts and receives the care being offered. '[R]ecognition of caring by the cared-for is necessary to the caring relation ... there is, necessarily, a form of reciprocity in caring', she wrote.[43] Similarly, the concern that care ethicists idealized the bond between mother and child seems difficult to maintain in light of Ruddick's prolonged discussion of what she called the 'struggle typical of maternal work' and the many frustrations caregiver might experience in their attempts to provide good enough care.[44] The critics of the care-ethical project did not always pick up on the intricacies present in this early care-ethical work.

Nevertheless, care ethicists did seem to take the objections levelled at them to heart. For example, Tronto[45] and Kittay,[46] both of whom published their landmark books on care ethics in the midst of the 'dependency debate', painstakingly explored the moral complexities of dependency relationships, such as the threat of domination and the significance of reciprocity. Tronto, not unlike Noddings, insisted that the process of care is not complete without 'care-receiving' – that is, the recognition of care by the care recipient. Good care, if not always reciprocal, at least requires that the care recipient responds to care, to ascertain that their need has been met and has been met adequately. The role of the care recipient thus gained theoretical prominence.

Tronto also began to stake out the fractured moral terrain of dependency relationships, analysing, for instance, the othering and paternalizing potential of caring following from asymmetries between the caregiver and care recipient.[47] Kittay, who continued to take the care relationship between a caregiver and her wholly dependent 'charge' as her 'paradigm case' of dependency, also attended in detail to problems of inequality, domination and vulnerability in such care relationships – a far cry from the alleged idealizing tendencies of early care-ethical thinking.[48] In these discussions, dependency becomes a multifaceted concept, a container of tensions between necessity and contingency and solicitude and abuse.

Notably, these authors pushed the ethics of care in a much more political direction; for instance, they considered at length how dependency relationships are patterned along lines of gender and race, as well as how caregivers are themselves tangled up in complex dependency relationships that secure the time and resources to care (Kittay's concept of 'nested' dependencies – see also below). In this vein, Tronto warned against the 'romanticisation of mother and child' that might follow from modelling philosophical concepts of care after the dyadic and (supposedly) necessary relationship between one mother and her infant – as she reminded us, even child-rearing itself is seldom a solitary pursuit.[49] Tronto sought to move beyond the mother–child blueprint to show how 'care can function socially and politically in a culture'. It is as though considering complex dependency relationships, beyond the (perhaps idealized) image of the mother–child relationship, brought care ethicists to attend in more detail to the social formations in which concrete care relations are nestled. Even if these authors did not always explicitly enter into dialogue with these feminist and disability critiques, we can read their work as responses to the concerns that had been raised against the earliest care ethicists.

3.3 FORAYS BEYOND DEPENDENCY

As the dependency debate swelled, so did the concept of dependency. Dependency transformed into a container of myriad ontological and ethical tensions: between the necessity of 'inevitable' dependency and the contingency of 'socially constructed' dependency; between the solicitude of care and the tyranny of domination; and between the passivity of 'helpless' dependents and the agency of subjects 'made' dependent.[50] These binary oppositions reflect just how polarized this debate was at its height.

Yet care ethicists and their interlocutors gradually started looking for some common ground as well. Some authors did this by looking for ways to reconcile the various tensions harboured by dependency.[51] Disability theorist Jenny Morris, for instance, sought to conceptualize dependency so that she could acknowledge both the inevitability of some dependencies for disabled people as well as the importance for autonomy within conditions of dependency.[52] Other authors tried to relieve the conceptual tensions within dependency by splitting it up in a set of sub-concepts.[53] Most famous, in this regard, is probably the distinction made by Nancy Fraser and Linda Gordon between 'economic', 'political', 'sociolegal' and 'moral/psychological' registers of dependency.[54] To this, Kittay later added a fifth register of 'inevitable human dependence'.[55]

At the same time, care ethicists also began to look beyond dependency as the conceptual anchor for the theory's moral claims. In this regard, three concepts stand out in particular: interdependence, vulnerability and precariousness. I will now go over each of these proposed supplements to dependency, explaining how they are defined by care ethicists and why (some) care ethicists believe they ought to sit at the moral heart of care ethics as a moral theory. Afterwards, I reflect on the merit of these proposals for care ethics.

3.3.1 Interdependence

The first concept care ethicists brought to the centre of care ethics is interdependence. Again, I turn to Miller for a helpful definition of the term.

> According to the care perspective, persons are not fundamentally independent. Rather, they are mutually dependent. Our unavoidable dependency means that if we are to survive, let alone thrive in leading lives that are recognizably human, others must respond to our dependent selves by meeting our needs through their caring actions ... But I am not solely a dependent being who needs others to bolster my well-being; others, in their inevitable dependence, also need my assistance, hence solidifying the mutuality of the relation.[56]

Interdependence thus underscores that dependencies are *mutual* and structure the social fabric of human societies; all of us have needs that can only be met by others, in various degrees, throughout our lifespan. There are two ways in which dependency can be said to be mutual according to care ethicists. First, human beings are interdependent in a *generational* sense: as an infant, all of us will rely on the care of others to survive – care which many of us will, in turn, provide for infants as we grow into adulthood. (As Kittay often put it idiomatically: 'we are all some mother's child'.) Second, human beings are also interdependent in a *societal* sense: we all rely on others to make our way in the world – on bakers, farmers, therapists, teachers, truck drivers, cleaners, refuse collectors and so on (the 'essential workers' I already mentioned above).

Truth be told, interdependence was never quite 'new' to care ethics. The idea of interdependence was used by care ethicists pretty much from the outset, to capture the idea of universal dependency: no human can be truly independent, as we all depend on others for care and services to varying degrees. Thus, even if the *term* interdependence did not always appear explicitly in the writing of scholars like Noddings and Ruddick, care ethicists like them were surely working in the *spirit* of the concept.

Yet when care ethicists began to take their project in a more outwardly political direction – a development, as I suggested, we can ascribe at least in part to their feminist and disability critics – the concept of interdependence increasingly became an explicit part of the care-ethical vocabulary. Tronto, for instance, insisted that a care perspective forced us to 'rethink our conceptions of human nature to shift from the dilemma of autonomy or dependency to a more sophisticated sense of human interdependence'.[57] For Tronto, then, interdependence was a crucial insight of the care-ethical project. Selma

Sevenhuijsen, another prominent 'political' care ethicist, similarly appreciated how interdependence exposed simplistic 'binary' thinking in terms of oppositions between autonomy and dependency or individual and community. For her, this was enough to deem interdependence the 'guiding principle of care ethics'.[58]

In my view, no care ethicist has considered the notion of interdependence as thoroughly as Kittay. As mentioned above, Kittay introduced the idea of 'nested' dependencies, referring to the way in which specific dependency relationships tend to generate new ones; for instance, to provide full-time care for a profoundly disabled child, a caregiver will have to rely on some form of support herself, be it from a partner, a state or otherwise. After all, those who spend time taking care have much less time to acquire resources needed for care – and to take care of themselves. For Kittay, this idea of nested dependency is an ontological fact, but it also functions normatively to anchor a set of public responsibilities. '[F]or the dependency worker to meet her responsibilities to another, it must be the responsibility of the larger social order to provide a structure whereby she, too, may be treated as a mother's child', she writes, meaning someone whose needs deserve to be met.[59] Without such structures, caregivers will be hindered in fulfilling their caregiving responsibilities, and the essential task of caregiving unfairly becomes a personal responsibility rather than a public good. Seeing as those caregivers will most likely be women, this is also a source of gender equality.

Interestingly, although 'nested dependencies' were obviously important for Kittay, she also insisted that dependency has analytical priority over interdependence: 'interdependence begins with dependence', she wrote.[60] Kittay believed that care-ethical analysis must start from the total dependency of an infant or a person with profound intellectual disabilities, because bracketing such dependencies would allow us to uphold the fiction of independence she sought to dispel – the fiction that 'interdependence is simply the mutual (often voluntary) cooperation between essentially independent persons'.[61] For Kittay, the care-ethical project could only be inclusive to the 'genuine needs and legitimate wants'[62] of those who are most dependent if it recognized asymmetrical relationships of total dependency as the foundation of human life. Thus, although Kittay significantly contributed to the development of the concept of interdependence, it did not become the linchpin of her care-ethical project.

The concept of interdependence has been taken up by various philosophers attempting to shed light on the complex interplay between dependency and autonomy that characterizes care relationships between people with disabilities and their caregivers.[63] It has also proven an acceptable compromise for disability critics looking to grapple with the care-ethical assertion that dependency is universal in light of their own intuition that dependency signals oppression.[64] In such work, interdependence is invoked to sidestep some of the more unwelcome connotations dependency carries, such as asymmetry, one-sidedness and submission. In this way, interdependence seems to help theorists resolve some of the core tensions harboured by the concept of dependency.

3.3.2 Vulnerability

Over the past few decades, vulnerability has become a central concept in (often feminist) philosophical and political-theoretical conversations about ethics and justice.[65] These conversations have not passed care ethicists by. Although vulnerability was always part of the care-ethical vocabulary – albeit often not clearly defined, nor demarcated from dependency – the past years have seen the concept drift ever closer to the core of care ethics, a trend visible in work by Estelle Ferrarese[66] and Sandra Laugier.[67] Amidst these philosophers, Daniel Engster has proposed to swap dependency for vulnerability as the definite theoretical backbone of care ethics.[68] To my mind, Engster is most self-aware about the theoretical shift towards dependency in care ethics. I will therefore now discuss his proposal in detail, to illustrate how and why vulnerability might 'replace' dependency as the theoretical foundation of the care-ethical project.

Let us start again with a definition of vulnerability. Engster does not provide a full-fledged definition, so I will turn to Martha Fineman's (herself not a care ethicist), whose account of vulnerability he largely follows.

> Vulnerability initially should be understood as arising from our embodiment, which carries with it the ever-present possibility of harm, injury, and misfortune from mildly adverse to catastrophically devastating events, whether accidental, intentional, or otherwise. Individuals can attempt to lessen the risk or mitigate the impact of such events, but they cannot eliminate their possibility. Understanding vulnerability begins with the realization that many such events are ultimately beyond human control.[69]

Fineman thus regards vulnerability as a 'state of constant possibility of harm'.[70] As such, it must be understood as a 'universal, inevitable, enduring aspect of the human condition'.[71] However, Fineman also underlines the particularity of vulnerability: 'it is experienced uniquely by each of us and this experience is greatly influenced by the quality and quantity of resources we possess or can command'.[72]

With this definition of vulnerability in hand, Engster begins to sketch its relationship to dependency. He sees dependency as a specific *form* of vulnerability: vulnerability is the more general category of which dependency is one instance. He approvingly cites Susan Dodds: 'Dependence is vulnerability that requires the support of a specific person (or people) – that is, care. To be dependent is to be in circumstances in which one must rely on the care of other individuals to access, provide or secure (one or more of) one's needs, and promote and support the development of one's autonomy or agency.'[73] For Engster, then, dependency denotes a vulnerability that requires a response from a concrete other, in the form of close personal care. (By contrast, other vulnerabilities might require a caring response not in the form of personal care, but less immediate institutional practices.) To Dodds's point, Engster adds two further characteristics that render dependency a specific form of vulnerability. First, Engster clarifies that dependency is a vulnerability that people cannot address on their own; dependents need *others* to take care of them, while people who 'by normal social standards take care of themselves' must also be considered vulnerable. Second, dependency requires a particularly urgent response; 'without some action on the part of others, harm, loss, or blight are highly probable and imminent'.[74]

Care, in Engster's framework, becomes a mitigating response to the broad state of vulnerability rather than to dependency, as most care ethicists would have had it. According to Engster, herein lies the greatest advantage of having vulnerability supplant dependency as the core of care ethics. Working with vulnerability allows care ethicists to broaden their conceptions of care, so that they come to include all kinds of institutional interventions that cannot be recognized as care when working with the dyadic model of close personal care. Some examples Engster mentions here are various forms of (state) protection, improving labour conditions and upholding personal liberties. These are responses to vulnerability, but not to dependency, at least not as Engster defines it. Intuitively, many care ethicists might have deemed such practices care, but it has not always been easy to justify this intuition; the picture of dyadic dependency held them captive, to paraphrase Wittgenstein. Placing vulnerability at the core of care ethics, then, 'redirects thinking about care away from a narrow focus on dyadic dependency relationships toward a broader, communal understanding' of care, suggests Engster.[75] And this allows care ethics to reverberate much more widely as a challenge to liberal theories of justice.

This relates to a second advantage Engster claims for a vulnerability-centred care ethics. With another nod to Fineman, Engster argues that challenges to liberal ethical and political theories on the basis of dependency can all too easily be dismissed by liberal theorists; such theorists can dismiss dependency as merely transitory and episodic and hence peripheral to politics. Moreover, the liberal public/private split also allows theorists to relegate dependency (and care) to the private realm: a personal responsibility resulting from a choice to be a parent, for instance. Vulnerability, meanwhile, is supposedly so undeniably universal that liberal theories must – and often already do – heed to it. In this way, where dependency fell short, vulnerability truly carries the potential of 'upending the dominant liberal discourse and mobilising broad support for a more responsive state'.[76] It is for these reasons that Engster pushes vulnerability to the centre of care ethics.

3.3.3 Precariousness

In recent years, precariousness has – like vulnerability – found its way into philosophy and political theory as a central concept of discussion.[77] And, like vulnerability, so precariousness (and its conceptual sibling, precarity) has been taken up in care ethics too.[78] Again, to explore how and why precariousness might have its place in the conceptual core of care ethics, I explore a specific proposal that makes this claim, this time Miller's. To be sure, Miller explicitly states she has no desire to replace dependency with precariousness: 'it is dependency, not vulnerability ... that serves as the ultimate ground of moral responsibility', she writes.[79] Yet insofar as Miller believes precariousness to be a significant addition to the care-ethical vocabulary, her proposal is worth exploring.

For Miller, precariousness makes up one-quarter of a 'constellation of care ethics' concepts ... comprising the substance of care ethics'.[80] The other concepts in the constellation are needs, vulnerability and dependency. Since uses of these terms tend to overlap, Miller attempts to define them in relation to each other. To grasp what she means by precariousness, it thus helps to briefly assess how she defines the other concepts in the constellation. *Need* 'indicates that which must be met or provided in order for humans to continue to live, to function as agents, and to thrive'. *Vulnerability* refers to an 'openness to the world and to other people ... over which we have little control'.[81] And *dependency*, finally, denotes our reliance on others to meet our needs and respond to our vulnerability. With these conceptualizations in mind, this is Miller's definition of precariousness:

> What precariousness adds to the moral landscape [of care ethics], and the feature of the overall human condition that it highlights, is attention to the fundamental instability and uncertainty that run through life. Our precariousness is embodied in the uncertainty of whether we can maintain a position where are our needs are met, where we do not actively and overtly need, where we are not currently being harmed. Articulated in the specific register of care ethics, precariousness brings us face to face with the uncertainty of whether we will be the consistent and abiding subject of others' care.[82]

Precariousness thus refers to the instability and uncertainty that mark human lives; of the presence of others, the solidity of social (infra)structures, of a responsive supporting state and so on. In this way, for care ethics, the concept of precariousness 'helps us to understand the extent to which care itself can be unstable'.[83]

Miller seems to take this concept of precariousness largely from Judith Butler's exploration of the term.[84] But, unlike Butler, Miller seeks to elucidate the role precariousness plays in the 'foundation, scope, and content of moral responsibility' in care ethics.[85] For Miller, precariousness constitutes one of four 'faces of human finitude' in which the source of moral responsibility for others lies – the other three being need, vulnerability and dependency. Dependency is the most critical of these: in what is quite a classic care-ethical argument, Miller argues that dependency must orient us morally because it reveals the essential role of caregiving in 'coming to be and continuing to exist as human beings with full agency and life'.[86] (Recall Kittay: the origin of moral responsibility is that 'dependents require care'.) Precariousness, meanwhile, points us at the uncertainty of such care being given or giving way, a risk all of us face indefinitely. 'If interdependence is the foundation of moral responsibility, then precariousness represents the ever-present call to attend to the care that others might need', Miller concludes.[87] In this 'constellation' of care-ethical concepts, precariousness becomes a significant, but not foundational, aspect of the moral demand of care.

3.4 DEPENDENCY AS THE RELATIONAL CORE OF CARE ETHICS

Dependency, as I have shown, has proven a contested concept in care ethics, a harbinger of moral tension, rife with internal contradictions. Given its ambiguities, dependency is perhaps an unlikely concept to tether a moral theory. No wonder, then, that care ethicists have looked beyond dependency to theorize the moral foundation of care ethics to interdependence, vulnerability and precariousness. What can we make of these proposals?

Interdependence, the insistence on *mutual* dependency, perhaps responds most directly to some of the concerns raised by critics in what I have called the dependency debate. Interdependence upholds the ethical primacy of (concrete or more abstract) relations of dependency but makes more conceptual space for reciprocity and symmetry, as it moves away from strictly dyadic accounts of caregiving towards what Kittay calls 'nested' dependencies. In this way, it relieves some of the moral anxieties from dependency's critics. Additionally, interdependence allows care ethicists to integrate care in social-political analyses, and also points towards a different conception of political equality, rooted not in our individual autonomy but in our relations to others.[88] In other words, interdependence can seem more acceptable ethically and more fruitful analytically than the much maligned dependency concept.

At the same time, Kittay's point surely still stands: 'interdependence begins with dependence'.[89] Interdependence can only anchor care ethics if dependency is acknowledged first. Without dependency, interdependence is emptied of its ethical significance, as it becomes just another way to describe the social-contractual relations of essentially independent individuals. We are all dependent, but some of us are more dependent than others, and these differences ought to matter to care theorists; precisely those differences generate responsibilities that go beyond those of a social contract. For this reason, interdependence can only make up the heart of care ethics in tandem with dependency. In this sense, interdependence does not so much challenge to replace dependency, but is rather an enrichment of the original care-ethical dependency concept.

The latter is not the case for vulnerability and precariousness, which are clearly different concepts that accentuate different aspects of the human condition. In a sense, then, these concepts do not so much resolve tensions contained in dependency, but rather look beyond them. Vulnerability signals our capacity to be touched, impinged upon; precariousness our proneness to uncertainty. Although, like Miller,[90] I consider these concepts relevant additions to the care-ethical vocabulary, I am sceptical that they can supplant dependency as the moral anchor of a care-ethical theory. This is because only dependency brings into relief our fundamental relationships to particular others and the responsibilities that emanate from these relationships. We can imagine vulnerability or precariousness without relationships, but not dependency; dependency *is* the relationship. If vulnerability or precariousness takes ontological and ethical precedence over dependency, this fundamental relationality – the core insight of care ethics – is no longer secure.

Let me explain with an example. Engster sees dependency as a particular *form* of vulnerability. The result is that dependency is no longer regarded as a core aspect of human existence. Vulnerability is the norm and dependency one instance of that norm. This is why Engster can differentiate between those who are 'truly' dependent and those who are 'merely' vulnerable, i.e. those who 'by normal social standards take care of themselves'.[91] I am reminded here of Silvers's attempt to differentiate those dependents who are 'truly' incompetent from those who merely 'profess' incompetence to receive care. Empirically, there is nothing wrong with this claim, of course. But on a conceptual level, we lose something important here: the sense in which we are always already thrown into relationships and that this fact has moral implications. If we take vulnerability or precariousness over dependency by casting the latter as a mere *instance* of the former, we can only do so at the expense of reducing dependency to an exclusively circumstantial condition: we are only *sometimes* dependent, or only some of us are *truly* dependent, and hence only *sometimes* rely on others. Such a move brings us awfully close to the liberal trope that we are essentially independent individuals, who perhaps sometimes just need a little bit of help – the very trope Engster himself sought to avoid. I do not think such a move serves care ethics.

'[C]are theorists have become prisoners of their own concepts', writes Engster about the care-ethical reliance on dependency as its foundation.[92] For him, thinking about care in terms of dependency leaves us with an overly narrow idea of what care can be, one that does not serve the care-ethical project. But concepts are not (just) prisons. They are lenses, directing our gaze to things that merit our attention. No doubt care ethicists do have much to learn from attending to interdependence, vulnerability and precariousness. But if it was not for a gaze steered by dependency – trained to see our particular relationships to others, and the network of responsibilities in which we find ourselves enmeshed as a result – what would those concepts show us? Without fundamental attention to dependency, a deep awareness of the fundamental relationality of existence, care ethics could not be what it now is; it could not show why, say, something like our vulnerability is ethically *relevant* for us.

This is why I think care ethicists are condemned to dealing with dependency at the core of care ethics. This is no easy fate, because dependency is an uncomfortable concept, a source of constant moral trouble for care ethicists. But these very qualities also render dependency a rich and fruitful concept, a constant source of moral reflection and theoretical renewal. It has been serving that role for decades now. In my view, there is still much more to learn.

NOTES

1. We face a difficult quandary here early on: *what is care ethics*? I cannot answer that question definitively, but I can say what I mean when I use the term. I regard care ethics as a moral theory, an ethical sensibility and as an interdisciplinary field of inquiry. As a moral theory, care ethics has its place in normative discussions in analytical moral philosophy (see: Sarah Miller, 'Need, Care and Obligation', *Royal Institute of Philosophy* Supplement 57 (2005): 137–60; and Stephanie Collins, *The Core of Care Ethics* (London: Palgrave Macmillan, 2015)). As an ethical sensibility, care ethics can inform and shed light on everyday moral practice (see: Sandra Laugier, *Politics of the Ordinary: Care, Ethics, and Forms of Life* (Leuven: Peeters, 2020)) – it is a manner of paying attention to things, in Iris Murdoch's sense (see: Iris Murdoch, *The Sovereignty of Good* (London and New York: Routledge, 1970)). Finally, as an interdisciplinary field of inquiry, care ethics investigates questions about 'good' care in concrete practices, by combining empirical and philosophical methods (see: Jeannette Pols, 'Towards an Empirical Ethics in Care: Relations with Technologies in Health Care', *Medicine, Health Care and Philosophy* 18, no. 1 (2015): 81–90; and Carlo Leget, Inge van Nistelrooij and Merel Visse, 'Beyond Demarcation: Care Ethics as an Interdisciplinary Field of Inquiry', *Nursing Ethics* 26, no. 1 (2017): 17–25). Since this chapter deals with concepts, I am mostly going to be concerned with care ethics as a moral theory. However, given that the conceptual frame of care ethics informs the care-ethical sensibility and interdisciplinary care-ethical research, the discussion inevitably bears on care ethics in these other senses too.
2. Simon van der Weele, 'Four Paradigm Cases of Dependency in Care Relations', *Hypatia* 36, no. 2 (2021): 338–59.
3. Collins, *The Core of Care Ethics*.
4. Selma Sevenhuijsen, *Citizenship and the Ethics of Care: Feminist Considerations on Justice, Morality, and Politics* (London and New York: Routledge, 1998).
5. Daniel Engster, 'Care Ethics, Dependency, and Vulnerability', *Ethics and Social Welfare* 13, no. 2 (2019): 100–14.
6. Sarah Miller, 'From Vulnerability to Precariousness: Examining the Moral Foundations of Care Ethics', *International Journal of Philosophical Studies* 28, no. 5 (2020): 644–61.
7. See: Judith Butler, *Precarious Life: The Powers of Mourning and Violence* (London and New York: Verso Books, 2004); Alyson Cole, 'All of Us Are Vulnerable, But Some Are More Vulnerable than Others: The Political Ambiguity of Vulnerability Studies, an Ambivalent Critique', *Critical Horizons* 17, no. 2 (2016): 260–77; Martha A. Fineman, 'The Vulnerable Subject: Anchoring Equality in the Human Condition', *Yale Journal of Law and Feminism* 20, no. 1 (2008): 1–23.
8. See: Judith Butler, *Frames of War: When Is Life Grievable?* (London: Verso Books, 2010); Isabell Lorey, *State of Insecurity: Government of the Precarious* (London and New York: Verso Books, 2015).
9. Nel Noddings, *Caring: A Feminine Approach to Ethics and Moral Education* (Berkeley: University of California Press, 1984).
10. Sara Ruddick, *Maternal Thinking: Toward a Politics of Peace* (Boston, MA: Beacon Press, 1989).
11. Virginia Held, *Feminist Morality: Transforming Culture, Society, and Politics* (Chicago, IL: University of Chicago Press, 1993).
12. For the notion of 'first' and 'second' generations of care ethicists, see Leget, van Nistelrooij and Visse, 'Beyond Demarcation'.

13. Joan C. Tronto, *Moral Boundaries: A Political Argument for an Ethic of Care* (London: Routledge, 1993).
14. Eva F. Kittay, *Love's Labor: Essays on Women, Equality, and Dependency* (New York: Routledge, 1999).
15. The metaphysics of dependency is by no means philosophically settled, even among care ethicists. I explore philosophical disagreement on the ontology of dependency in more detail in Van der Weele, 'Four Paradigm Cases of Dependency in Care Relations'.
16. Miller, 'Need, Care and Obligation', 140.
17. Tronto, *Moral Boundaries*, 145.
18. Kittay, *Love's Labor*, 34.
19. Tom Shakespeare, *Disability Rights and Wrongs Revisited* (London: Routledge, 2014).
20. Kittay, *Love's Labor*, 1.
21. Ibid.
22. Ibid.
23. Sara Ruddick, 'Care as Labor and Relationship', in *Norms and Values: Essays on the Work of Virginia Held*, ed. Joram G. Haber and Mark S. Halfon (Lanham, MD: Rowman & Littlefield, 1998), 20.
24. Noddings, *Caring*, 80.
25. Van der Weele, 'Four Paradigm Cases of Dependency in Care Relations'.
26. See: Martha Nussbaum, *Sex and Social Justice* (Oxford: Oxford University Press, 2000); Onora O'Neill, 'Justice, Gender and International Boundaries', *British Journal of Political Science* 20, no. 4 (1990): 439–59.
27. Claudia Card, 'Caring and Evil', *Hypatia* 5, no. 1 (1990): 101–8.
28. See: Alison Bailey, 'Mothering, Diversity, and Peace: Comments on Sara Ruddick's Feminist Maternal Peace Politics', *Journal of Social Philosophy* 26, no. 1 (1995): 162–82; María Lugones, 'On the Logic of Feminist Pluralism', in *Feminist Ethics*, ed. Claudia Card (Lawrence: University of Kansas Press, 1991), 35–44.
29. Diemut Bubeck, 'Justice and the Labor of Care', in *The Subject of Care: Feminist Perspectives on Dependency*, ed. Eva F. Kittay and Ellen K. Feder (Lanham, MD: Rowman & Littlefield, 2002), 160–85.
30. Sarah L. Hoagland, 'Some Concerns About Nel Noddings' *Caring*', *Hypatia* 5, no. 1 (1990): 110.
31. Anita Silvers, 'Reconciling Equality to Difference: Caring (F)or Justice For People With Disabilities', *Hypatia* 10, no. 1 (1995): 30–55.
32. Jenny Morris, 'Impairment and Disability: Constructing an Ethics of Care That Promotes Human Rights', *Hypatia* 16, no. 4 (2001): 1–16.
33. See: Mike Oliver, 'Disability and Dependency: A Creation of Industrial Societies', in *Disability and Dependency*, ed. Len Barton (London and New York: Routledge, 1989), 7–22; Michael Oliver, *The Politics of Disablement* (London: Macmillan Education, 1990).
34. Tom Shakespeare, *Help* (Birmingham: Venture Press, 2000).
35. Ibid., 17.
36. Silvers, 'Reconciling Equality to Difference', 40.
37. Ibid., 43.
38. Ibid., 40.
39. Ibid.
40. Ibid., 43.
41. Shakespeare, *Disability Rights and Wrongs Revisited*.

42. Simon van der Weele, 'The Moral Charge of Dependency: Contestations of Dependency in Care Theory and Care Practice' (PhD diss., Universiteit voor Humanistiek, 2022), 28.
43. Noddings, *Caring*, 71.
44. Ruddick, *Maternal Thinking*, 75.
45. Tronto, *Moral Boundaries*.
46. Kittay, *Love's Labor*.
47. Tronto, *Moral Boundaries*, 145.
48. Kittay, *Love's Labor*, 33–7.
49. Tronto, *Moral Boundaries*, 103.
50. Van der Weele, 'The Moral Charge of Dependency'.
51. See: Michael Fine and Caroline Glendinning, 'Dependence, Independence or Inter-dependence? Revisiting the Concepts of "Care" and "Dependency"', *Ageing and Society* 25, no. 4 (2005): 601–21; Teppo Kröger, 'Care Research and Disability Studies: Nothing in Common?', *Critical Social Policy* 29, no. 3 (2009): 398–420.
52. Morris, 'Impairment and Disability', 1–16.
53. See: Susan Dodds, 'Dependence, Care, and Vulnerability', in *Vulnerability: New Essays in Ethics and Feminist Philosophy*, ed. Catriona Mackenzie, Wendy Rogers and Susan Dodds (Oxford: Oxford University Press, 2014), 181–203; Jackie L. Scully, 'Disability and Vulnerability: On Bodies, Dependence, and Power', in *Vulnerability: New Essays in Ethics and Feminist Philosophy*, ed. Catriona Mackenzie, Wendy Rogers and Susan Dodds (Oxford: Oxford University Press, 2014), 204–21; Stacy C. Simplican, 'Care, Disability, and Violence: Theorizing Complex Dependency in Eva Kittay and Judith Butler', *Hypatia* 30, no. 1 (2015): 217–33.
54. Nancy Fraser and Linda Gordon, 'A Genealogy of Dependency: Tracing a Keyword of the US Welfare State', *Signs* 19, no. 2 (1994): 312.
55. Eva F. Kittay, 'Dependency', in *Keywords for Disability Studies*, ed. Rachel Adams, Benjamin Reiss and David Serlin (New York: New York University Press, 2015), 55.
56. Miller, 'Need, Care and Obligation', 140–1.
57. Tronto, *Moral Boundaries*, 101.
58. Selma Sevenhuijsen, 'The Place of Care: The Relevance of the Ethics of Care for Social Policy', in *Labyrinths of Care: The Relevance of the Ethics of Care Perspective for Social Policy*, ed. Selma Sevenhuijsen and Alenka Švab (Ljubljana: Peace Institute, 2003), 20.
59. Kittay, *Love's Labor*, 70.
60. Ibid., xii.
61. Ibid.
62. Eva F. Kittay, *Learning from My Daughter: The Value and Care of Disabled Minds* (New York: Oxford University Press, 2019), 174.
63. See: Laura Back, 'Private Dependence, Public Personhood: Rethinking "Nested Obligations"', *Hypatia* 30, no. 1 (2015): 115–31; Laura Davy, 'Between an Ethic of Care and an Ethic of Autonomy: Negotiating Relational Autonomy', *Angelaki* 24, no. 3 (2019): 101–14; Christine Kelly, 'Building Bridges with Accessible Care: Disability Studies, Feminist Care Scholarship, and Beyond', *Hypatia* 28, no. 4 (2013): 784–800.
64. See: Bill Hughes et al., 'Love's Labours Lost? Feminism, the Disabled People's Movement and an Ethic of Care', *Sociology* 39, no. 2 (2005): 259–75; Shakespeare, *Help*; Nick Watson et al., '(Inter)Dependence, Needs and Care: The Potential for Disability and Feminist Theorists to Develop an Emancipatory Model', *Sociology* 38, no. 2 (2004): 331–50.

65. See: Butler, *Precarious Life*; Cole, 'All of Us Are Vulnerable, But Some Are More Vulnerable than Others'; Dodds, 'Dependence, Care, and Vulnerability'; Fineman, 'The Vulnerable Subject'; Catriona Mackenzie, Wendy Rogers and Susan Dodds, eds, *Vulnerability: New Essays in Ethics and Feminist Philosophy* (Oxford: Oxford University Press, 2014).
66. Estelle Ferrarese, 'Vulnerability: A Concept with Which to Undo the World As It Is?', *Critical Horizons* 17, no. 2 (2016): 149–59.
67. See: Sandra Laugier, 'The Ethics of Care as a Politics of the Ordinary', *New Literary History* 46, no. 2 (2015): 217–40; Sandra Laugier, 'Politics of Vulnerability and Responsibility for Ordinary Others,' *Critical Horizons* 17, no. 2 (2016): 207–23.
68. Engster, 'Care Ethics, Dependency, and Vulnerability'.
69. Fineman, 'The Vulnerable Subject', 9.
70. Ibid., 11.
71. Ibid., 8.
72. Ibid., 10.
73. Dodds, 'Dependence, Care, and Vulnerability', 182–3.
74. Engster, 'Care Ethics, Dependency, and Vulnerability', 104.
75. Ibid., 110.
76. Ibid., 102.
77. See: Butler, *Frames of War*; Lorey, *State of Insecurity*; Guy Standing, 'The Precariat: Today's Transformative Class?', *Development* 61, no. 1–4 (2018): 115–21.
78. See: Maurice Hamington and Michael Flower, eds, *Care Ethics in the Age of Precarity* (Minneapolis: University of Minnesota Press, 2021); Eva F. Kittay, 'Precarity, Precariousness, and Disability,' *Journal of Social Philosophy* 52, no. 3 (2021): 292–309; Frans Vosman, *Surviving as a Form of Life: The Ethics of Care as a Critique of the Ideal of a Successful Life* (Utrecht: Eburon, 2023).
79. Miller, 'From Vulnerability to Precariousness', 653.
80. Ibid., 645.
81. Ibid., 646.
82. Ibid., 647.
83. Ibid.
84. See: Butler, *Frames of War*; Judith Butler, *The Force of Nonviolence: An Ethico-Political Bind* (London and New York: Verso Books, 2020); Simon van der Weele, 'Bridging Conversations: "Paradigm Cases" of Dependency in Eva Kittay and Judith Butler', in *Bodies That Still Matter: Resonances of the Work of Judith Butler*, ed. Annemie Halsema, Katja Kwastek and Roel V. Oever (Amsterdam: Amsterdam University Press, 2021), 103–12.
85. Miller, 'From Vulnerability to Precariousness', 651.
86. Ibid., 659.
87. Ibid.
88. See: Kittay, *Love's Labor*; Sevenhuijsen, *Citizenship and the Ethics of Care*; Joan Tronto, *Caring Democracy: Markets, Equality, and Justice* (New York: New York University Press, 2013).
89. Kittay, *Love's Labor*, xii.
90. Miller, 'From Vulnerability to Precariousness', 644–61.
91. Engster, 'Care Ethics, Dependency, and Vulnerability', 104.
92. Ibid., 107.

BIBLIOGRAPHY

Back, Laura. 'Private Dependence, Public Personhood: Rethinking "Nested Obligations"', *Hypatia* 30, no. 1 (2015): 115–31.

Bailey, Alison. 'Mothering, Diversity, and Peace: Comments on Sara Ruddick's Feminist Maternal Peace Politics', *Journal of Social Philosophy* 26, no. 1 (1995): 162–82.

Bubeck, Diemut. 'Justice and the Labor of Care', in *The Subject of Care: Feminist Perspectives on Dependency*, edited by Eva F. Kittay and Ellen K. Feder, 160–85. Lanham, MD: Rowman & Littlefield, 2002.

Butler, Judith. *Precarious Life: The Powers of Mourning and Violence*. London and New York: Verso Books, 2004.

Butler, Judith. *Frames of War: When Is Life Grievable?* London: Verso Books, 2010.

Butler, Judith. *The Force of Nonviolence: An Ethico-Political Bind*. London and New York: Verso Books, 2020.

Card, Claudia. 'Caring and Evil', *Hypatia* 5, no. 1 (1990): 101–8.

Cole, Alyson. 'All of Us Are Vulnerable, But Some Are More Vulnerable than Others: The Political Ambiguity of Vulnerability Studies, an Ambivalent Critique', *Critical Horizons* 17, no. 2 (2016): 260–77.

Collins, Stephanie. *The Core of Care Ethics*. London: Palgrave Macmillan, 2015.

Davy, Laura. 'Between an Ethic of Care and an Ethic of Autonomy: Negotiating Relational Autonomy', *Angelaki* 24, no. 3 (2019): 101–14.

Dodds, Susan. 'Dependence, Care, and Vulnerability', in *Vulnerability: New Essays in Ethics and Feminist Philosophy*, edited by Catriona Mackenzie, Wendy Rogers and Susan Dodds, 181–203. Oxford: Oxford University Press, 2014.

Engster, Daniel. 'Care Ethics, Dependency, and Vulnerability', *Ethics and Social Welfare* 13, no. 2 (2019): 100–14.

Ferrarese, Estelle. 'Vulnerability: A Concept with Which to Undo the World As It Is?', *Critical Horizons* 17, no. 2 (2016): 149–59.

Fine, Michael, and Caroline Glendinning. 'Dependence, Independence or Inter-dependence? Revisiting the Concepts of "Care" and "Dependency"', *Ageing and Society* 25, no. 4 (2005): 601–21.

Fineman, Martha A. 'The Vulnerable Subject: Anchoring Equality in the Human Condition', *Yale Journal of Law and Feminism* 20, no. 1 (2008): 1–23.

Fraser, Nancy, and Linda Gordon. 'A Genealogy of Dependency: Tracing a Keyword of the US Welfare State', *Signs* 19, no. 2 (1994): 309–36.

Hamington, Maurice, and Michael Flower, eds. *Care Ethics in the Age of Precarity*. Minneapolis: University of Minnesota Press, 2021.

Held, Virginia. *Feminist Morality: Transforming Culture, Society, and Politics*. Chicago, IL: University of Chicago Press, 1993.

Hoagland, Sarah L. 'Some Concerns About Nel Noddings' *Caring*', *Hypatia* 5, no. 1 (1990): 109–14.

Hughes, Bill, Linda McKie, Debra Hopkins and Nick Watson. 'Love's Labours Lost? Feminism, the Disabled People's Movement and an Ethic of Care', *Sociology* 39, no. 2 (2005): 259–75.

Kelly, Christine. 'Building Bridges with Accessible Care: Disability Studies, Feminist Care Scholarship, and Beyond', *Hypatia* 28, no. 4 (2013): 784–800.

Kittay, Eva F. *Love's Labor: Essays on Women, Equality, and Dependency*. New York: Routledge, 1999.

Kittay, Eva F. 'Dependency', in *Keywords for Disability Studies*, edited by Rachel Adams, Benjamin Reiss and David Serlin, 54–8. New York: New York University Press, 2015.
Kittay, Eva F. *Learning from My Daughter: The Value and Care of Disabled Minds*. New York: Oxford University Press, 2019.
Kittay, Eva F. 'Precarity, Precariousness, and Disability', *Journal of Social Philosophy* 52, no. 3 (2021): 292–309.
Kröger, Teppo. 'Care Research and Disability Studies: Nothing in Common?', *Critical Social Policy* 29, no. 3 (2009): 398–420.
Laugier, Sandra. 'The Ethics of Care as a Politics of the Ordinary', *New Literary History* 46, no. 2 (2015): 217–40.
Laugier, Sandra. 'Politics of Vulnerability and Responsibility for Ordinary Others', *Critical Horizons* 17, no. 2 (2016): 207–23.
Laugier, Sandra. *Politics of the Ordinary: Care, Ethics, and Forms of Life*. Leuven: Peeters, 2020.
Leget, Carlo, Inge Van Nistelrooij and Merel Visse. 'Beyond Demarcation: Care Ethics as an Interdisciplinary Field of Inquiry', *Nursing Ethics* 26, no. 1 (2019): 17–25.
Lorey, Isabell. *State of Insecurity: Government of the Precarious*. London and New York: Verso Books, 2015.
Lugones, María. 'On the Logic of Feminist Pluralism', in *Feminist Ethics*, edited by Claudia Card, 35–44. Lawrence: University of Kansas Press, 1991.
Mackenzie, Catriona, Wendy Rogers and Susan Dodds, eds. *Vulnerability: New Essays in Ethics and Feminist Philosophy*. Oxford: Oxford University Press, 2014.
Miller, Sarah. 'Need, Care and Obligation', *Royal Institute of Philosophy* Supplement 57 (2005), 137–60.
Miller, Sarah. 'From Vulnerability to Precariousness: Examining the Moral Foundations of Care Ethics', *International Journal of Philosophical Studies* 28, no. 5 (2020): 644–61.
Morris, Jenny. 'Impairment and Disability: Constructing an Ethics of Care That Promotes Human Rights', *Hypatia* 16, no. 4 (2001): 1–16.
Murdoch, Iris. *The Sovereignty of Good*. London and New York: Routledge, 1970.
Noddings, Nel. *Caring: A Feminine Approach to Ethics and Moral Education*. Oakland: University of California Press, 1984.
Nussbaum, Martha. *Sex and Social Justice*. Oxford: Oxford University Press, 2000.
Oliver, Mike. 'Disability and Dependency: A Creation of Industrial Societies', in *Disability and Dependency*, edited by Len Barton, 7–22. London and New York: Routledge, 1989.
Oliver, Michael. *The Politics of Disablement*. London: Macmillan Education, 1990.
O'Neill, Onora. 'Justice, Gender and International Boundaries', *British Journal of Political Science* 20, no. 4 (1990): 439–59.
Pols, Jeannette. 'Towards an Empirical Ethics in Care: Relations with Technologies in Health Care', *Medicine, Health Care and Philosophy* 18, no. 1 (2015): 81–90.
Ruddick, Sara. *Maternal Thinking: Toward a Politics of Peace*. Boston, MA: Beacon Press, 1989.
Ruddick, Sara. 'Care as Labor and Relationship', in *Norms and Values: Essays on the Work of Virginia Held*, edited by Joram G. Haber and Mark S. Halfon, 3–25. Lanham, MD: Rowman & Littlefield, 1998.
Scully, Jackie L. 'Disability and Vulnerability: On Bodies, Dependence, and Power', in *Vulnerability: New Essays in Ethics and Feminist Philosophy*, edited by Catriona Mackenzie, Wendy Rogers and Susan Dodds, 204–21. Oxford: Oxford University Press, 2014.
Sevenhuijsen, Selma. *Citizenship and the Ethics of Care: Feminist Considerations on Justice, Morality, and Politics*. London and New York: Routledge, 1998.

Sevenhuijsen, Selma. 'The Place of Care: The Relevance of the Ethics of Care for Social Policy', in *Labyrinths of Care: The Relevance of the Ethics of Care Perspective for Social Policy*, edited by Selma Sevenhuijsen and Alenka Švab, 13–41. Ljubljana: Peace Institute, 2003.
Shakespeare, Tom. *Help*. Birmingham: Venture Press, 2000.
Shakespeare, Tom. *Disability Rights and Wrongs Revisited*. London: Routledge, 2014.
Silvers, Anita. 'Reconciling Equality to Difference: Caring (F)or Justice For People With Disabilities', *Hypatia* 10, no. 1 (1995): 30–55.
Simplican, Stacy C. 'Care, Disability, and Violence: Theorizing Complex Dependency in Eva Kittay and Judith Butler', *Hypatia* 30, no. 1 (2015): 217–33.
Standing, Guy. 'The Precariat: Today's Transformative Class?', *Development* 61, no. 1–4 (2018): 115–21.
Tronto, Joan C. *Moral Boundaries: A Political Argument for an Ethic of Care*. London: Routledge, 1993.
Tronto, Joan C. *Caring Democracy: Markets, Equality, and Justice*. New York: New York University Press, 2013.
van der Weele, Simon. 'Four Paradigm Cases of Dependency in Care Relations', *Hypatia* 36, no. 2 (2021): 338–59.
van der Weele, Simon. 'Bridging Conversations: "Paradigm Cases" of Dependency in Eva Kittay and Judith Butler', in *Bodies That Still Matter: Resonances of the Work of Judith Butler*, edited by Annemie Halsema, Katja Kwastek and Roel V. Oever, 103–12. Amsterdam: Amsterdam University Press, 2021.
van der Weele, Simon. 'The Moral Charge of Dependency: Contestations of Dependency in Care Theory and Care Practice', PhD diss., Universiteit voor Humanistiek, 2022.
Vosman, Frans. 'Overleven Als Levensvorm: Zorgethiek Als Kritiek Op Het Ideaal van Het "Geslaagde Leven"', PhD diss., Universiteit voor Humanistiek, 2018.
Watson, Nick, Linda McKie, Bill Hughes, Debra Hopkins and Sue Gregory. '(Inter) Dependence, Needs and Care: The Potential for Disability and Feminist Theorists to Develop an Emancipatory Model', *Sociology* 38, no. 2 (2004): 331–50.

CHAPTER FOUR

A metaethics of care? Revisiting the normative authority of care ethics

MERCER E. GARY

INTRODUCTION

Is care ethics normative? If so, in what sense? Although these are longstanding questions, they have become newly salient: the wide variety of approaches to care scholarship, similarly varied interpretations of what make a theory 'normative', and increasing attention to metaethical issues in care all demand further answers about care ethics' normative structure. This chapter contributes to the contemporary conversation by reexamining the normative authority of care ethics. I begin by reviewing several of the competing concerns driving this debate. Clarifying my intent to speak across strands of care theoretical research, I first establish that care ethics should be normative but not perniciously normalizing. In the interest of generating broad appeal among care scholars, the bulk of the chapter returns to Margaret Urban Walker's *expressive-collaborative* model of moral reasoning, endorsed by several care ethicists who otherwise disagree with one another.[1] I argue that the contributions of Walker's account to care ethics are increased by the recent revisions proposed by Lisa Tessman. Specifically, I show that a Walker–Tessman approach to metaethical constructivism provides care ethics with: (a) a clarification and justification of a normative feminist project; (b) a maximally historical and social account of ethical subjects, contexts and ways of reasoning; (c) an appreciation of the non-rational apprehension of value; and (d) a process for collectively assessing, endorsing and rejecting ethical values and their applications. Although the goal of this chapter is to elaborate the positive contributions of this approach to constructivism for a range of thinkers of care, the final section identifies lingering questions in the approach that will require address in future research.

4.1 COMPETING PERSPECTIVES ON CARE'S NORMATIVITY

That care ethics should be concerned with metaethics at all was not a foregone conclusion. The early years of care ethics were marked by scepticism about the possibility of a genuinely feminist ethical project and warnings against feminists getting mired in metaethical debate. Though not a care ethicist herself, Marilyn Frye argued that the impulse towards the codification of rules of right conduct is a historically and politically situated one reflecting a need for validation and purity characteristic of middle-class white women who should instead dispense with this project altogether.[2] Frye's critique finds the basis of ethics to be ideological and its results to be actively harmful insofar as they reinforce existing hierarchies. Joan Tronto, for her part, did not reject the goal of determining standards of rightness altogether, but cautioned against the tendency for care ethics to become focused on abstract metatheoretical questions about grounding. Doubling down on the debate over the relative merits of care versus justice, 'prove[s] so unsatisfying and unresolved', Tronto argued, 'because the participants within the discussion presume ... that the question of metaethical adequacy is a question that can be resolved within the framework of philosophical discussion itself'.[3] Instead, both Frye and Tronto advocate for political, rather than ethical, interventions and, if not a rejection of normativity, at least a refusal to get caught up in theorizing its machinations.

More recently, care scholars drawing on other social theoretical resources have been even more skeptical of normative theorizing.[4] For instance, Maria Puig de la Bellacasa's more-than-human approach to care draws more heavily on feminist science and technology studies than on feminist moral philosophy, describing the obligations of care as 'anormative', or, occasionally, as evidencing a 'conjured normativity' unlike the prescriptive claims of mainstream ethics.[5] Part of her criticism is focused on the institutionalization of ethics in the form of review boards, but a more substantive challenge concerns the disciplining effects of normative theorizing noted by queer feminist theorists.[6] Such a rejection is not uncommon within feminist and queer scholarship on heteronormativity and cisnormativity, where definitions of queerness as necessarily opposed to all that is normative highlight a significant divide in understandings of the term.[7] Although both interpretations of normativity are broadly interested in the compulsion of behaviour – whether this be the fulfilment of ethical responsibility or the performance of gendered, racialized and ableist social norms – what that compulsion connotes differs significantly. Especially when arguing across disciplinary boundaries, then, care theorists must respond to the concern that their normative injunctions are merely reflections of the prevailing order. As I'll argue in the next section, there are compelling responses to these concerns – ones that mirror Margaret Urban Walker's response to Frye,[8] in which she insisted that not all normative ethics need take the form of mainstream moral theory.

But rather than completely rejecting normative theorizing, care ethicists have more typically disputed certain common features of mainstream normative theory. Indeed, part of the driving motivation of care ethics as a project comes from its critique of universal principles, of the idealization of ethical agents and contexts, and the necessity of impartiality to moral theory.[9] Carol Gilligan's landmark studies in moral psychology highlighted the congruence between these facets of moral theories and apparent gendered tendencies in moral reasoning, opening room to question parameters often accepted as the hallmarks of proper ethical inquiry. Each of the aspects of normative theory under critique by care ethicists – reliance on universal principles, idealization and impartiality – concerns the misrepresentation of ethical agents and the problems they respond to. In Walker's words, these tenets of mainstream normative theory 'can be insidiously misleading, covering over features of our human and social conditions that require us to be *morally* examined and challenged. They can become "ideological," enforcing patterns of thinking that make existing conditions and distributions of authority and power in human societies seem natural, inevitable, or normal when they are elaborately constructed.'[10] Though none of these criticisms disputed the normativity of care ethics per se, an open question remained about how many features of mainstream normative theorizing could be incorporated into an ethics of care without it thereby becoming precisely the kind of ethics it opposed.

At the same time, a number of care ethicists voiced concerns about rejecting some or all of the above-mentioned features of normative theories. On the one hand were worries that such a heterodox approach to ethical theorizing would play into sexist assumptions about women's intellectual and moral qualities: that women are less equipped to reason objectively and without emotion or that they are incapable of applying and consistently maintaining universal principles.[11] Although this may be the case – and it does seem true that care ethics' departures from mainstream moral theory have served as fuel for some ultimately misogynist dismissals of the scholarship – as Noddings agrees, this seems like an insufficient reason to back down from the criticisms care ethicists have levied. More compelling concerns have centred on the tools care ethics loses when it rejects, say, the use of universal principles. For instance, Sarah Clark Miller[12] has argued persuasively that, absent a concept of duty, care ethics confronts motivational and justificatory problems in cases where we are not driven by personal feeling for another. In order to maintain the moral responsibility of caring in certain circumstances where we lack the affective inclination to do so, Miller suggests duty as a supplement. Ensuring that care ethics contains adequate normative and metanormative tools is necessary, moreover, for responding to the criticism that the approach commits the naturalistic fallacy, deriving an *ought* from an *is*.[13] Rather than simply transgressing a rule of moral theorizing, falling into the naturalistic fallacy would effectively limit care ethicists to speaking about actually existing care relations.[14]

Instead of a comparative study of existing proposals for care ethics' normative architecture, the present chapter seeks to address a more basic question regarding care ethics' normative authority.[15] My contribution is geared towards a broad range of care theorists, including but not limited to those who understand themselves as care ethicists. I hope to show that care scholars of all theoretical backgrounds should be concerned about metatheoretical justification and can act on such concerns while maintaining their core commitments.

4.2 NORMATIVITY VERSUS NORMALIZATION IN FEMINIST THEORY

A metatheory of care that effectively responds to feminist ambivalence about normative theorizing must demonstrate the bindingness of its norms while defending against the charge that normative prescriptions are tools of domination. As noted above, such a defence is necessary given the scepticism of normative ethics that pervades interdisciplinary feminist theory, including some corners of feminist philosophy. By clarifying the difference between ethical normativity and pernicious normalization, this section establishes the possibility of an account that succeeds on both these levels. The 'normative question' with which I am primarily concerned is the one posed by Christine Korsgaard concerning the justification of moral authority, or 'why' behind moral requirements.[16] This is not the causal 'why' question of moral psychology, which asks how we come to be motivated to engage in ethical behaviour and deliberation, but rather the question of what it is about ethics that is binding, or how we justify our understanding of certain moral acts as not merely nice but necessary.[17]

Feminist theorist Alexis Shotwell offers a useful entry point into the defence of ethical normativity against concerns articulated elsewhere in feminist theory. Shotwell separates these two senses by differentiating between normativity and normalization: in her view, when queer theorists decry the violences of normativity, they are in fact speaking against normalization.[18] Shotwell, following Korsgaard, instead understands normativity as the process of valuing an object: deeming an action as wrong, a painting as beautiful, a relationship as good. Normativity operates not just at the level of explicit individual judgements, but also implicitly undergirds social life: our embodied habits while navigating a crowded sidewalk, for instance, enact norms of physical interaction with strangers. In ways both big and small, normativity provides us with frameworks for understanding and moving through the world. As Shotwell sees it, normativity is therefore central to the project of creating a life full of preferences, values and accountability, echoing Korsgaard's characterization of humans as normative animals.[19] Shotwell notes that there is no reason to assume that the normative valuing of an object implies a universal claim that others value it identically: 'there may be many recommended ways of being. Endorsing a way of being is distinct from endorsing the idea that everyone ought to be that way.'[20] Moreover, normativity in this sense is key to feminist projects working to both critique established standards and chart new ones.

For Shotwell, norms are a form of productive, rather than merely oppressive, power that regulates behaviour according to a common standard.[21] Social, aesthetic, epistemic, and ethical norms are alike, in that all are similarly constructed and none holds a particularly elevated status.[22] In clear contrast to a realist view of 'moral facts', Shotwell's account understands norms as both emerging from and being justified within particular local contexts rather than making a universal claim to truth. For Shotwell, norms are justified insofar as they enable greater possibilities of flourishing for all.

This general and unavoidable category of normativity should thus not be equated with *normalization*, which concerns the disciplinary processes by which normative standards are enforced.[23] As the target of Shotwell's critique,[24] normalization enforces standards 'delimiting and constraining the terrain of possibilities'.[25] Not all normativity is normalizing, in her view, in the sense that not all norms problematically narrow the possible paths for flourishing. According to Shotwell, then, mistaking the disciplinary efforts of normalization with the inevitable presence of normativity throws the evaluative and potentially transformative baby out with the subjectivizing bath water.

The problem I see in Shotwell's account is that what she characterizes as the (separable, pernicious) dynamic of normalization in fact attends all normative demands: even where it is aligned with the proliferation of possibilities for flourishing, norms involve the enforcement of a standard, albeit in varying ways. I take it that Shotwell agrees, given her citation of Korsgaard's definition of normativity as making claims on us.[26] That is, because normative statements make claims on us, they involve at minimum *encouragement* and potentially even *non-negotiable requirement*. The kind of enforcement operative within ethical normativity is precisely not legal or institutional, though these are the examples that Shotwell points to.[27] Instead, normative enforcement more often looks like external or internalized social pressure.[28] If we are interested in promoting opportunities for flourishing, then presumably we want to 'enforce' those opportunities in at least the minimal sense of encouraging them. Accordingly, not all 'enforcement' can be bad.

An injunction against murder, for instance, enhances possibilities for flourishing and therefore would be upheld on Shotwell's account. In order for the injunction to be meaningful, it would need to be enforced in some way, though only some forms of enforcement would be objectionable. An individual's internalization of this injunction, for instance, seems to be a desirable form of enforcement which could be made even less objectionable with the provision of resources for mental and physical health that guard against recourse to such violence. If we are to effectively defend the necessity of normative theorizing for feminist ethics, we must stand behind this compelling power of normativity. Without any kind of internal or external enforcement, the injunction not to murder would cease to be an injunction. Although I agree with Shotwell that creating more capacious norms is an important area for critical intervention, such shifts will mean less if we leave behind an understanding of norms as binding. Moreover, the intuition that normalization is not necessarily harmful is evident in popular calls to 'normalize' talking about taboo subjects like suicidal ideation. Such calls go beyond an endorsement of the practice of talking about suicidal thoughts, further encouraging those who struggle with such thoughts to express them and prompting others to listen nonjudgmentally. By promoting a norm that helps make it possible to live with suicidal ideation in a less isolated manner, we would be at minimum *suggesting* that others shift their behaviour in the direction of this norm. Care ethics would seem to want to make such claims, even as it also must remain alert to the problems of improperly imposing values and demands.

'Normalization' must therefore be understood to occur in the small, intersubjective moments of affirming or enacting ruling norms more so than through express institutional enforcement. This means that we cannot keep normativity while rejecting normalization, although we *can* differentiate between more and less pernicious forms of normalization. My arguments in this section serve two primary purposes. First, they show the possibility of meeting both demands of care ethics at the same time: we can, in principle, construe ethics as strongly normative and binding while guarding against the proliferation of pernicious norms supporting projects of domination. Second, in making these arguments via feminist and queer theory beyond the bounds of analytic ethics, I have demonstrated that retaining the bindingness of norms should be a priority for care theorists of many different stripes. What is needed now is an account that provides us with tools for differentiating between norms to embrace and norms to reject.

4.3 THE EXPRESSIVE-COLLABORATIVE MODEL'S CONTRIBUTIONS TO CARE ETHICS

First elaborated by Walker in the late 1980s, the expressive-collaborative model has found support among care theorists as varied in their approaches as Eva Feder Kittay[29] and Joan Tronto.[30] Their common endorsement suggests that Walker's model may prove useful for a range of care theorists and could potentially help to adjudicate differences between them. Interestingly, however, their remarks on the model have focused on rather different aspects. For her part, Kittay positively references Walker's account as an elaboration of the kind of naturalism to which care ethics should be committed: one that is responsive to empirical facts *and* social influence, avoiding unnecessary abstraction and idealization.[31] Kittay's nod to Walker emphasizes that care ethics is a non-ideal theory that retains normative purchase. Tronto, however, draws on Walker's understanding of moral responsibility as socially allocated, whose distribution among people and institutions should be the result of collective deliberation and decision rather than tradition, convenience or prejudice.[32] As we will shortly see, moral responsibility on Walker's account is a thoroughly social practice dependent on collectively adjudicated moral understandings; it therefore provides considerable support for Tronto's focus on the just distribution of moral and practical responsibilities for caregiving through democratic politics. Each founding thinker of care, then, finds something in Walker central to her own central project, divergent as these may be.

And yet, neither Kittay nor Tronto goes into depth about the expressive-collaborative model's approach to negotiating and justifying the norms of care ethics; I therefore make this the central focus of my chapter. Now is an especially productive time to revisit Walker's model following Lisa Tessman's recent[33] elaboration of it, which places Walker in the context of contemporary metaethical constructivist debates.[34] In what follows, I identify and flesh out four key contributions that the expressive-collaborative model offers care ethics. Though expansion in future research will be necessary, my arguments here indicate the productivity of Walker and Tessman's interventions for contemporary care ethics.[35]

To start, the expressive-collaborative model accords with the feminist position on normative theorizing I arrived at in the previous section. That is to say, it is able to account for ethics as normatively binding without sacrificing feminist attentiveness to the workings of power in moral theorizing. While eschewing universal, transhistorical conclusions, the expressive-collaborative model pursues confidence in our moral judgements and treats those that are validated as binding. Consider this *Contribution 1: a clarification and justification of feminist theorizing as a normative project*. My emphasis thus far on the collective generation and negotiation of norms that nonetheless continue to make demands on us suggests the promise of turning to constructivism. Broadly speaking, a constructivist approach to justification locates the bindingness of ethical claims in human practices of valuation and validation. Unlike the realist, the constructivist denies the existence of mind-independent moral truths. But in the absence of moral entities existing outside of human practices, constructivists do not thereby give up either the social presence of morality or its ability to make genuine claims upon us. For this reason, Korsgaard offers the label of 'procedural realism': ethical claims can have genuine normative weight, requiring us to perform certain actions and abstain from others, but this weight derives from a social process of validation. We can therefore obtain answers to ethical questions that are authoritative for everyday practice, but we must recognize that their authority comes from social processes of deliberation and validation, rather than any independent source. The resulting account might not strictly be considered a moral *theory*, given its lack of fixity and systematicity and it will, moreover, challenge our expectations of what kinds of answers ethics can provide. Given the perspectives I reviewed in the first section, this seems like a boon for care ethics.

The expressive-collaborative model differs from popular constructivist views in several ways that will be attractive to care-based critics of mainstream normative ethics. First, this feminist account is constructivist 'all the way down': all elements of ethical life and theorizing are made rather than assumed. This means that judgements, values, modes of apprehending moral claims and processes of justification themselves are all revisable products obtained through collective practices which endow them with a specifically moral authority.[36] Such a thoroughgoing constructivist account can be contrasted with the restricted constructivism of John Rawls. Rawls's view is specifically designed for use in well-ordered, liberal societies, rather than for morality as such, which means that he assumes rather than justifies a set of liberal democratic values and a thick concept of the person.[37] By committing to thoroughgoing constructivism, we refuse to assume such a conception of personhood and are thereby saved from the significant feminist objections to Rawls's ideal theory which 'assumes a mutual independence of persons and their desires that is false of all human beings ... [and] as much an idealisation of human social relations as an assumption of generalised altruism would be'.[38] Starting from the ground floor, therefore, helps to guard against the possibility of baking in an assumed hegemonic subject,[39] making this form of constructivism more suitable to feminist projects that have opposed the idealizing and ideological tendencies of liberal personhood. As much scholarship has noted, care ethics' focus on dependence and interdependence as characteristic of human life requires displacing the assumed independent subject of liberal theory. Moreover, care ethicists have emphasized the variations in caregiving practices and their organization across historical periods and political regimes.[40] Accounting for this variety requires both room for pluralism and attention to the scope of ethical claims. This point marks *Contribution 2: a maximally social and historical account of ethical subjects and situations.*

The expressive-collaborative model can accommodate further social and historical nuance by virtue of the fact that it is not Kantian, or at least not Kantian in the way that Korsgaard's is. Unlike Rawls, Korsgaard does intend to offer a constructivist account of morality in general, rather than one appropriate for use in liberal politics. For Korsgaard, the activity of valuing itself commits moral agents to the value of humanity. Any valuing creature, on this view, is bound to substantive moral commitments by virtue of their valuing at all. As with the Rawlsian position, Korsgaard's view commits her to determinate and universal values from the outset. But assuming these values implies both the existence of, and our general access to, a universal human nature which I am unwilling to grant. My unwillingness here stems from objections similar to those raised in the previous paragraph, which disputed both the accuracy and the unsubstantiated positing of the universal characteristics ascribed to humanity at large.

Greater flexibility is attainable through Tessman embrace of a Humean constructivism instead. This sort of account, as described by Sharon Street, 'den[ies] that the rabbit of substantive reasons can be pulled out of a formalist hat: to get substance out, we need to put substance in'.[41] That is to say, it is only from a particular valuing position, rather than the abstract position of valuing as such, that commitments to substantive values can be drawn. For instance, contingent aspects of human experience like our life expectancy will influence the evaluative standpoint: our values would be structured differently in an era where most people live to age ninety-five than they would be in a time when most live only to age forty. The Humean constructivist accepts that the activity of valuing is affected by empirical constraints that will dispose valuing creatures towards certain substantive moral conclusions and not others. Although some care ethicists seem inclined to endorse a more robust account of human nature, I find that the Humean constructivist position's sensitivity to our empirical constraints grants us as much of a sense of human nature as care ethics needs. That is, our finitude, embodiment, dependency and vulnerability necessarily structure our valuing position as we know it; no further claims about the essentialness of these qualities are necessary. Where care theorists have criticized the formalism of modern moral theory, an approach to constructivism that better accounts for the social and historical embeddedness of the valuing person provides a more attractive alternative.[42]

At the same time as Walker endorses a variety of naturalism, she is able to effectively counter the concerns raised by care ethicists about naturalized morality. Both Virginia

Held and Tove Pettersen have resisted a naturalized view of ethics on the grounds that such a move would reduce ethics to empirical analysis, limiting the possibility of care to be practised otherwise or to serve as a genuinely transformative value. Instead, Walker argues that 'to "naturalise" ethical thought in the right way is to avoid the pitfalls both of a scientistic reductionism about ethics and of an insistence on a pure nonempirical core of moral knowledge'.[43] Because the building blocks of ethical theory are the stuff of everyday life, Walker insists that theorists retain 'an obligation to inform themselves about diverse human lives through what scientific, artistic, and humanistic inquiries can teach us'.[44] But because the expressive-collaborative model's mechanism of transparency testing enables us to evaluate, endorse, or reject particular norms and practices of care, we need not accept all the gathered data as morally valid. On this point, the expressive-collaborative model is able to hold care theorists to their stated commitments to the lived realities of caregivers and care receivers without saying that the *oughts* of care ethics reduce to current, and frequently unjust, practices of care.

Because the constructivism of the expressive-collaborative model is thoroughgoing, neither proper modes of valuing nor the content of values themselves are predetermined. This leads to *Contribution 3: feminist constructivists need not require, or even prioritize, practical reason as a mode of apprehending and adjudicating ethical claims*. Here, the Walker–Tessman account differs from both Korsgaard and Street, who locate the force of their constructivist frameworks in the entailments of practical reason. On more mainstream accounts, values derive from the logical entailments of our starting positions, which are either purely formal (for Korsgaard) or substantive (for Street). Although they differ on whether practical reason itself can entail particular substantive moral judgements, both Street and Korsgaard understand the activity of valuing and the process of justification as essentially rational. However, this priority of practical reason within mainstream constructivist accounts seems to deny important non-rational aspects of moral experience, which have historically been points of emphasis within care ethics.

Tessman's revisions of Walker on this point are particularly instructive. Tessman's primary concern is making sense of values that are felt rather than reasoned and yet remain capable of issuing requirements as stringent as those that are rationally derived. Reframing frequent references to *Sophie's Choice* within introductory ethics courses, Tessman considers the possibility that the situation presents a genuinely insoluble moral dilemma that results in a persistent and haunting failure.[45] Moral failure is possible here because it need not be the case that one's competing requirements will both be rational and therefore, at least in principle, soluble. In such instances of unavoidable moral failure, contrary to the ought-implies-can principle, one is *required* to do something that one *cannot* do because one or more of the requirements in question is not rational. Sophie, under the threat of having both children murdered by Nazis, is required to choose one child to save. In this unimaginably gruelling situation, she experiences non-negotiable requirements to protect both children despite being practically able to fulfil only one of those requirements.

Such intuitively apprehended requirements appear to us through associations rather than logical inferences and are experienced as a feeling that we *ought* to do something. While a fuller examination of the social and psychological processes impacting the appearance and character of these associations is outside the scope of my discussion here, what is relevant for care ethics is that Tessman's[46] account is able to admit forms of obligation like those articulated by Nel Noddings[47] in her formulation of the '*I must*'.[48] When confronted with the vulnerability of a proximate other in need of care, Noddings (and Tessman) identify the attendant affective experience of being morally obligated by a call so strong that even questioning one's response would be unthinkable. Consistent with care ethics' appreciation of affect and emotion as sources of genuine moral insight, the '*I must*' can best be understood as an intuitively apprehended requirement.[49] That such experiences are both affective and embodied has marked a key point of intersection between care ethics and phenomenology, which has long emphasized the felt textures of ethical requirement.[50] The expressive-collaborative model gives care ethics resources for considering these experiences and values in processes of normative deliberation and justification.

The experience of relational attachment is not the only way of presenting values non-rationally. For instance, feminist critical theorist Amy Allen understands 'expressive/hermeneutic insight' or 'experiences of aesthetic world disclosure' as capable of posing challenges to or forming components of normative deliberation.[51] This same possibility is emphasized by Shotwell who finds aesthetic practices to provide uniquely productive sites for critical intervention into established norms.[52] She references the example of Sins Invalid, a performance collective of disabled people of colour that understands itself as providing '*new visions of sexuality and beauty*' that contravene prevailing societal norms.[53] The challenges made by the performers to existing standards that exclude disabled people from collective life proceed not through argumentation but rather through an 'aesthetic project … [that] aims to shift the grounds for judgment'.[54] Dance is transfigured when performed by Deaf artists whose relation to music and rhythm is not auditory, as it is when artists with mobility impairments transform ostensible 'assistive devices' like wheelchairs into dynamic props. This kind of aesthetic intervention repositions disabled people of colour as agents and creators in the public sphere. Shotwell describes these performances as challenging and uncomfortable, which I take to highlight how such an aesthetic experience can help audience members to identify exclusionary norms – such as those concerning how bodies should appear in public – to which they affectively, if not rationally, subscribe. Such an 'aesthetic world disclosure' posits an order of values distinct from what we encounter in the dominant culture, making our implicit commitments explicit and, potentially, putting them in question. Insofar as such aesthetic experiences involve an affective negotiation of values, they, too, provide relevant data to be included in normative construction.

By considering modes of valuing, as well as values themselves, to be objects of construction rather than givens, Tessman's[55] account admits these multiple forms of valuation.[56] By no means does this imply that *all* values must be perceived intuitively rather than arrived at through reason. Moreover, pluralism about modes of valuation does not entail that all instances of intuitively apprehended values can withstand scrutiny. What such pluralism *does* indicate, rather, is that the experience of the '*I must*' or aesthetic world disclosure likewise represents a potentially genuine source of moral insight that can enter into the process of construction, which can then be accepted, revised or rejected.[57] Particularly given the frequency with which intuited values appear in moral experiences, it is clear that any account that is truly constructivist all the way down cannot predetermine practical reason as the *only* means of apprehending values.

Displacing the role of practical reason in a feminist account of constructivism puts into question the role of rational coherence that usually governs constructivist justification. Rational coherence is taken by both Street and Rawls as the measure of successful construction, such that one can weed out untenable conclusions based on their conflicts with already validated conclusions. But both Tessman's commitment to value pluralism and her intent to make theoretical sense of the experience of irresolvable moral conflict lead her away from rational coherentism as the sole goal of moral construction. Instead of the Rawlsian approach to reflective equilibrium, which assesses rational coherence with a set of liberal values, Tessman develops a modified version of Walker's 'transparency test'.[58] This serves as *Contribution 4: the expressive-collaborative model's approach to justification through intersubjective deliberation*. That is, justification consists of:

> social negotiation in real time, where members of a community of roughly or largely shared moral belief try to refine understanding, extend consensus, and eliminate conflict among themselves. 'We' are the members of some actual moral community, motivated by the aim of going on together, preserving or building self and mutual understanding in moral terms ... we need *equilibrium between people* as well as within them.[59]

Holding constant one value in which they are confident, communities assess judgements in question in light of their considered values and affirm, reject or modify accordingly.

The difference in modes of assessing the authority of normative judgements reflects a difference in understanding of what poses the greatest threat to our confidence in those judgements. For both Walker and Tessman, the greatest threat is not abstract unfairness but the ideological shaping of our initial judgements, whether these result from the exercise of practical reason or the intuitive apprehension of a requirement. On this account, a moral claim stands as valid only when it is transparent, meaning that it does not pretend to be something other than it is by depending on obfuscation or coercion for its acceptance.[60] Transparency testing is therefore dependent on a plurality of perspectives and an acknowledgement of the shaping influence of power. In this light, care ethicists' criticisms of mainstream moral theory are themselves an example of transparency testing: is Kantian deontology, for instance, able to genuinely support human moral equality, or does this model of moral equality in fact rest on the exclusion of everyone but white, able men? The question for Walker then becomes whether a particular judgement, if made transparent, conflicts with other values or judgements in which we have confidence. It is an equilibrium between transparent judgements that a moral community is collectively working towards in their practices of justification.

Tessman modifies Walker's more rationally oriented account by making room for the justification of non-rational judgements. Here she follows empirical research in moral psychology on the dual-process model of moral judgement that understands normative judgements made intuitively to be unresponsive to reasoned reflection and deliberation.[61] Such judgements require intervention at an affective level, most effectively prompted by engagement with others who do not share the same sacralized values.[62] A transparency test for intuitively apprehended values looks much like the experience Shotwell describes of the audience member challenged by the performance of Sins Invalid.[63] Mobilizing aesthetic and affective experiences can illuminate and contest the non-transparency of one's values: for instance, that one's commitment to moral equality depends on racial homogeneity, or that one's belief in the right of all bodies to appear in public depends on those with non-normative bodies making themselves as unobtrusive as possible.

But if intuitively apprehended moral values can enter into the process of construction, how are they to be considered under a revised notion of reflective equilibrium? That is to say, how does transparency testing keep from collapsing into a rational coherentism?[64] Values apprehended at an intuitive level must also be modified at that level. Tessman thus considers the process of having such values – say, for instance, my confidence in the superiority of heterosexual monogamy – challenged by someone who does not share my value as capable of eliciting an affective experience that dislodges the value's sacredness and enables me to question it.[65] Although Tessman's understanding of automatic confidence introduces significant challenges for constructivism to confront – to which I will return in this chapter's final section – her account tracks the apparent intransigence of certain moral values and frequency with which their transformation depends on affective rather than reasoned intervention.

4.4 ASSESSING THE EXPRESSIVE-COLLABORATIVE MODEL: STRENGTHS AND LINGERING PROBLEMS

When we search for normative authority, what we are searching for is confidence that our normative judgements should be followed. That this confidence can wax and wane alongside changing background conditions, or can be shattered entirely, speaks to the sociality of normative authority in a way I take to be consonant with moral experience. Such mutability, however, is not equivalent with pernicious relativism: we can act on the basis of 'working theories' while still leaving them open to contestation and revision.

The expressive-collaborative model offers a mode of justification that remains distinct from the approaches of mainstream moral theory that feminists have critiqued. On this model, the morality of primary interest to feminists is an intersubjective practice rather than a static and rationally coherent theory. It pursues confidence in moral judgements rather than metaphysical truths without giving up commitments to binding moral obligation. Forgoing a metaphysical account of truth, the Walker–Tessman account instead pursues normative authority while denying that any particular authoritative judgement is absolute. Further, Tessman's revisions provide particular relevant resources for assessing the validity of claims based in attachment. While making sense of the moral experience that occurs when we intuitively apprehend our attachment to another as issuing a non-negotiable moral requirement, Tessman's expressive-collaborative model does not automatically grant all such intuitions as truths. Rather, this approach recognizes that intuitively held values will require a different form of intersubjective engagement in order to consider and validate since rational argumentation may be ineffective.

The expressive-collaborative model is especially suited to feminist projects because it grants a central place to the influence of domination on the construction of morality. With keen attention on the parts of both Walker and Tessman to the distorting effects of ruling ideology on moral judgements, individual knowledge is recognized to be partial and vulnerable to the influence of domination. Validation of judgements requires intersubjective engagement with stakes that are acknowledged to be quite high. Holding constant a commitment to non-domination, values or judgements under review can be examined for their transparency and fitness within a larger network of normative commitments. Here, the transparency test offers 'a strategy for moving from an initial evaluative state to an affirmation (or rejection) of the authority of this valuation ... that [is] attentive to the operations of power that gave rise to the initial evaluative state'.[66] Consideration of the impact of domination on initial moral intuitions is therefore built into this account's method of achieving reflective equilibrium.

While the expressive-collaborative model's strengths are significant, several lingering questions remain: first, the local and historical bounds of valid claims will be unappealing to some theorists, and especially those very concerned with relativism. Second, the composition of the moral community in question bears on the model's viability in a society that is not just pluralist but polarized. To expose the limits of the expressive-collaborative model from a mainstream perspective, I turn to a clear case where values that passed the transparency test at one time failed at a later one. Here, we must consider the overturning of the segregationist 'separate but equal' doctrine in *Brown* vs. *Board of Education*. Precedent in *Plessy* vs. *Ferguson* held that racial segregation was constitutionally permissible if the separate facilities for Black and white people were 'equal', legitimizing the widespread and enduring apartheid in the US South. Given the extension of apartheid throughout spheres of professional caregiving – including, but not limited to, education and healthcare – this doctrine affirmed the compatibility of segregation with projects of care. Even at the time of oral arguments before the Supreme Court in 1896, Albion Tourgée, council for the plaintiff, argued that segregation necessarily contradicted equality, since the alleged need for separation was dependent on an assumption of the racial inferiority of Black people. By appealing to an implicit judgement undergirding a supposedly just principle, Tourgée sought to make transparent a doctrine that masqueraded as something other than what it was, a doctrine that he believed could not withstand scrutiny once revealed. Of course, in 1896 the Court denied that Tourgée's attempt at 'transparency testing' was unsuccessful and upheld segregation for another sixty years.[67] Not until Thurgood Marshall's arguments in the 1954 *Brown* vs. *Board of Education* case was segregation effectively made transparent at the level of the US justice system: separate facilities demonstrably were not, and never could be, equal.[68]

The historical fact that transparency testing the same 'separate but equal' doctrine could fail in 1896 but then succeed in 1954 raises tough questions about the strength of the expressive-collaborative model as an approach to justification across communities and historical periods.[69] First, the difference between the *Plessy* and *Brown* rulings highlights the expressive-collaborative model's dependence on a critical moral epistemology. In the context of *Plessy*, Tourgée certainly was not the only one to see through the doctrine's purported accordance with equality. Indeed, even Justice John Marshall Harlan's dissenting opinion pointed to the exceptions to the separate but equal doctrine that proved its true intent: by allowing Black care workers to ride in whites-only train cars with their white charges, Harlan argued that Louisiana law revealed the intent of segregationist laws as specifically about subordinating Black people.[70] That white supremacist resistance to admitting the demonstrably discriminatory basis of segregationist laws prevented not just the rejection of the 'separate but equal' doctrine but also refused acknowledgement of its real basis clarifies the impact of epistemic blockages and wilful ignorance on this model of justification.

The expressive-collaborative model is a collective epistemological investigation in pursuit of ethical insight. This means that, in order to achieve its aim of shirking the influence of systems of domination over our moral judgements, the expressive-collaborative model will require significant critical knowledge practices in order to acknowledge and move through bias without being determined by it.[71] Given the pre-reflective level at which much prejudice lives, interventions into the perceptual and affective dimensions of moral experience will be necessary.[72] Even with such critical knowledge practices, taking even ostensibly critical narratives at face value, as Lorraine Code[73] points out, would be risky. I'm inclined to say, however, that feminists have substantial resources for attending to both the multi-party construction of narrative and the impossibility of fully accounting for ourselves in narrative (for instance, through thinkers as distinct as Hilde Lindemann and Judith Butler). With such tools in hand, the difficulty seems to lie less in the theory of justification than in the ongoing efforts of carrying out its everyday practice.

A second, related problem raised by the 1896 verdict concerns the bounds of the moral community under discussion. The expressive-collaborative model is intended as a local practice of justification, while still understanding this process to result in something more than a naïve relativism. Walker therefore notes that deliberation and transparency testing are best achieved in moral communities of largely or roughly shared views. But what does the deep disagreement, represented even among the Supreme Court justices and certainly extending far beyond them, imply for the bounds of a shared moral community capable of assessing normative judgements? Moreover, what are we to glean about the nature of moral authority from the shift that took place between 1896 and 1954? One response would be to say that moral claims across communities and across time periods are ones that the expressive-collaborative model is precisely not interested in.[74] The expressive-collaborative model is designed for the real-time negotiation and validation of moral commitments, rather than the generation of universal truths. For the expressive-collaborative model to work, we must hold constant some values while examining others; shared values that we have reasonable confidence in are the basis of inquiry. The gravest concern, however, centres on intractable contemporaneous disagreement.[75] For instance, it would seem that despite the disagreement among the 1896 Supreme Court justices about the ability of the separate but equal doctrine to pass the transparency test, the judgement in favour of segregation was, at least for a time, morally authoritative. Critical knowledge practices, affective interventions and recursive applications of the transparency test offer significant tools for the collective practice of moral inquiry, but still the problem of presenting moral judgements with some level of generality looms large.

CONCLUSION

What the revised expressive-collaborative model offers to care ethics is a mode of justification that accounts for feminist criticisms of mainstream constructivism by accommodating pluralism and attending specifically to the threat of domination influencing our values. Open questions regarding the expressive-collaborative model notwithstanding, further elaboration of feminist metaethical constructivism offers care ethicists both a way of accounting for their normative claims and active tools for negotiating the proposal and validation of judgements. Care ethicists can temporarily hold steady certain commitments in order to evaluate their compatibility with the new norms and values that emerge. Employing the strategy of the transparency test, we can remain alert to claims that gain traction by masquerading as something other than what they are.

NOTES

1. See: Eva F. Kittay, 'The Ethics of Philosophizing: Ideal Theory and the Exclusion of People with Severe Cognitive Disabilities', in *Feminist Ethics and Social and Political Philosophy: Theorizing the Non-Ideal*, ed. Lisa Tessman (Dordrecht: Springer Netherlands, 2009), 123–6, https://doi.org/10.1007/978-1-4020-6841-6; Joan C. Tronto, *Caring Democracy: Markets, Equality, and Justice* (New York: New York University Press, 2013), 52–4.
2. Marilyn Frye, 'A Response to Lesbian Ethics', *Hypatia* 5, no. 3 (1990): 132–7.

3. Joan C. Tronto, *Moral Boundaries: A Political Argument for an Ethic of Care* (New York: Routledge, 2020), 149, https://doi.org/10.4324/9781003070672.
4. This trend is partially representative of the widening of *care ethics* into a varied, interdisciplinary field better described as care *theory*. On this point, see Gary (2022). I refer to 'care ethics' throughout this chapter for the sake of simplicity, given the focus of the volume. I nonetheless take my arguments here to be consistent with much work in care theory as well.
5. Maria P. Bellacasa, *Matters of Care: Speculative Ethics in More than Human Worlds* (Minneapolis: University of Minnesota Press, 2017), 90–132.
6. Ibid., 132–5.
7. Alexis Shotwell, *Against Purity: Living Ethically in Compromised Times* (Minneapolis: University of Minnesota Press, 2016), 140–5.
8. Margaret Urban Walker, *Moral Contexts* (Lanham, MD: Rowman & Littlefield Publishers, 2002), 87–9.
9. See: Margaret Urban Walker, 'What Does the Different Voice Say?: Gilligan's Women and Moral Philosophy', *The Journal of Value Inquiry* 23, no. 2 (June 1989): 123–34, https://doi.org/10.1007/BF00137281; Annette Baier, *Moral Prejudices: Essays on Ethics* (Cambridge, MA: Harvard University Press, 1995); Tove Pettersen, *Comprehending Care: Problems and Possibilities in the Ethics of Care* (Lanham, MD: Rowman & Littlefield, 2008).
10. Walker, *Moral Contexts*, xii–xiv.
11. See: Nel Noddings, *Caring: A Feminine Approach to Ethics and Moral Education* (Oakland: University of California Press, 1984), 27.
12. Sarah Clark Miller, 'A Kantian Ethic of Care?', in *Feminist Interventions in Ethics and Politics: Feminist Ethics and Social Theory*, ed. Barbara S. Andrew, Jean Clare Keller and Lisa H. Schwartzman (Lanham, MD: Rowman & Littlefield, 2005), 111–27.
13. Pettersen, *Comprehending Care*, 38–40.
14. Virginia Held, *The Ethics of Care: Personal, Political, and Global* (Oxford: Oxford University Press, 2006), 39.
15. At this point, a number of care ethicists have put forward several ways of understanding different aspects of care ethics' normative architecture. In her reconstruction and philosophical elaboration of Gilligan's original arguments, Tove Pettersen proposes an 'expanded principle of not hurting' as the starting point for care ethics (see: Pettersen, *Comprehending Care*, 41–8). Her principle draws on both standard formulations of non-maleficence and beneficence, though differing from such accounts by demanding more positive intervention and refusing self-sacrifice. Stephanie Collins, by contrast, provides a mid-level principle ('dependency relations generate responsibilities') but shies away from more foundational discussions of justification (2015). Eva Feder Kittay's most recent work proposes a normative ideal of care and offers conditions under which real instances of caregiving practices can serve as exemplars of that ideal (see: Eva Feder Kittay, *Learning from My Daughter: The Value and Care of Disabled Minds* (New York: Oxford University Press, 2019)). Steven Steyl, however, constructs a virtue-based theory of right action for care ethics (see: Steven Steyl, 'A Care Ethical Theory of Right Action', *The Philosophical Quarterly* 71, no. 3 (2021): 502–23, https://doi.org/10.1093/pq/pqaa063; Steven Steyl, 'Caring Actions', *Hypatia* 35, no. 2 (2020): 279–97, https://doi.org/10.1017/hyp.2020.12). Collins and Steyl especially are cognizant that their proposals may not be appealing to some strands of care theorists, particularly those located outside the bounds of analytic ethics.

16. Christine M. Korsgaard, *The Sources of Normativity* (Cambridge and New York: Cambridge University Press, 1996).
17. Ibid., 8.
18. Shotwell, *Against Purity*, 145.
19. Korsgaard, *The Sources of Normativity*, 47.
20. Shotwell, *Against Purity*, 143.
21. See: Georges Canguilhem, *Le Normal et le Pathologique* (Paris: Presses Universitaires de France – PUF, 1984); Michel Foucault, *The Foucault Reader* (New York: Vintage, 1984), 144.
22. Shotwell, *Against Purity*, 143–4.
23. As will become clear, the question of what counts as 'enforcement' of norms is an important one.
24. Shotwell, *Against Purity*, 145.
25. Kittay is also careful to distance her normative account of care from restrictive definitions of the normal, similarly referencing Foucault and articulating a need for more capacious norms. (See: Kittay, *Learning from My Daughter*, 32–41.)
26. Shotwell, *Against Purity*, 143.
27. Ibid., 162–3.
28. See: Michel Foucault, *Discipline and Punish: The Birth of the Prison* (New York: Penguin, 1975); François Ewald, 'Norms, Discipline, and the Law', *Representations* 30 (1990): 153.
29. Kittay, 'The Ethics of Philosophizing'.
30. Joan C. Tronto, *Caring Democracy: Markets, Equality, and Justice* (New York: New York University Press, 2013).
31. See: Kittay, 'The Ethics of Philosophizing', 126; Tove, *Comprehending Care*, 38.
32. Tronto, *Caring Democracy*, 52–4.
33. Lisa Tessman, *Moral Failure: On the Impossible Demands of Morality* (Oxford: Oxford University Press, 2016).
34. See: Laura Engel, 'Layered Constructivism: The Plural Sources of Practical Reasons', *Philosophia* 50, no. 4 (September 2022): 1721–44, https://doi.org/10.1007/s11406-022-00505-z; Sharon Street, 'What Is Constructivism in Ethics and Metaethics?', *Philosophy Compass* 5, no. 5 (May 2010): 363–84, https://doi.org/10.1111/j.1747-9991.2009.00280.x; Sharon Street, *Constructivism in Practical Philosophy*, ed. James Lenman and Yonatan Shemmer (Oxford: Oxford University Press, 2012), 40–59.
35. I will refer to the 'expressive-collaborative model' generally, but will specify where individual points should be attributed to either Walker or Tessman in particular.
36. See: Street, 'What Is Constructivism in Ethics and Metaethics?'; Tessman, *Moral Failure*, 103–14.
37. John Rawls, 'The Law of Peoples', *Critical Inquiry* 20, no. 1 (1993): 36–68.
38. Onora O'Neill, *Constructions of Reason: Explorations of Kant's Practical Philosophy* (Cambridge: Cambridge University Press, 1990), 209, http://0-dx.doi.org.oasis.unisa.ac.za/10.1017/CBO9781139173773.
39. Charles W. Mills, '"Ideal Theory" as Ideology', *Hypatia* 20, no. 3 (2005): 165–83, https://doi.org/10.1111/j.1527-2001.2005.tb00493.x.
40. See: Tronto, *Caring Democracy*; Tronto, *Moral Boundaries*.
41. Street, 'What Is Constructivism in Ethics and Metaethics?', 370.
42. Joan C. Tronto, 'Beyond Gender Difference to a Theory of Care', *Signs* 12, no. 4 (1987): 644–63.
43. Walker, *Moral Contexts*, xvii.

44. Ibid.
45. Tessman, *Moral Failure*, 160–5.
46. Ibid., 226.
47. Noddings, *Caring*.
48. Though it merits more consideration than I can give here, it is important to at least note that Tessman's primary source for the intuitive apprehension of values is Jonathan Haidt's social intuitionist mode (see: Tessman, *Moral Failure*, 134–8). Here, I have tried to cast Tessman's view in broader terms to avoid dependence on Haidt, though a fuller demonstration that such a move is possible will come in future work.
49. As I'll indicate in the final section, whether these intuitively apprehended requirements should be understood as negotiable or not remains to be seen.
50. See: Noddings, *Caring*; Inge van Nistelrooij and Merel Visse, 'Me? The Invisible Call of Responsibility and its Promise for Care Ethics: A Phenomenological View', *Medicine, Health Care and Philosophy* 22, no. 2 (2019): 275–85; Maurice Hamington, 'Care Ethics and Engaging Intersectional Difference through the Body', *Critical Philosophy of Race* 3, no. 1 (2015): 79–100.
51. Amy Allen, *The End of Progress: Decolonizing the Normative Foundations of Critical Theory* (New York: Columbia University Press, 2017), 218.
52. Shotwell, *Against Purity*, 11.
53. Ibid., 157.
54. Ibid., 159.
55. Tessman takes this position to be more reflective of the Humean commitment to contingency than Street's account. That is, 'both the process and the product of construction [are] contingent not only on *what* one values, but also on *how* one values' (see: Tessman, *Moral Failure*, 117).
56. See: Engel, 'Layered Constructivism', 1721–44; Tessman, *Moral Failure*, 116–22; Lisa Tessman, 'Value Pluralism, Intuitions, and Reflective Equilibrium', *Philosophical Topics* 41, no. 2 (2013): 175–201.
57. For a discussion of sacralizing values badly, see: Tessman, *Moral Failure*, 127–9.
58. Even if, as Street claims, this is merely a heuristic, it is helpful for approaching some of the differences between these views (see: Street, 'What Is Constructivism in Ethics and Metaethics?').
59. Margaret Urban Walker, *Moral Understandings: A Feminist Study in Ethics* (New York: Routledge, 1998), 64.
60. See: Tessman, *Moral Failure*, 131–3; Walker, *Moral Contexts*, 109.
61. Tessman, *Moral Failure*, 134–8.
62. Ibid., 138.
63. Shotwell, *Against Purity*, 17.
64. Though I focus on Tessman's account here in order to specifically address intuitively apprehended values, I will note that Walker also wishes to distance her account from rational coherentism by pursuing reflective equilibrium on a community level. That is, through her concern with reflective equilibrium as established *between* people as well as within them, Walker's coherentism aspires to the achievement of sustainable social arrangements (see: Walker, *Moral Understandings*, 75).
65. Tessman, *Moral Failure*, 131–8.
66. Ibid.,132.
67. Erwin Cherminsky, 'The Court Should Not Let Politically Divided Times Affects Its Choices and Decisions', *William & Mary Law Review* 61 (2019): 971.

68. Contemporary arguments that formal racial equality has been achieved and has effectively eliminated racial domination can similarly rely on obfuscation for acceptance.
69. I treat this example as a moral argument so as to sidestep the complicating and not necessarily relevant questions of law.
70. Akhil R. Amar, '*Plessy v. Ferguson* and the Anti-Canon', *Pepperdine Law Review* 39 (2011): 75.
71. As a start, Walker cites feminist epistemologists and scholars of science Sandra Harding and Donna Haraway on their respective concepts of strong objectivity and situated knowledges (see: Walker, *Moral Understandings,* 58–9 and 201–25; Sandra Harding, '"Strong Objectivity": A Response to the New Objectivity Question', *Synthese* 104, no. 3 (1995): 331–49, https://doi.org/10.1007/BF01064504; Donna Haraway, 'Situated Knowledges: The Science Question in Feminism and the Privilege of Partial Perspective', *Feminist Studies* 14, no. 3 (1988): 575, https://doi.org/10.2307/3178066). Future work will need to attend to work in social epistemology, including: Patricia H. Collins, *Black Feminist Thought: Knowledge, Consciousness, and the Politics of Empowerment* (London: Routledge, 1990), 251–73; Mariana Ortega, 'Being Lovingly, Knowingly Ignorant: White Feminism and Women of Color', *Hypatia* 21, no. 3 (2006): 56–74; Nancy Tuana, 'The Speculum of Ignorance: The Women's Health Movement and Epistemologies of Ignorance', *Hypatia* 21, no. 3 (2006): 1–19; Kristie Dotson, 'Tracking Epistemic Violence, Tracking Practices of Silencing', *Hypatia* 26, no. 2 (2011): 236–57; and Kristie Dotson, 'Conceptualizing Epistemic Oppression', *Social Epistemology* 28, no. 2 (2014): 115–38.
72. See: Alia Al-Saji, 'A Phenomenology of Critical-Ethical Vision', *Chiasmi International* 11 (2009): 375–98; Alia Al-Saji, 'A Phenomenology of Hesitation', in *Living Alterities: Phenomenology, Embodiment, and Race*, ed. Emily S. Lee (Albany: State University of New York Press, 2014), 133–82.
73. Lorraine Code, 'Narratives of Responsibility and Agency: Reading Margaret Walker's Moral Understandings', *Hypatia* 17, no. 1 (2002): 156–73, https://doi.org/10.1111/j.1527-2001.2002.tb00685.x.
74. Walker, *Moral Understandings*, 221–2.
75. Claudia Card, 'Responsibility Ethics, Shared Understandings, and Moral Communities', *Hypatia* 17, no. 1 (2002): 141–55, https://doi.org/10.1111/j.1527-2001.2002.tb00684.x.

BIBLIOGRAPHY

Allen, Amy. *The End of Progress: Decolonizing the Normative Foundations of Critical Theory*. New Directions in Critical Theory. New York: Columbia University Press, 2017.

Al-Saji, Alia. 'A Phenomenology of Critical-Ethical Vision', *Chiasmi International* 11 (2009): 375–98. https://doi.org/10.5840/chiasmi20091170.

Al-Saji, Alia. 'A Phenomenology of Hesitation', in *Living Alterities: Phenomenology, Embodiment, and Race*, edited by Emily S. Lee, 133–72. Albany: State University of New York Press, 2014.

Amar, Akhil R. '*Plessy v. Ferguson* and the Anti-Canon', *Pepperdine Law Review* 39 (2011): 75–89.

Baier, Annette. *Moral Prejudices: Essays on Ethics*. Cambridge, MA: Harvard University Press, 1995.

Canguilhem, Georges. *Le Normal et le Pathologique*. Paris: Presses Universitaires de France – PUF, 1984.

Card, Claudia. 'Responsibility Ethics, Shared Understandings, and Moral Communities', *Hypatia* 17, no. 1 (2002): 141–55. https://doi.org/10.1111/j.1527-2001.2002.tb00684.x.

Cherminsky, Erwin. 'The Court Should Not Let Politically Divided Times Affects Its Choices and Decisions', *William & Mary Law Review* 61 (2019): 971–94.

Code, Lorraine. 'Narratives of Responsibility and Agency: Reading Margaret Walker's Moral Understandings', *Hypatia* 17, no. 1 (2002): 156–73. https://doi.org/10.1111/j.1527-2001.2002.tb00685.x.

Collins, Patricia H. *Black Feminist Thought: Knowledge, Consciousness, and the Politics of Empowerment*. London: Routledge, 1990.

Collins, Stephanie. *The Core of Care Ethics*. Basingstoke: Springer, 2015.

Dotson, Kristie. 'Tracking Epistemic Violence, Tracking Practices of Silencing', *Hypatia* 26, no. 2 (2011): 236–57. https://onlinelibrary.wiley.com/doi/abs/10.1111/j.1527-2001.2011.01177.x.

Dotson, Kristie. 'Conceptualizing Epistemic Oppression', *Social Epistemology* 28, no. 2 (2014): 115–38.

Engel, Laura. 'Layered Constructivism: The Plural Sources of Practical Reasons', *Philosophia* 50, no. 4 (2022): 1721–44. https://doi.org/10.1007/s11406-022-00505-z.

Ewald, François. 'Norms, Discipline, and the Law', *Representations* 30 (1990): 138–61.

Foucault, Michel. *Discipline and Punish: The Birth of the Prison*. New York: Penguin, 1975.

Foucault, Michel. *The Foucault Reader*. New York: Vintage, 1984.

Frye, Marilyn. 'A Response to Lesbian Ethics', *Hypatia* 5, no. 3 (1990): 132–7. https://onlinelibrary.wiley.com/doi/abs/10.1111/j.1527-2001.1990.tb00611.x.

Gary, Mercer E. "From Care Ethics to Pluralist Care Theory: The State of the Field." *Philosophy Compass* 17, no. 4 (2022), e12819.

Hamington, Maurice. 'Care Ethics and Engaging Intersectional Difference through the Body', *Critical Philosophy of Race* 3, no. 1 (2015): 79–100. https://doi.org/10.5325/critphilrace.3.1.0079.

Haraway, Donna. 'Situated Knowledges: The Science Question in Feminism and the Privilege of Partial Perspective', *Feminist Studies* 14, no. 3 (1988): 575–99. https://doi.org/10.2307/3178066.

Harding, Sandra. '"Strong Objectivity": A Response to the New Objectivity Question', *Synthese* 104, no. 3 (September 1995): 331–49. https://doi.org/10.1007/BF01064504.

Held, Virginia. *The Ethics of Care: Personal, Political, and Global*. Oxford: Oxford University Press, 2006.

Kittay, Eva F. 'The Ethics of Philosophizing: Ideal Theory and the Exclusion of People with Severe Cognitive Disabilities', in *Feminist Ethics and Social and Political Philosophy: Theorizing the Non-Ideal*, edited by Lisa Tessman, 121–46. Dordrecht: Springer Netherlands, 2009. https://doi.org/10.1007/978-1-4020-6841-6.

Kittay, Eva F. *Learning from My Daughter: The Value and Care of Disabled Minds*. New York: Oxford University Press, 2019.

Korsgaard, Christine M. *The Sources of Normativity*. Cambridge and New York: Cambridge University Press, 1996.

Miller, Sarah Clark. 'A Kantian Ethic of Care?', in *Feminist Interventions in Ethics and Politics: Feminist Ethics and Social Theory*, edited by Barbara S. Andrew, Jean Clare Keller and Lisa H. Schwartzman, 111–27. Lanham, MD: Rowman & Littlefield, 2005.

Mills, Charles W. '"Ideal Theory" as Ideology', *Hypatia* 20, no. 3 (2005): 165–83. https://doi.org/10.1111/j.1527-2001.2005.tb00493.x.

Noddings, Nel. *Caring: A Feminine Approach to Ethics and Moral Education*. Oakland: University of California Press, 1984.

O'Neill, Onora. *Constructions of Reason: Explorations of Kant's Practical Philosophy*. Cambridge: Cambridge University Press, 1989. http://0-dx.doi.org.oasis.unisa.ac.za/10.1017/CBO9781139173773.

Ortega, Mariana. 'Being Lovingly, Knowingly Ignorant: White Feminism and Women of Color', *Hypatia* 21, no. 3 (2006): 56–74. https://doi.org/10.1353/hyp.2006.0034.

Pettersen, Tove. *Comprehending Care: Problems and Possibilities in the Ethics of Care*. Lanham: Rowman & Littlefield, 2008.

Puig de la Bellacasa, Maria. *Matters of Care: Speculative Ethics in More than Human Worlds*. Minneapolis: University of Minnesota Press, 2017.

Rawls, John. 'The Law of Peoples', *Critical Inquiry* 20, no. 1 (1993): 36–68.

Shotwell, Alexis. *Against Purity: Living Ethically in Compromised Times*. Minneapolis: University of Minnesota Press, 2016.

Steyl, Steven. 'Caring Actions', *Hypatia* 35, no. 2 (2020): 279–97. https://doi.org/10.1017/hyp.2020.12.

Steyl, Steven. 'A Care Ethical Theory of Right Action', *The Philosophical Quarterly* 71, no. 3 (2021): 502–23. https://doi.org/10.1093/pq/pqaa063.

Street, Sharon. 'What Is Constructivism in Ethics and Metaethics?', *Philosophy Compass* 5, no. 5 (May 2010): 363–84. https://doi.org/10.1111/j.1747-9991.2009.00280.x.

Street, Sharon. *Constructivism in Practical Philosophy*, edited by James Lenman and Yonatan Shemmer. Oxford: Oxford University Press, 2012.

Tessman, Lisa. 'Value Pluralism, Intuitions, and Reflective Equilibrium', *Philosophical Topics* 41, no. 2 (2013): 175–201. https://doi.org/10.5840/philtopics201341221.

Tessman, Lisa. *Moral Failure: On the Impossible Demands of Morality*. Oxford: Oxford University Press, 2015.

Tronto, Joan C. 'Beyond Gender Difference to a Theory of Care', *Signs* 12, no. 4 (1987): 644–63.

Tronto, Joan C. *Caring Democracy: Markets, Equality, and Justice*. New York: New York University Press, 2013.

Tronto, Joan C. *Moral Boundaries: A Political Argument for an Ethic of Care*. New York: Routledge, 2020. https://doi.org/10.4324/9781003070672.

Tuana, Nancy. 'The Speculum of Ignorance: The Women's Health Movement and Epistemologies of Ignorance', *Hypatia* 21, no. 3 (2006): 1–19.

Van Nistelrooij, Inge, and Merel Visse. 'Me? The Invisible Call of Responsibility and its Promise for Care Ethics: A Phenomenological View', *Medicine, Health Care and Philosophy* 22, no. 2 (2019): 275–85. https://doi.org/10.1007/s11019-018-9873-7.

Walker, Margaret Urban. 'What Does the Different Voice Say?: Gilligan's Women and Moral Philosophy', *The Journal of Value Inquiry* 23, no. 2 (June 1989): 123–34. https://doi.org/10.1007/BF00137281.

Walker, Margaret Urban. *Moral Understandings: A Feminist Study in Ethics*. New York: Routledge, 1998.

Walker, Margaret Urban. *Moral Contexts*. Lanham: Rowman & Littlefield, 2002.

Walker, Margaret Urban. 'Morality in Practice: A Response to Claudia Card and Lorraine Code', *Hypatia* 17, no. 1 (2002): 174–82. https://doi.org/10.1111/j.1527-2001.2002.tb00686.x.

CHAPTER FIVE

Care ethics and phenomenology

CARLO LEGET

INTRODUCTION

Care is a complex phenomenon. Although it has been at the centre of care ethics and caring sciences as an interdisciplinary field of studies for more than forty years, we are still in the process of understanding better and deeper the many dimensions and complexities of what caring is. From the perspective of political science care has famously been defined as follows:

> On the most general level, we suggest that caring be viewed as a species activity that includes everything that we do to maintain, continue, and repair our 'world' so that we can live in it as well as possible. That world includes our bodies, our selves, and our environment ... all of which we seek to interweave in a complex, life-sustaining web.[1]

Although probably the most cited and influential definition of care, and despite its heuristic power to discover traces and indications of care in our world, it also raises questions. Is this 'everything we do' first and for all to be seen as a practice?[2] Or is it rather a virtue?[3] And what about those who see care as an emotion or something humans share with other animals?[4] Should a definition of care not be more explicitly related to the non-human world?[5] What about the meaning of care in our lives? Is care the fundamental category of relating to the world[6] or a heuristic category that leads us to what is existentially meaningful for a fulfilled life?[7] Is the importance of care as an inspiration and life fulfilling activity sufficiently addressed by a political view on care? And if not, how can we connect the different perspectives on care?

Care seems to be fundamental and omnipresent on the one hand, and multidimensional and elusive on the other. It is both a descriptive term and it has a normative dimension. From the level of ordinary language ('I do not care') to scientific analysis, speaking of care expresses what is important to us, and expresses somehow a view of 'the good life, with and for others, in just institutions'.[8] Although in education and research it is helpful to use a clear definition of care, in this chapter I will explore why it is important to continue to 'defrost' the concept of care according to whatever definition we use for it.[9] Both for the sake of the multidimensionality and elusiveness of care as a phenomenon, I will plea to always be ready to revisit our understanding of care by approaching it as an open question.

In this chapter I will argue that in philosophy there is one approach especially helpful in exploring the phenomenon of care as an open question: phenomenology. I consider phenomenology in the broad sense as the philosophical reflection on the way meaning structures appear in our consciousness. Rooted in both descriptive psychology[10] and philosophy,[11] phenomenology has taken an existential turn,[12] and developed into a range of methodologies that help us to understand caring practices better.[13] Just like care ethics, phenomenology has developed into a tree with many branches reaching out to different phenomena and using different approaches that are combined and integrated in many disciplines.[14] Without going into the differences between the phenomenological approaches I will introduce and illustrate different ways in which phenomenology can contribute to care ethics. Phenomenology can help to (1) develop a critical perspective on central concepts in care ethics; (2) analyse the lived experience of people; (3) develop empirical research methods in which the embodiment of knowledge is honoured; (4) give access to the non-discursive origin of meaning structures in caring; and (5) shed light on the foundations of normativity in care ethics.

5.1 PHENOMENOLOGY AND DEFROSTING CONCEPTS

In an insightful and thought-provoking paper, Cheryl Mattingly addresses the problem for critical theory – and I consider the mainstream of care-ethical literature in this tradition – that concepts can become canonical, training our way of looking without being questioned themselves. The paper explores a fundamental problem with language in general, 'for inevitably words obscure the impression and elusiveness of lived experience'.[15] On the other hand, of course, we need words and concepts to think discursively, analyse situations and communicate with each other. Mattingly is very clear in upholding the importance of different branches of critical theory in analysing and problematizing dominant societal discourses and exposing structures of power, inequality and violence. Although she does not mention care ethics in her paper, it is not difficult to see the shared programme with critical anthropology studying cultures with a both descriptive and normative interest. Her point, however, is that we also need a critical way of reflecting on the concepts that we use as lenses to look at reality.

For this aim, Mattingly builds on the work of Hannah Arendt who points to the fact that concepts are 'frozen thought', grouping together particulars that enable us to think swiftly, but also freezing them. Especially, political and ethical concepts that carry a substantial normative weight run the risk of becoming fixed ways of looking at the world, limiting our gaze, the abundance of meaning and potentiality inherent in every situation. For Arendt what protects us against evil is not the results of thinking as they can be crystallized in rules of practice or moral codes. It is the experience of uncertainty, the activity of not knowing that protects us. Building on her famous analysis of the banality of evil, she shows that it is doctrinal certainty that is a manifestation of non-thinking.

Mattingly situates her analysis of the potential role of phenomenology with regard to critical thinking in the broader developments of three lines of inquiry: phenomenological anthropology, anthropology's ethical turn and 'dark anthropology'.[16] What she calls 'critical phenomenology 1.0' refers to approaches that combine critical sociopolitical voices with traditions of phenomenological analysis. When phenomenology is also used to destabilize and unsettle the central critical concepts we work with ourselves, she calls it 'critical phenomenology 2.0'. This self-critical approach that defrosts central concepts brings us back to experience as an important way of unsettling theory. Phenomenology is an especially powerful resource here because – and here Mattingly refers to Michael D. Jackson – it (a) 'challenges the fetishization of the products of intellectual reflection'; (b) presumes that language is not sufficient to capture or contain the 'flux of experience'; and (c) 'absolutely prioritizes lived experience over practical knowledge'.[17]

Mattingly's call for using phenomenology not only to study lived experiences but also to reflect critically on the central concepts of the theoretical framework that is used, is practised by different authors in care ethics.[18] Empirical research and conceptual thinking can be developed in a dialectic of mutual critical reflection. On the one hand, critical insights from the theoretical framework of care ethics, like embodiment, relationality and vulnerability, can be used to direct one's attention during empirical research. On the other hand, the findings of the empirical research can help in developing new questions and viewpoints in the theoretical discussion about the same critical insights. Such a dialectical relation is principally open to develop infinitely, depending on new viewpoints and discoveries that inform the discussion.

Mattingly's paper gives food for thought for the critical role of phenomenology for care ethics. But how does it work in practice? What role can phenomenology play in a care-ethical analysis of societal debates? And how can such an open and non-judgemental approach to phenomena function in the context of a political debate? To develop this a little further guided by a concrete example we will look at the work of Els van Wijngaarden on the experience of a 'completed life' of older citizens in the Netherlands.

5.2 EXPLORING THE LIVED EXPERIENCE: THE CASE OF COMPLETED LIFE

In the Netherlands the debate about physician assisted dying has a long tradition, going back to the 1960s. Ten years before euthanasia and physician assisted suicide was regulated by law in 2002, a discussion in society started in which older people with no life-inhibiting or chronic medical condition who were tired of life asked for regulation that helped them to end their lives. At the time of writing, the euthanasia law that came into effect in 2002 still does not apply to being old and tired of life. But there are strong proponents of this option that are engaged in a citizen initiative 'Cooperatie Laatste Wil' ('Cooperation Last Will') putting pressure on the Dutch parliament to widen the criteria for physician assisted dying to also apply to older people who are tired of life. The discussion has been going on for thirty years now, regularly flaring up and raising major societal attention.

According to the proponents for widening the euthanasia criteria, the issue is relatively easy: people should have the opportunity to decide about their own life. The state should facilitate this, preferably by assigning medical assistance in the process, structuring the process in a civilized way, and preventing cruel self-inflicted deaths and unnecessary suffering or painful situations for family members. Basically, the argument is framed in terms of citizen rights and moral values as autonomy and prevention of suffering. Proponents present themselves as rational citizens being able to take responsibility for their own lives and make a rational decision about the value of their own life and death.

From a care-ethical perspective, however, this position raises many questions. Old age comes with many inconveniencies. Many older people suffer from physical problems, social isolation, a feeling of being of no use to society any longer, and older men without a life partner have significantly higher suicide rates. Could the idea that life is no longer worth living for a certain group of older people perhaps be internalized and amplified in them by a society that has difficulties in accepting vulnerability and decline, and is mainly interested in young and energetic people that help to sustain the economy? To what extent can we speak of a free decision to end one's life when the cultural developments of acceleration and isolation lead towards a marginalization of older people, abandoning them to their fate?

While one of the political parties in the Netherlands prepared for a widening of the euthanasia legislation, Van Wijngaarden conducted a qualitative, phenomenological interview study following Dahlberg's Reflective Lifeworld Approach.[19] She spoke extensively with twenty-five Dutch mentally competent elderly citizens (seventy+) who considered their life to be completed, were suffering from the prospect of living on, and at the moment of the interview had a reasonable death wish. Her research goals were: (1) to provide in-depth insight about what it means to feel 'life is completed and no longer worth living' as lived and experienced by elderly people who do not suffer from a life-threatening disease or a psychiatric disorder; and (2) to gain a deeper understanding of what it means to live with the firm intention to end life at a self-chosen moment.[20]

The twenty-five interviews were analysed and meaning units (coherent fragments of texts) were identified that partially described the phenomenon. Meaning units that were connected were clustered to form building blocks of the essence of the phenomenon of completed life. The essence of the experience that life is completed, and no longer worth living was described as: 'a tangle of inability and unwillingness to connect to one's actual life'. What is immediately clear from this essence is that the disconnectedness is partially a matter of not being able to and partially of not wanting to connect to one's actual life. This presents a different picture than the rational self-determining citizen, the individual expressing a rational and free choice, who appeared in the newspapers. Analysing the interviews it also became clear that next to its ambivalent nature, this experience of completed life was not permanent or stable: it reflected a process of experiencing both a will to live and a wish to die simultaneously, varying in intensity and balance over time.

Because of the unstable and ambivalent nature of the experience of completed life, the people interviewed in this study lived in a situation in-between intending and actually performing a self-chosen death. In van Wijngaarden's research, this paradoxical position was further explicated in the following tensions: detachment and attachment; rational and non-rational considerations; taking grip and losing grip; resisting interference and longing for support; and legitimacy and illegitimacy. In other words: the experience of 'completed life' is an unstable experience characterized by continuously navigating tensions rather than having a clear and fixed evaluation of one's life.

In her research, van Wijngaarden also found that underlying the experience of a completed life, there were five constituting elements: a sense of aching loneliness; the pain of not mattering; the inability to express oneself; multidimensional tiredness; and a sense of aversion towards feared dependence. By using a phenomenological analysis, the research was able to show that the concept of 'completed life' is a misleading term, painting a way too positive picture of a rational self-determining citizen, and leaving out the social and political context of the older people who were involved.

The phenomenological research on the concept of a completed life was discussed in the Dutch Parliament in November 2016, confirming the work of an independent governmental advisory committee that strongly recommended not to widen the legal criteria to obtain assisted dying. The care-ethical research by van Wijngaarden helped in clarifying the phenomenon by pointing to the ambiguities within the lived experiences of older people, the normative dimension of the political debate including different views on the nature of human beings and the ideal of flourishing, and the importance of understanding the pre-reflexive dimension of experiences when trying to understand the freedom of people to decide about life or death. It illustrates how phenomenological research in a care-ethical framework can be of political importance.

5.3 EMBODIMENT AND PHENOMENOLOGICAL RESEARCH IN CARE ETHICS

Like care ethics, phenomenology (both as a philosophical tradition and as a method for empirical research) focuses on understanding life as it is lived rather than through a predefined theoretical lens.[21] Els van Wijngaarden's work is one example of phenomenological research that focuses on the lived experience of citizens. Her methodology is based on the work of Karin Dahlberg, who – in a Husserlian tradition – has done important work to integrate phenomenology in healthcare research. Dahlberg's Reflective Lifeworld Approach, however, is not the only way phenomenological research can be integrated with care ethics. Generally speaking, there seem to be two ways in which care ethics and phenomenology are being combined: a theoretical and an empirical way.

First, there are the authors that draw upon phenomenology in a theoretical way when they reflect on central concepts in care ethics such as embodiedness, vulnerability and precarity, and use phenomenological sources to develop their care-ethical reflection. Good examples of this way of using phenomenology are the work of Patricia Benner and Maurice Hamington, who build on the work of Maurice Merleau-Ponty. Another example of this theoretical way is the work of care ethics as developed in Belgium by philosophers like Linus van Laere and Roger Burggraeve who are inspired by the phenomenology of Emanuel Levinas. The use of phenomenology to develop theoretical and conceptual reflections in care ethics is of great importance because it helps in deepening central concepts and informs methodological reflections. In this chapter, however, I will not so much dwell on this way of using phenomenology in care theory but focus on a second group of authors who do qualitative empirical research. In one of the rare edited volumes on care ethics and phenomenology that are available, Hanneke van der Meide points to the fact that although there is much agreement about the importance of bodiliness in care ethics, there is hardly any reflection on how phenomenology can help researchers in care ethics to address it in their studies.[22] She explains how in phenomenology the body is seen as not a mere object but a form of consciousness and quotes Merleau-Ponty who considers the body the general medium for experiencing the world as it is 'the horizon latent in all our experience and itself ever-present and anterior to every determining thought'.[23]

This view on the body has a great impact on understanding what meaning is. As human beings we are connected to the world by the invisible threads of meaning.[24] There is no way around this. These threads of meaning are co-constructed by the needs and possibilities of our body. Van der Meide gives the example of how the same bridge she admires walking through the city can become a big threshold or even obstacle when she reaches this bridge at the end of a marathon. The perception of the bridge is completely different as is its meaning. Thus, meaning is neither something subjective that belongs to me, nor objective that belongs to the bridge, and thus it rather belongs to the in-between structure of the lifeworld. Even the same experience can mean something different for the same person when the lifeworld is different due to a different place, context, past or future.

When we now think about empirical research from the perspective of this embodied view on knowledge, it is no longer possible to consider meaning as something present in a respondent that I can extract by interviewing and taking notes. Doing research, either by doing interviews or observations, is partaking in a situation and being enveloped in an atmosphere of emotional changes and moods.[25] Although this is an immediate bodily experience that we share when we meet each other in a situation, the meaning of our experiences will always be partly hidden. As soon as we begin to use words, we turn away from the immediate fresh experience, some form of reflection is involved and we are confronted with the differences in bodily needs, moods and histories.[26] Therefore, in phenomenology there is general agreement that we need to refrain from making judgements and open up in wonder to be led back ('phenomenological re-duction') to the moment of appearing of the phenomenon.[27] Suspending ('epochè') our mental acts that lead to a too quick understanding of the phenomenon is an important skill for researchers who use a phenomenological approach.

Van der Meide shows with two examples why bodiliness in empirical research is important and how it can be put into practice while doing empirical research. The first example regards older hospital patients.[28] Although it has been shown in many studies that being admitted to a hospital has great impact on older patients, the question of what it is like to be older and hospitalized is seldomly asked. Van der Meide chose a method from anthropology called shadowing as the preferred method of data collection, which means that she closely observed and followed older patients, as if she was their shadow. Her reasons for this methodology were both methodological and ethical: she did not want to exclude beforehand patients who did not have the ability to maintain focus on a phenomenon and or the narrative competence to give words to their experience in a structured and logical way. Moreover, shadowing can honour the bodiliness of both the researcher and the respondent. As meaning is also bodily expressed, it can help showing how something is experienced and enrich what is said by the other person. In her field notes, van der Meide described how she herself as a researcher was affected by the atmosphere in the hospital room and the mood of her shadowee. The shared experience of boredom in this case, was experienced bodily and was an entry point for the researcher to understand what the older patient was going through. But it also helped to build trust and familiarity that enabled the researcher to do research in a caring way, building on the development of a relationship.

The other example van der Meide gives focuses on the lived experience of patients with multiple sclerosis (MS). From a care-ethical perspective, there are two problematic sides to mainstream research on this group of patients. In the first place, they seem to consider living well with MS as an individual challenge, not addressing how individual experiences are a response to a social and cultural context and reflect this context as well. Second, most studies see the adjustment to living with MS as a task for the mind to deal with the body as meaningless material and thus show a mind–body dualism that installs a hierarchy of mind over body. From a phenomenological perspective, this dualism is unfortunate since it confirms by a theoretical approach the broken relation with their body experienced by MS patients, instead of exploring how to restore this relationship, acknowledging that the body is not just dead material but an ever-changing living reality.

In this research project on patients with MS, van der Meide used interviewing as the method of data collection, inviting the respondents to speak about how they experienced their body in different situations in everyday life. This time, the body was used in the analysis of the interviews, building on the work of phenomenologist philosopher Max van Manen. Van Manen considers writing a way of making contact with the world.[29] It is an embodied act through and through that can be used in the process of making contact with the data that were collected in the research. In a normal coding process, coding interview fragments is a series of cognitive acts that are performed using the data as raw material. At the end of the process of analysis there is a phase of writing down the results of the analysis. In van Manen's approach, writing is used and considered as a way of making contact with the data and bringing them to life again using our embodied awareness as a research skill.

Following van Manen and Finlay, van der Meide describes different steps in working towards a deeper understanding of the data that were collected by interviewing. The first phase consists of reading the transcripts, listening to the audio files and immersing oneself into the lived experiences that are accessible through the data. This is a bodily process, since those parts of the transcripts that resonate with us reveal something both about the lived experience of the interviewee and the preunderstanding that has been built up in our embodied experience and should be bracketed insofar as it contains preunderstandings that close us off from the phenomenon speaking to us. In the second phase, the 'rumble' in the manuscripts is removed and textual portrayals of the lived experiences are created that have an evocative character, allowing us to glimpse into the phenomenon. The textual portrayals are composed of sentences from the interviews and allow us to get an intuitive understanding of the phenomenon. In the last phase, the themes in the text are brought together into a structure for the final description in which the phenomenon is explicated, showing the ambiguities, and using sources from literature and philosophy to open up an understanding of the phenomenon that is provisional and partial, acknowledging that much has remained unsaid.

The examples of van der Meide are illustrative for what phenomenology can contribute to empirical research in care ethics: a humble understanding of the lived experience of phenomena that is embodied and open to the ambivalence and paradoxes of life. Klaartje Klaver adds some implications of acknowledging the critical role of phenomenology in care ethics: as everything is contextual, this also goes for the phenomenological researchers who try to bracket their preunderstandings; the lived experience of those whom we study will always escape researchers; honouring the otherness of the other will always limit our understanding of the phenomena we study; and the attention to and acknowledgement of otherness, ambiguity and power will enhance the quality of care-ethical research.[30]

5.4 PHENOMENOLOGY, MEANING AND CARE

From its early days, developing from descriptive psychology in the work of Dilthey and Husserl, phenomenology has focused on the way meaning structures appear in our consciousness. Martin Heidegger in the phenomenological analysis of being in *Being and Time* opened up a new approach in phenomenological research that can be called ontological or metaphysical. The radical newness of this approach lies in no longer viewing the meaning structures in human consciousness as things that can be studied as an objective reality from which the researcher is removed, as Husserl tried to develop; in Heidegger's view, this is impossible since human consciousness is not separated from the world it studies. The shift this brings about is best explained by the experience of being in wonder. As Finn Thorbjørn Hansen phrases it: 'in deep wonder, our consciousness is decentred from being the centre from which the world is being seen and understood, to a way of being, where the human consciousness seems to step aside as it were in order for the world itself to speak'.[31]

The Heideggerian turn has resulted in different interpretive phenomenological approaches in, for example, nursing research, developed by authors like Benner, Munhall and Conroy.[32] From a Heideggerian perspective, this tradition has been brought one step further by reflecting on the 'surplus of meaning' that is sometimes revealed in caring practices and that brings a completely new perspective on care. In the work of Sine Herholdt-Lomholdt, for example, moments in nursing are explored in which the subject–object dichotomy is suddenly cancelled and an overwhelming experience of fullness of meaning is experienced. In these moments it is as if caregivers are no longer in control, but something else calls and guides what is happening in the caring practice. These experiences raise many questions about the way healthcare is organized and caregivers are trained to focus their attention. In her work, Herholdt-Lomholdt calls for opening a space for otherness in the caring work we do, underlining the importance of developing a more receptive, listening and open attitude that enables a connection with the surplus of meaning in human encounters that is often inaccessible due to the great pressure of efficiency and targets that guide professional caring practices.[33]

The work of Herholdt-Lomholdt is inspired by Finn Thorbjørn Hansen's philosophical work on wonder and wonder-labs.[34] Building on the work of phenomenologists like Max van Manen and Steen Halling, Hansen has developed practical dialogical phenomenological practices that he calls 'wonder-labs' and that are used in various professional caring practices. Wonder-labs are a structured way of group work in which a moment of wonder is explored in a small group, bringing it into resonance with experiences of the group members but also with great works of art. The aim of these shared reflective moments is to open a different awareness to caring practices and be in touch with the surplus of meaning that is present in everyday caring practices. Although wonder-labs are meaningful in themselves and should not be instrumentalized, they add to more awareness of beauty and mystery, and help to develop a language to speak about it.

At the same time, wonder-labs are in a phenomenological tradition of research that honours the importance of not knowing. As Hans-Georg Gadamer has shown in *Truth and Method*, thinking is a creative process in which our unexpressed and inexpressible thoughts ('the inner word') are much richer than what we can express and what is solidified in language. As care ethicist Merel Visse expresses in a book chapter named after the first line of a poem by Emily Dickinson: 'your thoughts don't have words every day'.[35] This opens up a whole new field of phenomenologically inspired care studies that honour the non-rational and non-knowing aspects of caring as they are developed in arts-based research, for instance.[36] It also fuels reflections on how phenomenological forms of research can be developed in which research becomes part of living a question as opposed to the mainstream view of research as knowledge production.[37]

5.5 PHENOMENOLOGY AND THE FOUNDATION OF CARE ETHICS

If phenomenology can play an important role in exploring the freshness of a lived experience before it is related to the frozen concepts that structure our thinking and appreciation of reality, can it also be helpful for thinking about the normative foundation of care ethics? When we read the work of the women who helped to develop the moral approach that is known now as care ethics, there seems to be a congeniality in the way they felt the need for an alternative approach and how they tried to develop it. Carol Gilligan showed how the mainstream approach to moral development as it was coined by Lawrence Kohlberg, going all the way back to a Kantian deontology, obscured 'a different voice' of moral reasoning and development that was more relational, process-oriented and inductive.[38] Sara Ruddick wrote how as an academically trained philosopher she did not recognize anything of the problems she met in the practice of mothering reflected in her academic education.[39] Nel Noddings, following David Hume, wrote about natural caring as a universal response of mothers to the needs of their children, in whatever culture or context they find themselves.[40] In later years, Margaret Urban Walker's work on moral epistemology distinguished an expressive collaborative approach to morality from a theoretical-juridical model. She develops the idea that morality consists of practices of responsibilities, not theories, and moral theorizing needs to be freed from 'the impoverishing legacies of ideality and purity that make most of most people's lives disappear, or render those lives unintelligible'.[41]

There seems to be no doubt that according to these writers the foundation of the moral appeal in care ethics is not found in theory or categoric rules, but in the concrete practices people find themselves in. There is a naturalness and spontaneity in caring practices that seem to suggest that we are dealing with a premoral or non-moral practice. On the other hand, caring can be full of conflict or struggle, it can be smothering and harmful, it can be heroic and full of self-sacrifice.[42] From that perspective there is no doubt that caring is a practice with a moral dimension, like any other social practice. But what does this suggest about the foundation of care ethics as a moral theory? And in the context of this chapter: can phenomenology play a meaningful role in reflecting on this foundation?

When Nel Noddings, in her groundbreaking work, reflected on the foundation of an ethic of caring, she built on David Hume's idea that morality is founded upon and rooted in feeling.[43] Unlike Hume, however, she argued that morality requires two sentiments and not just one. The first sentiment she calls 'natural caring'. It is a very foundational way of doing that humans share with mammals: animals take care of their offspring and we do not call this ethical behaviour. This first sentiment can be followed by a second sentiment – an 'I must' – that is in response to remembering the first. Noddings calls this 'ethical caring' and it does have a moral dimension that can be developed in different ways. Interesting here is that in the foundation of an ethic of caring, the phenomenon appears as both natural and ethical, seemingly questioning or suggesting a parallel structure to the is–ought distinction. What role can phenomenology play in this discussion?

In an interesting chapter on phenomenology, care and the foundation of morality, Per Nortvedt discusses some fundamental similarities between care ethics and phenomenology concerning the foundation of morality. In the works of phenomenologists like Husserl, Løgstrup and Jonas, human beings have an innate and intuitive response to normative value. In care ethics there is a similar innate foundation in the relational ontology that views human beings as always embedded in relationships that have moral value.[44] Nortvedt discusses the work of various phenomenologists on the foundation of morality, including Levinas, for whom this foundation is not situated in pre-reflective consciousness, but in the radical otherness of the other. After a critical discussion of care-ethical literature, he concludes that both care ethics and phenomenology have a similar account of the foundation of morality but lack a solid empirical basis in moral psychology. The better we understand moral motivation, also from a psychological perspective, the better we understand the normative foundation of practices of caring.[45]

Nortvedt comes up with an interesting suggestion that can bridge the gap between accounts of moral foundation that are based on the pre-reflective, like care ethics and phenomenology, and accounts that are based on rational analysis, like mainstream moral theories such as deontology and consequentialism.[46] In the work of Lisa Tessman, we find a distinction between two systems of moral judgement that co-exist in the human brain. On the one hand, there is a controlled reasoning system that produces moral judgements and is mostly involved in reflection.[47] On the other hand, there is an automatic intuitive system that is deeply embedded and affect-based. According to this system, we encounter non-avoidable moral demands that have their own value and power – like, for instance, the demand of non-killing.

Discussing the role of phenomenology in reflecting on the moral foundation of care ethics is illustrative of both the strength and weakness of phenomenology and the nature of care ethics. Phenomenology is very helpful in exploring the lived experience of the topics care ethics reflects upon. It is also a great help in revealing meaning structures and articulating how phenomena may speak to us. For the discussion with other disciplines that are occupied with caring practices, however, other disciplines and epistemologies are needed as well. And this has everything to do with the reason why care ethics cannot be but an interdisciplinary field of study, based on the fact that care is a complex phenomenon.

CONCLUSION

In this chapter we have explored the importance and possibilities of phenomenological approaches in care ethics. Phenomenology can be helpful to defrost central concepts and develop critical appreciation of those concepts in our thinking that we take perhaps too much for granted. It can also be used to explore the lived experience of a phenomenon related to care, and help articulate the nuances, paradoxes and tensions inherent in lived experiences. Phenomenology can be used in an embodied way, either referring to the way empirical data are collected, or to the way data are analysed and interpreted. A phenomenological approach can bring us closer to lived experiences and their meaningfulness by realizing that there is a realm of life prior to verbalization, conceptualization and reasoning. It can open us to dimensions of care that are existential in nature. And, finally, phenomenology can play a role in the reflecting on the foundation of care ethics as a moral theory.

As an interdisciplinary (or even transdisciplinary) field of research, there are many traditions in philosophy and social sciences that can develop care ethics further. Phenomenology, in the broad sense, is one of them. Without claiming any completeness about the possible contributions phenomenology can make to care ethics, this chapter hopefully has given some insight into a valuable approach.

NOTES

1. Joan C. Tronto and Berenice Fisher, 'Toward a Feminist Theory of Caring', in *Circles of Care: Work and Identity in Women's Lives*, ed. Emily K. Abel and Margaret K. Nelson (Albany: State University of New York Press, 1990), 36–54.
2. See: Sara Ruddick, *Maternal Thinking: Toward a Politics of Peace* (Boston, MA: Beacon Press, 1989); Joan C. Tronto, *Moral Boundaries: A Political Argument for an Ethic of Care*

(New York: Routledge, 1993); Margaret Urban Walker, *Moral Understandings: A Feminist Study in Ethics* (New York: Oxford University Press, 2007).
3. Michael Slote, *The Ethics of Care and Empathy* (New York: Routledge, 2007).
4. Nel Noddings, *Caring: A Feminine Approach to Ethics and Moral Education* (Berkeley: University of California Press, 1984).
5. Maria Puig de la Bellacasa, *Matters of Care: Speculative Ethics in More Than Human Worlds*, vol. 41 (Minneapolis: University of Minnesota Press, 2017).
6. Martin Heidegger, *Being and Time* (New York: Harper and Row, 1962).
7. Carlo Leget, *Zorg om Betekenis. Over Zorgethiek en Spirituele Zorg, in Het Bijzonder in Relatie Tot de Palliatieve Zorg* (Amsterdam: SWP, 2013).
8. Paul Ricoeur, *Oneself as Another* (Chicago, IL: University of Chicago Press, 1992).
9. Cheryl Mattingly, 'Defrosting Concepts, Destabilizing Doxa: Critical Phenomenology and the Perplexing Particular', *Anthropological Theory* 19, no. 4 (2019): 415–39.
10. Wilhelm Dilthey, *Descriptive Psychology and Historical Understanding*, trans. R. M. Zaner and K. L. Heiges (The Hague: Martinus Nijhof, 1977).
11. Edmund Husserl, *Logical Investigations* (London: Psychology Press, 2001 [1900–01]).
12. See: Heidegger, *Being and Time*; Maurice Merleau-Ponty, *Phenomenology of Perception* (New York: Routledge, 1962); Simone de Beauvoir, *The Coming of Age*, trans. Patrick O'Brian (New York: Putnam, 1972 [1970]); Jean-Paul Sartre, *The Imaginary: A Phenomenological Psychology of the Imagination*, ed. Arlette Elkaïm-Sartre, trans. Jonathan Webber (London: Routledge, 2004 [1940]).
13. See: Karin Dahlberg, Helena Dahlberg and Maria Nyström, *Reflective Lifeworld Research* (Lund: Studentlitteratur, 2008); Finn Hansen, Solveig Eide and Carlo Leget, *Wonder, Silence and Human Flourishing: Toward a Re-Humanization of Health, Education, and Welfare* (Lanham, MD: Rowman & Littlefield, 2023); Ricoeur, *Oneself as Another*; Linda Finlay, 'Unfolding the Phenomenological Research Process', *Journal of Humanistic Psychology* 53, no. 2 (2012): 177–201; Jonathan A. Smith, '"Yes It Is Phenomenological": A Reply to Max Van Manen's Critique of Interpretative Phenomenological Analysis', *Qualitative Health Research* 28, no. 12 (2018): 1955–88, https://journals.sagepub.com/doi/10.1177/1049732318799577.
14. Max Van Manen, *Phenomenology of Practice: Meaning-Giving Methods in Phenomenological Research and Writing* (London and New York: Routledge, 2023).
15. Mattingly, 'Defrosting Concepts, Destabilizing Doxa', 423.
16. Sherry B. Ortner, 'Dark Anthropology and Its Others', *HAU: Journal of Ethnographic Theory* 6, no. 1 (2016): 47–73,https://www.journals.uchicago.edu/doi/10.14318/hau6.1.004.
17. Michael D. Jackson, *Things As They Are: New Directions in Phenomenological Anthropology* (Bloomington: Indiana University Press, 1996).
18. Carlo Leget, Inge van Nistelrooij and Merel Visse, 'Beyond Demarcation: Care Ethics as an Interdisciplinary Field of Inquiry', *Nursing Ethics* 24, no. 6 (2017): 673–82, https://doi.org/10.1177/0969733017707008.
19. Dahlberg, Dahlberg and Nyström, *Reflective Lifeworld Research.*
20. See: Els van Wijngaarden, Carlo Leget and Anne Goossensen, 'Ready to Give Up on Life: The Lived Experience of Elderly People Who Feel Life Is Completed and No Longer Worth Living', *Social Science & Medicine* 138 (2015): 257–64; Els van Wijngaarden, Carlo Leget and Anne Goossensen, 'Disconnectedness from the Here-and-Now: A Phenomenological Perspective as a Counteract on the Medicalisation of Death Wishes in Elderly People', *Medicine, Health Care and Philosophy* 19, no. 2 (2016): 265–73.

21. Hanneke van der Meide, 'Care Ethical Phenomenological Research: Bodiliness as a Central Feature', in *Care Ethics and Phenomenology: A Contested Kinship*, ed. Frans Vosman and Per Nortvedt (Leuven: Peeters, 2020), 35–52.
22. Frans Vosman and Per Nortvedt, 'Introduction', in *Care Ethics and Phenomenology: A Contested Kinship*, ed. Frans Vosman and Per Nortvedt (Leuven: Peeters Publishers, 2020).
23. Merleau-Ponty, *Phenomenology of Perception*, 106.
24. Merleau-Ponty, *Phenomenology of Perception*.
25. Hermann Schmitz, *Der Leib, der Raum und die Gefühle* (Bielefeld and Locarno: Edition Sirius, 2007).
26. Hans-Georg Gadamer, *Truth and Method* (London and New York: Continuum, 2004).
27. Hansen, Eide and Leget, *Wonder, Silence and Human Flourishing*.
28. Hanneke van der Meide, Gert Olthuis and Carlo Leget, 'Why Frailty Needs Vulnerability: A Care Ethical Perspective on Hospital Care for Older Patients', *Nursing Ethics* 22, no. 8 (2015): 860–9.
29. Van Manen, *Phenomenology of Practice*.
30. Klaartje Klaver, 'Being Attentive as a Researcher. The Value of Waldenfels's Phenomenology for My Care Ethical Empirical Study of Attentiveness in Healthcare', in *Care Ethics and Phenomenology: A Contested Kinship*, ed. Frans Vosman and Per Nortvedt (Leuven: Peeters Publishers, 2020), 13–34.
31. Hansen, Eide and Leget, *Wonder, Silence and Human Flourishing*, 4.
32. Margie Burns and Shelley Peacock, 'Interpretive Phenomenological Methodologists in Nursing: A Critical Analysis and Comparison', *Nursing Inquiry* 26 (2019): e12280, https://doi.org/10.1111/nin.12280.
33. Sine Maria Herholdt-Lomholdt, 'Invisible but Sensible Aesthetic Aspects of Excellence in Nursing', *Nursing Philosophy* 20 (2019): e12238, https://doi.org/10.1111/nup.12238.
34. Hansen, Eide and Leget, *Wonder, Silence and Human Flourishing*.
35. Merel Visse, 'Your Thoughts Don't Have Words Every Day: Poetic Quality and the Health Professions', in *Wonder, Silence and Human Flourishing: Toward a Re-Humanization of Health, Education, and Welfare*, ed. Finn Hansen, Solveig Eide and Carlo Leget (Lanham, MD: Rowman & Littlefield, 2023), 97–114.
36. Merel Visse, Finn Hansen and Carlo Leget, 'The Unsayable in Arts-Based Research: On the Praxis of Life Itself', *International Journal of Qualitative Methods* 18 (2019), https://doi.org/10.1177/1609406919851392.
37. Merel Visse, Finn Thuen Hansen and Carlo J. W. Leget, 'Apophatic Inquiry: Living the Questions Themselves', *International Journal of Qualitative Methods* 19 (2020), https://doi.org/10.1177/1609406920958975.
38. Carol Gilligan, *In a Different Voice: Psychological Theory and Women's Development* (Cambridge, MA: Harvard University Press, 1982).
39. Ruddick, *Maternal Thinking*.
40. Noddings, *Caring*.
41. Walker, *Moral Understandings*, 19.
42. Inge van Nistelrooij, *Sacrifice: A Care-Ethical Reappraisal of Sacrifice and Self-Sacrifice* (Leuven: Peeters, 2015).
43. Noddings, *Caring*, 79.
44. See: Virginia Held, *The Ethics of Care: Personal, Political, Global* (New York: Oxford University Press, 2006); Noddings, *Caring*; Tove Pettersen, *Comprehending Care: Problems and Possibilities in The Ethics of Care* (Lanham, MD: Lexington Books, 2008).

45. Per Nortvedt, 'Phenomenology and Care: Reflections on the Foundation of Morality', in *Care Ethics and Phenomenology: A Contested Kinship*, ed. Frans Vosman and Per Nortvedt (Leuven: Peeters, 2020), 133–61.
46. Ibid.
47. Lisa Tessman, *Moral Failure: On the Impossible Demands of Morality* (Oxford: Oxford University Press, 2014).

BIBLIOGRAPHY

de Beauvoir, Simone. *The Coming of Age*. Translated by Patrick O'Brian. New York: Putnam, 1972.

Burns, Margie, and Shelley Peacock. 'Interpretive Phenomenological Methodologists in Nursing: A Critical Analysis and Comparison', *Nursing Inquiry* 26 (2019): e12280. https://doi.org/10.1111/nin.12280.

Dahlberg, Karin, Helena Dahlberg and Maria Nyström. *Reflective Lifeworld Research*. Lund: Studentlitteratur, 2008.

Dilthey, Wilhelm. *Descriptive Psychology and Historical Understanding*. Translated by R. M. Zaner and K. L. Heiges. The Hague: Martinus Nijhof, 1977.

Finlay, Linda. 'Unfolding the Phenomenological Research Process', *Journal of Humanistic Psychology* 53, no. 2 (2012): 172–201.

Gadamer, Hans-Georg. *Truth and Method*. London and New York: Continuum, 2004.

Gilligan, Carol. *In a Different Voice: Psychological Theory and Women's Development*. Cambridge, MA: Harvard University Press, 1982.

Hansen, Finn, Solveig Eide and Carlo Leget. *Wonder, Silence and Human Flourishing: Toward a Re-Humanization of Health, Education, and Welfare*. Lanham: Rowman & Littlefield, 2023.

Held, Virginia. *The Ethics of Care: Personal, Political, Global*. New York: Oxford University Press, 2006.

Herholdt-Lomholdt, Sine Maria. 'Invisible but Sensible Aesthetic Aspccts of Excellence in Nursing', *Nursing Philosophy* 20 (2019): e12238. https://doi.org/10.1111/nup.12238.

Heidegger, Martin. *Being and Time*. New York: Harper and Row, 1962.

Husserl, Edmund. *Logical Investigations*. London: Psychology Press, 2001 [1900–01].

Jackson, Michael. *Things As They Are: New Directions in Phenomenological Anthropology*. Bloomington: Indiana University Press, 1996.

Klaver, Klaartje. 'Being Attentive as a Researcher. The Value of Waldenfels's Phenomenology for My Care Ethical Empirical Study of Attentiveness in Healthcare', in *Care Ethics and Phenomenology: A Contested Kinship*, edited by Frans Vosman and Per Nortvedt, 13–34. Leuven: Peeters Publishers, 2020.

Leget, Carlo. *Zorg om Betekenis. Over Zorgethiek en Spirituele Zorg, in Het Bijzonder in Relatie Tot de Palliatieve Zorg*. Amsterdam: SWP, 2013.

Leget, Carlo, Inge van Nistelrooij and Merel Visse. 'Beyond Demarcation: Care Ethics as an Interdisciplinary Field of Inquiry', *Nursing Ethics* 24, no. 6 (2017): 673–82. https://doi.org/10.1177/0969733017707008.

Mattingly, Cheryl. 'Defrosting Concepts, Destabilizing Doxa: Critical Phenomenology and the Perplexing Particular', *Anthropological Theory* 19, no. 4 (2019): 415–39.

Merleau-Ponty, Maurice. *Phenomenology of Perception*. New York: Routledge, 1962.

Noddings, Nel. *Caring: A Feminine Approach to Ethics and Moral Education*. Berkeley: University of California Press, 1984.

Nortvedt, Per. 'Phenomenology and Care: Reflections on the Foundation of Morality', in *Care Ethics and Phenomenology: A Contested Kinship*, edited by Frans Vosman and Per Nortvedt, 133–61. Leuven: Peeters Publishers, 2020.

Nortvedt, Per, and Frans Vosman. 'Introduction', in *Care Ethics and Phenomenology: A Contested Kinship*, edited by Frans Vosman and Per Nortvedt, 1–20. Leuven: Peeters Publishers, 2020.

Ortner, Sherry B. 'Dark Anthropology and Its Others', *HAU: Journal of Ethnographic Theory* 6, no. 1 (2016): 47–73. https://doi.org/10.14318/hau6.1.004.

Pettersen, Tove. *Comprehending Care: Problems and Possibilities in The Ethics of Care*. Lanham, MD: Lexington Books, 2008.

Puig de la Bellacasa, Maria. *Matters of Care: Speculative Ethics in More Than Human Worlds*. Minneapolis: University of Minnesota Press, 2017.

Ricoeur, Paul. *Oneself as Another*. Chicago, IL: University of Chicago Press, 1992.

Ruddick, Sara. *Maternal Thinking: Toward a Politics of Peace*. Boston, MA: Beacon Press, 1989.

Sartre, Jean-Paul. *The Imaginary: A Phenomenological Psychology of the Imagination*, edited by Arlette Elkaïm-Sartre. Translated by Jonathan Webber. London: Routledge, 2004 [1940].

Schmitz, Hermann. *Der Leib, der Raum und die Gefühle*. Bielefeld and Locarno: Edition Sirius, 2007.

Slote, Michael. *The Ethics of Care and Empathy*. New York: Routledge, 2007.

Smith, Jonathan A. '"Yes It Is Phenomenological": A Reply to Max Van Manen's Critique of Interpretative Phenomenological Analysis', *Qualitative Health Research* 28, no. 12 (2018): 1955–8. https://doi.org/10.1177/1049732318799577.

Tessman, Lisa. *Moral Failure: On the Impossible Demands of Morality*. Oxford: Oxford University Press, 2014.

Tronto, Joan C. *Moral Boundaries: A Political Argument for an Ethic of Care*. New York: Routledge, 1993.

Tronto, Joan C., and Berenice Fisher. 'Toward a Feminist Theory of Caring', in *Circles of Care: Work and Identity in Women's Lives*, edited by Emily K. Abel and Margaret K. Nelson, 36–54. Albany: State University of New York Press, 1990.

Van Manen, Max. *Phenomenology of Practice: Meaning-Giving Methods in Phenomenological Research and Writing*. London and New York: Routledge, 2023.

Van der Meide, Hanneke. 'Care Ethical Phenomenological Research: Bodiliness as a Central Feature', in *Care Ethics and Phenomenology: A Contested Kinship*, edited by Frans Vosman and Per Nortvedt, 35–52. Leuven: Peeters, 2020.

Van der Meide, Hanneke, Gert Olthuis and Carlo Leget. 'Why Frailty Needs Vulnerability: A Care Ethical Perspective on Hospital Care for Older Patients', *Nursing Ethics* 22, no. 8 (2015): 860–9.

Van Nistelrooij, Inge. *Sacrifice: A Care-Ethical Reappraisal of Sacrifice and Self-Sacrifice*. Leuven: Peeters, 2015.

Van Wijngaarden, Els, Carlo Leget and Anne Goossensen. 'Ready to Give Up on Life: The Lived Experience of Elderly People Who Feel Life Is Completed and No Longer Worth Living,', *Social Science & Medicine* 138 (2015): 257–64.

Van Wijngaarden, Els, Carlo Leget and Anne Goossensen. 'Disconnectedness from the Here-and-Now: A Phenomenological Perspective as a Counteract on the Medicalisation of Death Wishes in Elderly People', *Medicine, Health Care and Philosophy* 19, no. 2 (2016): 265–73.

Visse, Merel. 'Your Thoughts Don't Have Words Every Day: Poetic Quality and the Health Professions', in *Wonder, Silence and Human Flourishing: Toward a Re-Humanization of Health, Education, and Welfare*, edited by Finn Hansen, Solveig Eide and Carlo Leget, 97–114. Lanham, MD: Rowman & Littlefield, 2023.

Visse, Merel, Finn Hansen and Carlo Leget. 'The Unsayable in Arts-Based Research: On the Praxis of Life Itself', *International Journal of Qualitative Methods* 18 (2019). https://doi.org/10.1177/1609406919851392.

Visse, Merel, Finn Thuen Hansen and Carlo J. W. Leget. 'Apophatic Inquiry: Living the Questions Themselves', *International Journal of Qualitative Methods* 19 (2020). https://doi.org/10.1177/1609406920958975.

Walker, Margaret Urban. *Moral Understandings: A Feminist Study in Ethics*. New York: Oxford University Press, 2007.

CHAPTER SIX

Necessary care, moral practices and the cultivation of competent carers

MATILDA CARTER

INTRODUCTION

One of the most potent insights that has emerged from the work of care ethicists is one that is so obvious that no reasonable person could object to it: there is not a single one of us who has not depended on another for care. Human infants are born in a state of profound helplessness, being unable to move independently, feed themselves or protect themselves from threats. They also develop slowly, taking much longer than other newborn primates to reach their maximum brain size.[1] Without care, none of us would have survived infancy, let alone been in a position to reflect on ethical and political questions. What is perhaps less appreciated by those working outside of care ethics, however, is that proper acknowledgement of this fact has wide-ranging implications for our moral practices.

Most if not all views within care ethics, as I demonstrate in Section 6.1, draw on a concept of *necessary care*, referring to a set of practices, the successful performance of which is an often unacknowledged precondition of a vast array of moral prescriptions. Drawing attention to the necessity of care for the survival of infants helps to build the care ethicist's case against moral frameworks that make insufficient space for dependency relationships. It would be a mistake, however, to interpret the concept of necessary care this narrowly – or so I argue in Section 6.2. Mere survival is not sufficient for shaping infants into moral agents, nor for cultivating the sort of carers capable of facilitating moral development. Human moral life is dependent, in this sense, on much thicker, socially inculcated practices of caring. Building on this point, in Section 6.3 I examine the state of affairs in contemporary Western societies and briefly discuss the prospects of a policy of universal access to psychotherapy for addressing deficits in the social provision of necessary care.

6.1 INTRODUCING NECESSARY CARE

As in any flourishing school of thought, there are significant internal disagreements among care ethicists. Some, like Virginia Held,[2] conceive of care as grounding a distinct moral framework, while others, like Eva Feder Kittay[3] and Daniel Engster,[4] seek to reformulate justice in the image of care. Some, like Raja Halwani,[5] interpret the view as a form of virtue ethics, whereas others, like Maureen Sander-Staudt,[6] firmly reject that notion. There is unity, nevertheless, around the charge that moral and political philosophy in the analytic tradition has largely neglected inevitable dependencies and the caring obligations they engender.

In bringing attention to its absence in dominant frameworks, care ethicists have revealed the extent to which the successful delivery of care is a *practical presupposition* of the conclusions to which many of those working within them come. Drawing on the work of prominent scholars in the field, in this section I explore this notion of necessary care: care that is necessary, that is, because its performance is a background condition of the securing of morally good, politically just, or otherwise ethically valuable outcomes. As I here argue, this concept plays a crucial role within the structure of care ethics as a theory, aiding in building its case against atomistic views of the person and contributing to the shaping of its substantive demands.

6.1.1 Presupposing the successful delivery of care

Given no infant could survive to adulthood without it, it is striking that Western moral and political philosophy has historically had relatively little to say about care. In Held's view, this neglect is symptomatic of the centring of male experience in and the impact of the gendered division of labour on philosophical thought. For most of Western history, women have been expected to take sole responsibility for the care of infants and have been denied access to the public sphere on the same terms as men. It is unsurprising, then, that what she describes as 'the dominant moral theories' in the Western philosophical tradition – namely, Kantianism and utilitarianism – were developed with little significant input from those women who provided the overwhelming majority of care to dependents.[7] This is a thought echoed by Joan Tronto, who concludes that these theories 'cannot accommodate those aspects of life that are usually associated with women'.[8]

While they rarely discuss the matter of care for dependents explicitly, however, the successful delivery of that care is very often a practical presupposition of their prescriptions. Any conclusion about what we ought to do that requires the continual existence of the human species implicitly assumes that at least some care must be delivered and, as Kittay rightly points out, that caring work must be done by *someone*.[9] Failing to discuss this explicitly has the effect of both placing the expectation that women take on the responsibility for care beyond the scope of moral debate and imbuing it with the weight of a moral duty.

Now, to state that moral prescriptions intended to apply to humans usually assume that human society should exist and the practices necessary to continue its existence should be performed might appear glib. Neither the Kantian nor the utilitarian would be likely to be astounded by this observation, and it may not be immediately obvious that it offers much of a challenge to the frameworks they adhere to. Necessary care could, for instance, be conceived of as one among many burdens of social cooperation that ought to be fairly distributed between Kantian autonomous agents. The utilitarian, likewise, could argue that any world in which necessary care is not performed will evidently contain less utility than one in which it is.

It may also seem unclear why anyone with more than a passing commitment to feminist aims should be struck by this observation. That men have taken for granted the labour they historically expected women to perform is hardly a revelation and neither, it might be thought, is the fact that this exploitation has influenced the development of moral philosophy in the West. Abandoning these frameworks in favour of a care ethics approach is one strategy for addressing this issue, but it might not be obvious to the feminist why such a drastic response is needed. There is a tradition within feminist thought that aims to reformulate existing moral frameworks to better incorporate a commitment to gender equality, and it might be thought that a project of this kind would be sufficient to address this issue of the occlusion of care.

Merely bringing attention to the unacknowledged role of necessary care in the carrying out of moral prescriptions, however, has an impact that goes beyond drawing attention to gender inequality. From the vantage point of care ethics, the hitherto dominant moral frameworks seem mistakenly atomistic in the way they conceive both of the person and of society more broadly. Their substantive demands, likewise, often seem unsuitable for a species whose lives are characterized by inevitable dependencies and necessary interdependence. Even were the division of caring labour to be made more equal among the genders, there are areas in which these theories conflict with care ethics that would remain. It is in part because of the concept of necessary care, therefore, that care ethics can be understood as a *rival* moral theory, rather than solely a feminist critique of those that have dominated Western thought.

6.1.2 Persons, preferences and society

By far the most influential Kantian in the past century of political philosophy is John Rawls, whose 1971 monograph *A Theory of Justice* is widely credited with reviving interest in the social contract tradition. His predecessors, most notably Thomas Hobbes[10] and John Locke,[11] developed principles for the governance of social and political life by imagining life outside of formal social and political institutions. Understanding why persons would choose to leave the freedom of the 'state of nature' and agree to be bound by rules, at least on one prominent interpretation of this tradition, was thought to be crucial to understanding the shape those rules should take. Rawls, by contrast, develops his principles of justice by imagining what persons would choose when participating in a procedure that is *fair* – not just in the absence of formal social and political institutions, but in the absence of knowledge about their individual circumstances and the positions they would take up once their 'veil of ignorance' is lifted.[12]

Altering the initial choice situation, from a care ethicist's perspective, is a wise move. Whether depictions of the state of nature are intended to be historically accurate or not, some measure of realism is required to give them argumentative force; it is unclear what compelling reasons we would have to grant weight to implausible visions of life beyond the state when shaping the principles we choose to govern us. We should reject, therefore, any construction that cannot explain how and why necessary care would be delivered before negotiations over the social contract began, because there would be no parties capable of negotiating in its absence. Likewise, we should regard any depiction of life outside of the state as violent, distrusting or solitary as dubious – both in terms of its accuracy and its relevance to how we live within the state – given the compelling biological and anthropological evidence that, as Engster has argued, strongly suggests that the disposition to care is innate, rather than socially inculcated.[13]

Unlike with the Hobbesian and Lockean states of nature, there is no serious discussion to be had about whether the Rawlsian original position is intended to be *historically* accurate; there has never been a time at which persons became ignorant of their own identities and social positions in advance of drafting a contract to govern social cooperation. A significant amount of its argumentative force, nevertheless, would seem to depend on whether persons under a veil of ignorance really would behave as Rawls suggests. This is a point that has been made by John C. Harsanyi, who argues that rational decision making always involves the assigning of subjective probabilities, and that parties to the social contract could not arrive at Rawls's principles unless they irrationally assumed they were guaranteed or near-guaranteed to take up the position of the worst off in the resulting society.[14] Others have doubted that parties to the contract would even be capable of making a choice, given they lack the most basic knowledge of their own values and goals. Indeed, Michael Sandel suggests that Rawls's contracting situation is not really a matter of choosing at all, but a matter of placing persons under conditions in which they will be guaranteed to acknowledge the validity of his principles of justice.[15]

For the care ethicist, however, it is not the rationality of the parties to the contract nor the impact of the veil of ignorance on their capacity for choice that is most damaging for the Rawlsian picture. It is, rather, the suggestion that the appropriate principles for governing a society can be found in an agreement made between mutually disinterested individuals, with no knowledge of their relationships with others – even if they would behave as Rawls suggests. As Kittay points out, because he does not include the inevitability of dependency within his set of basic facts about society that parties remain aware of behind the veil of ignorance, there is no guarantee that they will imagine themselves as dependents or carers when negotiating, making the representation of their concerns a contingent matter.[16] Worse, because he models the parties as rational, fully functioning persons with roughly equal powers, she argues that Rawls constructs the original position such that dependency and the care of dependents are rendered deviations from the normal condition of human beings and, thus, concerns that are extraneous to the fundamental questions of how the social order ought to be designed. She concludes, therefore, that any principles chosen behind the veil of ignorance will be skewed in favour of those who *can* function independently and *are not* responsible for dependents, even if some parties try in earnest to represent the interests of dependents and those that care for them.[17]

For the care ethicist, the influential Rawlsian approach incorporates a conception of the person that is mistakenly atomistic. As none of us could have survived infancy without care, let alone gone on to reason about the basic principles for social cooperation, we are fundamentally born in relation to others. In light of this they urge a rejection of the idea that persons are disinterested individuals in favour of a conception of the person as, in the words of Held, 'an embodied nexus of relations'.[18] From this perspective, it is likewise a mistake to conceive of social life as a cooperative venture among atomized persons, regulated by principles that would be endorsed by persons so conceived under the Rawlsian veil of ignorance. As Kittay has pointed out, care of dependents is demanding, time-consuming work: work that impairs the ability of those who are delivering it to apprise themselves of the resources they need to do so. Humans are also prone to illness and periods of incapacity, meaning successful care of dependents usually requires an ability to temporarily transfer responsibilities to others.[19] None of us, therefore, would have survived infancy without a wider set of social relations surrounding the care relationship into which we were born, rendering (at least some basic level of) social cooperation an obligatory feature of human life, rather than one that is voluntary. At the root of both of these argumentative moves is an appeal to the concept of necessary care.

Utilitarianism is, in one sense, far less atomistic in its outlook than its rival moral framework. In fact, one of Rawls's enduring criticisms of it concerns what he perceives as a failure to 'take seriously the distinction between persons'.[20] For the care ethicist, nevertheless, it remains atomistic in the way it conceives of the relations between persons. This is particularly true of preference utilitarianism, a view distinguished by its aim of promoting the highest overall satisfaction of individual interests within a population. Much care, as Held points out, cannot be delivered successfully without the carer suspending their interests in favour of those of their charge, and very often the interests of both become enmeshed.[21] The preference utilitarian might try to accommodate the phenomenon of enmeshed interests by counting them twice – once for the carer and once for the cared for – but it is not clear how they can account for personal interest suspension in a way that gives due weight to necessary care.

Other forms of utilitarianism fare somewhat better; when a caregiver sacrifices the pursuit of their preferences in order to direct energy towards a dependent, it is plausible to think that either total or average utility in the population will be increased. Nevertheless, these sorts of aggregating views, because they do not incorporate respect for the separateness of persons, still struggle to give necessary care its due weight. If we are seeking total utility, then we must arrive at the conclusion that a small population in which the care needs of all dependents are met is worse off than a much larger population in which they are not – a variation on Derek Parfit's 'Repugnant Conclusion'.[22] If we are seeking average utility, however, we must conclude that a society would be better off not meeting the needs of its dependents if the utility gains on the part of the caregivers abdicating their duties outweighed the losses of their charges. Either approach strips necessary care of its importance, relegating it to one set of acts among many that may increase or decrease utility, rather than a fundamental component of human existence.

By invoking the concept of necessary care, care ethics stakes out positions on persons, preferences and society that differ from both of these frameworks. As Held notes, the successful delivery of necessary care requires valuing its recipients for their own sake, rather than as a means to the end of preference satisfaction or overall utility maximization.[23] Without consistency and reliability, there is no guarantee that care needs will be met, and caregivers that did not recognize persons as having separate and incommensurable value would have no reasons, in cases in which these acts would lead to increased total or average utility in their society, to avoid abandoning one dependent in favour of another or suddenly renouncing their duties. Nevertheless, because the successful delivery of necessary care requires some degree of enmeshment of interests, a caregiver cannot consider *themselves* entirely separate from the dependent they are charged with supporting. As Kittay has argued, identification of one's own good and self-respect with the interests of the dependent one is caring for is part of what it means to be a responsible caregiver; without it, caregivers would lack the strong moral imperative to meet the needs of their dependents and press their claims in social settings when doing so requires sacrifice of wellbeing or the pursuit of interests on their own part.[24]

Under care ethics, in sum, persons are of separate, incommensurable value but, because none could exist without the provision of necessary care and the relations that support it, they are also fundamentally (and pre-politically) social.[25] Necessary care involves an enmeshment of preferences that is fundamentally anti-individualistic, but the need for it to be consistent and reliable makes it incompatible with aggregating models of welfare maximization. Invoking necessary care establishes in care ethics, in short, an approach to these fundamental features of an ethical framework that is genuinely *relational*.

6.1.3 Shaping substantive demands

Alongside helping to establish it as a distinct ethical framework, appeals to the concept of necessary care also play a crucial role in shaping the substantive demands of care ethics. Individual theorists differ in their conclusions, but most (if not all) draw on the inevitably dependent nature of human beings to reach them. While I cannot consider every variation here, a survey of some of the key figures within the school of thought will be sufficient to illustrate the link between necessary care and the substantive demands of care ethicists.

Let us begin with Engster, a representative example of a justice-based care ethicist. In shaping what he thinks of as the substantive demands of care ethics, he makes explicit appeal to necessary care. Going further than merely noting that the delivery of necessary care is a practical presupposition of moral life, he argues that all of us presuppose a weighty moral norm that 'capable human beings ought to care for human beings in need'.[26] This is so, because anybody who has survived infancy has made an implicit demand to be cared for by others that has been treated as legitimate. Invoking a principle of non-contradiction, he concludes that anyone can rationally justify a demand for care from another (who is reasonably well positioned to meet it) by grounding it in the same norm to which that person themselves has implicitly appealed in the past.[27]

Kittay, though she does not use the language of presupposition, is similarly explicit in linking the substantive demands of her theory to the concept of necessary care. Having argued that the Rawlsian principles of justice cannot satisfactorily capture the concerns of dependents and those that care for them, she suggests an additional principle of *doulia* – from the term *doula*, referring to a person charged with caring for the primary caregiver of a newborn – that would mandate a sense of social responsibility for care and the development of institutions tasked with supporting those that deliver it.[28] Incorporating the observation that no person would survive infancy without being cared for, she states the principle in the following form: 'just as we have required care to survive and thrive, so we need to provide conditions that allow others – including those who do the work of caring – to receive the care they need to survive and thrive'.[29]

For Joan Tronto, the centrality of care to human life requires a rethinking of a number of assumptions made about human nature. We are not (and never can be) fully autonomous, we are beings of profound need, not just possessors of interests, and we are deeply morally engaged with one another, not beings of detached self-interest. This account of human nature, transformed by appeal to the concept of necessary care, entails in Tronto's view the need to renegotiate the moral boundary between public and private life and to make the question of who provides care to whom central to political discussion.[30]

Finally, Held, who defends an account of care and justice as two separate moral frameworks, uses the concept of necessary care to undergird explorations of core questions in political theory. Of particular note is her discussion on rights, which she argues cannot be secured without a presumption that people care enough about each other to protect them. We must establish then, in her view, a form of civil society that fosters appreciation for practices of and demands for care, grounded in the universal experience of being cared for and the necessity of care for the survival of societies.[31]

Necessary care, in sum, is a concept that plays a number of crucial roles within care ethics. The observation that no one would survive infancy, let alone develop a capacity to engage in moral reflection, reveals the extent to which traditional moral frameworks presuppose the delivery of care and places pressure on their underlying elements. As well as operating as a powerful tool for critique, the concept is also appealed to to distinguish care ethics as an ethical framework from those that have preceded it and to shape its substantive demands. Which caring practices ought to fall under the definition of necessary care, therefore, is a highly consequential question – one that I will provide an answer to in the next section.

6.2 NECESSARY CARE AS THE FOSTERING OF EMOTIONAL MATURITY

Survival is the starting point of any plausible account of necessary care. None of us would be here if we had not received the basic level of care needed to survive infancy, including nutritional support and protection from external threats. In this section, however, I argue that the concept should be defined far more broadly than this, because moral reasoning presupposes the existence of moral agents. For this reason, any plausible account of necessary care (plausible in the sense that it can bear the weight placed on it by the structure of the care-ethical framework) must include those practices that are necessary to rear infants into capable-enough moral agents. With reference to psychological research on child development, here I defend the view that these must include those practices necessary to guide an infant to emotional maturity.

6.2.1 Raising moral agents

Whenever we assert moral claims about how others ought to behave, we make two types of assumption that indicate our presupposition of the importance of necessary care. The first type involves assumptions about ourselves as moral reasoners: chiefly, that we have the standing to make claims on others – that we have what Stephen Darwall calls 'second-personal authority' – or, if reasoning from a third-person standpoint, that we have a moral sense that is sufficiently developed to come to legitimate conclusions about how others should behave in the pursuit of morally good outcomes. The second involves assumptions that we make about those we are addressing: chiefly, that they have the capacity to recognize the claims we make on them as reasons to act – that they have what Darwall calls 'second-personal competence' – or, when they are being asked to consider third-personal claims, that they have the moral sense to understand why the conclusions we make about morally good outcomes are legitimate.[32]

Coupled to both sorts of assumptions, as the care critique of the traditional moral frameworks makes plain, is a presupposition of the successful delivery of necessary care. Helpless infants cannot morally reason and do not have the capacity to consider or recognize claims on their conduct as legitimate. Some degree of maturity is required to play both sorts of roles, and that maturity will not be reached without the receipt of some care. These prescriptions could neither be made nor carried out, therefore, without the delivery of those care practices necessary to ensure infant survival.[33]

Mere survival, however, is not sufficient to maintain the existence of moral agents. For one thing, no single carer will be able to rear an infant into maturity without assistance from others. This is true both because it is near impossible to acquire the means to care for an infant alone at the same time as providing that care and because, being human, carers are prone to periods of sickness and incapacity during which their care duties must be temporarily fulfilled by others. There is therefore, in Kittay's words, 'a matrix of practices, roles, and understandings'[34] surrounding the successful performance of necessary care whose existence we presuppose when asserting moral claims that bear on the conduct of others.

Once we recognize that carers need to be cared for, the scope of necessary care becomes a lot wider. What is involved in ensuring the basic survival of an infant differs from what is involved in supporting someone engaging directly in that endeavour. More than just being able to feed, water and protect the recipient of care from threats, the persons in the matrix of social relations surrounding the care relationship need to be able to acquire resources for care and be disposed to share them with the person doing the caring. They also need to have the baseline level of emotional intelligence necessary to recognize signs of stress, fear, or worry from the primary carer as signals that they need support or may be at risk of becoming indisposed. All of these sorts of practices, therefore, need to be brought under the umbrella of necessary care.

What is crucial to recognize, moreover, is that the more advanced kinds of caring skills exhibited by those supporting a provider of care also need to be exhibited by the carer themselves. There would be no persons capable of supporting carers for infants had they not been raised to possess these skills, which implies that the persons caring for them also possessed them to some minimal degree, along with the skills necessary to imbue them in their charges. Necessary care, in short, must include that which is necessary to pass on caring skills and practices without losing that which was necessary to pass them on in the first place. They may not look the same from generation to generation, but our moral life is dependent on a robust transfer of caring practices because we could not have moral agents without it.

6.2.2 Motivation, maturity and moral agency

There is a strongly rationalist interpretation of moral agency that is adopted by some scholars working within the dominant frameworks of Kantian liberalism and utilitarianism. In the Kantian tradition, at least on one common interpretation, the ability to act morally simply *is* the ability to act according to reason, such that one is capable of valuing things for their own sake rather than satisfying one's instincts.[35] Similarly, Peter Singer has argued that rationality is a key strength of utilitarianism, in the sense that its conclusions bypass initial intuitive responses to moral quandaries that evidence from evolutionary psychology suggests we should distrust.[36]

There is no doubt that the capacity to *act* morally does depend in part on the capacity to act rationally; even under sentimentalist approaches, such as Michael Slote's distinct empathy-based version of care ethics,[37] persons still require some degree of rational agency to devise and carry out actions that meet the demands of their emotional responses. Acknowledging the concept of necessary care, nevertheless, requires us to rethink the relationship between rationality and the emotions. If the moral claims we assert that bear on the conduct of others assume the existence of a robust and transferable set of caring practices, then they also assume that those who are engaging in care are acting morally by doing so (and would be acting immorally if they intentionally gave insufficient care or chose to abandon their charges). Moreover, because necessary care involves the transmitting of the capacity to rear moral agents from generation to generation, any instance of moral reasoning presupposes that a carer would be acting immorally if they intentionally refused to transmit that caring capacity, even if their charge were capable of comprehending and acting upon some moral reasons. Whatever emotional capacities are required to successfully rear moral agents, therefore, are prerequisites for possessing that agency in its fullest form, in the sense that persons, in their absence, cannot act in accordance with moral demands to deliver necessary care.

To get a sense of what the relevant emotional capacities are, it is helpful to start with a clear picture of what care looks like in their absence. Carers can ensure their charges survive infancy without much sophistication in their emotional development; merely being able to feed, water and protect infants from threats requires little more than a bare minimum of physical and intellectual competence. Carers can even ensure that their charges are themselves capable of ensuring the survival of *their* infants without much emotional development; all they need are the capacities necessary to pass these intellectual and physical competencies on. Without the ability to recognize an infant as someone whose survival matters for *their own sake*, however, carers would only be motivated to care out of self-interest, and so not guaranteed to provide what is necessary to pass on the underlying components of moral agency.

One way to ensure that providing survival care is in the interest of some humans is to threaten them with violence. We can reasonably assume that all humans value their own continued existence in the absence of pain, even if sometimes the desire to avoid pain can outweigh the desire to survive. Accordingly, credible threats of painful or fatal consequences if an infant is not provided with care would motivate compliance in most if not all humans on the receiving end of them, in the sense that few if any other interests they had could possibly outweigh their interest in avoiding pain and death.

Aside from the appalling nature of such a proposal, the key problem that would be faced by a society intending to replicate itself by threatening violence against those who fail to care for infants is that it is unclear why the persons issuing those threats would be motivated to do so. All in a position to demand that infants are cared for under pain of death would have been raised under the same, bare minimal caring practices, such that they did not themselves have the underlying capacities necessary to care about others for their own sake. Consequently, they too could only draw on self-interest as motivation, and it is not immediately clear why ensuring the survival of infants (or, for that matter, ensuring those infants can one day keep *their* infants alive) would be of such great interest that they would divert energies they could be using to pursue their own goals towards forcing others to provide care.

Perhaps, emotionally undeveloped persons might desire the survival of humanity in order to preserve their own legacy. They might view their own offspring as extensions of themselves, such that their influence on the world can be maintained long after their death by the survival of their infants. Powerful others might, alternatively, consider it in their interests for there to be a continuing supply of human labour that they can readily exploit to their own ends. Even if these were strong enough self-interested reasons for persons to provide or force others to provide care, however, the resulting society would not be one hospitable to the development of a moral sense, nor to the acceptance of moral demands made by some on others. This is because any moral framework, including those used by the crudest forms of libertarianism, presupposes that persons care about what happens to others for reasons external to their own self-interest: either because they value them for their own sake, or because they have some sense of 'the greater good'.

Now, it is rare in our contemporary societies for persons to entirely lack an underlying moral sense; even the common belief that there exist true psychopaths who are incapable of understanding moral reasons is contested in the relevant psychological literature.[38] Nevertheless, it would be wrong to assume that moral agency is an innate feature of human adults, such that the *quality* of care received by an infant bears no significant influence upon their development. It is one thing to understand moral reasons as such, but quite another to be motivated to *act* on them or afford them significant weight when deliberating about what to do. While an infant might be able to survive bare minimal care with the former capability intact, we have good reasons to think that the latter is dependent on how well-developed their emotional capacities are.

A useful model of the concept of emotional maturity comes from clinical psychologist Lindsay C. Gibson. Emotionally immature people, in her view, adopt rigid and single-minded approaches to problems, deal with stress badly, tend to make decisions based on what feels good in the moment, struggle to assess situations through anything other than their own sense of what feels right or wrong, have little respect for differences in values or opinions, are egocentric, preoccupied and self-involved, focus excessively on themselves while struggling to be genuinely self-reflective, and, crucially, have a low capacity for empathy.[39] While these qualities do not suggest an inability to understand moral reasons as such, they do point to a difficulty in giving them priority over narrow self-interest, such that those who possess them are impaired in their ability to act upon them.

When emotionally immature persons become parents, Gibson argues, they fail to cultivate emotional intimacy in their relationships with their children, often promoting a kind of role reversal such that they position *themselves* as the dependent in need of support from their charge.[40] If a child complies with this role reversal, she goes on, they tend to develop a strong sense of empathy as adults, but pair it with a suppressed sense of their own self-interest such that they neglect their own needs and become overly invested in those of others. If they reject it, however, they tend to develop a strong sense of their own self-interest but constantly demand that others meet their needs because they do not know how to do so themselves. These internalizing and externalizing tendencies, which are often exhibited by the same person in a fluctuating pattern, are symptoms of the same underlying paucity of emotional regulation skills that lead to emotionally immature parenting styles.[41]

Gibson's observations on emotional maturity and its relationship with parenting are supported in the wider psychological literature. A 2019 meta-analysis found that children had poorer emotional regulation skills when they were emotionally maltreated by their parents, who in turn self-reported lower levels of emotional regulation skills than those that did not subject their children to this form of abuse.[42] Likewise, a meta-analysis of fifty-three studies published between 2000 and 2020 found that parents with better emotional regulation skills tended to pass them on to their children, who in turn exhibited far fewer internalizing symptoms – though they found the link with externalizing symptoms less well-evidenced.[43] Similar conclusions were drawn from a recent study of children in Beijing but, interestingly, the authors only found a strong intergenerational effect between maternal childhood emotional neglect and poor emotional regulation, with the emotional neglect of fathers seemingly exhibiting no effect on the emotional regulation or parenting styles of their adult children. As the authors themselves suggest, the traditional view of the mother as the primary caregiver of the child likely explains much of this difference in effect, with mothers typically spending more time with their children and thus being more directly involved in their upbringing.[44]

It is clear from the psychological evidence, then, that emotional dysregulation is predictably passed on by parents to their children. The two types of coping styles developed by emotionally dysregulated persons, moreover, represent direct impairments to the kind of moral sense needed for moral agency. An internalizer with a high degree of empathy may be capable of recognizing the needs of others, but being motivated to meet them because of a desperate need to receive the emotional nourishment they lacked as a child is not the same as being motivated by moral reasons, and they may find it difficult to distinguish between morally salient and purely self-interested demands made by others. Indeed, Gibson observes that internalizers often enter into abusive relationships as adults, exerting great energy to meet the needs of partners who offer little in return.[45] Externalisers, on the other hand, may sometimes respond to moral demands, but their relentless focus on pursuing their self-interest and having their needs met by others suggests that they will be unlikely to do so without a clear sense of what they will gain.

If, as I have argued in this section, the proper purpose of necessary care is to rear moral agents, a sufficient degree of emotional maturity on the part of the carer is required. Without it, their children will be impaired in the capacities underlying moral agency through the transmission of emotional dysregulation. They, in turn, will be likely to pass this on to their children, leading to a population that is capable of ensuring the survival of infants but incapable of cultivating the moral sense that is presupposed in any act of moral reasoning. Emotional maturity, in short, is a necessary background condition of our moral life.

6.3 CULTIVATING EMOTIONAL MATURITY THROUGH ACCESS TO PSYCHOTHERAPY

Recognizing that the concept of necessary care includes the transmission of emotional maturity has practical implications for the society governed by principles of care ethics. The matrix of overlapping relations that supports the rearing of infants into moral agents evidently includes material and physical support for the primary carer, but it ought to be clear that these relations must provide the background conditions for the cultivation of emotional maturity. In an ideal world, all primary caregivers and their supporting relations would possess strong emotional regulation skills, and therefore be able to pass them on from generation to generation. In our non-ideal world, however, emotionally mature parenting is not so common. Indeed, the global prevalence of emotional maltreatment by parents has been estimated to be greater than its physical equivalent, with a 2014 meta-analysis of self-reports finding a rate of 363/1000 for emotional abuse and 184/1000 for emotional neglect.[46]

Any transition from our world to a society governed by care ethics, therefore, would require a substantial degree of intervention to improve the emotional regulation skills of adults. Where we lack the robust and transferable set of practices, as well as their underlying social norms and support mechanisms, we must look to the structures that already exist for aid. From within the hyper-individualized Western structures of care and care support, the best prospects for cultivating the background emotional conditions for moral life can be found in the field of psychotherapy.

Improved emotional regulation is a well-evidenced outcome of successful psychotherapeutic intervention,[47] with some suggestion that long-term psychodynamic therapy is particularly useful when dysfunction is complex.[48] Such therapy, however, is often inaccessible for those that are most in need of it, given the unavoidably high costs of long-term therapeutic work and the preference of publicly funded healthcare systems for briefer, cheaper alternatives. Addressing this accessibility gap, then, seems like a crucial priority for transitioning to a world that better supports the flourishing of moral agency necessary for moral life.

The robust and transferable practices necessary for the cultivation of moral agency will, of course, be difficult to maintain without extensive structural changes to better support them. Widespread and effective systems of social support for parents, well-funded child welfare services, and an end to the chronic resource insufficiency that puts care-disrupting pressure on poor and subordinated groups are all the sorts of policies that a society seeking to transition to governance by care ethics ought to pursue. I have raised the importance of psychotherapy here, however, because it is a practice whose potential for disrupting the inhibition of care from within our currently existing social structures is underappreciated. There are further ethical issues that must be dealt with, including the relative merits of different modalities, how to ensure an ethical relationship between therapist and client, and how the caring society ought to respond to those emotionally dysregulated persons who refuse the intervention. Care ethicists may disagree about the right answers to these further questions, but it seems clear that all should accept the opportunities associated with widening *access*.

CONCLUSION

In this chapter, I have explored the concept of necessary care and its importance for the structure of care ethics as a distinct moral framework. I have argued that this set of practices, whose delivery is presupposed by any act of moral reasoning, must include those that confer emotional maturity to children, as this is a necessary underpinning of the capacities required for moral agency. I have also discussed the practical implications of including the practices aimed at developing emotional maturity within the definition of necessary care, concluding that widespread access to psychotherapy is a promising avenue for transitioning to the caring society.

NOTES

1. Karen R. Rosenberg, 'The Evolution of Human Infancy: Why It Helps to Be Helpless', *Annual Review of Anthropology* 50, no. 1 (2021): 424–30.
2. Virginia Held, 'Care and Justice, Still', in *Care Ethics and Political Theory*, ed. Daniel Engster and Maurice Hamington (Oxford: Oxford University Press, 2015), 18–36.
3. Eva F. Kittay, 'A Theory of Justice as Fair Terms of Social Life Given Our Inevitable Dependency and Our Inextricable Interdependency', in *Care Ethics and Political Theory*, ed. Daniel Engster and Maurice Hamington (Oxford: Oxford University Press, 2015), 51–71.
4. Daniel Engster, *The Heart of Justice: Care Ethics and Political Theory* (Oxford: Oxford University Press, 2007), 2.
5. Raja Halwani, 'Care Ethics and Virtue Ethics', *Hypatia* 18, no. 3 (2003): 161–92.

6. Maureen Sander-Staudt, 'The Unhappy Marriage of Care Ethics and Virtue Ethics', *Hypatia* 21, no. 4 (2006): 21–39.
7. Virginia Held, *The Ethics of Care: Personal, Political, and Global* (New York: Oxford University Press, 2005), 23–4.
8. Joan C. Tronto, *Moral Boundaries: A Political Argument for an Ethic of Care* (London: Psychology Press, 1993), 56.
9. Eva F. Kittay, *Love's Labor: Essays on Women, Equality, and Dependency* (London: Psychology Press, 1999), 16.
10. Thomas Hobbes, 'Leviathan', in *Leviathan: With Selected Variants from the Latin Edition of 1668*, ed. Edwin Curley (Indianapolis, IN: Hackett Publishing, 1994), 74–233.
11. John Locke, 'The Second Treatise', in *Locke: Two Treatises of Government, Student Edition*, ed. Peter Laslett (Cambridge: Cambridge University Press, 1988), 269–78.
12. John Rawls, *A Theory of Justice* (Cambridge, MA: Belknap Press, 1999), 102–60.
13. Daniel Engster, 'Care in the State of Nature: The Biological and Evolutionary Roots of the Disposition to Care in Human Beings', in *Care Ethics and Political Theory*, ed. Daniel Engster and Maurice Hamington (New York: Oxford University Press, 2015), 226–51.
14. John C. Harsanyi, 'Review: Can the Maximin Principle Serve as a Basis for Morality? A Critique of John Rawls's Theory', *The American Political Science Review* 69, no. 2 (June 1975): 598–600.
15. Michael J. Sandel, *Liberalism and the Limits of Justice* (New York: Cambridge University Press, 1982), 122–32.
16. Kittay, *Love's Labor*, 83–6.
17. Ibid., 90–3.
18. Held, *The Ethics of Care*, 48.
19. Kittay, 'A Theory of Justice as Fair Terms of Social Life Given Our Inevitable Dependency and Our Inextricable Interdependency', 55–8.
20. Rawls, *A Theory of Justice*, 24.
21. Held, *The Ethics of Care*, 157.
22. Derek Parfit, *Reasons and Persons* (New York: Oxford University Press, 1984), 381–90.
23. Held, *The Ethics of Care*, 82.
24. Kittay, *Love's Labor*, 94–5.
25. That this is the case is in part because the view of personhood within care ethics is fundamentally relational. Strongly rationalist views of personhood might allow for the possibility that artificial intelligence models could reach the threshold of personhood without the receipt of care, but care ethicists do not typically think of possessing this status as solely a matter of a being's internal attributes.
26. Engster, *The Heart of Justice*, 48.
27. Ibid., 45–54.
28. Kittay, *Love's Labor*, 106–13.
29. Ibid., 107.
30. Tronto, *Moral Boundaries*, 161–77.
31. Held, *The Ethics of Care*, 132.
32. Stephen Darwall, *The Second-Person Standpoint: Morality, Respect, and Accountability* (Cambridge, MA: Harvard University Press, 2006), 3–38.
33. This is, at the very least, true of humans, who are the only known beings with the capacity for moral subjecthood in this world at this time. A sufficiently advanced artificial general intelligence might attain the ability to make moral claims and recognize claims on its conduct as legitimate via an alternative route. The same could be true of bio-enhanced

humans or aliens from far-off galaxies who spawn fully cognitively formed. Moral life in worlds that contain such beings would be different in many ways from moral life in this one, so it is unsurprising that the presupposition of the successful performance of necessary care would not necessarily apply. Nevertheless, in keeping with the commitment of care ethicists to keeping particular contexts in focus, rather than aspiring to universality, I set aside this issue in this chapter. My thanks to Nicolas Côté for pressing me on this point.

34. Eva F. Kittay, 'At the Margins of Moral Personhood', *Ethics* 116, no. 1 (2005): 111.
35. Christine M. Korsgaard, 'Kant's Formula of Humanity', *Kant-Studien* 77, no. 1–4 (1986): 184.
36. Peter Singer, 'Ethics and Intuitions', *The Journal of Ethics* 9, no. 3–4 (2005): 349–51.
37. Michael A. Slote, *The Ethics of Care and Empathy* (London: Psychology Press, 2007), 55.
38. Jarkko Jalava and Stephanie Griffiths, 'Philosophers On Psychopaths: A Cautionary Tale in Interdisciplinarity', *Philosophy, Psychiatry, & Psychology* 24, no. 1 (2017): 4–6.
39. Lindsay C. Gibson, *Adult Children of Emotionally Immature Parents: How to Heal from Distant, Rejecting, or Self-Involved Parents* (Oakland, CA: New Harbinger Publications, 2015), 7–36.
40. Ibid.
41. Ibid., 88–122.
42. Meredith A. Gruhn and Bruce E. Compas, 'Effects of Maltreatment on Coping and Emotion Regulation in Childhood and Adolescence: A Meta-Analytic Review', *Child Abuse & Neglect* 103 (2020): 104446.
43. Melanie J. Zimmer-Gembeck et al., 'Parent Emotional Regulation: A Meta-Analytic Review of its Association with Parenting and Child Adjustment', *International Journal of Behavioral Development* 46, no. 1 (2021): 63–82.
44. Xinyi Yu et al., 'Intergenerational Effects of Childhood Maltreatment: The Relationships Among Parental Childhood Emotional Neglect, Emotional Expressiveness and Children's Problem Behaviors', *Child Abuse & Neglect* 140 (2023): 106147.
45. Gibson, *Adult Children of Emotionally Immature Parents,* 116–22.
46. Marije Stoltenborgh et al., 'The Prevalence of Child Maltreatment across the Globe: Review of a Series of Meta-Analyses', *Child Abuse Review* 24, no. 1 (2014): 37.
47. Nils M. Sønderland et al., 'Emotional Changes and Outcomes in Psychotherapy: A Systematic Review and Meta-Analysis', *Journal of Consulting and Clinical Psychology*, 2023.
48. Falk Leichsenring and Sven Rabung, 'Effectiveness of Long-term Psychodynamic Psychotherapy', *Journal of the American Medical Association* 300, no. 13 (2008): 1551–65.

BIBLIOGRAPHY

Anderson, Elizabeth. 'The Fundamental Disagreement between Luck Egalitarians and Relational Egalitarians', *Canadian Journal of Philosophy* 40, no. 1 (2010): 1–23.

Bubeck, Diemut E. *Care, Gender, and Justice*. Oxford: Oxford University Press, 1995.

Carter, Matilda. 'The Indirect Approach: Towards Non-Dominating Dementia Care', *Res Publica* 28, no. 3 (2021): 467–80.

Darwall, Stephen. *The Second-Person Standpoint: Morality, Respect, and Accountability*. Cambridge, MA: Harvard University Press, 2006.

Engster, Daniel. *The Heart of Justice: Care Ethics and Political Theory*. Oxford: Oxford University Press on Demand, 2007.

Engster, Daniel. 'Care in the State of Nature: The Biological and Evolutionary Roots of the Disposition to Care in Human Beings', in *Care Ethics and Political Theory*, edited by Daniel Engster and Maurice Hamington, 226–51. New York: Oxford University Press, 2015.

Fisher, Berenice, and Joan C. Tronto. 'Toward a Feminist Theory of Care', in *Circles of Care: Work and Identity in Women's Lives*, edited by Emily Abel and Margaret Nelson, 35–62. Albany: State University of New York Press, 1991.

Gibson, Lindsay C. *Adult Children of Emotionally Immature Parents: How to Heal from Distant, Rejecting, or Self-Involved Parents*. Oakland, CA: New Harbinger Publications, 2015.

Gruhn, Meredith A., and Bruce E. Compas. 'Effects of Maltreatment on Coping and Emotion Regulation in Childhood and Adolescence: A Meta-Analytic Review', *Child Abuse & Neglect* 103 (2020): 104446.

Halwani, Raja. 'Care Ethics and Virtue Ethics', *Hypatia* 18, no. 3 (2003): 161–92.

Harsanyi, John C. 'Review: Can the Maximin Principle Serve as a Basis for Morality? A Critique of John Rawls's Theory', *The American Political Science Review* 69, no. 2 (1975): 594–606.

Held, Virginia. *The Ethics of Care: Personal, Political, and Global*. New York: Oxford University Press, 2005.

Held, Virginia. 'Care and Justice, Still', in *Care Ethics and Political Theory*, edited by Daniel Engster and Maurice Hamington, 18–36. New York: Oxford University Press, 2015.

Hobbes, Thomas. 'Leviathan', in *Leviathan: With Selected Variants from the Latin Edition of 1668*, edited by Edwin Curley, 74–233. Indianapolis, IN: Hackett Publishing, 1994.

Jalava, Jarkko, and Stephanie Griffiths. 'Philosophers On Psychopaths: A Cautionary Tale in Interdisciplinarity', *Philosophy, Psychiatry, & Psychology* 24, no. 1 (2017): 1–12.

Kittay, Eva F. *Love's Labor: Essays on Women, Equality, and Dependency*. London: Psychology Press, 1994.

Kittay, Eva F. 'At the Margins of Moral Personhood', *Ethics* 116, no. 1 (2005): 100–31.

Kittay, Eva F. 'A Theory of Justice as Fair Terms of Social Life Given Our Inevitable Dependence and Our Inextricable Interdependency', in *Care Ethics and Political Theory*, edited by Daniel Engster and Maurice Hamington, 51–71. New York: Oxford University Press, 2015.

Korsgaard, Christine M. 'Kant's Formula of Humanity', *Kant-Studien* 77, no. 1–4 (1986): 183–202.

Leichsenring, Falk, and Sven Rabung. 'Effectiveness of Long-term Psychodynamic Psychotherapy', *Journal of the American Medical Association* 300, no. 13 (2008): 1551–65. https://doi.org/10.1001/jama.300.13.1551.

Locke, John. 'The Second Treatise', in *Locke: Two Treatises of Government Student Edition*, edited by Peter Laslett, 265–428. Cambridge: Cambridge University Press, 1988.

Parfit, Derek. *Reasons and Persons*. New York: Oxford University Press, 1984.

Rawls, John. *A Theory of Justice*. Cambridge, MA: Belknap Press, 1999.

Rosenberg, Karen R. 'The Evolution of Human Infancy: Why It Helps to Be Helpless', *Annual Review of Anthropology* 50, no. 1 (2021): 423–40.

Sandel, Michael J. *Liberalism and the Limits of Justice*. New York: Cambridge University Press, 1982.

Sander-Staudt, Maureen. 'The Unhappy Marriage of Care Ethics and Virtue Ethics', *Hypatia* 21, no. 4 (2006): 21–39.

Slote, Michael A. *The Ethics of Care and Empathy*. London: Psychology Press, 2007.

Singer, Peter. 'Ethics and Intuitions', *The Journal of Ethics* 9, no. 3–4 (2005): 331–52.

Sønderland, Nils M., Ole A. Solbakken, Dag E. Eilertsen, Magnus Nordmo and Jon T. Monsen. 'Emotional Changes and Outcomes in Psychotherapy: A Systematic Review and Meta-Analysis', *Journal of Consulting and Clinical Psychology*, 2023. https://doi.org/10.1037/ccp0000814.

Stoltenborgh, Marije, Marian J. Bakermans-Kranenburg, Lenneke R. Alink and Marinus H. Van Ijzendoorn. 'The Prevalence of Child Maltreatment across the Globe: Review of a Series of Meta-Analyses', *Child Abuse Review* 24, no. 1 (2014): 37–50.

Tronto, Joan C. *Moral Boundaries: A Political Argument for an Ethic of Care*. London: Routledge, 1993.

Yu, Xinyi, Ting He, Yuxin Tan, Peilian Chi and Xiuyun Lin. 'Intergenerational Effects of Childhood Maltreatment: The Relationships Among Parental Childhood Emotional Neglect, Emotional Expressiveness and Children's Problem Behaviors', *Child Abuse & Neglect* 140 (2023): 106147.

Zimmer-Gembeck, Melanie J., Julia Rudolph, Jessica Kerin and Gal Bohadana-Brown. 'Parent Emotional Regulation: A Meta-Analytic Review of its Association with Parenting and Child Adjustment', *International Journal of Behavioral Development* 46, no. 1 (2021): 63–82.

CHAPTER SEVEN

Freedom to care, for women of colour

ASHA LEENA BHANDARY

7.1 EVALUATING THE SYSTEM OF CARE THROUGH INTERSECTIONAL LIBERALISM[1]

Mainstream political philosophy has been shaped by people who occupy a social position from which they receive care without a concomitant expectation to provide hands-on care to others. Their location in the *system of care* is not merely a component of their location in extractive and exploitative systems of wealth acquisition. Instead, the *system of care* includes micro-units of care like the family, extended families and community-based networks of care, as well as large scale societal systems of care, which include broader dynamics and trends that cut across these units, with variables including gender, race, caste, sexuality, gender identity and class. As empirical research about global care chains confirms,[2] caregivers flow globally, and relations of care are often racialized or organized by caste when paid. Various forms of paid caregiving debunk the myth that units like the family are self-contained. Systems of care, thus, are social structures that overlap with other varieties of oppression, with the division of labour, and with the bounds of belonging.[3]

In the theories written by these political philosophers, the fact that they had received care was invisible, and therefore the social worlds they justified could not be criticized through the tools of their theories. Understood through the hermeneutical resources of these theories, care for the men of an elite class was assumed to be 'appropriate', such that it did not warrant justification or remark. Consequently, material and emotional caregiving was not tracked as a burden of social cooperation. The corresponding model of rationality embedded in the mainstream philosophical tradition has been shaped by the ease with which these men accessed care, the lack of any felt debt to their caregivers, and their facility at grafting the substance of others[4] onto themselves.

Feminist philosophers and care ethicists debunked the falsehoods embedded in the image of human life that had been dominant in political philosophy. Working against the ideological invisibility of care,[5] care ethicists clarified the facts of care, its value and its role in the gendering of (white) women in the second half of the twentieth century.[6] By 'care ethics', I mean the moral and political doctrine according to which care takes priority in the competition among values governing human life.[7] According to care ethics, the caring person is the ideal moral agent,[8] and a caring society is the primary social ideal.[9] Work in care ethics made possible a critique of liberal political theory that revealed its lacunae.[10] My theory of liberal dependency care builds from selected premises in care ethics to develop a new liberalism, one that articulates how liberalism can, and must, address the facts of dependency care.[11]

I employ the term '*care theory*' as a category for political theories which hold that the human need for care must be addressed, but which remain agnostic or critical of several more robust tenets of care ethics.[12] Thus, *care theories* are intellectually indebted to care ethics, while nonetheless disagreeing with care ethics about whether, and when, care has priority over other values in a normative theory governing social cooperation. *Care theories*,[13] therefore, may evaluate the subject of care from an alternative framework, as do liberal theories of care,[14] Marxist theories of care,[15] and care theories based on the capabilities approach.[16]

My *care theory* is embedded in a *critical liberalism, which establishes a structure of justification that builds on my argument that* care must be included in our theories of distributive justice, relying on minimal premises that derive from the logic of the Humean–Rawlsian circumstances of justice.[17] My *theory of liberal dependency care* (LDC)[18] prioritizes the autonomy and freedom of the individual within the constraints required for fair social cooperation, where receiving material caregiving must be included as a basic need of social cooperation.[19]

According to my *critical liberalism*, the *philosophical* doctrine of liberalism is conceptually distinct from the *actual* Western societies where the doctrine has been developed. With social structures permeated by racism and gender oppression, these societies have never conformed to its ideals.[20] Therefore, by advancing a new form of liberalism, I do not also defend the actual societies where the liberal tradition originated. On the contrary, my critical liberalism requires radical departures from the habituation of privileged persons in status quo social forms. In addition, it requires subjecting the content and implementation of laws and policies involving governmental intervention to standards of scrutiny from the domain of nonideal theory to capture phenomena such as differential enforcement. Critical liberalism thus gives rise to *intersectional* liberalism, which theorizes about the necessity and role of care in ways that are explicitly informed by the intersectional social position of a minority woman in the United States, thereby integrating care theory, liberalism and women of colour feminism(s).[21]

Critical liberalism evaluates the justice of a society where the subject of justice is the system of practices,[22] which must include caregiving arrangements. The *arrow of care map* concept plays an essential role in identifying and evaluating caregiving arrangements.[23] The arrow of care map is a conceptual scaffold with which to track who receives care, and from whom, in ways that evaluate system-wide patterns of inequality. It dictates that patterns of caregiving and of care receiving should be filtered using variables based on a variety of salient social groups, simultaneously recognizing that there may be unexplored social categories and patterns of care that are not captured by the dominant understandings of social groups in a society.

The flexibility of the arrow of care map enables ongoing evaluations about how new and emerging social groups become linked to structures of care exploitation. The assessment of racialized distributions of caregiving must include the questions: (1) Do people of colour *provide* disproportionate amounts of care? (2a) Which social groups have their needs *met* at the highest levels? and (2b) Are these needs met within practices that are self-contained within the group? (2c) Alternatively, are the group's needs for care met through structures and processes that exploit the caregiving of others?

When evaluating patterns of care, the smallest unit of evaluation is the individual human. Although the basic units of analysis in the arrow of care map are individual human beings, the arrow of care map is not committed to a metaphysical view of the self as atomistic and fundamentally individuated from other human beings. Individual human beings are modelled as the smallest unit for the purpose of a political philosophy aimed at tracking distributive injustice. The theory within which the arrow of care map is embedded is compatible with metaphysical views of the self that assert the ontological relationality of selves. Furthermore, it leaves entirely open that people may have conceptions of the self and lives of value according to which they are deeply intertwined with other people. Neither does it recommend self-understandings founded in 'rational' and self-interested bargaining. Instead, it is a model conception for identifying distributive imbalances; to identify the gendered inequality and concomitant vulnerabilities women regularly experience in virtue of maternal roles, we must be able to track the disadvantages these individual women experience.

When we track care in a way that does not already assume the legitimacy of existing relations of care, local patterns of caregiving and globalized care relations become evident. Tracking quantities of hands-on caregiving in intensity and duration, the map yields information about how care practices are arranged within and across societies. The arrow of care map methodology enables bracketing people's relationships, and in doing so it provides an independent source of data, one that does not embed background inequalities into its justification. Understanding our care relations through the data as it is organized by this concept is necessary for a comprehensive evaluation of the justice of the system of practices. It brings into view the way that, for instance, in the United States – where emotional care, social cohesion and material care are invisible and undervalued – these forms of labour are often assigned to the intersectional groups with the least social power, namely, women of colour and people who are legally vulnerable without the security of citizenship status. The inclusion of caregiving practices in our systems of social organization thus unearths a form of labour that coincides with subordinate status in many social hierarchies.

To identify the distributive inequalities in the system of caregiving is to reveal the *de facto* standing of members of different social groups. This is because, as I will argue in the next section, receiving care is a form of *status recognition*, conveying that the person who receives the care is worthy of attention. Minimal status recognition occurs when a claim to life receives uptake.

7.2 RECEIVING CARE IS AN ACT OF MINIMAL STATUS RECOGNITION

By receiving care, a person is recognized as one who can claim the attention and care of others. A minimal form of status recognition is present when a person's social standing is recognized as sufficient to impel caregiving by others. There are no guarantees that 'mothers' will receive the necessary support for good starting conditions for their child.[24] The many cases of people who are deprived of the conditions for continued life, when persecuted in war, liminally stranded in refugee camps, or restricted and thwarted in a social form hostile to their existence, clarify that status recognition is not guaranteed for every human. The first instance of status recognition is conferred by the gestational body who brings the child to life, and this form of recognition itself occurs within a social practice which confers the birthing person more or less status and agency. Therefore, to receive care is to have a place in a society, where that place is often created by one's parents, and informed by the mother's standing in broader society, or by the presence of a familial network. Clearly, that a person's life chances are informed by the wealth of their family and the social standing of the mother is inconsistent with egalitarianism's normative aim to secure equal standing for all persons.[25]

Whereas receiving care at all denotes minimal status recognition, the type of care we receive, the control we have as we receive care, and the publicity of that care demonstrate varying degrees of status recognition.[26] An idea that can be traced to the work of Jean-Jacques Rousseau,[27] the need for *recognition* is based on the human need for recognition in a social system.[28] Care differs in both quality and the level of care one receives. In addition, and significantly for this account, the attitudinal and affective components of care convey the regard with which the caregiver holds the recipient of care and/or the social standing of the recipient of care. Thus, deference intersects with care. Deference also intersects with subordination, so that to be a caregiver coincides with a subordinate social role in some societies.

If a care recipient has firm social standing, such as the nation-level standing of white men in public spaces and the standing men achieve within private families in patriarchy, then even a caregiver who cares very little for that man but who is socially assigned as one who should provide care, will nonetheless perform *material caregiving*,[29] or acts of caregiving. Moreover, material caregiving can give rise to affective caregiving, and by living in a society in which it is expected that they perform the care, the subjectivity of the caregiver may become shaped to include affectively caring for the wellbeing of that high-status individual for whom they provide material caregiving. This type of shaping of subjectivity is more likely when a counter-discourse is absent.

Societies structured by rigid guilds and castes, where identities were linked to forms of work, conferred social standing in explicitly hierarchical forms. The Enlightenment's discourse of egalitarianism asserted the equal status of each individual, but it also displaced social structures in which kinship legitimated claims to care[30]. Consequently, an explicit and public commitment to the value of universal equality was accompanied by loss of identity categories and the erosion of the kinship structures which supply care.[31] Losses in the social goods of care and belonging were collateral damage. In the absence of new social structures to guide care, much care today occurs in ways that are heavily shaped by markets and capitalist social modes of organization. The result is that many societies that purport to be committed to universal and impartial ideas of moral obligation in fact revert to status hierarchies, and race and gender have replaced other formal hierarchies and group-based identities.[32] Thus, the social structures guiding the distribution of care remain obscure, and they have yet to be thoroughly subjected to the scrutiny that is required for transparency.

To have actual status rather than normative-theoretical but unrealized status, we need to be treated in certain ways, as someone who counts. The recognition of status as a claimant is demonstrated through visual markers, social interactions and social policies. For instance, in Finland, with robust social policies and low birth rates, the message that nearly every baby counts, is materially affirmed by the state in the form of a gift that includes a snowsuit and diapers which arrive in a cardboard box which can itself be made into a crib. Expectant maternal persons must have a prenatal exam in order to receive the box, which has been provided since 1938.[33] This practice displays the way in which a general state policy to support children secures their status recognition.

An alternative approach to securing the status recognition of individuals occurs within the unit of a community as a subgroup. So, for instance, societal subgroups make it clear that children are members of their group. In South Asian Bunt communities, children are embedded in relationships with relational names, where belonging within the community means that one will be well cared for. Some other South Asian communities, such as Brahmin Iyengar communities, have longstanding traditions of branding their members to indicate membership. In addition to the boundaries of the group, which assert one's status as counting, one's status within the group varies. For instance, in patriarchal Brahmin communities, males receive more care and attention, with higher levels of needs-satisfaction.[34] In the United States, although the needs for belonging and care were long overlooked as matters of national concern, immigrant communities, neighbourhoods and families are examples of units of belonging within which care can take place in ways that are not dominated by market norms.[35]

When caregiving is invisible, as it is in liberal social forms with a public–private divide that naturalizes and minimizes the labour of care, caregivers are typically disadvantaged as measured by their share of the core primary goods. Therefore, a vital step to remedy the disadvantage is to identify arrangements, thereby making them transparent. However, in the process of making our own practices transparent, we will find them deeply flawed, for, as decades of feminist scholarship have identified, obfuscating norms make women's work as caregivers invisible or, alternatively, justified as natural.[36] Therefore, liberal theorists of care should also look to practices of care that exist or that have existed in a wide range of societies because every existing society utilizes some set of practices to meet their care needs. These arrangements cross public, private and commercial domains. For example, in the private sphere, gender norms assigning caregiving to girls and women serve as internal organizing principles within families, which then shape expectations about who will care for whom.[37] Although gendered norms and arrangements are not always formalized in legal statutes or policies, they are nonetheless enforced using a variety of mechanisms, which include gender norm enforcement through teasing and social pressure, media depictions, and outright violence against people who do not meet the requirements of the categories and tropes, such as people who are transgender.

The private nuclear family is a core caregiving institution in the United States,[38] and the idea that women will supply care appears in many cultural narratives, norms and tropes.[39] It is therefore unsurprising that literature about gendered inequality in marriage has dominated feminist discussions about care. However, we must go beyond the family and gender when we theorize about care. The concepts I have developed to theorize about care extend beyond assumptions of the family as the primary source of care. In addition to the arrow of care map, already discussed as enabling a systems-level understanding of caregiving arrangements, *customary care practices* are a companion concept with which to identify public and private practices that secure care within a given social form.[40]

7.3 CUSTOMARY CARE PRACTICES

Whereas the presence of a caregiving arrangement is a universal feature of every human society, the details of those arrangements differ. I call the practices that secure care within a given social form 'customary care practices' (or CCPs). Actual caregiving arrangements exist as combinations of numerous kinds of 'customary care practices'.[41] CCPs include principles specifying the people who are connected in the caring practices as well as the norms and values that shape their expectations and actual practices.

CCPs are comprised of:

1. Unit delineating principles. These principles are often implicit, and they specify who is in the right kind of relationship with each other to count as fellow 'persons' in a caring unit.
2. Norms and values that shape expectations within the actual practice, thereby specifying the division of labour within that unit.

For instance, CCPs include marital practices shaping entry conditions and the meaning of the family, such as arranged marriage versus romantic love marriage, as well as conceptualizations of family units as nuclear families, extended families, chosen families and other alternatives. The principles that govern the creation of these units are marriage law, socialization norms, family law, social recognition of families as in invitations to events that involve bringing one's 'family'. They also include explicitly designed institutions for care, such as daycare and elder-care institutions and in-home care, state-provided care and communes. The implicit norms and values within these institutions will distribute how care is provided internally within these CCPs, usually occurring along the lines of gender, birth order for children or social vulnerability.[42]

Including CCPs within the subject of justice enables theorizing about micro-level practices of care in ways that make these practices' functional role their most salient feature. For instance, a particular form of the family, like a nuclear family, may be re-described as a CCP.[43] The concept of the CCP is therefore a concept for cross-cultural theoretical work that gives us a way of talking about the broad range of existing and possible practices that serve the functional role of meeting care needs.

Many CCPs rely on the appropriation of the labour and bodies of 'outsiders'. Let us call them 'the appropriated'. For example, when caregivers are not mothers, their labour may become invisible even while it remains essential to the functioning of society.[44] Thus, their labour is appropriated even while they are excluded from social recognition. Their substance is grafted by their employers, for instance, and the care is received without identification. In cases where the employer characterizes the caregiver as a member of the family, the superficiality of that characterization becomes evident quickly when the needs of the caregiver conflict with those of their employer.

7.4 CARE WORK AND THE SOCIAL ONTOLOGY OF 'WOMEN OF COLOUR'

In the United States, de facto entitlements to receive care are intimately linked to categories of race and ethnicity, both of which play important roles in an informally structured system of social inequality and role designations. As vital components of society's system of practices, caregiving arrangements are shaped by norms, family and child welfare laws, and socialization practices that create the social ontological categories boy/girl, woman/man, designating a binary gender logic with corresponding roles in practices of caregiving. The system of care also creates a functional category for women of colour, who do not share histories, but who are placed together in Western cognitive schemas as those who are not full claimants, and who are thus construed as ready to meet the needs of others.

When the 'sight lines'[45] of care responsibilities are not visible, social groups who can be made invisible are subsumed into the caregiving system as vessels for the needs of others. In numerous 'liberal' societies, including the United States and countries in Europe, this invisible group is women of colour. As our labour is grafted onto the selves of others,[46] the energy we can devote to our most meaningful relationships is diminished.

Correspondingly, the intimate and familial relationships women of colour prioritize are challenged by societies where we are expected to attend and respond to the 'needs' white entitlement creates. What can tracking the sight lines of care in late capitalist and avowedly liberal societies like the United States tell us about who counts? Undervalued labour that is feminized, such as daily acts of bodily repair and maintenance, is socially assigned to people of colour, immigrants and women of colour.[47] This labour is 'justified' via a conceptual schema that places upon women of colour a universal maternal social role which correspondingly denies us social allowances for our own intimate relationships, thereby revealing the ideological function of this maternal trope.

Social arrangements are structured around expectations for care upon which group-based identities supervene, and which are continuous with histories of care labour. As these social arrangements interact with the social categories relevant to a particular society, a new social ontology emerges, according to which an individual's position in the caregiving arrangement creates social expectations, and where these social positions are shaped by one's place in the map of care, overlapping with, and adding to, known social categories, including gender, race, ethnicity and sexuality.

Our social positions in the map of care impact our social affordances, and thus they significantly impact the terrain for agency. However, because social spaces are varied, and people's facility in navigating them will depend on their autonomy skills, the aspects of their social positions that matter will also vary. Sometimes, they may not matter much at all, leaving instead individual subjectivity, commitments and horizons of concern. It is therefore vital to maintain flexibility in the social ontology while including diagnostic techniques to identify what matters, where and when.[48] Nonetheless, due to the strong connection between a social location as tender to others and non-white women's social positions in the United States, theorizing from and about this broader category is needed to unstitch the connection between this group identity and being a resource for others. Consequently, theorizing about 'women of colour' as a social group that is contrastive with white women, where women of colour are located in the system of care as receptacles for the care needs of others, should contribute to the demise of its ontological significance.

To achieve the normative aim of *freedom to care,*[49] the relationship between the invisibility of care in theories of distributive justice and 'women of colour' as a social position must be analysed. Because the longstanding invisibility of care work in societies enables the accretion of social inequality, a philosophical analysis of the relationship between varieties of inequality, practices of care, and social group categories identifying the functional roles served by these social groups in our system of social organization is long overdue.[50] Only then may we transform them into egalitarian relations through durable change.

Although the histories, stereotypes and norms applied to women in various non-white groups are highly differentiated, the social category 'women of colour', defined to include the set of all non-white women, serves an important function in the context of the injustice of caregiving arrangements in white dominant societies. It serves this important function as a concept in a theory of distributive justice, even while recognizing that 'women of colour' is not a description of shared history across identity groups, nor does it describe commonalities across experiences for many women who are included in the category. Instead, I define the term 'woman of colour' in relation to the structure of a society, which is analysed in a theory of distributive justice as defining the parameters of the just distribution of benefits and burdens of social cooperation.[51] On this view, distributive justice applies to the social entity defined by the Greek term 'Oikos', which translates as the 'economy' understood as the cooperative unit and arrangement within which human needs are met.[52]

Therefore, if we are to evaluate existing social inequalities, we must include care in our theories of distributive justice. In the absence of considered practices for care, *women of colour*, as those who are disadvantaged in formal structures, occupy a social position that is not a full claimant position; and we are instead interacted with as substance to be used, appropriated or grafted onto others.[53] Therefore, when women of colour act in accordance with our own priorities, these actions are too often received with resistance and anger. Furthermore, when women of colour prioritize the needs of our own families, asserting a domain for privacy, intimacy, and care against the societal presumption that our caregiving is the property of society and of impersonal others in society more broadly understood, we encounter additional resistance.

I argue that it follows from a recognition of the social and relational nature of human beings and the assertion that all humans are full claimants, that each person/human/claimant should (1) have access to their children, (2) be able to maintain relationships with their elders, and (3) be able to secure a domain for core interpersonal relationships with minimal outside interference.[54]

Extrapolating from the relationships listed above results in a list of several freedoms. The first freedom, also serving as a normative criterion for a political theory is *freedom to care* indexed to women of colour. Let us call this nonideal theoretical principle of justice *freedom to care for women of colour*. It means that women of colour should have effective freedom to provide material and emotional caregiving for the people they care about. The assertion of this freedom is necessary because one of the ways individual human beings are denied full claimant status is through deficits in this vital social good.

Full claimant status is thus linked to status recognition. Whose child gets recognized as one worthy of care? Because every person is someone's child, the child's minimal status recognition is impacted by the mother's location in the social practices. In cases where a parent rejects the child, as in cases of homophobic parents of LGBTQIA+ children, the child must seek alternative sources of care.[55]

7.5 FREEDOM TO CARE, FOR WOMEN OF COLOUR

From these claims about differential status, the connection between receiving care and status, and the way the social group women of colour can serve as an all-purpose bucket for the needs of others in society that are not met through visible and valued modes of cooperation, it follows that for women of colour, freedom to care for the people we care about is a radical act and a goal for a radically transformed just society. My *intersectional liberalism* for a caring and just society places the autonomy of women of colour at the centre, with other changes to the social form driven by this goal.[56] Women of colour are the social group supplying undervalued and invisible caregiving to impersonal others, often to the detriment of their own sphere of intimate others. For this reason, a theory beginning from the normative concerns and perspectives of this diverse social group will better promote justice than a theory beginning with the white cis man whose interests and perspectives masqueraded as neutral in these theories even while he was their normative subject. Moreover, because women of colour are often denied the effective entitlements that should accompany full claimant status, 'intersectional liberalism' assesses personal autonomy in relation to our social affordances.

7.5.1 Living counterfactually[57]

Women of colour who claim the formal and informal entitlements standardly granted to others, and who go beyond that to occupy domains of intellectual authority *live counterfactually* – we live in ways that are not licensed for us, acting as if affordances were present when they are not there. Consequently, living autonomously, as a woman of colour, is a radical act, one that summons the burdens that come from acting against affordances, where conflict with the social world makes its way into the body as stress.

We encounter interference in forms both overt and insidious. Construed as a resource for others, we are expected to be available to them, rather than granted domains for privacy and sovereignty. In the United States context, prioritizing our own families makes us unavailable to serve as nannies and in other readily appropriated labour roles. In the workplace, living counterfactually means we are unavailable for the mammified labour the organizations expect. We are denied latitude to act upon our commitments, so that guiding our lives to be available to the people we care about, so that our life energy can be a resource for them, is violently wrested from us, repeatedly, and through broader social systems. Respect for autonomy, then, can be understood as a second personal attitude of respect for the authority of a person over her own life's energy. Correspondingly, insisting that our families are a domain of negative liberty, or non-interference, is a radical assertion.[58] Overall, because caregiving arrangements claim and appropriate the life energy of women of colour, asserting one's agency as a full claimant illuminates the distributions of the social form.

7.5.2 Social hierarchy and deference

We can now see the complementarity of the claims of this chapter. When existing social forms are evaluated through a lens that understands care to be a form of status recognition, it becomes clear that women of colour asserting freedom to care for the people we care about is a radical act. The assignment of caregiving to people with less social power means that many needs for care are met, but that they are met in ways that are linked to relationships of hierarchy, entailing the appropriation of their labour.

7.6 INTERSECTIONAL LIBERALISM

For women of colour to be liberated from the social role of universal caregiver, societies' care needs must be met, and they must be met with systems that are transparent and fair. The invisibility of care results in intuitions that are linked to the ideological invisibility of care's importance,[59] and which also fail to identify how it is secured in existing society.[60]

Because care is the spine of culture,[61] these intuitions about care are then connected to other deeply felt self-understandings and expectations for others. Consequently, the ways we are habituated in relation to care are connected to how we understand the world, our embodiment and our social access to others for our needs and desires. It is unsurprising, then, that many of the people who assert a commitment to equality in a cool and calm moment will not sustain that commitment in their bodily habit and comportment when their needs for care are at stake. A reason for failing to sustain such a commitment is due to a lack of self-knowledge and awareness, including the absence of meta-lucidity. They will not know how they assume care, attendance and attention from women of colour. The 'rogue emotions'[62] will reveal to them that it is irksome when women of colour are not available or accessible – physically, emotionally and intellectually.[63]

This is why a procedure that abstracts away from real relationships of care, thereby defamiliarizing our expectations of others, is a necessary element of avoiding the reification of those very hierarchies. The theory of liberal dependency care (LDC) defends a variety of constructivism that makes explicit the background distributive patterns of caregiving. Rendering these practices transparent will modify our intuitions as to what counts as a 'reasonable' claim and way of life.

LDC's structure of justification consists of an abstract form of evaluation to assess what we would agree to if we did not know our social position in society and in a requirement for autonomy skills in the real world. The first aspect is a version of the Rawlsian idea of hypothetical acceptability that embraces his earlier formulation of its subject of justice[64] as the 'system of practices'.[65] LDC, like John Rawls's account of liberalism, is a form of constructivism. It embraces an iterative process of justification, whereby the intuitions employed are reflexively assessed in light of the account of justice that results. However, although the model of the person in Rawls's account of the original position is purportedly neutral, the way persons are understood in this model is, in fact, informed by assumptions about what a reasonable life includes in social forms where caring labour has been invisible.[66]

Theorizing from the perspective of a woman of colour, I insist on the enduring need to prioritize autonomy in a society with just care practices, and to maintain a conceptual distinction between autonomy and care.[67] For example, embedding a requirement of responsiveness to others, or of caring into a conception of autonomy would inevitably translate into more epistemic leaning and deference from people of colour. Therefore, if we are to understand the nature of a liberal society with just caregiving practices, we must begin with the autonomy of women of colour, for doing so reveals the hidden nature of Western 'liberal' social forms and the determinate content embedded in abstract accounts of accountability, entitlements, needs, care and equality. To diagnose caregiving injustice through the lens of a woman of colour is to present new reasons in defence of a liberal constructivism. This constructivism must interrogate (1) the relational nature of entitlements, (2) the distributive backdrop that shapes whether a claim is understood as a need or a preference, and (3) how accountability can be evaded by perpetrators of violence, particularly when the victim acts in ways that contravene assigned roles in dominant cultural constructions. I have taken a few steps toward explicating each of these three components, thereby demarcating the outlines of a care theory of justice that begins from social understandings as a woman of colour. These are the beginnings of the theory that I call 'intersectional liberalism'.

In *Freedom to Care*, my defence of autonomy skills is as a legitimacy condition for two-level contract theory, which identifies how a theorist is connected to the world, but it does not offer a full account of the requirements for a theorist of justice. There, I write that 'my focus is not to identify criteria for the theorist; that is a separate project for social epistemology'.[68] I have, since then, added a variety of dialogical responsiveness as requirement for the theorist in my modifications to contract theory. This requirement is prompted by Andrea Westlund's argument that theorists of justice need to have skills with a 'dialogical or relational structure, and include skills involved in theorists' responsiveness to other perspectives, as well'.[69]

Many of the existing systems of practices that appear to meet the care needs of their members rely on a public understanding that 'justifies' the arrangement by conceptualizing the members of some group as naturally caring such that they simply want to care for others, or by denying them full claimant status. For example, a system of practices may rely on the falsehood embedded in the mammy stereotype, or on the social role of the daughter-in-law as caregiver to the family. In these cases, the Black woman in the United States or the Indian daughter-in-law in a patriarchal schema is expected to meet others' care needs, where demands for their caregiving are not limited by their own health needs, wellbeing or choices. Consequently, it is essential to determine who incurs responsibility for meeting care needs.

In the *theory of LDC*, the needs of caregivers and people in social groups who are assumed to be caregivers take centre stage. The demand to receive care, and the demand to provide it, are too often coded into social class, caste, race and gender groups. Maintaining a steady supply of caregivers has involved naturalizing women as caring, the overt coercion and violence of domestic abuse, as well as moral pressure such as shaming people who do not want to provide care. It is for these reasons that LDC holds that an ideal that specifies a threshold of care received cannot be asserted without simultaneously asserting conditions of freedom for caregivers. I characterize the agents of construction in the original position as self-interested in order to prevent absorbing the life energy of some people into the schema as a whole at the most foundational level of theory. If individuals are not recognized as distinct at that level, we cannot discern when interests should be combined. When contract theory advances a construction of persons to achieve certain pragmatic ends, as I do in liberal dependency care, that construction is not a description of real people.

Of course, real-world forms of 'cooperation' to secure care have often included prescriptive socialization, so that what seems (to some) to be a cooperative schema also includes a variety of coercive measures, including outright violence, microaggressions and status hierarchies. Our cooperative schemas have typically relied on some subset of the community displacing their own needs in favour of the needs of others.

Rejecting the subsumption of some individuals into the cooperative schema as a whole, my theory of distributive justice establishes, at the abstract level of theory design, that each person counts as one, thereby providing conceptual and practical resources for identifying the exploitation of individual caregivers. To this foundation, I add a device for evaluating systemic patterns in care. A theory that begins with the claim that we should each *receive* the care we need, while neither acknowledging the possibility of scarcity of care provision, nor tracking inequalities in care *received* across populations, fails to yield adequate anti-racist conceptual resources. In the absence of a requirement for transparency of caregiving arrangements, and a flexible concept that can be used to track a variety of characteristics, we will not be able to find out whether some racial groups' needs are assessed as legitimate more often than those of others, nor will we be able to assess whether there are vast racial inequalities in the population of caregivers. Therefore, we need resources at the level of theory to identify who is receiving care, and how much, and to critically assess the legitimacy of needs. For example, LDC's evaluation of care provision at the level of system-wide patterns allows us to ask whether the needs for survival and flourishing of a white child with significant disabilities are met more often than the needs of a Black or brown child with the same disabilities.[70]

My view is that a just society can have many forms, and that there will be a wide array of social practices that are compatible with a society that is just with respect to care. We must imaginatively evaluate caregiving arrangements in ways that do not assume the immutability of capitalism or of our particular gendered and racialized constructions of care. The arrow of care map creates conceptual space for imagining a range of practices that could be compatible with a just society, to be evaluated by three metrics: respect for the autonomy of individuals, the fairness of the distribution of caregiving labour, and the degree to which society meets its members' legitimate needs for care.[71]

Along with the need to modify and design caregiving practices, an ameliorative virtue is needed to continually adjust away from injustice in the current, nonideal world. This ameliorative virtue, 'interpersonal reciprocity', is needed to rectify the care-based social position women of colour occupy.

7.7 INTERPERSONAL RECIPROCITY

The underlying social inequalities that shape existing Western liberal relationships of caregiving and care receiving make it the case that only through a virtue and a social norm of interpersonal reciprocity can individuals unsettle, and thereby avoid perpetuating, these harms.[72] *Interpersonal reciprocity* is an active disposition towards the person from whom one receives care, but its target is not limited to that person. In particular, when people are embedded within a close-knit community, interpersonal reciprocity includes long-term overlapping relationships such that people take on responsibility for the community.

When a person develops an understanding of the value of interpersonal reciprocity, that person develops a disposition to contribute as a response to receiving generosity and care from others. The person with interpersonal reciprocity thinks, 'How can I return the care that was shown to me?' Its structure is like a virtue, in that the person has a disposition to respond in a certain way. As discussed previously, practices that cultivate interpersonal reciprocity have the value of preventing the formation of a subjectivity that is shaped by entitlement, for these practices prevent people from experiencing the world as one that is simply oriented towards them. Interpersonal reciprocity is thereby also a regulative ideal for individual behaviour. A person who is cared for by others seeks to return it to the people who have rendered it to them; they also consider it to be a broader responsibility to their community, but not as a universal and impartial responsibility.

The virtue of interpersonal reciprocity is one vital component of a social system that achieves and maintains fair caregiving arrangements. Interpersonal reciprocity incorporates several goods. However, community-based interpersonal reciprocity might not be accessible in highly globalized social forms responding to capitalist economies. The geographic mobility in these social forms present challenges for delimiting the scope of a community or to keep extended family members in close geographic proximity. Moreover, the idea that caregiving should take place in the context of other forms of work is also more difficult to apply to these economies, when caregiving is one among few in-person interactions in these economies. In Western liberal societies with capitalist economies, many goods are produced far from the people who use them. When our lives occur among the passage of mass-produced goods travelling great distances, it is more challenging to find a way to make reciprocity personal. In contrast, the land-based systems Kim Anderson describes for native communities in Canada had systems of care labour that were thoroughly intertwined with other forms of work within smaller communities.[73] For these reasons, a CCP that is shaped by the value of interpersonal reciprocity may be difficult to achieve in a social form like the mainstream United States. Despite these difficulties, diasporic conceptions of community and global remunerances demonstrate the agentic responses people have to maintain ties with the people they care about.

When people learn the value of interpersonal reciprocity, one of the things they learn is what they should *not* do – they should *not* receive care and generosity from others without reciprocating in some way. Consequently, a person who has this value can avoid damaging others through his entitlement.[74]

CONCLUSION

I have argued that to be a member of a society, a person must receive care, and these acts then constitute their status recognition as a claimant. Human beings do not already arrive in the world counting as persons. Instead, we become members of the society, recognized as such, through a range of social practices. When children are presented as well-groomed, for instance, it asserts to the broader social world that they count, and that a parent, often a mother, grandparent or a community is asserting their value as one who matters.[75] In this way, and in others, social practices indicate membership in ways that signify overall social belonging or specific subgroup belonging.

A person's status may vary as indexed to family, community or nation. Crucially, it is not the case that subordinate national status is merely compounded at the family and community levels. Instead, a person who is devalued in nation-level value systems can have their status, and thus, sense of self-worth, reasserted at the family and/or community level. Immigrant communities, for instance, are often sources of robust material caregiving, affective care, and narratives of worth for their members. LGBTQIA+ spaces are also locations for care and status recognition for their members, who are too often devalued in the broader society, or cast out of their family of origin. Therefore, community, family and nation are each independent domains within which a person can have the status to impel care. For each of them, belonging is a condition for receiving care, and it is also reasserted through that care. Belonging and social hierarchy are embedded in the micro-practices of care that I define as 'customary care practices'.

One's status as worthy of care is doubly relational. For adults, the relata are the individual and a family, community, country or world. However, for a person arriving in the world, the status the broader social world confers in their maternal parent greatly impacts the life of the child, and the experiences of the gestating mother that predate the existence of the child also influence their life. Furthermore, a parent's ability to provide care is dependent on their own social status. Social status should be understood as a relational property, where the relata are within a family, community, country or world. Unqualifiedly high status is affirmed globally, such as the status of straight white affluent men, and is also embedded in philosophical theories in the form of universal status of a full claimant. Clearly, though, philosophical theories of care and justice should not assume that everyone has this de facto standing.

While the project of arriving at just practices of care is an ongoing and perpetual task, one with practical and philosophical implications, the task for the unjust meantime[76] is to continually correct away from the hierarchical and racialized structures that inform our systems of care. Interpersonal reciprocity can guard against the worst forms of exploitation, and thus it is an essential stopgap for liberal egalitarian, and just, systems of care. For these reasons, *interpersonal reciprocity* is a vital virtue in *intersectional liberalism*.

NOTES

1. Material in this section is adapted from Asha Bhandary, 'Caring for Whom? Racial Practices of Care and Liberal Constructivism', *Philosophies* 7, no. 4 (2022): 78.
2. Arlie Hochschild, 'Global Care Chains and Emotional Surplus Value', in *On the Edge: Living with Global Capitalism*, ed. Anthony Giddens and Will Hutton (London: Jonathan Cape, 2000), 130–60.
3. Asha Bhandary, *Freedom to Care: Liberalism, Dependency Care, and Culture* (London: Routledge, 2020).
4. I discuss 'grafting the substance of others' in Section 7.4.
5. Joan C. Tronto, *Moral Boundaries: A Political Argument for an Ethic of Care* (New York: Routledge, 1993).
6. See: Carol Gilligan, *In a Different Voice: Psychological Theory and Women's Development* (Cambridge: Harvard University Press, 1982); Sara Ruddick, *Maternal Thinking: Toward a Politics of Peace* (Boston, MA: Beacon Press, 1989).
7. Virginia Held makes this claim about priorities most clearly, see: Virginia Held, *The Ethics of Care: Personal, Political, and Global* (Oxford: Oxford University Press, 2006). See also: Eva F. Kittay, *Love's Labor: Essays on Women, Equality and Dependency* (London: Routledge, 1999).
8. Held, *The Ethics of Care*.
9. Tronto, *Moral Boundaries*.
10. Kittay, *Love's Labor*.
11. See: Asha Bhandary, 'Dependency in Justice: Can Rawlsian Liberalism Accommodate Kittay's Dependency Critique?', *Hypatia* 25, no. 1 (2010): 140–56; Asha Bhandary, 'Liberal Dependency Care', *Journal of Philosophical Research* 41 (2016): 43–68; Asha Bhandary, 'The Arrow of Care Map: Abstract Care in Ideal Theory', *Feminist Philosophy Quarterly* 3, no. 4 (2017); Asha Bhandary, 'Arranged Marriage: Could It Contribute to Justice?', *Journal of Political Philosophy* 26, no. 2 (2018): 193–215; Bhandary, *Freedom to Care*; Bhandary, 'The Theory of Liberal Dependency Care'; Bhandary, 'Caring for Whom?'.
12. For this definition of care theory, see: Bhandary, 'Caring for Whom?', 1–2.
13. For a range of liberal approaches to care, see: Asha Bhandary and Amy R. Baehr, eds, *Caring for Liberalism: Dependency and Liberal Political Theory* (London: Routledge, 2021). Because questions about care have overlapped with debates about women's labour and socialization, the liberal tradition of evaluating care has been shaped by Susan Okin's feminist liberalism (Susan Okin, *Justice Gender and the Family* (New York: Basic Books, 1989)). See also: Ann Cudd, *Analyzing Oppression*.
14. Bhandary, *Freedom to Care*.
15. Diemut Bubeck, *Care, Gender, and Justice* (Oxford: Clarendon Press, 1995).
16. See: Daniel Engster, *The Heart of Justice: Care Ethics and Political Theory* (New York: Oxford University Press, 2007); Ingrid Robeyns, 'Gender and the Metric of Justice',

in *Measuring Justice: Primary Goods and Capabilities*, ed. Harry Brighouse and Ingrid Robeyns (Cambridge: Cambridge University Press, 2010), 215–35.
17. See: Bhandary, 'Dependency in Justice'; Bhandary, *Freedom to Care*.
18. Bhandary, *Freedom to Care*.
19. See: S. A. Lloyd, 'Toward a Liberal Theory of Sexual Equality', in *Varieties of Feminist Liberalism*, ed. Amy R. Baehr (Lanham, MD: Rowman & Littlefield, 2004), 65. See also: John S. Mill, 'On Liberty', in *On Liberty and Other Writings*, ed. Stefan Collini (Cambridge: Cambridge University Press, 1989); John Rawls, 'Justice as Fairness', *The Philosophical Review* 67, no. 2 (1958): 164–94; and Bhandary, 'The Arrow of Care Map'.
20. See: Bhandary, 'The Theory of Liberal Dependency Care'; Domenico Losurdo, *Liberalism: A Counter-History* (Bologna: Verso Books, 2006); Charles W. Mills, *Black Rights/White Wrongs: The Critique of Racial Liberalism* (New York: Oxford University Press, 2017).
21. I advance this intersectional liberalism in my manuscript in progress: *Being at Home: Living Autonomously in an Unjust World*. For women of colour feminisms, see: Audre Lorde, *Sister Outsider: Essays and Speeches* (New York: Crossing Press, 1984); bell hooks, 'Racism and Feminism: The Issue of Accountability', in *Ain't I a Woman: Black Women and Feminism* (London: Routledge, 2014); and María Lugones, *Pilgrimages/Peregrinajes: Theorizing Coalition Against Multiple Oppressions* (Lanham, MD: Rowman & Littlefield, 2003). For decolonial feminisms, see: Gayatri Spivak, 'Can the Subaltern Speak?', in *Marxism and the Interpretation of Culture*, ed. Cary Nelson and Lawrence Grossberg (London: Macmillan, 1988): 267–310; Uma Narayan, *Dislocating Cultures: Identities, Traditions, and Third World Feminism* (New York: Routledge, 2013); and Serene Khader, *Decolonizing Universalism: A Transnational Feminist Ethic* (New York: Oxford University Press, 2019). For a feminist discussion of autonomy in conditions of oppression, see: Shay Welch, *Existential Eroticism: A Feminist Approach to Understanding Women's Oppression-Perpetuating Choices* (Lanham, MD: Lexington Books, 2015).
22. Rawls, 'Justice as Fairness'.
23. See: Bhandary, 'The Arrow of Care Map'; Bhandary, *Freedom to Care*.
24. See reproductive justice scholars, particularly Dorothy Roberts, and research on racial differences in maternal care, as well as the phenomenon of obstetric violence.
25. For an analysis of the different forms of equality at stake in debates about egalitarianism, including Young and Anderson's relational egalitarianism in relation to Rawls's distributive paradigm, see my student Timothy Sommers's dissertation (Timothy Sommers, 'What is the Point of Equality?' (PhD diss., University of Iowa, 2021), ProQuest).
26. On the politics of recognition, see: Axel Honneth, *The Struggle for Recognition: The Moral Grammar of Social Conflicts* (Cambridge, MA: MIT Press, 1996); Charles Taylor, 'The Politics of Recognition,' in *Multiculturalism: Examining the Politics of Recognition*, ed. Amy Gutmann (Princeton, NJ: Princeton University Press, 1994).
27. Jean-Jacques Rousseau, *Discourse on the Origin of Inequality* (Amsterdam: Marc-Michel Rey, 1755).
28. Taylor, 'The Politics of Recognition'.
29. Elizabeth Brake, *Minimizing Marriage: Marriage, Morality, and the Law* (New York: Oxford University Press, 2012).
30. see also Arendt.
31. Tronto, *Moral Boundaries*, ch. 4.
32. See: Taylor, 'The Politics of Recognition'.
33. This practice occurs in the context of a relatively homogenous population.

34. See also Amartya Sen's Nobel prize-winning work on nutritional deficits.
35. On market norms, see: Elizabeth S. Anderson, 'What Is the Point of Equality?', *Ethics* 109, no. 2 (1999): 287–337.
36. See: Sandra Bartky, *Femininity and Domination: Studies in the Phenomenology of Oppression* (New York: Routledge, 1990); Diana T. Meyers, *Gender in the Mirror: Cultural Imagery and Women's Agency* (New York: Oxford University Press, 2002).
37. Bartky, *Femininity and Domination.*
38. Martha A. Fineman, *The Autonomy Myth: A Theory of Dependency* (New York: New Press, 2004).
39. Meyers, *Gender in the Mirror.*
40. Bhandary, 'The Theory of Liberal Dependency Care'.
41. Ibid.
42. This paragraph is adapted from Asha Bhandary, 'Interpersonal Reciprocity', in *Caring for Liberalism: Dependency and Liberal Political Theory*, ed. Asha Bhandary and Amy R. Baehr (New York: Routledge, 2021), 148–9.
43. See Tamara Metz's proposal for 'intimate caregiving union status' (Tamara Metz, *Untying the Knot: Marriage, the State, and the Case for Their Divorce* (Princeton, NJ: Princeton University Press, 2010)). Elizabeth Brake's 'minimal marriage' (Brake, *Minimizing Marriage*) and Martha Fineman's account of the family (Fineman, *The Autonomy Myth*) also make the connection between care and family explicit and reconceptualize family in ways that prioritize its functional role.
44. I am indebted to a conversation with Diana Tietjens Meyers about the nature of social exclusion. The type of oppression experienced by these caregivers can be contrasted with Iris Marion Young's account of marginals, defined as people the system cannot use. For Young, marginalization is a way of being excluded from the system of social cooperation (see: Iris M. Young, *Justice and the Politics of Difference* (Princeton, NJ: Princeton University Press, 1990)].
45. Margaret U. Walker, *Moral Understandings: A Feminist Study in Ethics* (New York: Oxford University Press, 2007).
46. See: Marilyn Frye, *The Politics of Reality: Essays in Feminist Theory* (Berkeley, CA: Crossing Press, 1983); María Lugones, *Pilgrimages/Peregrinajes: Theorizing Coalition Against Multiple Oppressions* (Lanham, MD: Rowman & Littlefield, 2003).
47. See: Ann Ferguson, *Blood at the Root: Motherhood, Sexuality and Male Dominance* (London: Pandora Press, 1989). For a recent study, see Emma Dowling, *The Care Crisis: What Caused It and How Can We End It?* (New York: Verso Books, 2021).
48. For sophisticated discussions of these phenomena, see Chela Sandoval's account of agency across contexts as engaging a 'clutch' (Chela Sandoval, *Methodology of the Oppressed*, Minneapolis: University of Minnesota Press, 2013)) and Mariana Ortega's account of the multiplicitous self. See also Chapter 5 of this book, for a discussion of María Lugones.
49. Bhandary, *Freedom to Care.*
50. For other accounts of social groups, see: Amie L. Thomasson, 'The Ontology of Social Groups,' *Synthese* 196, no. 12 (2019): 4829–45; and Sally Haslanger, *Resisting Reality: Social Construction and Social Critique* (New York: Oxford University Press, 2012).
51. Lloyd, 'Toward a Liberal Theory of Sexual Equality'.
52. Maxine Eichner, 'The Free-Market Family. Liberalism, Families, and the Government's Responsibility to Regulate the Market', in *Caring for Liberalism: Dependency and Liberal Political Theory*, ed. Asha Bhandary and Amy R. Baehr (New York: Routledge, 2021), 238–65.

53. Of course, the extent to which others assume we are available to them depends on the context, the location, the specific racial group and other factors, such as whether we are socially understood to be mothers. See: Bhandary, *Freedom to Care*; Bhandary, 'The Theory of Liberal Dependency Care'; Bhandary, 'Caring for Whom?'. See also Lugones on grafting in her world-travelling Hypatia article.
54. See my book in progress, *Being at Home*, for this argument. For a human rights-based argument that relationship goods are essential to our wellbeing, see: Kimberley Brownlee, *Being Sure of Each Other: An Essay on Social Rights and Freedoms* (Oxford: Oxford University Press, 2020).
55. I am indebted to Helga Varden for conversations on this topic.
56. See my draft monograph, *Being at Home*.
57. See Bhandary, 'The Theory of Liberal Dependency Care' for further discussion. Parts of this section are reprinted from that article.
58. For a discussion of those US policies that create family separation, theorized through the lens of reproductive justice see: Dorothy Roberts, *Shattered Bonds: The Color of Child Welfare* (New York: Basic Books, 2002).
59. Tronto, *Moral Boundaries*.
60. Bhandary, 'The Arrow of Care Map'.
61. See: Bhandary, *Freedom to Care*. Bhandary, 'The Theory of Liberal Dependency Care'.
62. Bartky, *Femininity and Domination*.
63. For instance, middle-class professionals in the UK who bemoaned their sudden loss of professional childcare and cleaning services during the pandemic (including white feminist columnists who spoke of it as an issue of gender equality) were tacitly bemoaning the loss of access to women of colour to attend to their needs. Many thanks to Matilda Carter for this example.
64. Rawls, 'Justice as Fairness'.
65. See Bhandary, 'Interpersonal Reciprocity'. For a feminist defence of hypothetical acceptability, see also: Cynthia A. Stark, 'Hypothetical Consent and Justification', *The Journal of Philosophy* 97, no. 6 (2000): 313–34.
66. Bhandary, *Freedom to Care*, ch. 4.
67. Bhandary, 'Interpersonal Reciprocity'.
68. Bhandary, *Freedom to Care*, 97.
69. Andrea Westlund, 'Education for Autonomy, and for Care: A Comment on Asha Bhandary's *Freedom to Care*', *Critical Review of International Social and Political Philosophy* 25, no. 6 (2022): 820–6. For discussion, see Bhandary, 'The Theory of Liberal Dependency Care'.
70. Some of the sections above are reprised from my reply to critics in *CRISPP*, 2021.
71. Bhandary, *Freedom to Care*, 160.
72. Bhandary, 'Interpersonal Reciprocity', 152–3.
73. Kim Anderson, *Life Stages and Native Women: Memory, Teachings, and Story Medicine* (Winnipeg: University of Manitoba Press, 2011).
74. Although the community basis for interpersonal reciprocity may be rare in mainstream Western societies, it is alive and well in a number of non-Western societies. This section is adapted from Bhandary, 'Interpersonal Reciprocity'.
75. When white children appear unkempt without incurring negative consequences, it attests to the security of white social standing in the US. This phenomenon seems to be an outlier and does not generally track with privileged social groups in a number of other societies.
76. This term is borrowed from Alison Jaggar.

BIBLIOGRAPHY

Anderson, Elizabeth. 'What Is the Point of Equality?' *Ethics* 109, no. 2 (1999): 287–337.
Anderson, Kim. *Life Stages and Native Women: Memory, Teachings, and Story Medicine*. Winnipeg: University of Manitoba Press, 2011.
Bartky, Sandra. *Femininity and Domination: Studies in the Phenomenology of Oppression*. New York: Routledge, 1990.
Bhandary, Asha. 'Dependency in Justice: Can Rawlsian Liberalism Accommodate Kittay's Dependency Critique?', *Hypatia* 25, no. 1 (2010): 140–56.
Bhandary, Asha. 'Liberal Dependency Care', *Journal of Philosophical Research* 41 (2016): 43–68.
Bhandary, Asha. 'The Arrow of Care Map: Abstract Care in Ideal Theory', *Feminist Philosophy Quarterly* 3, no. 4 (2017): Article 5.
Bhandary, Asha. 'Arranged Marriage: Could It Contribute to Justice?', *Journal of Political Philosophy* 26, no. 2 (2018): 193–215.
Bhandary, Asha. *Freedom to Care: Liberalism, Dependency Care, and Culture*. London: Routledge, 2020.
Bhandary, Asha. 'Interpersonal Reciprocity', in *Caring for Liberalism: Dependency and Liberal Political Theory*, edited by Asha Bhandary and Amy R. Baehr, 145–67. New York: Routledge, 2021.
Bhandary, Asha. 'The Theory of Liberal Dependency Care: A Reply to my Critics', *Critical Review of International Social and Political Philosophy* 25, no. 6 (2021): 843–57.
Bhandary, Asha. 'Caring for Whom? Racial Practices of Care and Liberal Constructivism', *Philosophies* 7, no. 4 (2022), 78.
Bhandary, Asha. *Being at Home: Liberal Autonomy in an Unjust World*. Draft monograph in progress, n.d.
Bhandary, Asha, and Amy R. Baehr, editors. *Caring for Liberalism: Dependency and Liberal Political Theory*. London: Routledge, 2021.
Brake, Elizabeth. *Minimizing Marriage: Marriage, Morality, and the Law*. New York: Oxford University Press, 2012.
Brownlee, Kimberley. *Being Sure of Each Other: An Essay on Social Rights and Freedoms*. Oxford: Oxford University Press, 2020.
Bubeck, Diemut. *Care, Gender, and Justice*. Oxford: Clarendon Press, 1995.
Cudd, Ann E. *Analyzing Oppression*. New York: Oxford University Press, 2006.
Dowling, Emma. *The Care Crisis: What Caused It and How Can We End It?* New York: Verso Books, 2021.
Eichner, Maxine. 'The Free-Market Family. Liberalism, Families, and the Government's Responsibility to Regulate the Market', in *Caring for Liberalism: Dependency and Liberal Political Theory*, edited by Asha Bhandary and Amy R. Baehr, 238–65. New York: Routledge, 2021.
Engster, Daniel. *The Heart of Justice: Care Ethics and Political Theory*. New York: Oxford University Press, 2007.
Ferguson, Ann. *Blood at the Root: Motherhood, Sexuality and Male Dominance*. London: Pandora Press, 1989.
Fineman, Martha A. *The Autonomy Myth: A Theory of Dependency*. New York: New Press, 2004.
Frye, Marilyn. *The Politics of Reality: Essays in Feminist Theory*. Berkeley, CA: Crossing Press, 1983.

Gilligan, Carol. *In a Different Voice: Psychological Theory and Women's Development*. Cambridge, MA: Harvard University Press, 1982.
Hannah Arendt, The Human Condition, Chicago and London: University of Chicago Press, published in 1958, with a new foreword by Danielle Allen, 2018.
Haslanger, Sally. *Resisting Reality: Social Construction and Social Critique*. New York: Oxford University Press, 2012.
Held, Virginia. *The Ethics of Care: Personal, Political, and Global*. Oxford: Oxford University Press, 2006.
Hochschild, Arlie. 'Global Care Chains and Emotional Surplus Value', in *On the Edge: Living with Global Capitalism*, edited by Anthony Giddens and Will Hutton, 130–46. London: Jonathan Cape, 2000.
Honneth, Axel. *The Struggle for Recognition: The Moral Grammar of Social Conflicts*. Cambridge, MA: MIT Press, 1996.
hooks, bell. 'Racism and Feminism: The Issue of Accountability', in *Ain't I a Woman: Black Women and Feminism*, 2nd ed., 119–58. London: Routledge, 2014.
Khader, Serene. *Decolonizing Universalism: A Transnational Feminist Ethic*. New York: Oxford University Press, 2019.
Kittay, Eva F. *Love's Labor: Essays on Women, Equality and Dependency*. London: Routledge, 1999.
Lloyd, S. A. 'Toward a Liberal Theory of Sexual Equality', in *Varieties of Feminist Liberalism*, edited by Amy R. Baehr, 63–84. Lanham, MD: Rowman & Littlefield, 2004.
Lorde, Audre. *Sister Outsider: Essays and Speeches*. New York: Crossing Press, 1984.
Losurdo, Domenico. *Liberalism: A Counter-History*. Bologna: Verso Books, 2006.
Lugones, María. *Pilgrimages/Peregrinajes: Theorizing Coalition Against Multiple Oppressions*. Lanham, MD: Rowman & Littlefield, 2003.
Metz, Tamara. *Untying the Knot: Marriage, the State, and the Case for Their Divorce*. Princeton, NJ: Princeton University Press, 2010.
Meyers, Diana T. *Gender in the Mirror: Cultural Imagery and Women's Agency*. New York: Oxford University Press, 2002.
Mill, John S. 'On Liberty', in *On Liberty and Other Writings*, edited by Stefan Collini, 1–116. Cambridge: Cambridge University Press, 1989.
Mills, Charles W. *Black Rights/White Wrongs: The Critique of Racial Liberalism*. New York: Oxford University Press, 2017.
Narayan, Uma. *Dislocating Cultures: Identities, Traditions, and Third World Feminism*. New York: Routledge, 2013.
Okin, Susan. *Justice, Gender and the Family*. New York: Basic Books, 1989.
Rawls, John. 'Justice as Fairness', *The Philosophical Review* 67, no. 2 (1958): 164–94.
Roberts, Dorothy. *Shattered Bonds: The Color of Child Welfare*. New York: Basic Books, 2002.
Robeyns, Ingrid. 'Gender and the Metric of Justice', in *Measuring Justice: Primary Goods and Capabilities*, edited by Harry Brighouse and Ingrid Robeyns, 215–35. Cambridge: Cambridge University Press, 2010.
Rousseau, Jean-Jacques. *Discourse on the Origin of Inequality*. Amsterdam: Marc-Michel Rey, 1755.
Ruddick, Sara. *Maternal Thinking: Toward a Politics of Peace*. Boston, MA: Beacon Press, 1989.
Sandoval, Chela. *Methodology of the Oppressed*. Minneapolis: University of Minnesota Press, 2013.
Sommers, Timothy. 'What is the Point of Equality?', PhD diss., University of Iowa, 2021. ProQuest.

Spivak, Gayatri. 'Can the Subaltern Speak', in *Marxism and the Interpretation of Culture*, edited by Cary Nelson and Lawrence Grossberg, 267–310. London: Macmillan, 1988.
Stark, Cynthia A. 'Hypothetical Consent and Justification', *The Journal of Philosophy* 97, no. 6 (2000): 313–34.
Taylor, Charles. 'The Politics of Recognition', in *Multiculturalism: Examining the Politics of Recognition*, edited by Amy Gutmann, 25–73. Princeton, NJ: Princeton University Press, 1994.
Thomasson, Amie L. 'The Ontology of Social Groups', *Synthese* 196, no. 12 (2019): 4829–45.
Tronto, Joan C. *Moral Boundaries: A Political Argument for an Ethic of Care*. New York: Routledge, 1993.
Walker, Margaret U. *Moral Understandings: A Feminist Study in Ethics*, 2nd ed. New York: Oxford University Press, 2007.
Welch, Shay. *Existential Eroticism: A Feminist Approach to Understanding Women's Oppression-Perpetuating Choices*. Lanham, MD: Lexington Books, 2015.
Westlund, Andrea. 'Education for Autonomy, and for Care: A Comment on Asha Bhandary's Freedom to Care', *Critical Review of International Social and Political Philosophy* 25, no. 6 (2022): 820–6.
Young, Iris M. *Justice and the Politics of Difference*. Princeton, NJ: Princeton University Press, 1990.

CHAPTER EIGHT

Political perspectives on care

What can we learn from Nancy Fraser?

CHRISTINE NOËL LEMAITRE

INTRODUCTION

The ethics of care assumes a conception of persons as relational beings, rather than as the self-sufficient independent individuals of the dominant moral theories, which has significant consequences on its conception of politics. Care has been introduced in the field of politics, especially by Joan Tronto in the 1990s. According to her, feminist theories have not led to effective political change. Arguments based on 'women's morality' have proved ineffective, and care has remained confined to the private sphere, a domain attributed to women, and relegated to the rank of secondary activities. Since Machiavelli's thought, politics has been situated outside the domain of morality. Morality and politics are considered as two separate (but not necessarily opposite) orders and the specific virtue of politicians cannot be only assessed in the light of moral standards. The history of the relationship between morality and politics is indeed characterized by two different tendencies. For the first tradition, eminently illustrated by Platonic philosophy, politics must be conceived as a kind of enlarged morality. The aim of the politician must be to guarantee an organization that favours fair behaviour. For a second tradition initiated by Machiavelli, politics and morality are distinguished both by their ends and by their means. Since Machiavelli, philosophers have questioned the complexity of the links between politics and morality, opening up a range of theoretical positions, from the reduction of politics to a simple technology for exercising power (a position exemplified by Michel Foucault) to the development of institutions capable of sustaining pluralist democracy on the basis of a cross-referenced consensus (for Rawls). Fitting into the Aristotelian framework where morality and politics are closely intertwined, Tronto proposes a concept of care having the capacity to describe a moral and political version of the good life, thus escaping the dilemmas of seeing these as separate spheres. She points out that care can play both the role of a moral value and politically found a good society, and unpacks political implications of the ethics of care, seeing care as a political as well as moral ideal. The need for care would be 'the highest social goal'.[1] Following Tronto, Bubeck, Kittay and others argue that care must be seen as a public concern and not only relegated to the private responsibility of women or the arbitrariness of private charities.

However, if politics and morality must not be considered as separated areas of life and should become closely linked, if care is both a moral and a political concept, what does that imply? The thought of the American contemporary philosopher, Nancy Fraser, can help us to have a better understanding of the political stakes of the ethics of care. Nancy Fraser is the author of an abundant body of work, often produced in collaboration with others. Our contribution aims to offer a reading of the key concepts of Nancy Fraser's philosophy that could shed light on a conciliation between her thought and the theory of care under its political dimensions. Nancy Fraser teaches and develops research in political philosophy at the New School for Social Research in New York. Her work is rooted in the critical theory exemplified by Jürgen Habermas and Theodore Adorno. It is characterized by a wide range of themes, focuses on the political and social issues at stake in major contemporary debates, such as gender and feminism, diversity, the transnationalizing of the public sphere and comparisons between contemporary French and German philosophy. Her position is both militant (she has taken a stand in favour of feminism, against American intervention in the Vietnam War and in opposition to American imperialist policy) and theoretically productive, leading her to engage in dialogue with the founding texts of the history of philosophy and to renew its concepts. Criticizing the immobilism of 'armchair philosophers' who wish to remain outside contemporary political and social struggles, Nancy Fraser uses international comparisons to draw attention to the diversity of forms injustice takes, and the political responses that can be made to it.

8.1 NANCY FRASER, A CHEEKY PHILOSOPHER

Born in the United States, Nancy Fraser grew up in Baltimore, where her father came from an Eastern European Jewish family who emigrated to the United States, and her mother from an Irish family. She was a high-school student when the Civil Rights Act was passed, prohibiting discrimination on the basis of race or gender. Her parents, whom she describes as progressive liberals, made her aware of the problem of injustice. Nancy Fraser presented her choice to study philosophy as a way of rebelling against the 'superficial consumerism' that characterized the United States in the late 1960s. She entered the University in the midst of the Vietnam unrest, from 1965 to 1969, and immersed herself in activism, subscribing to Marxist thought. She recounts how, convinced that the great authors of the history of philosophy belonged to the bourgeois ideology against which she was in revolt, she decided, in a fit of anger, to sell all the philosophy books she had bought for her studies, and for five years threw herself into activism.

At the end of these five years, Nancy Fraser decided to come back to her studies and finished her studies in philosophy at New York University. She wrote her dissertation in the philosophy of history under the supervision of Peter Caws, a teacher interested in continental philosophy, structuralism and existentialism, in an American academic world largely dominated by analytic philosophy. Influenced by the work of Richard Rorty, she obtained several opportunities with his help to make her work better known. She wrote and published an abundant body of work: books as well as academic articles.

Nancy Fraser appears first as a feminist philosopher. She uses the term 'feminism' in a very broad sense. According to her, feminism refers to any 'thought or activism that defines itself as aiming to overcome: sexism, the subordination of women, male domination, patriarchy'. She thus opposes a sectarian definition of feminism insofar as what should count is that everyone can find the best way to advance the feminist cause, whatever path they choose. In *Fortunes of Feminism: From State-Managed Capitalism to Neoliberal Crisis*, Nancy Fraser analyses the different shapes of the feminist imaginary that have clashed since the 1950s. Her reading of American feminism unfolds in three acts.[2] The first act is an insurrectionary feminism that strives to make gender inequalities visible in order to combat them more effectively. The second act begins in the early 1980s with the emergence of neoliberalism and the questioning of policies for the redistribution of goods and resources. From this time onwards, feminists abandoned the economic dimension of gender justice to focus on identity-based demands, demanding recognition of their difference and embracing a neoliberal dynamic. Nancy Fraser characterizes this second act as a troubled period, during which feminism seems to have been tamed, so to speak. The third and final act in the history of feminism opens up new perspectives. The neoliberal crises of the 2000s are said to have prompted feminist movements to reinvest in the economic field, articulating their demands in this area with those unfolding in the cultural dimension of lack of recognition.

In her historical reading, Nancy Fraser discusses the arguments put forward by feminists, notably Julia Kristeva and 'culturalist feminists'. In her view, culturalist feminism comes up against three pitfalls. Firstly, culturalist feminists, who identify the majority of gender injustices from the symbolic order, would be locked into a narrow feminism. Furthermore, by focusing on the question of women's identity and subjectivity, they tend to overlook the many relations of domination that combine with the question of gender. Finally, by abandoning the economic explanation of social injustices in favour of a cultural reading, they have enabled neoliberals to recuperate certain feminist demands in order to legitimize the outdated nature of the welfare state.

We will synthesize in this chapter the main concepts used by Nancy Fraser to set up political consequences of the ethics of care: the androgenism of state capitalism, public space and the links between social justice and the need for recognition and parity.

8.2 ANDROGENISM AND STATE CAPITALISM

Nancy Fraser does not define *a priori* criteria for what is fair or unfair. She seeks to identify the causes that generate inequality and injustice by preventing the equitable distribution of resources. She sets out to unpack the grammar of social struggles. Her conception of social justice has its roots in the critical theory of Marx and the Frankfurt School. Critical theory aims to shed light on social relations of domination and exploitation, in order to foster the emancipation of dominated and exploited groups. Nancy Fraser contrasts critical theory with traditional theory in that it is guided by a practical and emancipatory interest. The focal point of her philosophy is the critique of institutionalized injustice.

From this perspective, she describes the institutionalization of androcentric views of family and work in state capitalism. Nancy Fraser points out that state capitalism has turned the male worker belonging to the ethnic majority into the average citizen: a head of household with a wife and children. It was also widely accepted that this worker's salary was his family's main income and often the only one. The gendered construction of the 'male family wage' had a dual function: to keep women out of public space and to legitimate male domination. In the 1950s and 1960s, however, the ideal of the family wage still served to define gender norms and call to order those who broke them, since it reinforced authority inside and outside. The political culture of state capitalism has in the same way concealed the social extent of unpaid care and reproductive work. One of the consequences of this culture has been to naturalize gender injustices and remove them from the realm of political contestation.

8.3 PUBLIC SPACE

Public space is the place where social identities are formed and expressed. Nancy Fraser criticizes the conception of public space as forged by the critical school and Jürgen Habermas in particular. Elaborated in 1962 in *Strukturwandel der Öffentlichkeit*, and reworked on numerous occasions by Habermas, the notion of public space refers to a network for communicating opinions. In the public sphere, communication flows are filtered and synthesized to form public opinions.[3] The image of a public space where citizens express themselves without any constraint because they live in a democracy is far too naive for Nancy Fraser. According to her, the problem lies not only in Jürgen Habermas's idealization of bourgeois public space, but also in his neglect of the study of other competing, non-liberal, non-bourgeois public spaces, leading him to idealize bourgeois public space, which remains his only point of reference. Taking the example of women and ethnic minorities, she points out that Habermas's conception of public space is dominated by bourgeois ideology, and thus characterized by underlying elementary forms of domination that are invisible at first glance. In this sense, she argues that 'the official public space was – and remains – the first institutional site for the construction of consent defining the new, hegemonic mode of domination'. As an alternative to this bourgeois public space, Nancy Fraser proposes another vision of public space that would include a plurality of parallel publics designated as 'subaltern counterpublics', producing as many counter-discourses of contestation to the dominant publics. These counter-discourses would constitute a necessary condition for the effectiveness of parity of participation.

The notion of public space appears to Fraser as a relevant instrument for analysing politics and the access of each type of citizen to the expression of their own views and interests. But she criticizes the way Habermas idealised bourgeois public space, and the way he doesn't see how this public space could exclude from its scope a set of actors such as women, who were deprived of the right to speak. Public space refers to a space within modern societies where political participation is mediated by language. Here, citizens can debate their common affairs. It is an institutionalized place of communicative interaction that differs from the state in that the discourses produced and exchanged can be critical of the state. The heart of Fraser's critique focuses on the work of historians and sociologists such as Joan Landes or Mary Ryan who consider that Habermas's interpretation tends to idealize public space, overlooking the exclusions in spite of which it functioned.

Joan Landes points out that the main axis of exclusion from public space was gender, since women's voices were not heard in this space. Women had no place there. Fraser picks up on Landes's analysis that the ethos of the new republican public space in France was deliberately constructed in opposition to the ethos of a more women-friendly 'salon culture', which republicans denounced as 'artificial', 'effeminate' and 'aristocratic'. This critique was accompanied by the promotion of an austere type of public discourse and behaviour, deemed 'rational', 'virtuous' and 'virile'. Thus, gendered and masculinist mental constructs were integrated into the very conception of republican public space, which had the effect, at the height of the Jacobin period, of officially excluding women from public life.[4] Fraser's common etymology of the terms 'public' and 'publicity' bears witness to the ancestral separation of the public and femininity. Indeed, in ancient times, it was necessary to have a penis in order to speak in public (incidentally, 'testimony' and 'testicle' also share a common etymology).

Fraser also draws on Mary Ryan's analyses, which highlight how nineteenth-century North American women from diverse classes and ethnic groups were able to gain access to public life despite their exclusion from the official public sphere.[5] Mary Ryan's works enable Fraser to show that the bourgeois public was never the public, and that the nineteenth century saw the emergence of a multitude of competing counterpublics: that of the nationalists, that of elite women and that of the working class.

Generally speaking, recent historiography suggests a much darker vision of the bourgeois public sphere than the one reflected in Habermas's work. The exclusions and conflicts that appeared in Habermas's work as incidental features now appear to be constitutive. The result is a shift that modifies the very meaning of public space. We can no longer assume that his liberal model was a utopian ideal that could not be realized; it was also an ideological notion that legitimized the emergence of class (and racial) domination. Fraser does not entirely invalidate the Habermasian reading of recent historiography. For her, contemporary work does not discredit 'the' concept of public space per se, but it does call into question his conception of public space. By pointing out the mechanisms by which opinion is produced in the public arena, Nancy Fraser highlights the obstacles faced by the dominated in making their voices heard. The dominated are not always directly prevented from expressing their opinion, but they can also become convinced that they have no opinion worthy of public expression. Care therefore means becoming aware of these multiple forms of exclusion so that everyone can free their voice.

8.4 SOCIAL JUSTICE

Social justice unfolds in three distinct spheres: the economic order, where it concerns the distribution of resources; the cultural order, where it takes the form of recognition; and the political order, where it concerns representation. Within each order, inequalities take the form of specific injustices. Economic injustices result from inequitable distribution, which can take various forms, such as exploitation or the appropriation of surplus value by the dominant class,[6] marginalization, which means being relegated to back-breaking, low-paid jobs, or destitution, which is the absence of sufficient resources to live decently. Cultural injustice refers to cultural domination, i.e. the imposition of a cultural model that differs from one's culture of origin, and non-recognition, which renders certain people invisible to dominant groups. Lastly, political injustices are generated by a denial of representation, which can result in the inadequate representation of certain minorities who are not allowed to participate fully in political life, or in the exclusion of certain people due to political frameworks limited to the national territory.

According to Nancy Fraser, social justice refers less to the equal distribution of material wealth than to the participation of all concerned in debates for the design and implementation of an equitable distribution of wealth within society, as well as the recognition and representation of the diversities involved. Working for social justice means fighting on three fronts to remove the institutionalized obstacles that give rise to inequitable distribution, denial of recognition and lack of representation. These obstacles deprive the people concerned of resources, recognition and the opportunity to express themselves. They are placed in a position where they cannot fully participate in the debates that lead to the recognition of their claims.

According to Nancy Fraser, the fundamental injustice characterizing contemporary society is no longer the exploitation of one class over another but cultural domination. Economic and social injustice has, according to her, been supplanted by symbolic injustice, which consists in seeking to impose a social model on a diversity of actors. 'Claims for economic equality are less salient today in the knowledge society than in the Fordist heyday of the Keynesian welfare state.'[7] This reading of Nancy Fraser could lead us to regard her as naive and out of touch with reality. Can she really ignore the fact that, even in developed countries, between 10 and 20 per cent of the population is forced to live below the poverty line? Can she ignore the fact that the globalized world economy functions thanks to the exploitation of a large, if not majority, part of the population located in developing countries, where child labour is permitted and the exploitation of wage earners the law? Nancy Fraser does not claim that our world is free from all forms of economic exploitation but that the need for recognition has transformed the nature of the political and social demands of our time. Victims of injustice would sometimes suffer as much from economic injustice as from a denial of recognition.

8.5 THE NEED FOR RECOGNITION AND PARITY

Nancy Fraser argues that recognition is a matter of justice and that its denial is 'a matter of public and verifiable manifestations of obstacles to full membership in society imposed on some people, and these obstacles are morally indefensible, whether or not they distort subjectivity'.[8]

The need for recognition can lead actors who feel aggrieved or unrecognized to claim their specificity in order to assert their right to break away from the social model or norms (this is the case, for example, with women who may wish to realize their potential outside the dominant model of the accomplished mother) or, on the contrary, to deny their specificity insofar as it may be stigmatizing (this is the case with homosexual couples claiming the right to benefit from adoption or medically assisted procreation possibilities in the same way as heterosexual couples). Moreover, the same actor may want to both claim and deny his or her specificity, depending on whether it deprives him or her of the freedom to exist as he or she wishes, or deprives him or her of certain rights. To overcome this tension, Nancy Fraser proposes associating recognition with status rather than identity. What should be recognized in the public space is not so much individual or collective identity, but rather the status of a full partner. Recognizing the other as my partner in a social interaction means considering them as my peer in the public space, and that they should not be prevented from participating in social life.

To remedy injustice, barriers to participation must be removed. Parity of participation also requires certain conditions to be met: (1) objective conditions, relating to the distribution of material resources ensuring 'participants independence and the opportunity to express themselves'; (2) intersubjective conditions, embodied in cultural models characterized by 'equal respect for all participants and ensuring equality of opportunity in the pursuit of social esteem'; and (3) political conditions that include all those affected by injustices, subject to specific deliberations, which must take place according to fair.[9]

While many countries have taken up the issue of parity, and in particular gender parity, by imposing quotas designed to promote the balanced participation of women in various private bodies (such as boards of directors) or public bodies (such as certain institutions) not only for reasons of justice and equity, but also to ensure that women's voices are heard, Nancy Fraser proposes an alternative approach of parity, more qualitative. According to her, parity is not a matter of numbers. Requiring women to make up half of electoral lists is not the alpha and omega of parity. Parity cannot just be about representation. Thinking about an integration of care into politics should lead us to take into account three dimensions of domination: economic distribution, cultural and legal recognition, and political representation. And it should be applied to all aspects of social life, not just political institutions (from labour markets, sexual relations, family life, public spheres and also civil society associations).

According to Sandra Laugier and Pascale Molinier, '*care* has thus introduced ethical issues into politics, undermining the apparently obvious link between an ethics of justice and political liberalism'.[10] Care ethics are based on the concept of an ontologically vulnerable and relational moral subject. While care theories emphasize the moral importance of concern for others, the effectiveness of care ethics depends on importing concern for others, including their weakness and vulnerability, into the political sphere as part of the preservation of a shared world. Nancy Fraser's work thus contributes to the integration of the principles of care into politics. This integration presupposes a rethinking of the notion of social justice, the notion of recognition and the very organization of the public arena, so that voices stifled or minoritized by gender, social class, health condition or race can express themselves and be heard. If, since the Greeks, politics has meant speaking out and exchanging freely formed opinions, concern for others must lead us to ensure the conditions for a political debate in which every voice counts. Nancy Fraser's work is part of this drive to alert us to the transformations needed to ensure that the ethic of care does not remain wishful thinking.

NOTES

1. Joan C. Tronto, *Moral Boundaries: A Political Argument for an Ethic of Care* (New York: Routledge, 1993), 175.
2. Nancy Fraser, *Fortunes of Feminism: From State-Managed Capitalism to Neoliberal Crisis* (London: Verso, 2013).
3. Jürgen Habermas, *Strukturwandel der Öffentlichkeit: Untersuchungen zu einer Kategorie der bürgerlichen Gesellschaft* (Frankfurt am Main: Suhrkamp, 1962).
4. Joan B. Landes, *Women and the Public Sphere in the Age of the French Revolution* (Ithaca, NY: Cornell University Press, 1988).
5. See: Mary P. Ryan, *Women in Public: Between Banners and Ballots, 1825–1880* (Baltimore, MD: Johns Hopkins University Press, 1990); Mary P. Ryan, 'Gender and Public Access: Women's Politics in Nineteenth-Century America', in *Habermas and the Public Sphere*, ed. Craig Calhoun (Cambridge, MA: MIT Press, 1992), 259–88.
6. Nancy Fraser, 'From Redistribution to Recognition? Dilemmas of Justice in a "Post-Socialist" Age', *New Left Review* 212 (1995): 68–93.
7. Nancy Fraser, 'Social Justice in the Knowledge Society: Redistribution, Recognition, and Participation', paper presented at the Gut zu Wissen Conference, Heinrich Böll Stiftung, 2001.
8. Nancy Fraser, 'Social Justice in the Age of Identity Politics: Redistribution, Recognition, and Participation', in *Culture and Economy after the Cultural Turn* (SAGE Publications, 1999), 25–52.

9. See: Fraser, 'Social Justice in the Age of Identity Politics'; Nancy Fraser, 'Reframing Global Justice', *New Left Review* 36 (2005): 69–88.
10. Sandra Laugier and Pascale Molinier, 'Politiques du care', *Multitudes* 37–38, no. 2–3 (2009): 74.

BIBLIOGRAPHY

Fraser, Nancy. 'From Redistribution to Recognition? Dilemmas of Justice in a "Post-Socialist" Age', *New Left Review* 212 (1995): 68–93.

Fraser, Nancy. 'Social Justice in the Age of Identity Politics: Redistribution, Recognition, and Participation', in *Culture and Economy after the Cultural Turn*, 25–52. SAGE Publications, 1999.

Fraser, Nancy. 'Social Justice in the Knowledge Society: Redistribution, Recognition, and Participation', paper presented at the Gut zu Wissen Conference, Heinrich Böll Stiftung, 2001.

Fraser, Nancy. 'Reframing Global Justice', *New Left Review* 36 (2005): 69–88.

Habermas, Jürgen. *Strukturwandel der Öffentlichkeit: Untersuchungen zu einer Kategorie der bürgerlichen Gesellschaft*. Frankfurt am Main: Suhrkamp, 1962.

Landes, Joan B. *Women and the Public Sphere in the Age of the French Revolution*. Ithaca, NY: Cornell University Press, 1988.

Laugier, Sandra, and Pascale Molinier. 'Politiques du care', *Multitudes* 37–38, no. 2–3 (2009): 74–5.

Ryan, Mary P. *Women in Public: Between Banners and Ballots, 1825–1880*. Baltimore, MD: Johns Hopkins University Press, 1990.

Ryan, Mary P. 'Gender and Public Access: Women's Politics in Nineteenth-Century America', in *Habermas and the Public Sphere*, edited by Craig Calhoun, 259–88. Cambridge, MA: MIT Press, 1992.

Tronto, Joan C. *Moral Boundaries: A Political Argument for an Ethic of Care*. New York: Routledge, 1993.

CHAPTER NINE

Care, justice and equality

COSTANZA PORRO

INTRODUCTION

The relationship between care and justice has been at the centre of the literature on the ethics of care since its very beginning. Care ethics was originally conceived and presented by some of its most prominent advocates as an alternative to the justice perspective, namely as an approach centred around considerations other than those usually foregrounded by traditional, mostly liberal, approaches to moral and political theory. In this chapter, I provide a conceptual map of the relationship between care and justice as it has been understood by care theorists. From the initial opposition between care and justice, in recent scholarship there have been a number of more conciliatory proposals, including attempts to provide care-centred accounts of justice, often drawing on the framework of John Rawls's theory of justice. In reconstructing the relationship between care and justice, I also shed light on care theorists' understanding of the notion of justice. Another aim of this chapter is to reflect on the relationship between care and equality. As equality is typically understood as one of the core values of the justice perspective, care and equality have also often been seen in opposition to each other. Theorists of care, with the notable exception of Eva Kittay, have not paid sufficient attention to the relationship between care and equality. In the final part of this chapter, drawing from Kittay's work on care and equality, I identify some new directions of inquiry that those interested in developing an integrated approach to care, justice and equality should pursue.

9.1 CARE AS AN ALTERNATIVE TO JUSTICE

The ethics of care was initially presented as an alternative to what theorists of care called the justice approach.[1] As the original focus of theorists of care was moral theory, early theorists of care aimed to show that care ethics was bringing to the forefront a set of concerns which had traditionally been neglected in moral theorizing. It was, in other words, a distinctive and distinct approach to moral theory. The idea of the ethics of care as an alternative to the ethics of justice was originally developed starting from the observations of psychologist Carol Gilligan,[2] who identified a distinctive approach to moral theory in many of the women she interviewed for her studies.[3]

Before looking at the way in which early theorists of care conceived the relationship between care and justice, it is worth discussing their understanding of the justice approach. First, early theorists of care often refer to justice meaning an ethics of justice, as a particular approach to moral theory. Under the heading of the justice approach, they grouped together two different families of moral theories: deontological and especially

Kantian approaches, and consequentialist and utilitarian approaches. These were the dominant approaches to moral theory at the time and remain very influential today. Rather than focusing on the differences between these two families of theories, which was the object of much discussion in moral philosophy, theorists of care pointed out their similarities, the elements that they have in common that the ethics of care rejected, or at least de-emphasized.

The core idea defended by theorists of care was not that the ethics of care and the ethics of justice are opposites or mirror-images of one another, with justice uncaring and care unjust. Instead, these perspectives embody different ways of organizing the basic elements of morality and moral judgement: self, others and the relationship between them. The ethics of justice is a rationalistic ethics which regards moral reason as the best guide in our moral decision making. On the contrary, the ethics of care values the role that emotions have in the process of trying to understand what would be morally best for us to do and be. Relatedly, traditional moral theories endorse a style of reasoning that is abstract: moral theory is organized around universal principles that apply in all the relevant cases. This is seen as helpful for making sure that our moral decision making is impartial, as impartiality is a core value for these theories. The ethics of care recommends instead that we choose in a situated and contextual manner and regards the claims of particular others with whom we share actual relationships as paramount. For an ethics of care, meeting the needs of particular others that we are responsible for has primary moral salience and relationships are the source of our main moral obligations.

So far, we have mainly focused on moral theory; however, it is not hard to see how many of these considerations are also relevant for political theory. While, as we have seen, the theorizing on care started in moral philosophy, in recent decades an increasing number of care theorists have shifted their focus to political theory, arguing that care and the care perspective should be seen as having a central role in how we think about politics. A similar dichotomy between care and justice also arose in the domain of political theory; here, the main targets are traditional liberal theories of justice. Proponents of the ethics of care endorse a different conception of the person that the one traditionally endorsed by liberalism. For the ethics of care, individuals are not self-sufficient equal parties to a social contract primarily concerned with their own interests and freedoms understood in negative terms, as in their description of the liberal model. Instead, individuals are understood as relational beings, enmeshed in relationships with others, on which they depend and for which they have responsibility. The revaluing and the focus of relationality and dependence is related to a longstanding preoccupation of feminist philosophy to dispose of the liberal distinction between the private and the public domain to bring to the foreground and address some of the most pressing gender inequalities, especially in caregiving.

The picture of the self attributed to liberal theorists by early proponents of the ethics of care might seem an unfair characterization of, at least some, contemporary liberal theories of justice. This criticism is in part valid; however, two points are worth making as partial replies to it. First, contemporary theories of justice have benefited from cross pollination with the ethics of care and other approaches in feminist philosophy and other traditions such that, compared to the state of the literature in the 1980s and 1990s, they are much more hospitable to some of the concern of the ethics of care around, for instance, relationality and vulnerability.[4] Thus, the early criticisms of the liberal tradition were more fitting at the time than they are now. Further, and despite this, some elements of this picture, such as the idea of the social contract and society as a fair and mutually beneficial enterprise of social cooperation among free and equal citizens, do remain true for many contemporary liberal theories of justice. Precisely for this reason, as I will discuss in more detail in Section 9.3.1, these remain the object of discussion and potential criticism for those aiming to develop a liberal theory of justice with care at its centre.

In this section, we have seen how theorists of care initially understood the care perspective as a distinctive and separate approach from traditional moral and political theories. In what follows, I discuss the subsequent developments in the relationship between care and justice in political philosophy.

9.1.1 Subsuming justice under care

So far, we have seen how proponents of the ethics of care originally conceived their approach to moral and political philosophy as distinct from traditional liberal theories. For these theories, care cannot be simply incorporated by justice. Further, they argue that the care perspective is in some ways superior to the justice approach as it is more truthful to the human experience and captures moral and political considerations that are more pressing and significant. For some theorists, especially in the early days of ethics of care, care should replace justice altogether as the central concept of morality because an ethics of care would be sufficient on its own.[5] Not many care theorists share this view and argue that the justice perspective should have no place in our theorizing; however, they often see the care approach as in some sense more fundamental.

Arguing that the care perspective should replace the justice perspective is not the only way to articulate the superiority of care over justice. Another possibility is to suggest that the care approach is superior because many of the considerations of justice can be subsumed under the heading of care. Hence, the care approach is more capacious than the justice perspective. Going even further, one might argue that many concerns that are typically understood under the lens of justice can be better dealt with by care ethics.[6] In other words, we can better make sense of some of our existing commitments that we often articulate in liberal terms using the resources of care theory. This in many cases will also allow to develop a normatively superior version of such commitments. Michael Slote argues that this is the case by presenting an ethics of care centred around empathy, which, he maintains, is not necessarily limited to those who are near and dear but can be cultivated to be directed towards those who are distant from us. First, Slote claims that one of the core commitments of liberal justice, that to respect, is better understood as a form of emphatic understanding of others and their perspective rather than mere liberal toleration regardless of how repugnant one finds other people's views to be. Further, he contends that commitment such as that to the welfare of the worst off or democracy are best conceived as grounded in empathy. Finally, and he takes this to be the strongest argument in favour of his view, Slote argues that care ethics gives us better answers than liberalism on a range of important issues hence providing a better account of the foundations of justice. Discussing cases as diverse as free speech and restraining orders Slote claims that the liberal focus on autonomy and basic liberties leads to incorrect responses to these issues which would not follow from an empathy-based care perspective which focuses on people's welfare.

In presenting this view, it is important to distinguish it from another view that is sometimes defended by care theorists which I will discuss in Section 9.3, namely the idea that justice is in some senses grounded in care because it is the fact that we care for others that is the reason why we are committed to justice in the first place. Slote also endorses this claim but goes a step further claiming that our political commitments are not just motivated or grounded in care – empathy in his terminology – but rather than our whole approach to politics is better understood and should be refashioned under a care ethics framework. Possible objections to this approach include pointing out that even if we grant that all of our political concerns could be captured by the care perspective, it seems more natural to understand them as grounded in a variety of different values, some of which belonging to the justice perspective. For instance, concerns around freedom of speech appear to be more naturally grounded in the value of freedom, rather than that of care. It is true that freedom is not the only value to be taken into account when thinking about questions of freedom of speech, including limits to freedom to speech, and other values such as respect and concern for others should also play a role. However, it is precisely this commitment to pluralism that might make us wary of Slote's approach. While empathy and care can help us in understanding and grounding a variety of our concerns, it might be hard to believe that they can alone be the basis of all our commitments.

9.2 THE SEPARATE DOMAINS APPROACH

The idea that the liberal approach to justice does not have much to offer and that all our justice commitments are best understood under the care framework is rejected by many of the more recent contributions to this debate, which often attempt to, at least partly, reconcile the two perspectives in a way that does not reduce all the concerns of justice to the care approach. They argue that the justice perspective has its own contribution to make and values such as fairness and equality cannot simply be translated in the language of care. The importance of justice is acknowledged not only in general terms but also by reflecting on the relevance that this perspective and of concepts and values such as equality, rights and autonomy have for feminist philosophy in dealing with gender injustice, including in the domain of caregiving.[7] This was partly the result of learning from other traditions within feminist moral and political philosophy which heavily draw on the resources of the liberal justice perspective.

An interesting attempt in the direction of combining care and justice has been proposed by Virginia Held.[8] Held maintains that care and justice are compatible. For her, like for other theorists of care, care is the most basic value as it is the very precondition of human life and the continuation of society. She argues that a lot of human life, and good human life too, goes on without justice but could not go on without care. While the ethics of care is the more comprehensive moral framework and network, justice can be the chief value in some domains, such as the law. The idea is that different domains have different chief values, which does not mean that the other value cannot play any role, but it is always the former that has priority in that domain. In this way, against the background of a net of caring relationships, which are crucial for justice, it is possible to construe some of our political ideals and demands, and some of the ways in which we relate to each other, using the resources of liberal theories of justice.

Importantly, contrary to what some critics of Held have argued,[9] this does not amount to saying that justice is the chief value in the public sphere and care in the private one, thereby following the problematic distinction between private and public that many feminist theorists wish to abandon. After all, Held is one of the main proponents of the idea that care is a public value and caring attitudes and concerns should inform a variety of relationships and domains beyond the intimate realm. To give an example, for Held, relationships of care in civil society play a crucial role in shaping our societies and are a precondition of justice. More broadly, the care perspective recommends rethinking the primary aim of our societies, moving from a model mainly preoccupied with economic gain and individual interests to one in which the promotion of care and caring relationships are our chief concerns. Caring considerations might be a better guide than considerations of justice in deciding, for instance, how extensive markets should be.[10] Against this backdrop, however, there is still a role for (liberal) justice to play.

A possible criticism to Held's idea that justice and care occupy a primary role in different domains is that it is in tension with one of the most attractive aspects of Held's proposal, the idea that care considerations can be brought to bear in domains that are usually not seen as domains in which care plays a significant role, such as the law, policing and the military. It is not clear which role considerations of care can play in domains in which justice is the chief value and whether considerations of justice should always prevail when the two are in tension. The separate domains approach makes it rather difficult to establish the relative weight of different values in different domains. More broadly, keeping the two values separate prevents us from seeing that they should be brough to bear on each other, as argued by a number of other theorists of care.

9.3 THE ENMESHING OF CARE AND JUSTICE

While recognizing the importance of justice, at least in some domains, Held's approach does not seek to truly combine care and justice but considers them separate approaches. Other theorists of care have instead opted for a different approach to the relationship between the two perspectives arguing, first, that care and justice are essential to each other and, second, that they can be combined in a unitary theory.

Starting with the first claim, different authors have argued that justice and care, rather than belonging to different domains, are essential for each other. Care is instrumental to justice in a variety of ways. First, care is essential for the creation of citizens, as without care children cannot grow up into fully fledged members of the community, as well as for looking after existing citizens. Second, care is also central for the development and sustaining of moral virtues necessary for being a member of a political community.[11] This is the case, first and foremost, if we think about care for children which is an exercise aimed at their moral development, including their acquisition of these virtues. However, this is also true of wider relationships of care between adults, including relationships of care in civil society, which promote attitudes such as trust and cohesion, which are key for the functioning of our societies and the promotion of justice.[12] It has also been argued that care is not only instrumental but also constitutive of justice. First, this is the case because people's willingness to do what justice requires even in the face of significant sacrifice can only be ensured if people are committed to a certain degree of caring for others. This is an argument which looks at care and empathy as background moral motivation for justice. Further, it has also been suggested that, for the models of justice which, like John Rawls's theory of justice, rely on the idea of deliberation on the principles of justice under conditions of ignorance about one's social position and one's other socially salient features, care and the ability to emphatically imagine others' situation is essential for making deliberation possible in the first place.[13] Finally, care might also play a constitutive role in justice when it comes to applying principles of justice to specific situations as this requires a form of contextual and situated moral deliberation as well as attitudes such as sensitivity and attentiveness to other people's needs, the very same skills and attitudes which are central to the ethics of care.[14]

If, as we have seen, care is essential to justice, there are various ways in which care relies on justice. A fair distribution of resources and burdens in society, which also applies to the resources needed for caring for others and the burden of caregiving, are essential for caregivers to be put in the best conditions to provide care while at the same time being able to care for themselves.[15] Further, injustice tends to injure caring because as socialization is part of caring, especially of caring for children, caring in unjust circumstances often requires caregivers to impose on those who they take care of unfair expectations as these are in line with prevailing social norms. Finally, justice can make care better because regarding those we care for also as autonomous agents, or at least as autonomous agents in the making, might rein in the tendency of care towards excessive paternalism.[16]

While what has been said so far is helpful in providing a fuller picture of the relationship between care and justice, it does not yet amount to developing an integrated political theory in which care and justice both play a role. After a brief discussion of the nature of care, I dedicate the rest of this section to the discussion of some such attempts.

9.3.1 What Is care?

Before presenting different approaches to combining justice and care, it is worth briefly discussing different understandings of care adopted by those reflecting on the relationship between justice and care. One of the most significant divides is that between those who adopt a narrow and those who opt for a broad definition of care. The former focus on dependency care: care aimed at meeting the needs of dependents. This kind of care is hands-on care for those who cannot meet their basic needs on their own and with whom we stand in relationships of dependence.[17] Paradigmatic examples of this are care for babies and children, care for those who are ill or live with severe disabilities and, in case they require it, the elderly. The lack of this kind of care typically results in significant and immediate harm as those who receive it depend on it for meeting the most basic needs. Proponents of the narrow understanding of care argue that dependency care is the kind of care that we should focus on when thinking about the role of care in our political arrangements for three main reasons. First, they rightly see this kind of care as a matter of basic survival rather than only flourishing.[18] While dependency care is also essential for the development of capacities and for people's flourishing, the significance of this care is first and foremost grounded in the fact that its recipients cannot meet their basic needs without it. Second, they argue that this kind of care, especially when it comes to care for babies and children, is necessary for the continuation of society over time, and hence is key from a societal point of view. Thirdly, they argue it is key in the promotion of justice. Fourth, because this is the kind of care which is most crucial for care receivers and most burdensome for caregivers, they argue dependency care arrangements are the source of the most urgent inequalities, both when it comes to who receives and who provides care, as providers of dependency care typically come from the same, and otherwise disadvantaged, social groups, such as women, and especially working-class, migrant and racialized women.[19] Many of the proponents of liberal accounts of care that we will discuss in Section 9.3.3 endorse a narrow definition of care.

Proponents of the broad account of care agree on the political significance of dependency care but argue that the exclusive focus on it is problematic because it misses some other care-related normatively significant phenomena that are often neglected but should be captured by political theorists. Many political theorists of care aim to show that care is not just important in the domain of close relationships where most dependency care takes place but in more distant ones as well and that the care perspective should be brought to bear to very different domains of society.[20] Further, proponents of the broad account worry that such a narrow definition of care makes it more easily dismissible as episodic, as it only affects people at discrete stages of their lives, such as infancy, and in particular conditions, such as illness. This, together with the fact that it is most commonly carried out in the private domain of the home, makes it easier to think of dependency care as a private responsibility of individuals and families, rather than a common responsibility.[21] Theorists in this camp do not share a common definition of care but present different alternatives. Two of the most prominent ones are Tronto and Fisher's and Engster's accounts of care. Tronto and Fisher define caring 'as a species activity that includes everything that we do to maintain, continue, and repair our "world" so that we can live in it as well as possible. That world includes our bodies, ourselves, and our environment, all of which we seek to interweave in a complex, life-sustaining web.'[22] In his recent work,[23] Engster defines care as a response to vulnerability, understood as susceptibility to harm, need, loss, coercion, domination and other unwanted ills.[24] One of the problems of such broad definitions of care, according to their critics, is that they are excessively broad to the point of losing sight of the distinctiveness of care. Further, one might worry that these definitions of care end up capturing normative considerations that are better accounted for by other values. For instance, Engster's account of care includes concerns and phenomena like susceptibility to domination and coercion that might be better understood as concerns of equality or freedom.

9.3.2 Care as the heart of justice

The first way to combine care and justice in a unitary theory that I will discuss has been proposed by Daniel Engster.[25] In his earlier work, Engster understands care as 'everything we do directly to help individuals meet their vital biological needs, develop and maintain their basic capabilities, and avoid or alleviate unnecessary and unwanted pain and suffering, so that they can survive, develop and function in society'.[26] This definition of care is narrower than the one centred around vulnerability discussed in the last section but still broader than the notion of dependency care as it is not exclusively focused on those with whom we stand in relationships of dependency. This narrower definition is in line with Engster's approach to the relationship between care and justice. He argues that care is integral to liberal justice because it is its core, its heart. Attending to the needs of care is central to the functioning of society and the aims and virtue of caring precede and underlie all theories of justice. Society should be organized first and foremost around the goal of supporting care practices and ensuring adequate care for all. Care represents the most minimal, and hence pressing, core of justice; there is more to justice than care because the care perspective only establishes a minimal set of moral principles that apply to all and are targeted at the meeting of basic needs, the development of basic capabilities and the alleviation of unwanted suffering. If we imagine the metaphor of concentric circles, care represents the inner one which is contained by the wider circle of justice. The wider circle of justice contains other principles and commitments, including those of the liberal tradition but also feminist concerns that go beyond the care. Because of his emphasis on care creating a set of minimal requirements, Engster understands his view of the relationship between care and justice as closer to the theorizing on needs, rather than as a comprehensive and perfectionist approach. From his account of the relationship between care and justice, Engster derives a set of principles that a caring government must follow as well as implications for domains like economic justice and international relations.

Compared to other accounts of the role of care in the political domain, such as Held's approach, Engster is more minimalistic. Precisely because of this, it can be criticized for failing to see how taking care seriously can lead to a much more profound rethinking of our societies beyond the principle of meeting vital biological needs and developing basic capacities.[27]

9.3.3 Liberal care: Rawls and the primary goods

Engster's account of care as the heart of justice has not been the only attempt to combine justice and care in a unitary theory. Other authors have also aimed to show that care is integral to justice. Proponents of this approach argue that care should be added to the list of goods that should be provided to people as a matter of justice, which would already amount to a significant reshaping of existing theories of justice. Many such proposals have focused on a particularly influential liberal theory of justice: John Rawls's account. Famously, Eva Kittay presents a series of challenges to Rawls's theory, based on his failure to take care, and especially dependency care, into account in his theory of justice.[28] Among her main worries is the exclusion from the boundaries of justice of dependents and those who live with significant cognitive disability in light of, respectively, their inability to contribute to society and the lack of certain capacities, necessary, for Rawls, to qualify as a person. For Rawls, individuals are free and equal in virtue of the possession of the two moral powers: the capacity for a conception of the good, i.e. the capacity to form, revise and pursue one's conception of what a worthwhile human life is; and the capacity for a sense of justice, i.e. the capacity to understand, apply and be moved to act from the principles of justice. Further, Rawls fails to acknowledge the dependencies and vulnerabilities experienced by caregivers in virtue of their role, precisely because he does not centre care and its proviso in his analysis. Kittay is also critical of the way in which liberal justice is grounded in the social contract model understood as a voluntary association. The voluntariness of our obligations does not reflect the nature of our obligations towards others, especially when it comes to relationships of care. Despite the significant criticisms, Kittay argues that Rawls's theory can be revised to incorporate issues of care and proposes two main amendments to his theory. First, she argues that next to the two moral powers we should introduce a third moral power – the capacity to care – as part of the conception of the person. Second, and following from this, she adds a sixth primary good besides the ones identified by Rawls – the primary good of care, understood as being cared for when unable to care for oneself as well as the means to meet the dependency needs of others without unduly sacrificing oneself. These amendments lead to a profound revision of Rawls's theory when it comes to the conception of the person and of society, including his idea of cooperation as mutual benefit.

Questions have been raised as to whether such amendments combined with other commitments of Rawls's account constitute a coherent theory and are overall desirable.[29] For Bhandary, Kittay's addition of a third moral power is misguided as it is in tension with the core Rawlsian idea of the representative of the parties being mutually disinterested. Further, Bhandary sees Kittay's criticism of the Rawlsian notion of a person being the source of self-authenticating valid claims as problematic because it concedes too much to the idea that caregivers' independent needs are largely eclipsed by those of their dependents. Bhandary contends that this is a state of affairs which often is the result of the caregivers' role but is not one that a theory should endorse. The criticism of Kittay's rejection of the idea of individuals as self-authenticating sources of valid claims echoes other sound critiques of Kittay's model of the transparent self.[30] Bhandary's commitment to this element of Rawls's theory is motivated by her concern for people's autonomy and the exploitation to which caregivers are often subjected. From this starting point, she presents her own view of how Rawlsian liberal justice can incorporate many of the concerns of care theory. She proposes two main amendments to the Rawlsian framework: the addition of care as a basic human fact that characterizes the circumstances of justice because it is a core interest of all of us to receive care; and of a sixth primary good which, unlike Kittay's, is focused only on the receipt of care. The fact that society needs to be organized in such a way that it can provide care for all already leads to a substantial rethinking of justice. Further, Bhandary proposes a number of principles aimed at ensuring that, first, those who care for others are not disadvantaged as a result of their role and, second, that those who occupy caregiving roles are not coming from the same, and often otherwise disadvantaged, social groups. These principles reflect her concern not only for the conditions of caregivers but also for the ways in which the allocation of caregiving roles in our societies reflects and exacerbates gender, racial, class and other inequalities. Overall, Bhandary's account is closer to Rawls as she wishes to preserve many of its core features, such as the commitment to reciprocity and productive contributions and the exclusion of those with significant cognitive disabilities from the original position in virtue of their lack of certain capacities as well as the modelling of the parties of the original position as mutually disinterested. Her commitment to the idea of reciprocity is motivated by a concern about existing care arrangements in our society and especially the observation that those belonging to privileged social groups believe they are entitled to care without needing to reciprocate it. Overall, her intention to maintain the normative focus on individuals and their needs, rather than reducing it to relations situates her theory squarely in the liberal tradition.

Elizabeth Brake goes even a step further and suggest that it is possible to incorporate considerations of care within Rawls's framework with very little modification to it.[31] She argues that care should be seen as one of the primary goods insofar as it is needed to pursue one's life plans and for developing and exercising the moral powers. Brake contends that that is the case not only when it comes to dependency care, and especially care for children, which can be easily seen as key in developing the moral powers, but also when we take into account caring relationships between independent adults because a small number of stable caring relationships are crucial for our mental health and our self-respect which in turn are essential for the moral powers. Amy Baher also proposes to amend Rawls's theory to include considerations of care.[32] Her amendments are more in line with Kittay's approach and hence more substantial than those suggested by Bhandary and Brake.

While all these four authors believe that a liberal Rawlsian account of justice, albeit altered, can incorporate considerations of care, their disagreements reflect different understandings of which elements of the theory can and should be kept when developing a care-based account of liberal justice.

9.4 CARE AND EQUALITY

So far, we have seen different ways to understand the relationship between justice and care. In what remains of the chapter, I explore the relationship between care and equality. The question of the relationship between care and equality has not attracted much attention among care theorists for a number of reasons. First, equality is understood as one of the core values of the justice perspective; hence, if one thinks of care and justice as alternative approaches, it follows that one would regard equality and care as distinct if not in tension with each other. Second, care theorists conceive of relationships often not as relationships between independent equals but rather as relationships between interdependent unequals, modelled on care relationships.[33] As we have seen, they criticize what they consider the liberal fiction of a society of equals for masking the unavoidable dependency and need of care that we all experience at difference points of our lives. Further, they stress that inequalities of power and in certain cases capacities are ubiquitous in relationships of care which points to a different model of the person than the independent self-sufficient equal. Does it follow from this fact that we should refrain from regarding people as equals in moral status, if not power and capacities, as well as understanding equality as a key concept and consideration for care theorists?

That conclusion is rather too hasty. After all, a number of theorists of care, especially those who aim to develop a care-centred theory of justice, do discuss issues of equality, especially when it comes to questions of inequalities related to the allocation of caring responsibilities.[34] However, they often limit their discussion to these kinds of issues. In line with his minimal approach discussed in Section 9.3.2, Engster argues that care theory should not be seen as supporting a fully egalitarian society; in his view, questions of women's equality, let alone equality more generally, will be addressed by care theory only when they concern the allocation of care responsibilities and the social recognition of care.[35] In other words, Engster does not believe that a more systematic account of the relationship between equality and care, or an integrated approach to care and equality, should be developed. In line with her separate domains approach, Held defends a similar conclusion.[36] Among care theorists, Eva Kittay is the only one who has developed a more systematic account of the relationship between care and equality.[37]

9.4.1 Kittay's approach to equality

Kittay starts her reflection on the relationship between care and equality from two main ideas. First, as I have in part anticipated in Section 9.3.3, there is the idea that dependency care should be central to our understanding of justice but is obscured by the liberal understanding of a society of independent equals. Second, she argues that we should not abandon the normative aspirations of equality as it is key to any progressive movement. In other words, while the descriptive claim that we are all equals in our capacities, power and ability to contribute regardless of our different care needs and care responsibilities is incorrect and misleading, the normative commitment to treat each other as equals should not be abandoned. In her work, she aims to square this apparent paradox. She develops her conception of equality, the idea of connection-based equality, on the basis of her dependency critique of prevalent understandings of equality. Instead of starting from the interests of an independent self equipped with the moral powers and the equal right to the conditions and resources to form and pursue one's conception of the good, Kittay assumes a fundamental need for relationships and derives claims that are due to us in virtue of our relationships of care with others. The idea of connection-based equality explains why people are entitled to be treated as equals, contributing to answering the question about the basis or grounds of moral equality.[38] Kittay uses the metaphor of 'being some mother's child' to make sense not only of the grounds of these entitlements but also their content. These entitlements are first and foremost to be cared for, and, second, to the social conditions to be able to care for one's dependents without harming one's own wellbeing.

9.4.2 *Towards an Integrated Approach to Care, Justice and Equality*

We have seen the two roles that the idea of connection-based equality has in Kittay's work: first, as an account of the grounds of moral equality and, second, as an understanding of the demands of equality as a political ideal. For her, the answer to the latter question is tightly connected to her understanding of what justice demands.

One of the lessons of Kittay's writing about care and equality regards the conception of moral equality that those interested in developing an integrated approach to care, justice and equality should adopt. Many approaches to justice and equality have tended to draw on rationality-based conceptions of the grounds of moral equality, and, relatedly, conception of the person, often spelled out in Rawlsian terms as the possession of the two moral powers. This perspective remains the predominant one in contemporary egalitarianism.[39] Despite the attempts to incorporate considerations of care in the Rawlsian framework that we discussed in Section 9.3.3, there are a number of reasons to be sceptical that that project can be successful. It is doubtful whether proposals like Brake's or Bhandary's can incorporate all the forms of care and caring relationships that should be accounted for as a matter of justice. These include care for those with significant cognitive impairments, who would not be included in the Rawlsian framework, as well as forms of care that are not strictly required to develop and maintain the moral powers, such as care among 'independent' adults beyond the small core of intimate long-term caring relationships discussed by Brake.[40] Even when a link between care and the moral powers can be articulated, there is a question as to whether we should rely on the sometimes contingent, and not very straightforward, connection with the moral powers to justify the entitlements to care. The fundamental problem with such approaches is that they do not start from care, and our nature as caring and needy beings, but rather attempt to bring it in at a later stage. This invites us to rethink the relevant conception of the person we should adopt when reflecting on issues of care and justice. However, Kittay's relational account of moral equality, especially when combined with her idea of the transparent self whose needs are eclipsed by those of their dependents, risks sacrificing too much of our autonomy and individuality on the altar of care and relationships.[41] One of the challenges that those interested in developing a theory of care, justice and equality face is to propose a conception of moral equality, and the person, which can be truly inclusive of all and can account for our need to receive and provide care, while at the same time being able to capture important aspects of the liberal tradition, such as respect for autonomy. This is particularly important if one contends that the account of moral equality in question should be able to ground our care-related entitlements as well as other aspects of justice, including the idea that people should be treated as equals in society.

Moving then to equality as a political ideal, we need to go back to the problem mentioned at different points in this chapter, namely whether equality and care are in some sense in tension with each other. In replying to this question, I will adopt a relational understanding of equality. Among the most influential contemporary approaches to equality, relational egalitarianism maintains that equality does not concern the distribution of certain goods but instead the quality of social relations. For people to be equals to each other they need to be able to stand in relationships of equality with others, and to related to each other as such.[42] The enemies of equality are not primarily unequal distributions, even though relational egalitarians mount a number of mostly indirect criticisms to them, but unequal relationships of power and status, including relationships of subordination, domination, oppression, stigmatization and exclusion. The task of the state is to express the equality of its citizens through its action[43] and create the conditions such that they are able to stand as equals in society.

The question under examination here is whether it is truly possible for those who stand in relationships of care to relate to each other as equals. Even if we abandon the much-criticized liberal fiction of a society of independent equals, as we should, we are faced with this problem because relationships of care are often characterized by profound inequalities of power and capacities, especially in the context dependency care. An egalitarian might be worried about such significant inequalities of power and the risk of domination in those relationships, especially when the potentially dominated party has little resources to resist that domination.[44] At the same time, however, it would be a problematic feature of relational egalitarianism if it opposed such relationships of care on the grounds that they cannot be relationships among equals, considering how morally and politically fundamental and valuable such care relationships are. While egalitarians can and do argue that there are different ways to reduce the vulnerability of one of the parties to the other and hence reduce the chances of domination in the relationships, in some relationships of care, especially dependency care, it is impossible to eliminate these imbalances altogether. Think, for instance, about the relationship between parents and young children, or that with those who live with profound cognitive disabilities. This, however, should not make us conclude that there is a fundamental incompatibility between care and equality. On the contrary, relational egalitarians should reflect further on the conditions that should obtain within these relationships of care, when it comes to the structure of the relationship and the attitudes of the parties, as well as the broader societal conditions that need to be in place for the parties to enjoy equal status. In so doing, they can address the apparent incompatibility between care and equality, and attempt to make sense of the fact that not all relationships of care in which one of the parties has the power to dominate the other are necessarily relationships among unequals which egalitarians should object to.[45] In other words, thinking about care could stimulate relational egalitarians to delve deeper into the nature of egalitarian relationships and the social conditions that sustain them. On the other hand, this could help address an important problem that theorists of care have rightly been criticized for neglecting, namely the problem of power and domination in caring relationship.

Much more needs to be said about what the relationship between care, justice and equality and about what individuals are owed when it comes to care as a matter of justice and equality. This project of reflecting on care, equality and justice is one that is worth embarking on – however, before doing so, it is necessary to address some of these fundamental questions about the conception of moral equality that this account should adopt as well as whether there is a fundamental tension between care and equality.

CONCLUSION

In this chapter, I have provided a conceptual map of the different understandings of the relationship between care, justice and equality. My reconstruction started with earlier theorists of care who conceive the care perspective as an alternative to the justice perspective, understood as the traditional approach to moral theory and, in political philosophy, as liberal theorizing on justice. I then discussed Held's approach which sees the care perspective as more fundamental, yet the two mainly belonging to different domains.[46] I also explored different attempts to combine care and justice, including those based on an analysis of Rawls's account of justice. Throughout the chapter, I have also highlighted the different understandings of care adopted by different theorists and how that impact their view of the connection between care, justice and equality. In the last part of the chapter, I moved to explore the relationships between care and equality, first analysing Kittay's dependency care-based approach to the grounds and the content of equality.[47] I then identified some new directions of inquiry for theorists interested in developing an integrated approach to equality, justice and care.

NOTES

1. See: Carol Gilligan, *In a Different Voice: Psychological Theory and Women's Development* (Cambridge, MA: Harvard University Press, 2003); Nel Noddings, *Caring: A Feminine Approach to Ethics and Moral Education* (Oakland: University of California Press, 1984).
2. Gilligan, *In a Different Voice*.
3. Importantly, this was not presented as an essentialist claim about care ethics being women's perspective on morality grounded in women's nature but rather an approach to morality most commonly articulated by women and most likely based on their gendered roles, including that of caregivers.
4. One of the most significant examples of this is the growing popularity of the idea of relational autonomy in liberal political philosophy. See: Catriona Mackenzie and Natalie Stoljar, eds, *Relational Autonomy: Feminist Perspectives on Autonomy, Agency, and the Social Self* (New York: Oxford University Press, 2000).
5. Noddings, *Caring*.
6. Michael Slote, 'Care Ethics and Liberalism', in *Care Ethics and Political Theory*, ed. Daniel Engster and Maurice Hamington (Oxford University Press, 2015), 37–50, https://doi.org/10.1093/acprof:oso/9780198716341.003.0003.
7. Virginia Held, *The Ethics of Care: Personal, Political, and Global* (Oxford/New York: Oxford University Press, 2006), ch. 4.
8. Ibid.
9. Slote, 'Care Ethics and Liberalism'.
10. Held, *The Ethics of Care*, ch. 2.
11. Held, *The Ethics of Care*.
12. Annette Baier, *Moral Prejudices: Essays on Ethics* (Cambridge, MA: Harvard University Press, 1996).
13. Susan Moller Okin, 'Reason and Feeling in Thinking about Justice', *Ethics* 99, no. 2 (1989): 229–49.
14. Anca Gheaus, 'Care and Justice: Why They Cannot Go Together All the Way' (PhD diss., Central European University, 2005) (Academia.edu).
15. Eva Feder Kittay, *Love's Labor: Essays on Women, Equality, and Dependency* (New York: Routledge, 1999).
16. Gheaus, 'Care and Justice'.
17. See: Amy R. Baehr, 'Political Constructivism and Justice in Caregiving', in *Caring for Liberalism: Dependency and Liberal Political Theory*, ed. Asha Bhandary and Amy R. Baehr (New York: Routledge, 2022), 187–212; Asha Bhandary, *Freedom to Care: Liberalism, Dependency Care, and Culture* (New York: Routledge, 2021); Kittay, *Love's Labor*.
18. See: Bhandary, *Freedom to Care*; Kittay, *Love's Labor*.
19. Bhandary, *Freedom to Care*.

20. See: Held, *The Ethics of Care*; Joan C. Tronto, *Moral Boundaries: A Political Argument for an Ethic of Care* (New York: Routledge, 1993).
21. Martha Fineman, 'The Vulnerable Subject and the Responsive State', *Emory Law Journal* 60, no. 2 (2010): 251–75.
22. Tronto, *Moral Boundaries*, 103.
23. In his earlier work, which I will discuss in the next section, Engster adopts a definition of care that is different from the one just presented.
24. Daniel Engster, 'Care Ethics, Dependency, and Vulnerability', *Ethics and Social Welfare* 13, no. 2 (2019): 100–14, https://doi.org/10.1080/17496535.2018.1533029.
25. Daniel Engster, *The Heart of Justice: Care Ethics and Political Theory* (Oxford: Oxford University Press, 2007), https://doi.org/10.1093/acprof:oso/9780199214358.001.0001.
26. Ibid., 28–9.
27. Anca Gheaus, '*The Heart of Justice: Care Ethics and Political Theory*, by Daniel Engster', *European Journal of Philosophy* 18, no. 4 (2010): 619–23, https://doi.org/10.1111/j.1468-0378.2010.00429.x.
28. Kittay, *Love's Labor*.
29. Bhandary, *Freedom to Care*.
30. See: Shiloh Y. Whitney, 'Dependency Relations: Corporeal Vulnerability and Norms of Personhood in Hobbes and Kittay', *Hypatia* 26, no. 3 (2011): xx, https://onlinelibrary.wiley.com/doi/abs/10.1111/j.1527-2001.2011.01188.x; Catriona Mackenzie, 'Three Dimensions of Autonomy: A Relational Analysis', in *Autonomy, Oppression, and Gender*, ed. Andrea Veltman and Mark Piper (New York: Oxford University Press, 2014), 15–41.
31. Elizabeth Brake, 'Fair Care: Elder Care and Distributive Justice', *Politics, Philosophy & Economics* 16, no. 2 (2017): 132–51, https://doi.org/10.1177/1470594X15600831.
32. Baehr, 'Political Constructivism and Justice in Caregiving'.
33. Baier, *Moral Prejudices*.
34. Bhandary, *Freedom to Care*.
35. Engster, *The Heart of Justice*, ch. 1.
36. Held, *The Ethics of Care*.
37. Kittay, *Love's Labor*.
38. Kittay also discusses the problem of the grounds of moral equality in later work, developing a distinctive relational approach to the problem. See: Eva Feder Kittay, 'At the Margins of Moral Personhood', *Ethics* 116, no. 1 (2005): 100–31.
39. See: Elizabeth S. Anderson, 'What Is the Point of Equality?', *Ethics* 109, no. 2 (1999): 287–337; Ronald Dworkin, *Sovereign Virtue* (Cambridge, MA: Harvard University Press, 2000); Samuel Scheffler, 'What Is Egalitarianism?', *Philosophy & Public Affairs* 31, no. 1 (2003): 5–39, https://doi.org/10.1111/j.1088-4963.2003.00005.x; Christian Schemmel, *Justice and Egalitarian Relations*, Oxford Political Philosophy (New York: Oxford University Press, 2021).
40. Daniel Engster, 'Just Add Care and Stir? The Limits of Mainstream Liberal Theory for Taking on Dependency Care', *Critical Review of International Social and Political Philosophy* 25, no. 6 (2022): 827–34, https://doi.org/10.1080/13698230.2021.1922862.
41. A further fundamental question about this account is whether it can explain why these relationships are normatively significant when it comes to moral equality and able to ground duties that all human beings have towards each other, rather than only those who stand in more direct caring relationships.
42. See: Anderson, 'What is the Point of Equality?'; Samuel Scheffler, 'The Practice of Equality', in *Social Equality*, ed. Carina Fourie, Fabian Schuppert and Ivo Wallimann-Helmer (Oxford: Oxford University Press, 2015), 20–44.

43. Schemmel, *Justice and Egalitarian Relations.*
44. Some have also suggested that there is a tension between an attitude of respect, which is typically considered a core aspect of relating to others as equals, and the attitudes that constitute care. I find this objection much less troubling for egalitarians interested in care.
45. For some contributions in this direction, see: Matilda Carter, 'The Indirect Approach: Towards Non-Dominating Dementia Care', *Res Publica* 28, no. 3 (2022): 467–80, https://doi.org/10.1007/s11158-021-09540-1; and Daniel Sharp, forthcoming, 'Asymmetric Vulnerability without Subordination: Reconciling Value-Enabling Vulnerability with Relational Equality', in *Vulnerability and Relational Equality*, ed. Costanza Porro and Christine Straehle (Cambridge: Cambridge University Press).
46. Held, *The Ethics of Care.*
47. Kittay, *Love's Labor.*

BIBLIOGRAPHY

Anderson, Elizabeth S. 'What Is the Point of Equality?' *Ethics* 109, no. 2 (1999): 287–337.

Baehr, Amy R. 'Political Constructivism and Justice in Caregiving', in *Caring for Liberalism: Dependency and Liberal Political Theory*, edited by Asha Bhandary and Amy R. Baehr, 187–212. New York: Routledge, 2022.

Baier, Annette. *Moral Prejudices: Essays on Ethics*. 3rd printing. Cambridge, MA: Harvard University Press, 1996.

Bhandary, Asha. *Freedom to Care: Liberalism, Dependency Care, and Culture*. New York: Routledge, 2021.

Brake, Elizabeth. 'Fair Care: Elder Care and Distributive Justice', *Politics, Philosophy & Economics* 16, no. 2 (2017): 132–51. https://doi.org/10.1177/1470594X15600831.

Carter, Matilda. 'The Indirect Approach: Towards Non-Dominating Dementia Care', *Res Publica* 28, no. 3 (2022): 467–80. https://doi.org/10.1007/s11158-021-09540-1.

Dworkin, Ronald. *Sovereign Virtue*. Cambridge, MA: Harvard University Press, 2000.

Engster, Daniel. *The Heart of Justice: Care Ethics and Political Theory*. Oxford: Oxford University Press, 2007. https://doi.org/10.1093/acprof:oso/9780199214358.001.0001.

Engster, Daniel. 'Care Ethics, Dependency, and Vulnerability', *Ethics and Social Welfare* 13, no. 2 (2019): 100–14. https://doi.org/10.1080/17496535.2018.1533029.

Engster, Daniel. 'Just Add Care and Stir? The Limits of Mainstream Liberal Theory for Taking on Dependency Care', *Critical Review of International Social and Political Philosophy* 25, no. 6 (2022): 827–34. https://doi.org/10.1080/13698230.2021.1922862.

Fineman, Martha. 'The Vulnerable Subject and the Responsive State', *Emory Law Journal* 60, no. 2 (2010): 251–75.

Gheaus, Anca. 'Care and Justice: Why They Cannot Go Together All the Way', PhD thesis, Central European University, 2005 (Academia.edu).

Gheaus, Anca. '*The Heart of Justice: Care Ethics and Political Theory*, by Daniel Engster', *European Journal of Philosophy* 18, no. 4 (2010): 619–23. https://doi.org/10.1111/j.1468-0378.2010.00429.x.

Gilligan, Carol. *In a Different Voice: Psychological Theory and Women's Development*. 38th printing. Cambridge, MA: Harvard University Press, 2003.

Held, Virginia. *The Ethics of Care: Personal, Political, and Global*. Oxford and New York: Oxford University Press, 2006.

Kittay, Eva Feder. *Love's Labor: Essays on Women, Equality, and Dependency*. New York: Routledge, 1999.

Kittay, Eva Feder. 'At the Margins of Moral Personhood', *Ethics* 116, no. 1 (2005): 100–31.

Mackenzie, Catriona. 'Three Dimensions of Autonomy: A Relational Analysis', in *Autonomy, Oppression, and Gender*, edited by Andrea Veltman and Mark Piper, 15–41. New York: Oxford University Press, 2014.

Mackenzie, Catriona, and Natalie Stoljar, eds. *Relational Autonomy: Feminist Perspectives on Automony, Agency, and the Social Self*. New York: Oxford University Press, 2000.

Noddings, Nel. *Caring: A Feminine Approach to Ethics and Moral Education*. Oakland: University of California Press, 1984.

Okin, Susan Moller. 'Reason and Feeling in Thinking about Justice', *Ethics* 99, no. 2 (1989): 229–49.

Scheffler, Samuel. 'What Is Egalitarianism?' *Philosophy & Public Affairs* 31, no. 1 (2003): 5–39. https://doi.org/10.1111/j.1088-4963.2003.00005.x.

Scheffler, Samuel. 'The Practice of Equality', in *Social Equality*, edited by Carina Fourie, Fabian Schuppert and Ivo Wallimann-Helmer, 20–44. Oxford: Oxford University Press, 2015.

Schemmel, Christian. *Justice and Egalitarian Relations*. Oxford Political Philosophy. New York: Oxford University Press, 2021.

Sharp, Daniel. Forthcoming. 'Asymmetric Vulnerability without Subordination: Reconciling Value-Enabling Vulnerability with Relational Equality', in *Vulnerability and Relational Equality*, edited by Costanza Porro and Christine Straehle. Cambridge: Cambridge University Press.

Slote, Michael. 'Care Ethics and Liberalism', in *Care Ethics and Political Theory*, edited by Daniel Engster and Maurice Hamington, 37–50. Oxford University Press, 2015. https://doi.org/10.1093/acprof:oso/9780198716341.003.0003.

Tronto, Joan C. *Moral Boundaries: A Political Argument for an Ethic of Care*. New York: Routledge, 1993.

Whitney, Shiloh Y. 'Dependency Relations: Corporeal Vulnerability and Norms of Personhood in Hobbes and Kittay', *Hypatia* 26, no. 3 (2011): 554–74. https://doi.org/10.1111/j.1527-2001.2011.01188.x.

CHAPTER TEN

Care ethics and structural injustice

STEPHANIE COLLINS

INTRODUCTION

Philosophical interest in structural injustice has risen sharply since the publication of Iris Marion Young's *Responsibility for Justice*.[1] In short, a structural injustice occurs when social, economic or political processes operate to produce an unjust outcome, where those processes cannot be reduced to identifiable wrongs perpetrated by isolatable agents (regardless of whether those agents are individuals or collectives, such as governments or corporations).[2] Paradigm examples of structural injustices include widespread homelessness and exploitative labour practices – both of which are examples analysed by Young.

As Young explains, an individual might end up without a home – or might end up working under terrible conditions – through no fault of any individual (or even collective) agent. This is because all agents operating in the system that produces such outcomes are constrained by what the system makes possible. The system might be set up to produce such outcomes, regardless of the choices of agents operating within the system. In such cases, the standard 'liability model' for distributing responsibility goes silent: the liability model of responsibility demands that each unjust outcome must be traced to the culpable actions of identifiable agent(s), yet there are no identifiable agent(s) that can be singled out as the sole perpetrators of structural injustice. The primary task of theorists, then, has been to develop *alternative models for assigning responsibility* for structural injustices.

In this chapter, I suggest that care ethics offers useful resources for developing alternative models of responsibility in the face of structural injustice. I begin in Section 10.1 by providing an overview of what structural injustice is and of the 'forward-looking' models of responsibility that have been developed by theorists for dealing with it. These forward-looking models stand in contrast to the 'liability model' described above. My goal in Section 10.1 is not to expose any specific limitations of these existing forward-looking models: I believe they are on the right track. My claim, therefore, is not that care ethics offers an incompatible alternative to the existing forward-looking models. My goal in Section 10.1 is to outline what structural injustice theorists have said thus far, so that subsequent sections can reveal what care ethics is able to add as a complement to these theories.

In Section 10.2, I give an overview of (my interpretation of) care ethics. This will reveal several points of resonance between care ethics and existing forward-looking theories of responsibility for structural injustice. In short, I view care ethics as concerned with *human dependency*. In the care-ethical framework, forward-looking responsibilities arise out of this dependency. The forward-looking responsibilities of care ethics call upon us to engage in practices of care, where these practices include both actions and attitudes, and where care is an ongoing and open-ended process that necessarily includes contributions from the care recipient. The paradigm examples of care occur within personal human relationships – such as between friends and family. Yet care ethics is obviously not limited to such contexts, instead calling upon agents to bring a caring orientation to other forms of interdependency – including the economic, political and social interdependencies that are at issue in structural injustices.

In Section 10.3, I weave these two threads together, explicitly enumerating several care-ethical insights that can be brought to bear on forward-looking theories of responsibility for structural injustice. For example, in my care-ethical approach, responsibilities can arise regardless of the behaviours one has performed in the past or present. Also, the care-ethical approach emphasizes context-specificity and the importance of foregrounding the voices of those who are negatively affected by problematic social arrangements, including structural injustice.

Throughout, I will use the example of climate change as a case study. I am not the first to theorize climate change as a structural injustice (see, for example, Eckersley,[3] Godoy,[4] Larrère[5] and Sardo[6]). Yet I am not aware of any work that brings *care ethics* specifically to bear on climate change as a structural injustice.[7] In this way, my argument reveals how three areas of normative concern – care ethics, structural injustice and climate ethics – can be mutually informative.

10.1 STRUCTURAL INJUSTICE

10.1.1 What is structural injustice?

According to Young, structural injustice exists

> when social processes put large groups of persons under systemic threat of domination or deprivation of the means to develop and exercise their capacities, at the same time that these processes enable others to dominate or have a wide range of opportunities for developing and exercising capacities available to them. Structural injustice is a kind of moral wrong distinct from the wrongful action of an individual agent or the repressive policies of a state. Structural injustice occurs as a consequence of many individuals and institutions acting to pursue their particular goals and interests, for the most part within the limits of accepted rules and norms.[8]

Young's characterization is largely compatible with other, more recent, analyses. For example, Sally Haslanger defines structural injustice as follows:

> Structural injustice occurs when the practices that create the structure – the network of positions and relations – (a) distort our understanding of what is valuable, or (b) organize us in ways that are unjust/harmful/wrong, e.g., by distributing resources unjustly or violating the principles of democratic equality. Systemic injustice occurs when an unjust structure is maintained in a complex system that is self-reinforcing, adaptive, and creates subjects whose identity is shaped to conform to it.[9]

Thus, Haslanger distinguishes between a 'structure' and a 'system'. A 'structure' is an abstract array of positions and relations between those positions. A 'system' is a specific instantiation of a structure. For example, the 'structure' of a carbon-based economy includes roles or positions such as 'coal extractor', 'coal burner' and so on, where these positions are related by economic relations such as the 'sells coal to' relation or the 'buys coal from' relation. Such structures can be unjust – for example, by giving too much power to those who own the means of production, or by not including positions and relations that hold the powerful in check. Meanwhile, a *specific* carbon-based economy – for example, the global economy in the twenty-first century – is a 'system', insofar as it instantiates the more general 'structure' of a carbon-based economy. A specific system can be unjust in ways that are not necessarily reflected in the abstract structure – for example, because of how that system is embedded historically or environmentally.

For our purposes, we need not be concerned with the differences between Young's and Haslanger's accounts, or with the intricate differences between systemic and structural injustice. It is more illuminating to focus on the similarities between Young and Haslanger, and between systemic and structural injustice. As Lisa Herzog puts it, what we can generally take from these accounts of structural and systemic injustice is the importance of focusing on the 'social *positions* that individuals can end up in, emphasizing that these should neither be understood as the result of personal failure nor as caused by unhappy circumstances for which no one is responsible'.[10] That is: structures and systems are maintained and instantiated by people; they are therefore not merely 'unhappy circumstances'. Yet structures and systems often are not the result of identifiable actions of any particular agents within the structure/system; they are therefore not simply 'the result of personal failure'.

Likewise, Robin Zheng employs the concept of 'unendorsed structural wrongs' to refer to 'actions of an otherwise morally unobjectionable type that harm others by forming part of unjust social-structural processes – usually without the agent's knowing, willing, or desiring to do so'.[11] As Zheng puts it, 'the primary source of their wrongness is located in the overarching *system* of domination as a whole and only very derivatively in the individual acts themselves'.[12] When applied to a harm such as climate change, it seems clear that many agents are 'knowing' in the sense that they know their actions form part of harmful social-structural processes. Yet these harms are not a matter of agents 'willing' or 'desiring' to cause these harms; instead, we operate in a social-economic structure that leaves us little choice.

More generally, whether we are using Young's, Haslanger's, Herzog's or Zheng's characterization of structural injustice, it's fairly easy to see how climate change will count as a structural injustice. In the climate change case, the relevant 'social processes' (following Young and Zheng) or 'practices' (following Haslanger) or 'positions' (following Herzog) rely on *the burning of fossil fuels*. These processes, practices and positions deprive some people within the structure of the means to exercise their capacities (namely, those people who suffer climate harms), at the same time as others within the structure reap benefits (for example, fossil fuel companies and their executives). This distributes resources unjustly, so there is an injustice at play.

Yet the actions that contribute to this injustice are, in Zheng's words, 'otherwise morally unobjectionable'. There is nothing inherently wrong with heating one's home, driving one's car or flying to visit one's relatives. While we might be able to attribute *some* (what Herzog calls) 'personal failure' to actors within the system – most glaringly, to fossil fuel companies – arguably the level of personal failure that can be attributed to such actors is not *proportionate* to the enormous scale of the injustice. They can be attributed liability for their own choices and plans, but these identifiably culpable choices and plans do not 'add up' to the full extent of the structural injustice. As Young puts it, all actors in the structure 'operate under serious structural constraints',[13] making it difficult for them to do otherwise than act so as to maintain the system. The *system itself* is the locus of the injustice.

10.1.2 Responsibility for structural injustice

Given these features of structural injustice, what kind of responsibility can be attributed? In answer to this question, Young advocates the 'social connection model' of responsibility. Within this model, 'responsibility' is understood as a *forward-looking* imperative, rather than a *backward-looking* assessment of culpability or blameworthiness (as under the liability model sketched in the introduction to this chapter). Young writes:

> The social connection model of responsibility says that individuals bear responsibility for structural injustice because they contribute by their actions to the processes that produce unjust outcomes. Our responsibility derives from belonging together with others in a system of interdependent processes of cooperation and competition through which we seek benefits and aim to realize projects ... All who dwell within the structures must *take* responsibility for remedying injustices they cause, though none is specifically liable for the harm in a legal sense. Responsibility in relation to injustice thus derives ... from participating in the diverse institutional processes that produce structural injustice. (emphasis added)[14]

The responsibility at issue here is not a matter of morally assessing what agents have done in the past, so as to assess these actions as culpable, reckless, negligent or otherwise wrongful. Instead, the 'responsibility' is something one must *take* into the future. Young thus eschews a *backward-looking* lens in favour of a *forward-looking* lens. Roughly, the backward-looking lens examines the past, asking which agents produced the structural injustice in a manner that is culpable or blameworthy. The forward-looking lens examines the future, asking which agents can take up responsibility for ameliorating the structural injustice.

Some theorists have vigorously argued – contra Young – that there is much backward-looking responsibility in the context of structural injustice.[15] Indeed, one might think that the assertion of forward-looking responsibility makes little sense if agents will not, in the future, become blameworthy should they fail to adequately perform their forward-looking responsibilities. But I shall leave these points about the viability of backward-looking responsibility to one side. My goal is ultimately to bring care ethics to bear on structural injustice. Care ethics (in my rendering) shares Young's emphasis on the forward-looking over the backward-looking. Yet care ethics need not deny that backward-looking considerations also apply, as we will see. I will therefore consider the forward-looking aspects of Young's account, while leaving open the possibility that backward-looking responsibility also has a place in normative analyses of structural injustice.

Young's forward-looking account of responsibility for structural injustice delineates four 'parameters of reasoning', which Young recommends agents use when deciding how to perform their forward-looking responsibilities. The four parameters of reasoning are power, privilege, interest and collective ability. As Young puts it, the 'power' parameter states that '[w]hen individuals and organizations do not have sufficient energy and resources to respond to all of the structural injustices to which they are connected, they should focus on those where they have a greater capacity to influence structural processes'.[16]

The 'privilege' parameter applies to those who benefit from the structural injustice; these people also have 'greater responsibilities than others to take actions to undermine injustice'.[17] The 'interest' parameter picks out those whose 'self-interest may coincide with promoting justice'.[18] Here, Young[19] singles out victims of structural injustice as having special responsibilities, since '[i]t is they who know the most about the harms they suffer'.[20] Finally, the 'collective ability' parameter identifies agents who 'are in positions where they can draw on the resources of already organized entities and use them in new ways for trying to promote change'.[21] On Young's account, agents should consider these parameters when acting to alleviate structural injustice.

Before turning to care ethics, it is worth considering some other, more recent, accounts of forward-looking responsibility for structural injustice. Like Young's, these more recent accounts can also be complemented by the care-ethical approach that I will develop. One such account is that of Robin Zheng, who has developed a 'role-ideal model' of responsibility for structural injustice.[22] In Zheng's model, each agent occupies various social roles – such as their professional, familial, cultural and religious roles. Each role brings in train a number of expectations about behaviour and ways of being in the world. According to Zheng, we each have the responsibility to push the boundaries of our roles in ways that might ameliorate structural injustice. Thus, the nature of one's forward-looking responsibility is shaped by and situated within the roles one finds oneself in, according to Zheng's theory.

Another recent theory is that of Maeve McKeown, who argues that forward-looking responsibility for structural injustice is created by the fact that agents *reproduce* structural injustice through their actions.[23] To use an example related to climate change: driving a car might not *cause* climate change (since the climate is already changing and will change regardless of whether one drives one's car), but driving one's car does help *reproduce* the processes that lead to climate change. McKeown suggests that such social and economic reproduction is the basis of agents' forward-looking responsibility. Unlike Zheng's account, then, we can see McKeown's account as a theory of the *basis* of forward-looking responsibility, without so much specifying the *content* of those responsibilities.

Finally, Corwin Aragon and Alison M. Jaggar suggest that forward-looking responsibility for structural injustice is grounded not in a broad notion of 'connection' as Young contended, nor in the specific 'parameters of reasoning' that Young distinguished, but rather in agents' *complicity* in structural injustice. Their theory, like McKeown's, thus concerns the *basis* (not so much the *content*) of our forward-looking responsibilities. Of course, for agents to count as 'complicit' in structural injustice, we will need a concept of complicity that does not require intentions: most agents who act in ways that perpetuate structural injustice do not *intend* to do so. Thus, Aragon and Jaggar develop a concept of 'structural complicity', which they argue is the basis of agents' forward-looking responsibility to ameliorate structural injustice. This concept of structural complicity allows agents to be unintentionally complicit.[24]

These accounts from Zheng, McKeown, and Aragon and Jaggar all emphasize the *embeddedness* of agents within structural injustice. For Zheng, our *roles* embed us within unjust systems and shape what we should do to act on those systems; for McKeown, our actions that *reproduce* the injustice embed us in unjust processes and justify our forward-looking responsibility for changing those processes; for Aragon and Jaggar, our *complicity* embeds us in structural injustice and justifies our forward-looking responsibility to respond. I take these accounts to be broadly compatible and not necessarily competitors: it might be that our forward-looking responsibilities are grounded in our contributions[25] and our roles[26] and our reproduction[27] and our complicity,[28] while we should act in ways shaped by our parameters[29] and our roles.[30] As we will see, this general emphasis on our embedded agency has important resonances with care ethics. Care ethics is, therefore, a promising place to turn in further fleshing out this picture of our forward-looking responsibility for structural injustice. I turn to this next.

10.2 CARE ETHICS

There are many different care-ethical theories. Depending on which theory one chooses, one will get slightly different results for theorizing responsibility for structural injustice. In this section, I will lay out my own preferred version of the theory.[31]

Care ethics starts from a specific vision of human life: humans are unavoidably entangled in webs of dependency relations with others. We all depend on particular others, in various ways, and have particular others who depend on us, in various ways. This includes more personal relationships (such as the dependence of a child on their parent, or dependence of spouses on one another) and more distant relationships (such as the dependence of those who grow our food on our purchase of that food). Because dependence is pervasive and present from the start of life, ethical decisions are inevitably made in the context of this entanglement, not in the abstract.

Care ethics takes the phenomenology of actual decision making as crucial data for ethical theorizing. When deciding what we should do in a given circumstance, we typically take account of the particularities and complexities of the relationships between the unique persons in the dilemma. We do not normally apply abstract rules or perform regimented calculi. These decision-making processes often strike us as coldly lacking in moral qualities or not quite suitable for the given situation. Rather, we remain focused on the concrete world, which contains an intricate web of connections that call on us to make a moral response.

Early care ethicists developed these themes – contextual particularity, the uselessness of general principles, and webs of relationships extended over time – from their presentation in Carol Gilligan's *In A Different Voice,*[32] which focused on the moral experience of women.[33] Gilligan found that many of her interview subjects did not appeal to general principles or make categorical assertions about right and wrong. They instead used 'the responsibility conception', which 'focuses on the limitations of any particular resolution and describes the conflicts that remain'.[34] This ambivalence was a result of subjects' perception that each dilemma involved many conflicting responsibilities. Paradigmatically, Gilligan described 'Amy', a subject who saw a particular dilemma as 'a narrative of relationships that extends over time' in 'a world that coheres through human connection rather than through systems of rules'.[35] Gilligan asserted that this 'orientation toward relationships and interdependence implies a more contextual mode of judgment and a different moral understanding' than one that focuses on universal ethical principles.[36]

Building on these insights, in my view, care ethics asserts: that responsibilities derive directly from relationships between particular people, rather than from abstract rules and principles; that deliberation should be empathy-based rather than duty- or principle-based; that personal relationships have a moral value that is often overlooked by other theories; that at least some responsibilities aim at fulfilling the particular needs of vulnerable persons (including their need for empowerment), rather than the universal rights of rational agents; and that morality demands not just one-off acts, but also certain ongoing patterns of interactions with others and certain general attitudes and dispositions. Most importantly, care ethicists claim that morality demands actions and attitudes of *care*, in addition to those of respect, non-interference, and tit-for-tat reciprocity (which care ethicists generally see as over-emphasized in other normative ethical and political theories).

Not all care ethicists hold all these views; different theorists define them differently, and different theorists emphasize different ones. Nonetheless, this loose cluster of claims gives us some sense of what care ethicists believe matters. What's more, most care ethicists accept that care must be in some way fused or combined with its early opponent, justice, where 'justice' can be understood as primarily concerned with liberty and reciprocity.[37] Care ethicists thus task themselves with pointing out important ethical truths that have been neglected by other theories. But they need not claim that other theories get nothing right. This allows that backward-looking blameworthiness – and the 'liability model' of responsibility – does indeed have a place in our moral assessments. But, like Young in her analysis of structural injustice, care ethics does not emphasize the backward-looking notions employed by the liability model. It seeks to turn our attention elsewhere.

As I view it, the core normative claim of care ethics is that *dependence relationships generate moral imperatives to provide care.*[38] (Call this 'the care imperative'.) The care imperative is 'normative' in the straightforward sense it involves an 'ought': the 'ought' of a moral imperative. This normative claim therefore differs from the descriptive claims of care ethics, such as the claim that humans are inevitably interdependent and that moral reasoning inevitably happens in the context of that interdependency. Nonetheless, there is a close connection between these descriptive claims and the care imperative: if it is true, as a matter of fact, that humans are interdependent and reason from the context of this interdependence, then it would stand to reason that such interdependence should form the basis of forward-looking moral imperatives.

In my view, dependence relationships hold when: (1) there is an *important interest* that is unfulfilled; (2) an agent is *sufficiently capable* of fulfilling that interest; and (3) the agent's most efficacious measure for doing so is *not too costly*. These three components generate a 'well-placed' dependency responsibility – that is, a responsibility that is grounded in one's being well-placed to fulfil another's important interests. Some relationships instead generate a 'best-placed' dependency responsibility: a dependency responsibility grounded in one's being best-placed to fulfil another's important interests. Best-placed dependency responsibilities arise when a fourth component is present: (4) the agent's fulfilling the interest would be the *least costly* of any agent's doing so.[39]

My account has affinities with others in the literature. For the purposes of this chapter, it is not necessary to choose between my account and these other ones: what matters is that all these accounts endorse (something like) the care imperative identified above. For example, Eva Feder Kittay gives a compelling account of the pervasiveness of dependence in human life, before using that descriptive account to argue for the following 'principle of social responsibility for care', which has strong resonances with the care imperative: '*[t]o each according to his or her need for care, from each according to his or her capacity for care, and such support from social institutions as to make available resources and opportunities to those providing care, so that all will be adequately attended in relations that are sustaining*'[40] (emphasis in original).[41] Similarly, Daniel Engster states that '[i]n claiming care from others, we *imply* that capable human beings ought to help individuals in need when they are able to do so consistent with their other caring obligations' (emphasis added).[42] On Engster's theory of care ethics, then, something very much like the care imperative derives from the fact that all humans have experienced receiving care from others in times of dependency. The important point here is that care ethics includes the care imperative; it is less important whether one endorses a justification and specification of that imperative that comes from myself, Kittay, Engster or a different theorist.

Care ethics is thus an essentially *relational* theory: the fundamental basis of moral requirements is found in relations between people. For care ethics, these are *relations of dependence*. 'Dependence', in this context, is not a matter of mere psychological reliance or trust. We can be dependent on each other without knowing it and without being disposed to act in any way on that basis. Instead, dependence is a matter of objective vulnerability: it's a matter of our most important interests being such that they can be fulfilled only (or most effectively, efficiently or usefully) by certain behaviours or attitudes from others, who thereby acquire forward-looking moral responsibilities. By emphasizing relations between particular persons, the care imperative differs from typical 'cosmopolitan-utilitarian' or 'humanitarian' accounts of responsibility. (This is important, because Young explicitly distinguishes her account of responsibility from injustice from such accounts,[43] and I seek to follow her in this.)[44]

The care imperative requires deep contextual sensitivity in its application, which ties it to the concrete particulars of interrelated human lives. The question of what to do, feel or judge in a given situation cannot be answered in abstraction from the particular persons – and particular relations – at issue.[45] For this reason, most care ethicists are resistant to general moral principles, instead advocating a contextual, embedded and empathetic mode of reasoning, outlined above.[46]

Does this scepticism about general moral principles mean we should reject the care imperative, since it is a moral principle? I don't think so. The care imperative is a matter of the *justificatory* grounds of our forward-looking responsibilities, rather than a matter of the method we should use for *deliberating* about those responsibilities. To foreshadow the next section: Young grounds our forward-looking responsibilities in our *connections*, McKeown grounds them in our *reproduction*, and Aragon and Jaggar ground them in our *complicity*; in complement to these, my care-ethical approach grounds our forward-looking responsibilities for structural injustice in our *dependence relationships*. This 'grounding' relation is an objective justificatory relation. But it doesn't mean that we should think about dependence constantly while responding to structural injustice: the imperative to provide care is not necessarily an imperative to think about dependence all the time. Dependence relations *justify* our responsibilities. Yet the *content* or *deliberative procedure* required by those responsibilities might be something quite different.

Indeed, the care imperative is not silent on the required content or deliberative procedure. It states that dependence relationships generate moral imperatives to provide *care*. Thus, *care* is the content or deliberative procedure that is recommended by care ethics. But what is care? In my view, care includes both attitudes and actions – where the latter, importantly, are usually not one-off performances, but rather require ongoing practices, habits and dispositions. More specifically, I have argued that, concerning caring attitudes:

> Care ethics sometimes calls for agents to have *caring attitudes*, that is, attitudes that: (i) have as their object something that has *interests*, or something that might affect something that has interests; and that (ii) are a *positive response* (e.g. promoting,

> respecting, revering) to those interests; and that (iii) lead the agent's *affects, desires, decisions, attention*, or so on to be influenced by how the agent believes things are going with the interest-bearer. (emphasis added)[47]

And further, concerning caring actions:

> Care ethics sometimes calls for agents to perform [caring] actions (i) that are performed under the (perhaps tacit) *intention of fulfilling (or going some way to fulfilling) interest*/s that the agent perceives some moral person (the recipient) to have; (ii) where the strength of the demand is a complex function of the value of the intention, the likelihood that the action will fulfil the interest, and the extent to which the interest is appropriately described as a 'need.' (emphasis added)[48]

It is important that these precepts of care ethics – precepts requiring agents to hold caring attitudes and perform caring actions – are not simple duties or obligations that can be fully 'discharged'. Both caring attitudes and caring actions are a matter of ongoing and open-ended processes and orientations towards the world. This is also how Young uses the term 'responsibility' in contrast to 'duty' or 'obligation': unlike duties and obligations, responsibilities are open-ended and potentially insatiable.[49]

In fact, care is perhaps better viewed as an *interpersonal process*, rather than a personal attitude or action – even of the ongoing or open-ended kind. By viewing caregiving as an interpersonal process, the care recipient becomes a much more active player in successful caring. On this view of caring, care arises out of interactions between the caregiver and care recipient. This can be contrasted with a view on which care is entirely a matter of certain attitudes and actions on the part of caregiver, wherein the care recipient is relegated to the role of passive receptacle.

A useful version of the 'interpersonal process' view of caring is Joan Tronto's four-stage theory of caring. Tronto's formulation makes the care recipient active in the final stage of successful caregiving – which turns care into more of an interpersonal process than a personal attitude or action. Tronto's four stages of caring are: (1) attentiveness, which can be understood as a proclivity or disposition to become aware of need; (2) responsibility, which is a willingness to respond and take care of need; (3) competence, which is the skill of providing good care to those in need whom one can help; and finally (4) responsiveness, which includes consideration of the position of others as they see it and recognition of the potential for abuse in care.[50]

Tronto's fourth phase can be further enriched by adding what Kittay calls 'the completion of care'.[51] This is a stage of caring in which the care recipient 'takes up' and responds to the actions of the caregiver. For an infant, this might mean ceasing to cry. For someone with advanced dementia, this might mean acting at ease. Kittay goes so far as to say that the care recipient has an obligation to receive care graciously, if they are able to bear obligations at all. Similarly, Virginia Held says that care is 'more the characterization of a social relation than the description of an individual disposition, and social relations are not reducible to individual states'.[52] The suggestion from all these thinkers is that successful caregiving actively involves both the caregiver and care recipient. For the purposes of this chapter, it is not necessary to choose between the accounts of Tronto, Kittay or Held: what matters is that all three accounts include a strong role for the care recipient. I will put this role to work in the next section, when I bring care into conversation with structural injustice theorists. (For competing definitions of the 'care' at issue in care ethics, see for instance Bubeck[53] and Engster.[54])

A final point about my preferred version of care ethics concerns the role of personal relationships within the theory. Personal relationships are those in which the participants value one another non-fungibly – that is, the other participants in the relationship could not simply be replaced by another person, even if the replacement person had all the same properties or features as the person being replaced. According to my preferred version of care ethics: 'To the extent that they have value to individuals in the relationship, [personal] relationships ought to be (a) treated as moral paradigms, (b) valued, preserved, or promoted (as appropriate to the circumstance at hand) and (c) acknowledged as giving rise to weighty duties.'[55] To treat personal relationships as 'moral paradigms' is to take them to be a model to emulate in other, less personal contexts. This means approaching other relationships as we do our personal relationships, at least to some extent – for example, by approaching those less personal relationships with empathy, attention to complex particularities, and a view towards the open-ended thriving of all parties to the relationship. In the next section on care-ethical lessons for structural injustice, I will focus on part (a) of the above precept, since parts (b) and (c) concern the treatment of personal relationships themselves, which are not so much at issue in cases of structural injustice.

With this sketch of care ethics on the table, we can turn to consider the ways in which it enriches and complements the theories of responsibility for structural injustice that were outlined in Section 10.1.

10.3 CARE-ETHICAL RESPONSIBILITY FOR STRUCTURAL INJUSTICE

A first point to note is that care ethics agrees with the forward-looking focus of Young and the other forward-looking responsibility theorists. Care ethics' forward-looking orientation can easily be deduced from the distinction that is typically drawn between care and justice. Although almost all care ethicists recognize the importance of combining the insights of care theories and justice theories,[56] it's still true that care ethics is not so much concerned with attributing blame or liability for wrongs that occurred in the past, as is typical within backward-looking theories. Instead, care ethics – and, more specifically, the care imperative that I outlined in the previous section – is concerned with the question of who should do what in the future. It is, in this sense, a forward-looking theory of responsibility for structural injustice.

Yet care ethics suggests both a different *foundation*, and a different *content*, for these responsibilities than is envisioned by the structural injustice theorists outlined in Section 10.1. First, let us consider the *foundation* of responsibility. Care-ethical responsibilities are founded on dependency: we have a responsibility to care for those whose needs are dependent on our care (or the care of groups to which we belong). This differs from the justificatory bases provided by Young, McKeown, and Aragon and Jaggar. For Young, as we saw above, responsibility for structural injustice is grounded in one's contribution to structural injustice. Yet, as Zheng points out, in Young's contribution-based approach 'individuals can try to avoid responsibility by denying that they have any backward-looking causal connections or forward-looking ability to control structural processes'.[57] In my care-ethical approach, by contrast, our responsibility is grounded in the fact that others in the structure are dependent on our choices. This is not a matter of having caused structural injustice or having the ability to control structural injustice taken as a whole.

The care-ethical approach likewise differs from, while resonating with, Young's four 'parameters of reasoning'. Recall that these parameters are power, privilege, interest and collective ability. The parameter of 'power' has much in common with the care imperative. Those with power are those who have a 'greater capacity' to alleviate structural injustice.[58] Similarly, the care imperative says a person has a responsibility to care if another's important interests are vulnerable to the person's care, which will at least partly be a matter of the person having a 'greater capacity'. Yet the relation of 'dependence' includes more than just 'greater capacity'. A relation of 'dependence' holds when one person is either best-placed, or simply well-placed, to fulfil another's important interest, using a measure that is not too costly. Thus, a dependence relation can hold even if one does not have a 'greater capacity' than others in a *comparative* sense: on the care imperative, one might have a responsibility simply by being *well-placed*, even if one is not *better-placed* than others. Additionally, as explained in the previous section, my preferred notion of 'dependence' includes the condition that one can act at not too much cost; thus, considerations of 'over-demandingness' are internal to the care imperative, in a way they are not internal to Young's notion of 'power'.

When it comes to Young's other three parameters of reasoning – privilege, interest and collective ability – it is clearer how the care imperative is distinct. The care imperative differs from 'privilege' in that it might produce responsibilities regardless of whether one *benefits* from structural injustice. It differs from 'interest' in that it produces responsibilities even when one's *own wellbeing* is not at stake. And it differs from 'collective ability' in that it calls for action even beyond the confines of *already-established organizations*. Yet, the care imperative encapsulates much of what is appealing about these three parameters of reasoning: arguably, those with privilege, those with interest (such as victims), and those with collective ability, should each act on structural injustice precisely *when and because others depend on them*. (In the case of victims, those who depend on them are *other victims*; this generates victim-to-victim responsibilities, as argued by Ashwini Vasanthakumar.[59]) The care imperative can thus unify and explain Young's four parameters of reasoning, without displacing them in the practical deliberative process of actual agents.

What about the approaches of McKeown, and of Aragon and Jaggar? On McKeown's approach, forward-looking responsibility is grounded in the fact that one *reproduces* structural injustice. In arguing for her approach, McKeown critiques 'dependent connection' as a potential basis for forward-looking responsibilities to ameliorate structural injustice. McKeown's critique deserves consideration, since dependent connection has seeming similarities to my care-ethical approach. On the dependent connection approach critiqued by McKeown, responsibilities are generated by the fact that the responsibility-bearer is dependent on those towards whom they have responsibilities. For example, I might have responsibilities to victims of climate harms, since my high-emissions lifestyle 'depends' on these people being harmed. This dependence approach is the *reverse* of the care-ethical approach. On the care-ethical approach, responsibilities are generated by the fact that the responsibility-bearer *is depended upon* by those who are vulnerable to the attitudes and actions of the responsibility-bearer – not the fact that the responsibility-bearer *depends upon* others. This avoids many of the critiques forwarded by McKeown.[60]

That said, McKeown states that responsibility for structural injustice is 'a responsibility to ensure that the structures in which we act are just, not a direct responsibility for the well-being of particular others'.[61] She also objects to 'the familiar way of thinking about global injustice: that the rich have obligations toward the poor'.[62] These two critiques might seem to apply to the care-ethical approach. Yet the care-ethical approach handles both of these critiques. By noting that caring actions are always contextually embedded, we allow that caring actions in the context of structural injustice require acting to improve structures, rather than merely targeting others' wellbeing directly. Also, the care-ethical approach does not assume that 'the poor' are dependent on 'the rich'. Those who are well-placed or best-placed to provide care in a particular structural context will not often be 'the rich'. It is an open question as to who is well-placed or best-placed to provide care within a particular structural injustice – but care is often best provided at local levels, within communities. It is only in these contexts that particularized empathy and deliberation can occur. Affluent allies might have a responsibility to provide material resources through democratically accountable channels. But community-led action will often be best, particularly in the third of Tronto's four phases, which involves 'the skill of providing good care to those in need whom one can help'.

As opposed to dependent connection, McKeown advocates responsibility that is grounded in *reproducing* structural injustice. As she puts it: 'when I go to a high-street shop, the structural injustice of sweatshop labor already exists, but when I purchase clothes, I reproduce the practice. Structures are the preconditions for our actions, but we also reproduce unjust structures when we act.'[63] Such reproduction produces responsibilities, on McKeown's account.

The care-ethical approach adds to this reproduction-based approach, because the care imperative can apply even in contexts where reproduction does not occur. McKeown herself mentions 'the bottom billion' – that is, those 'who make little or no contribution to the global economy, living subsistence lives'.[64] It's unclear how any of my actions *reproduce* structures that maintain the radical inequality between such people and the global 1 per cent; after all, 'the bottom billion' are defined by non-participation in global economic structures. Yet this inequality is undoubtedly a structural injustice: it results from economic and social systems, without being part of those systems. It seems we need something other than the reproduction of structures to ground responsibility in this context.

The care-ethical approach produces responsibilities for those who are well-placed or best-placed to fulfil the important interests of 'the bottom billion'. As noted above, this does not imply that 'the rich' must 'save' 'the poor': the rich are often ignorant about how to do so, and their meddling may be unhelpful, because they are incapable of the kind of sensitive contextual deliberation that care ethics champions. Often those who are distant cannot usefully engage in the kind of empathetic, particularized and open-ended orientation that is required by care. Yet they can act in ways that facilitate such care by others. The point is that the care-ethical approach allows that responsibilities can arise without the kind of reproduction McKeown points to. Thus, care ethics can complement the reproduction-based approach, offering an alternative foundation for forward-looking responsibilities.

Similar remarks apply to Aragon and Jaggar's approach. According to them, forward-looking responsibility is grounded in the fact that one is *complicit* in structural injustice. Like Young's 'contribution' and McKeown's 'reproduction', Aragon and Jaggar's 'complicity' requires that one has performed some positive actions in the past: it 'links our present responsibilities with our past and present exercise of agency, providing a moral grounding for these responsibilities'.[65] Unlike other theories of complicity (for example, that of Kutz[66]), Aragon and Jaggar's conception of complicity does not require any particular state of mind on the part of complicitous people. Instead, '[p]eople are structurally complicit when they exercise their agency in ways that reinforce the unjust social structures in which they participate, regardless of their conscious intentions'.[67]

My care-ethical approach differs from this in that it does not require any actions or omissions of complicity: one can acquire responsibility for structural injustice without necessarily acting in ways that reinforce that injustice. Likewise, not all who act complicitously will acquire responsibilities on my account. To take the example of climate change, most people in the world are complicit, in the sense that most people participate in the global economy in ways that reinforce the carbon-based economic structure that has unjust effects on the victims of climate harms. Yet not all these people are best-placed or even well-placed to perform actions or adopt attitudes that will fulfil the important interests of victims of climate harms. On Aragon and Jaggar's approach, it seems such people would nonetheless have (pro tanto and overridable) responsibilities. My account takes a more targeted approach to responsibilities.

Finally, the care-ethical approach complements Zheng's role-based approach. For Zheng, one has a forward-looking responsibility to push the boundaries of one's roles in a way that ameliorates the structural injustices in which those roles are enmeshed. Yet one's role itself cannot be what justifies one's responsibility to push the boundaries of one's role. After all, roles themselves do not contain the justifications for their own alteration; if they did, such alteration would not be 'alteration' or 'boundary pushing' at all, since those actions would also be included within the role. Therefore, the justification for altering a role must come from *outside* the role itself.

The question thus arises: why should one push the boundary of one's role – say, the role of 'oil company executive' – in this way rather than that way? Zheng's theory does not – as she notes[68] – provide us with a normative theory that tells us *when* we should work to overthrow our roles, or *in what direction* we should push the boundaries of our roles. The care-ethical approach fills this gap: it points out that others' need-fulfilment is *vulnerable to* or *dependent on* how we push the boundaries of our roles; therefore, we should work to change our roles in ways that fulfil the needs (including the need for autonomy and empowered agency) of those who depend on us.

The discussion in this section thus far has mostly concerned the foundations, grounds or justifications for forward-looking responsibility for structural injustice. Yet care ethics also has insights concerning the *content* of forward-looking responsibilities. Under conditions of structural injustice, the care imperative demands attitudes and actions of *care*, where these require particularized empathetic deliberation and include open-ended habits, practices and dispositions. Care is both individual and structural: it needn't be only a matter of face-to-face interaction with particular others, but rather can include acting on social processes, procedures and practices with a view to the needs of particular others. In this way, one can care for distant others.[69] But what does care look like in practice, in the context of structural injustice?

Here it is important that care ethics takes a situated and particularistic approach to moral decisions. Deliberation about how to act in a given situation requires close attention to the particularities of one's relations to others in that situation. This applies as much to structural injustice as to personal life. Recall that care ethics takes personal relationships as *moral paradigms*, which means that even the non-personal relationships at issue in structural injustice should be approached with empathy, attention to complex particularities, and a view towards the open-ended thriving of all parties to the relationship. It is difficult to generalize.

Nonetheless, a few points can be made. A first point is that care is oriented towards the perspective of those who are disadvantaged by structural injustice. Care starts from their perspective and their needs, and those who are disadvantaged have an essential role to play in defining 'successful' care. This is the insight of Tronto's 'responsiveness' and Kittay's 'the completion of care'. Taking climate change as an example, this might mean starting from the perspective of people who are particularly affected by structural injustice – for example, Indigenous peoples. Extreme and unpredictable weather, and receding ice, has already impacted the lives of Inuit peoples in ways that disrupt their use of traditional knowledge and practices. Climate change has made it more difficult to hunt for food, disrupted generations of cultural traditions, and negatively impacted mental health.[70] In a care-ethical approach to the structural injustice of climate change, such perspectives would be central.

A second point is that care-ethical approaches to structural injustice will engage in what Daniel Engster calls 'the principle of subsidiarity'. On this principle, 'we should shift the actual delivery of care whenever possible to the most local and personal levels. We should care for others whenever possible by enabling them to care for themselves.'[71] This principle follows from the fact that care ethics aims to fulfil needs, in combination with the acknowledgement that needs are particular and contextual – and, therefore, that those who are in a situation know best what needs are at stake in a situation.[72] In the climate change context, this might mean working to alleviate structural injustice by acting within one's own community or own's own part of the supply chain, rather than trying to intervene unilaterally at the other end of a supply chain.

More specifically, in the context of climate change, the principle of subsidiarity might be respected by taking action at the local level. Indeed, economists have argued that smaller governance units might have an important role to play in building the trust required to adequately reduce carbon emissions.[73] When many different such units are combined – operating in overlapping and interactive ways – the result would be a polycentric system that overall responds to the demand for mitigation of climate change, adaption to climate change, and responses to claims of loss and damage from climate change. Such a polycentric system is arguably already beginning to exist in response to the climate crisis – for example, in cooperation between local and regional governments, non-governmental organizations, and even corporations (Andonova, Betsill and Bulkeley;[74] Bäckstrand et al.;[75] and Aragon and Jaggar[76] make similar proposals for polycentric action on the structural injustice of migrant domestic labour, but my account still differs from theirs regarding the foundations of responsibility).

CONCLUSION

Care ethics is a rich and diverse moral tradition. In this chapter, I do not claim to have captured the full richness and diversity. I rather hope to have revealed what one specific understanding of care ethics can contribute to debates about forward-looking responsibility for structural injustice. On that understanding of care ethics, the core normative claim of care ethics is that *dependence relationships generate moral imperatives to provide care*. This provides a different justification for responsibilities than recent theories of structural injustice, while also saying something about the content of those responsibilities. I hope this demonstrates the more general point that care ethics has much to contribute to ongoing and emerging topics in social and political theory.

NOTES

1. Iris Marion Young, *Responsibility for Justice* (Oxford: Oxford University Press, 2011).
2. One might think 'mainstream' theories of justice – notably, John Rawls (see: John Rawls, *A Theory of Justice* (Cambridge, MA: Harvard University Press, 1971)) – have always been concerned with structural injustice; after all, Rawls argued that the ideal of justice applies to the 'basic structure' of society. Yet Rawls's ideal-theoretic approach contrasts with the concerns of structural injustice theorists like Young, who start with injustices in the here and now, such as homelessness and sweatshop labour. Moreover, Rawls's theory (and that of other mainstream justice theorists) concerns mostly the 'formal' institutions of the basic structure, rather than the largely uncodified social systems and practices analysed by Young.
3. Robin Eckersley, 'Responsibility for Climate Change as a Structural Injustice', in *Oxford Handbook of Environmental Political Theory*, ed. Teena Gabrielson, Cheryl Hall, John M. Meyer and David Schlosberg (Oxford: Oxford University Press, 2016), 346–61.
4. Eric S. Godoy, 'What's the Harm in Climate Change?', *Ethics, Policy, and Environment* 20, no. 1 (2017): 103–17.
5. Catherine Larrère, 'Responsibility in a Global Context: Climate Change, Complexity, and the "Social Connection Model of Responsibility"', *Journal of Social Philosophy* 49, no. 3 (2018): 381–92.
6. Michael Christopher Sardo, 'Responsibility for Climate Justice: Political, Not Moral', *European Journal of Political Theory* 22, no. 1 (2020): 26–50.
7. Mara Marin provides a somewhat care-ethical approach to structural injustice (not climate change specifically), but she conceives of care ethics very differently from me. Marin's core notion is *commitment*, such as the commitments found in personal relationships with friends, spouses and so on. Marin argues that individuals are committed to social structures in similar ways to how they are committed to personal relationships. According to Marin, this commitment both generates obligations to change social structures and can motivate individuals to engage in solidary action. (See: Mara Marin, *Connected by Commitment: Oppression and Our Responsibility to Undermine It* (Oxford: Oxford University Press, 2017).) As we will see, commitment is not the basis of obligations (or forward-looking responsibilities) under my conception of care ethics. Another recent theorist who has examined care through the lens of structural injustice is Hee-Kang Kim. Kim examines how structural injustices oppress those engaged in caring relationships, paradigmatically children and their women carers. Kim's analysis, therefore, does not use care ethics so much as a normative theory to conceptualize responsibility for resolving structural injustice, as an analytic theory to conceptualize gendered care work as an instance of structural injustice. See: Hee-Kang Kim, 'Care Ethics as Challenge to the Structural Oppression Surrounding Care', *Ethics and Social Welfare* 15, no. 2 (2021): 151–66.
8. Young, *Responsibility for Justice*, 52.
9. Sally Haslanger, 'Systemic and Structural Injustice: Is There a Difference?', *Philosophy* 98, no. 1 (2023): 22.

10. Lisa Herzog, 'What Could Be Wrong with a Mortgage? Private Debt Markets from a Perspective of Structural Injustice', *Journal of Political Philosophy* 25, no. 4 (2016): 414.
11. Robin Zheng, 'Moral Criticism and Structural Injustice', *Mind* 139, no. 518 (2021): 517.
12. Ibid., 518.
13. Young, *Responsibility for Justice*, 132.
14. Ibid., 105.
15. See, for example: Martha Nussbaum, 'Foreword', in *Responsibility for Justice*, by Iris Marion Young (Oxford: Oxford University Press, 2011); Christian Barry and Luara Ferracioli, 'Young on Responsibility and Structural Injustice', *Criminal Justice Ethics* 32, no. 3 (2013): 247–57; Farid Abdel-Nour, 'Responsibility for Structural Injustice', *Ethics & Global Politics* 11, no. 1 (2018): 13–21; Valentin Beck, 'Two Forms of Responsibility: Reassessing Young on Structural Injustice', *Critical Review of International Social and Political Philosophy* 26, no. 6 (2020): 918–41; and Christian Barry and Robert E. Goodin, 'Responsibility for Structural Injustice: A Third Thought', *Politics, Philosophy & Economics* 20, no. 4 (2021): 339–56. I agree with these authors that backward-looking considerations might deserve more of a place than Young gives them in her theory; however, my contribution will be to supplement the forward-looking part of Young's theory.
16. Young, *Responsibility for Justice*, 144.
17. Ibid., 145.
18. Ibid., 146.
19. See also: Tamara Jugov and Lea Ypi, 'Structural Injustice, Epistemic Opacity, and the Responsibilities of the Oppressed', *Journal of Social Philosophy* 50, no. 1 (2019): 7–27.
20. Young, *Responsibility for Justice*. 146.
21. Ibid., 147.
22. Robin Zheng, 'What Is My Role in Changing the System? A New Model of Responsibility for Structural Injustice', *Ethical Theory and Moral Practice* 21, no. 4 (2018): 869–85.
23. Maeve McKeown, 'Iris Marion Young's "Social Connection Model" of Responsibility: Clarifying the Meaning of Connection', *Journal of Social Philosophy* 49, no. 3 (2018): 484–502.
24. Corwin Aragon and Alison M. Jaggar, 'Agency, Complicity, and the Responsibility to Resist Structural Injustice', *Journal of Social Philosophy* 49, no. 3 (2018): 439–60.
25. Young, *Responsibility for Justice*.
26. Zheng, 'What Is My Role in Changing the System?'
27. McKeown, 'Iris Marion Young's "Social Connection Model"'.
28. Aragon and Jaggar, 'Agency, Complicity, and the Responsibility to Resist', 439–60.
29. Young, *Responsibility for Justice*.
30. Zheng, 'What Is My Role in Changing the System?'
31. I argued for roughly the following version of care ethics in: Stephanie Collins, *The Core of Care Ethics* (London: Palgrave Macmillan, 2015).
32. Carol Gilligan, *In a Different Voice* (Cambridge, MA: Harvard University Press, 1982).
33. In my view, theorists such as Joan Tronto convincingly separated the ethics of care from 'women's ethics.' (See: Joan C. Tronto, 'Beyond Gender Difference to a Theory of Care', *Signs* 12, no. 4 (1987): 644–63.) I will therefore put to one side care ethics' association with feminism and 'the feminine', on the assumption that care ethics' status as a cause, effect, help or hindrance to the various (contested) goals of feminism(s) can be separated from care ethics' commitments as a normative ethical and political theory. This assumption

is not uncontentious (for example, Virginia Held rejects it (see: Virginia Held, *The Ethics of Care: Personal, Political, and Global* (Oxford: Oxford University Press, 2006), 20).

34. Gilligan, *In a Different Voice*, 22.
35. Ibid., 28–9.
36. Ibid., 29.
37. See: Virginia Held, 'Taking Care: Care as Practice and Value', in *Setting the Moral Compass: Essays by Women Philosophers*, ed. C. Calhoun (Oxford: Oxford University Press, 2004), 65–8; Held, *The Ethics of Care*, 15–17; Eva Feder Kittay, 'Human Dependency and Rawlsian Equality', in *Feminists Rethink the Self*, ed. Diana T. Meyers (Boulder, CO: Westview Press, 1997), 219–66; Eva Feder Kittay, *Love's Labor: Essays on Women, Equality and Dependency* (New York: Routledge, 1999); Fiona Robinson, *Globalizing Care: Ethics, Feminist Theory, and International Relations* (Boulder, CO: Westview Press, 1999), 23ff; Sara Ruddick, 'Care as Labor and Relationship', in *Norms and Values: Essays on the Work of Virginia Held*, ed. J. C. Haber and M. S. Halfon (Lanham, MD: Rowman & Littlefield, 1998), 3–25; Tronto, 'Beyond Gender Difference to a Theory of Care', 167.
38. Collins, *The Core of Care Ethics*.
39. I lay out these conditions in: Collins, *The Core of Care Ethics*, 97.
40. Kittay, *Love's Labor*, 133.
41. Kittay leads up to this principle with the following observations: 'If we were to amend the theory of justice as fairness to include the social position of the participants in the dependency relation, it would most likely give rise to a [principle that] in contrast to the others, would not be based on our equal vulnerability, nor on our possession of rationality, a sense of justice, and a vision of our own good. Instead, it would be based on our unequal vulnerability in dependency, on our moral power to respond to others in need, and on the primacy of human relations to happiness and well-being.' (See: Kittay, *Love's Labor*, 133.) This demonstrates how (what I have called) the care imperative derives from the descriptive facts of human interdependency, including unequal dependency.
42. Daniel Engster, *The Heart of Justice: A Political Theory of Caring* (New York: Oxford University Press, 2007), 48.
43. Young, *Responsibility for Justice*, 104–5.
44. For more on how care ethics' relational focus makes it different from utilitarianism, see: Stephanie Collins, 'The Ethics of Care as a Normative Ethical Theory', forthcoming in *Oxford Handbook of Normative Ethics*, ed. David Copp, Tina Rulli and Connie Rosati (Oxford: Oxford University Press).
45. See: Held, *The Ethics of Care*, 80; Kittay, 'Human Dependency and Rawlsian Equality', 236; Fiona Robinson, *The Ethics of Care: A Feminist Approach to Human Security* (Philadelphia, PA: Temple University Press, 2011), 4; Sara Ruddick, 'From Maternal Thinking to Peace Politics', in *Explorations in Feminist Ethics*, ed. E. Browning-Cole and S. Coultrap-McQuin (Bloomington: Indiana University Press, 1992), 152.
46. See: Daniel Engster, 'Care Ethics and Natural Law Theory: Toward an Institutional Political Theory of Caring', *The Journal of Politics* 66, no. 1 (2004): 114; Diana T. Meyers, 'The Socialized Individual and Individual Autonomy: An Intersection between Philosophy and Psychology', in *Women and Moral Theory*, ed. Eva Feder Kittay and Diana T. Meyers (Totowa, NJ: Rowman & Littlefield, 1987), 142; Selma Sevenhuijsen, *Citizenship and the Ethics of Care: Feminist Considerations on Justice, Morality, and Politics* (New York: Routledge, 1998), 57; Sarah Clark Miller, 'Need, Care and

Obligation', *Royal Institute of Philosophy* 80, *Supplement 57* (2005): 139; Nel Noddings, *Caring: A Feminine Approach to Ethics and Moral Education* (Oakland: University of California Press, 1984), 85; Joan C. Tronto, *Caring Democracy: Markets, Equality, and Justice* (New York: New York University Press, 2013), 53–5.
47. Collins, *The Core of Care Ethics*, 64.
48. Ibid., 80.
49. Young, *Responsibility for Justice*, 143.
50. Joan C. Tronto, *Moral Boundaries: A Political Argument for an Ethic of Care* (London: Routledge, 1993), 126–36.
51. Eva Feder Kittay, 'The Completion of Care – With Implications of a Duty to Receive Care Graciously', in *Care Professions and Globalization*, ed. Ana Marta Gonalez and Craig Iffland (Basingstoke: Palgrave Macmillan, 2014), 33–42.
52. Held, *The Ethics of Care*, 42.
53. Diemut Bubeck, *Care, Gender and Justice* (Oxford: Clarendon Press, 1995), 127.
54. Engster, *The Heart of Justice*, 28.
55. Collins, *The Core of Care Ethics*, 145–6.
56. See: Held, *The Ethics of Care*, 15–17; Tove Pettersen, *Comprehending Care: Problems and Possibilities in the Ethics of Care* (Lanham, MD: Lexington Books, 2008), ch. 6.
57. Zheng, 'What Is My Role in Changing the System?', 874.
58. Young, *Responsibility for Justice*, 144.
59. Ashwini Vasanthakumar, 'Epistemic Privilege and Victims' Duties to Resist Their Oppression', *Journal of Applied Philosophy* 35, no. 3 (2018): 465–80.
60. McKeown, 'Iris Marion Young's "Social Connection Model"', 489–91.
61. Ibid.,, 492.
62. Ibid., 493.
63. Ibid., 497.
64. Ibid., 491.
65. Aragon and Jaggar, 'Agency, Complicity, and the Responsibility to Resist', 447.
66. Christopher Kutz, *Complicity: Ethics and Law for a Collective Age* (Cambridge: Cambridge University Press, 2000).
67. Aragon and Jaggar, 'Agency, Complicity, and the Responsibility to Resist', 449.
68. Zheng, 'What Is My Role in Changing the System?', 883.
69. See: Held, *The Ethics of Care*; Tronto, *Caring Democracy*.
70. Glen Mercer, '"Sea, Ice, Snow … It's All Changing": Inuit Struggle with Warming World', *The Guardian*, 30 May 2018.
71. Engster, *The Heart of Justice*, 58.
72. This point has some resonances with Young's 'interest' parameter, which underlines the idea that the care imperative can be used to unify Young's four parameters.
73. Elinor Ostrom, 'Beyond Markets and States: Polycentric Governance of Complex Economic Systems', *American Economic Review* 100, no. 3 (2010): 641–72.
74. Liliana N. Andonova, Michele Betsill and Harriet Bulkeley, 'Transnational Climate Governance', *Global Environmental Politics* 9, no. 2 (2009): 52–73.
75. Karin Bäckstrand, Jonathan W. Kuyper, Björn-Ola Linnér and Eva Lövbrand, 'Non-State Actors in Global Climate Governance: From Copenhagen to Paris and Beyond', *Environmental Politics* 26, no. 4 (2017): 561–79.
76. Aragon and Jaggar, 'Agency, Complicity, and the Responsibility to Resist', 453–4.

BIBLIOGRAPHY

Abdel-Nour, Farid. 'Responsibility for Structural Injustice', *Ethics & Global Politics* 11, no. 1 (2018): 13–21.

Andonova, Liliana N., Michele Betsill and Harriet Bulkeley. 'Transnational Climate Governance', *Global Environmental Politics* 9, no. 2 (2009): 52–73.

Aragon, Corwin, and Alison M. Jaggar. 'Agency, Complicity, and the Responsibility to Resist Structural Injustice', *Journal of Social Philosophy* 49, no. 3 (2018): 439–60.

Bäckstrand, Karin, Jonathan W. Kuyper, Björn-Ola Linnér and Eva Lövbrand. 'Non-State Actors in Global Climate Governance: From Copenhagen to Paris and Beyond', *Environmental Politics* 26, no. 4 (2017): 561–79.

Barry, Christian, and Luara Ferracioli. 'Young on Responsibility and Structural Injustice', *Criminal Justice Ethics* 32, no. 3 (2013): 247–57.

Barry, Christian, and Robert E. Goodin. 'Responsibility for Structural Injustice: A Third Thought', *Politics, Philosophy & Economics* 20, no. 4 (2021): 339–56.

Beck, Valentin. 'Two Forms of Responsibility: Reassessing Young on Structural Injustice', *Critical Review of International Social and Political Philosophy* 26, no. 6 (2020): 918–41.

Bubeck, Diemut. *Care, Gender and Justice*. Oxford: Clarendon Press, 1995.

Collins, Stephanie. *The Core of Care Ethics*. London: Palgrave Macmillan, 2015.

Collins, Stephanie. Forthcoming. 'The Ethics of Care as a Normative Ethical Theory', in *Oxford Handbook of Normative Ethics*, edited by David Copp, Tina Rulli and Connie Rosati. Oxford: Oxford University Press.

Eckersley, Robin. 'Responsibility for Climate Change as a Structural Injustice', in *Oxford Handbook of Environmental Political Theory*, edited by Teena Gabrielson, Cheryl Hall, John M. Meyer and David Schlosberg, 346–61. Oxford: Oxford University Press, 2016.

Engster, Daniel. 'Care Ethics and Natural Law Theory: Toward an Institutional Political Theory of Caring', *The Journal of Politics* 66, no. 1 (2004): 113–35.

Engster, Daniel. *The Heart of Justice: A Political Theory of Caring*. New York: Oxford University Press, 2007.

Gilligan, Carol. *In a Different Voice*. Cambridge, MA: Harvard University Press, 1982.

Godoy, Eric S. 'What's the Harm in Climate Change?' *Ethics, Policy, and Environment* 20, no. 1 (2017): 103–17.

Haslanger, Sally. 'Systemic and Structural Injustice: Is There a Difference?' *Philosophy* 98, no. 1 (2023): 1–27.

Held, Virginia. 'Taking Care: Care as Practice and Value', in *Setting the Moral Compass: Essays by Women Philosophers*, edited by C. Calhoun, 59–71. Oxford: Oxford University Press, 2004.

Held, Virginia. *The Ethics of Care: Personal, Political, and Global*. Oxford: Oxford University Press, 2006.

Herzog, Lisa. 'What Could Be Wrong with a Mortgage? Private Debt Markets from a Perspective of Structural Injustice', *Journal of Political Philosophy* 25, no. 4 (2016): 411–34.

Jugov, Tamara, and Lea Ypi. 'Structural Injustice, Epistemic Opacity, and the Responsibilities of the Oppressed', *Journal of Social Philosophy* 50, no. 1 (2019): 7–27.

Kim, Hee-Kang 'Care Ethics as Challenge to the Structural Oppression Surrounding Care', *Ethics and Social Welfare* 15, no. 2 (2021): 151–66.

Kittay, Eva Feder. 'Human Dependency and Rawlsian Equality', in *Feminists Rethink the Self*, edited by Diana T. Meyers, 219–66. Boulder, CO: Westview Press, 1997.

Kittay, Eva Feder. *Love's Labor: Essays on Women, Equality and Dependency*. New York: Routledge, 1999.

Kittay, Eva Feder. 'The Completion of Care – With Implications of a Duty to Receive Care Graciously', in *Care Professions and Globalization*, edited by Ana Marta Gonalez and Craig Iffland, 33–42. Basingstoke: Palgrave Macmillan, 2014.

Kutz, Christopher. *Complicity: Ethics and Law for a Collective Age*. Cambridge: Cambridge University Press, 2000.

Larrère, Catherine. 'Responsibility in a Global Context: Climate Change, Complexity, and the "Social Connection Model of Responsibility"', *Journal of Social Philosophy* 49, no. 3 (2018): 381–92.

Marin, Mara. *Connected by Commitment: Oppression and Our Responsibility to Undermine It*. Oxford: Oxford University Press, 2017.

McKeown, Maeve. 'Iris Marion Young's "Social Connection Model" of Responsibility: Clarifying the Meaning of Connection', *Journal of Social Philosophy* 49, no. 3 (2018): 484–502.

Mercer, Glen. '"Sea, Ice, Snow … It's All Changing": Inuit Struggle with Warming World', *The Guardian*, 30 May 2018.

Meyers, Diana T. 'The Socialized Individual and Individual Autonomy: An Intersection between Philosophy and Psychology', in *Women and Moral Theory*, edited by Eva Feder Kittay and Diana T. Meyers, 139–53. Totowa, NJ: Rowman & Littlefield, 1987.

Miller, Sarah Clark. 'Need, Care and Obligation', *Royal Institute of Philosophy* 80, *Supplement 57* (2005): 137–60.

Noddings, Nel. *Caring: A Feminine Approach to Ethics and Moral Education*. Oakland: University of California Press, 1984.

Nussbaum, Martha. 'Foreword', in *Responsibility for Justice*, by Iris Marion Young. Oxford: Oxford University Press, 2011.

Ostrom, Elinor. 'Beyond Markets and States: Polycentric Governance of Complex Economic Systems', *American Economic Review* 100, no. 3 (2010): 641–72.

Pettersen, Tove. *Comprehending Care: Problems and Possibilities in the Ethics of Care*. Lanham, MD: Lexington Books, 2008.

Rawls, John. *A Theory of Justice*. Cambridge, MA: Harvard University Press, 1971.

Robinson, Fiona. *Globalizing Care: Ethics, Feminist Theory, and International Relations*. Boulder, CO: Westview Press, 1999.

Robinson, Fiona. *The Ethics of Care: A Feminist Approach to Human Security*. Philadelphia, PA: Temple University Press, 2011.

Ruddick, Sara. 'From Maternal Thinking to Peace Politics', in *Explorations in Feminist Ethics*, edited by E. Browning-Cole and S. Coultrap-McQuin, 141–55. Bloomington: Indiana University Press, 1992.

Ruddick, Sara. 'Care as Labor and Relationship', in *Norms and Values: Essays on the Work of Virginia Held*, edited by J. C. Haber and M. S. Halfon, 3–25. Lanham, MD: Rowman & Littlefield, 1998.

Sardo, Michael Christopher. 'Responsibility for Climate Justice: Political, Not Moral', *European Journal of Political Theory* 22, no. 1 (2020): 26–50.

Sevenhuijsen, Selma. *Citizenship and the Ethics of Care: Feminist Considerations on Justice, Morality, and Politics*. New York: Routledge, 1998.

Tronto, Joan C. 'Beyond Gender Difference to a Theory of Care', *Signs* 12, no. 4 (1987): 644–63.

Tronto, Joan C. *Moral Boundaries: A Political Argument for an Ethic of Care*. London: Routledge, 1993.
Tronto, Joan C. *Caring Democracy: Markets, Equality, and Justice*. New York: New York University Press, 2013.
Vasanthakumar, Ashwini. 'Epistemic Privilege and Victims' Duties to Resist Their Oppression', *Journal of Applied Philosophy* 35, no. 3 (2018): 465–80.
Young, Iris Marion. *Responsibility for Justice*. Oxford: Oxford University Press, 2011.
Zheng, Robin. 'What Is My Role in Changing the System? A New Model of Responsibility for Structural Injustice', *Ethical Theory and Moral Practice* 21, no. 4 (2018): 869–85.
Zheng, Robin. 'Moral Criticism and Structural Injustice', *Mind* 139, no. 518 (2021): 503–35.

CHAPTER ELEVEN

Normative questions, empirical burdens and global justice

Perspectives from care ethics

FIONA ROBINSON

INTRODUCTION

In this chapter, I interrogate the relationship of 'the empirical' and 'the normative' in the context of global ethics, focusing on the contributions of the ethics of care. Normativity, in philosophy, marks a distinction not between the good and the bad, but rather 'between the good-bad … on the one hand, and the actual, possible, or usual, on the other'.[1] Many strands of moral philosophy reject the claim that empirical 'data' – such as exercises in public engagement or deliberation – can, in themselves, lead to any normative conclusions.[2] In so doing, they would claim, further, that any transition from claims about what is to claims about 'what ought to be done' requires 'additional premises and arguments' in order to avoid the 'naturalistic fallacy'.[3] On Kant's view, for example, empirical principles cannot ground moral laws because whereas these laws bind all rational beings universally, necessarily and unconditionally, the authority of empirical principles, by contrast, depends on contingent aspects of human nature.[4]

Within the study of international politics or international relations (IR), this distinction has long been upheld by the dominant theoretical frameworks – realism, often understood as *realpolitik*, and idealism, often dismissed by realists as 'moralism'.[5] Constructivists in IR have challenged the dominance of 'realism versus idealism', proposing a research programme for theorizing 'moral limit and possibility' in world politics that systematically considers the empirical when asking 'the normative question' – 'how are we to act?'.[6] In 2021, Brooke Ackerly and colleagues sought to highlight the under-recognized work of those engaged in 'grounded normative theory' (GNT), which is 'marked by shared commitments to incorporating original empirical data or analysis in a recursive process of theory development striving for accountability to persons in empirical contexts'.[7]

While these developments are promising, I argue that they tend to keep in place the distinction between the normative and the empirical, thus failing to see clearly how ethics operate in and through the political. Care ethics, by contrast, can challenge this distinction in two ways: first, through an understanding of our subjectivities – moral and otherwise – as relational; and, second, through a view of morality as operating in and through sociopolitical life, emphasizing the need for critical interrogation of the distribution of responsibility and care and the effects of this on people's lives and wellbeing. As a feminist understanding of morality, moreover, care ethics foregrounds gendered relations of power, offering a critique of the way that mainstream, masculinist moral philosophy represents moral life; in so doing, it puts the 'authority and credibility of representative claims about moral life under harsh light, and challenges epistemic and moral authority that is politically engineered and self-reinforcing'.[8]

The term 'empirical burden' in the chapter's title is taken from the work of feminist philosopher Margaret Urban Walker who argues, in her 1998 book, that ethics must bear a 'far greater descriptive and empirical burden, in pursuing details of actual moral arrangements, than is commonly thought'.[9] While Walker does not label her view of morality 'care ethics', her 'expressive-collaborative' approach has informed the thinking of many care ethicists, and her arguments on feminist ethics resonate strongly with several accounts of feminist care ethics (including my own).[10] For this chapter, I turn to Walker's key claims about the nature of morality and consider these with respect to the relationship between the normative and the empirical. I argue that Walker's account of morality as consisting in practices of responsibility is particularly instructive for working through what it actually means for ethics to take on this 'descriptive and empirical burden'. Once we no longer see morality as something to be 'applied' to sociopolitical life, but operating in and through it, ethics – and care ethics in particular – becomes an important resource for addressing questions of global injustice. Indeed, Walker offers a template for thinking about global ethics when she calls for 'detailed and situated descriptions of the expectations and negotiations surrounding assignments of responsibility'.[11] This approach provides global ethicists with capacity not simply to consider the empirical context, but to offer the 'critical methods and reflexive techniques' to make visible 'unshared and unequal powers' within and among communities.[12]

Relying primarily on Walker's work, I argue that feminist care ethics is thus uniquely positioned to reveal sites and stories of global injustice, as well as provide a normative orientation towards their amelioration. Importantly, the belief that morality consists of practices, rather than principles, rules or theories, does not amount to claiming that we should simply 'attribute normative significance to existing social practices'.[13] Indeed, care ethics eschews the strong normativity of rationalist moral theories. Rather, following Walker, care ethics focuses attention on practices of responsibility that implement commonly shared understandings about 'who gets to do what to whom and who is supposed to do what for whom'.[14] This guided question not only provides a focus for our attention to the (potentially overwhelming) 'empirical' world, but also ensures a critical edge that encourages us to investigate who is deemed responsible and whether or not those responsibilities are being upheld. This method draws our attention to a range of socio-economic and political practices and structures in global politics that may actively prohibit our ability to care – such as the crises in welfare provisioning or availability of human and material resources to respond to care needs. But it also highlights the ideational power of structures and norms – including the neoliberalization of feminism and structures of patriarchy – that simultaneously feminize and devalue care while constructing it as a burden, and promote what Joan Tronto has called 'privileged irresponsibility' for men, and white, Western women of privilege.[15] A critical, feminist ethics of care interrogates practices of global (ir)responsibility, shining a light on our collective failure to care for ourselves and our planet.

This chapter proceeds in three parts. In the first part, I explore the relationship between the normative and the empirical in moral and political philosophy and in international political theory. I set out the limitations in this regard of both traditional 'rationalist' approaches to ethics and 'constructivists' in IR who claim to offer a way of mediating between the demands of 'moral principles' and 'the real world' through careful empirical research, as well as recent innovations in 'grounded normative theory' which aim to bring together the work of scholars using empirical research to make claims about global justice, and establish it as a distinctive mode of theorizing. In the second part, I trace the development of thinking on the relationship between the normative and the empirical in the literature on care ethics, focusing on the persuasive and influential contribution of Margaret Urban Walker. Finally, in the third section, I consider these insights from care ethicists in the context of questions of global injustice. To illustrate the contribution of care ethics here, I turn to two examples of recent work in feminist IR scholarship, which reveal the importance of practices of care in the struggle towards post-conflict social rebuilding and the social reproduction of daily life. Importantly, this work does not idealize care, but recognizes its operation in and through relations of power, theorizing both the deleterious consequences of 'depletion', and depoliticized discourses of care and love.

11.1 THE NORMATIVE AND THE EMPIRICAL, ETHICS AND POLITICS

The distinction between what 'is' and what 'ought to be' often features in public discourse and everyday conversation; this reflects its important place in the Western canon on ethics. Both Hume and Kant agreed that there is no legitimate logical connection or transition between 'is' and 'ought'; while Kant gave us the 'naturalistic fallacy', Hume offered what R. M. Hare called 'Hume's Law' – that no ought-judgement may be correctly inferred from a set of premises expressed only in terms of is. Indeed, this is taken to be a kind of 'common sense' argument by many when addressing questions of ethics, especially in public/political contexts. Although Hume's precise meaning is widely debated, the standard interpretation takes Hume to be asserting here that no set of nonmoral premises can entail a moral conclusion.[16] This interpretation has taken on a life of its own, with the claim that an 'ought cannot be derived from an is' being regularly invoked when addressing questions of ethics, especially in public/political contexts.

A range of dominant perspectives in global ethics – including Kantian deontological, utilitarian and contractualist ethics – adhere to this strict separation of the normative and the empirical. Kimberly Hutchings helpfully groups these together as 'rationalist approaches', emphasizing that, for all of them, different forms of rationality play an important part in providing the basis for the authority of ethical claims, and for differentiating ethical claims from the claims of pure self-interest or subjective feeling.[17] Moral epistemology here – what Hutchings calls 'the authority of moral claims' rests on some form of rationality, either 'self-legislating' or 'instrumental' reason. For these rationalist approaches, the empirical realm plays no part in either the creation or the 'grounding' of normative claims. In moral and political theory, the widespread commitment to rationalism has resulted in the predominance of 'ideal theory' – which sets out moral principles of what is good and right and, by implication, prescribes how we ought to live. This type of theory can be developed in isolation from any reference to actual or empirical lives or worlds, but can also, secondarily, be *applied* to those lives and worlds. Theories of justice derived from Kantian, neo-Kantian and contractualist principles are ideal theories of this kind – the most well-known example being, of course, Rawls's *A Theory of Justice*.

Of course, not all moral and political theorists accept this dichotomy. As Brooke Ackerly and colleagues point out, there is a growing family of political theory calling for more attention to empirical politics in theory development. Predominant within this family has been the work of so-called political realists, such as Bernard Williams, Raymond Geuss and James Tully, who argue that political philosophy must start from and be concerned with not only how people ought ideally (or ought 'rationally') to act, but rather with the 'way the social, economic, political, etc., institutions actually operate in some society at some given time'.[18] Geuss has been particularly scathing in his critique of the 'empirical abstemiousness' of much contemporary political theory, especially Kantianism. Indeed, he rejects the claim that there is, or could be, such a thing as a separate discipline called Ethics, which 'assumes that one can study this subject matter without constantly locating it within the rest of human life, and without unceasingly reflecting on the relations one's claims have with history, sociology, ethnology, psychology, and economics'.[19]

Notably, while Geuss's philosophical realism is characterized by his critique of the separation between ethics and politics, it is widely understood that realism in the theory of international relations (IR) is committed to an 'explanatory agenda that largely excludes normative theorising as the terrain of "political theory", "normative theory" or "philosophy"'.[20] Many scholars view realist IR theory, in its many forms, as not only adhering to a separation of the normative and the empirical, but sidelining or bracketing the normative altogether. As international justice scholar Charles Beitz put it, one of the foundational assumptions of realism in IR is that 'moral judgements have no place in discussions of international affairs or foreign policy'.[21] 'Normative theorists' in IR, such as Beitz, have, by contrast, followed in the footsteps of their 'ideal theory' colleagues in political theory, constructing liberal cosmopolitan theories of justice for the global context.[22]

This gap between the 'real' and the 'ideal' in global politics has been addressed by constructivist IR scholars. Notably, Richard Price's 2008 book, *Moral Limit and Possibility in World Politics*, begins with a question: 'At what point, if any, is one to reasonably concede that the "realities" of world politics require compromise from cherished principles or moral ends, and that what has been achieved is ethically justified?'[23] Price goes on to accuse both liberal and critical theories of IR of laying claim to the moral high ground and, in so doing, being open to charges of utopianism.[24] His analysis builds to the following central argument:

> Since social constructivist analyses of the development and effects of moral norms entail theoretical and empirical claims about the conditions of possibility and limits of moral change in world politics, that agenda should provide insightful leverage on the ethical question of 'what to do' insofar as one accepts that a responsible answer depends not just on what one judges as right in the abstract, but also what one may have some reasonable expectation of working, and thus prescribing as a course of action or judgement.[25]

Later, Price details six major contributions of constructivism to addressing global ethical dilemmas, including 'attention to the relation between the ethical and empirical, including providing a way to help adjudicate the empirical bases of ethical positions'.[26] The emphasis here is on what Price sees as the possibilities *actually available* in any given context.

Lived experiences and social practices vary considerably around the world, and are shot through with wide-ranging, diverse and often conflicting norms of social organization and forms of power. Constructivist scholars are interested in 'normative change' in world politics, and seek to build a bridge between the normative and the ethical in the study of international relations; it is on these grounds that they advocate for 'careful empirical research' in order to demonstrate the limits and possibilities of moral progress.[27] But the 'constructivist solution' is ultimately of little use in navigating the tension between the empirical and the normative – or the 'real world' and the 'ideal' – because it keeps in place the dichotomous distinction between them. Indeed, as I argued in 2009,

> Resolving this tension demands sustained attention to questions of moral epistemology, the possibility of moral judgment, and how both of these relate to the book's stated (and crucial) concerns about the role of power. It may also involve interrogating how existing moral discourses and normative structures serve to exclude, oppress and in other ways hurt some individuals and groups and not others, and consideration of better and worse alternatives, within specific contexts, that may begin to transform those discourses and structures so that they may lead to less exclusion and suffering.[28]

A more promising development in addressing the relationship between the empirical and the normative in political (and international political) theory is the recent identification of an umbrella term to capture the method shared by a range of empirically engaged political theory. Grounded normative theory (GNT) is marked by shared commitments to incorporating original empirical data or analysis in a recursive process of theory development striving for accountability to persons in empirical contexts.[29] While the authors discuss and cite a diverse set of works that, they suggest, would qualify as works of GNT, most notable, to my mind, is their reference to Coulthard and Simpson's work on grounded normativity. For Coulthard and Simpson, grounded normativity refers to the ethical frameworks provided by Indigenous place-based practices and associated forms of knowledge.[30] They are particularly critical of the modernist, Eurocentric, developmentalist ontology that treats the 'locatedness of land, culture and place as material and ideational impediments to the formation of broader coalitions and, in turn, posits them as factors that need to be abandoned for the sake of our own emancipation'.[31] For Coulthard and Simpson, grounded normativity houses and reproduces the practices and procedures, based on deep reciprocity, that are inherently informed by an intimate relationship to place.[32] Importantly, that normativity is not only grounded in land and place, but foregrounds the settler colonial frame, which is characterized by diverse configurations of power which produce a host of violences, in the form of white supremacy, heteropatriarchal domination and class exploitation and inequality.[33] As I will argue below, this acute recognition of, and attention to, forms of power is crucial for empirically aware moral thinking.

11.2 THE NORMATIVE, THE EMPIRICAL AND THE ETHICS OF CARE

Political realism, constructivist theory and GNT aim to offer different but related approaches to bringing the empirical into normative political (and international political) theory. But, as I argued above, constructivism is limited by its commitment to what we might have a 'reasonable expectation' of working, as well as a lack of onto-epistemological reflexivity on the empirical 'reality' – the world or worlds that are to be examined as a prelude to making normative claims. GNT, in its methodological commitment to attentiveness and recursivity, comes closer to the approach of feminist care ethics, especially those versions that pay close attention to context, place, relationality and power. In what follows here, I argue that feminist ethics, and care ethics in particular, provides a unique and particularly useful approach to the relationship between the normative and the empirical; it does this through: (1) a thin normative commitment to radical moral-social transformation that is rooted in the everyday care practices of relational subjects; and (2) a methodological commitment to interrogating practices of responsibility (or irresponsibility) in specific social-moral contexts in order to reveal patterns of injustice. Before I address this method in more detail, I will trace the development of thinking on the relationship between the normative and the empirical in the literature on care ethics.

The 'different voice' of care ethics – as identified by Carol Gilligan in her groundbreaking 1982 book[34] – stands in contrast to dominant, rationalist, masculinist, justice-based moral reasoning. The ethics of care focuses not on the principled grounds for moral judgement, but rather on the relational and contextual (and often messy) everyday process of working through moral-social life in the context of webs of relations and responsibilities of care. Indeed, care ethics starts from a thoroughgoing relational ontology; moral subjects are understood as deeply relational subjects who consider questions of 'how to act' amidst thick contexts of interdependence with others. Care itself may be understood as a response to need through attentiveness and responsiveness – 'being there' for others with whom we exist in relationship. Patience, trust, attentive listening and focused attention are skills that must be cultivated in order to respond with care; these practices are often difficult and must be learned and practised. Responding with care to others may involve 'juggling', struggle, worry and failure. The needs of others must be weighed and balanced, and we often must confront the danger of 'losing' our own sense of self in the process of caring for others. There are no rational principles for good care – instead, what is good, true and beautiful is revealed through caring itself. As relational moral subjects, we become morally better through slow and often painful processes of learning and unlearning, as we nurture our relationships and struggle to see and know others as they wish to be seen and understood.

Care ethics scholars have emphasized the importance of concrete contexts – rather than abstract dilemmas – for making moral judgements. Nel Noddings echoes Gilligan's research when she refers to hypothetical moral dilemmas and the need to 'know more', in order to 'form a picture more nearly resembling real moral situations'.[35] As she puts it, '[m]oral decisions are, after all, made in *real* situations; they are qualitatively different from the solution of geometry problems' (italics added).[36] For Noddings, like Gilligan, this is a specifically feminine approach to morality, based on women's social-moral positionality or what she refers to as 'our experience as women': '[w]omen, in particular, seem to approach moral problems by placing themselves as nearly as possible in concrete situations and assuming personal responsibility for the choices to be made'.[37] It is this process of 'concretization', rather than 'abstraction', that is key to Noddings's account here. Virginia Held reinforces this line of argument when she states that 'the method of moral inquiry I advocate relies on actual rather than hypothetical moral experience'.[38] She stresses the need to consider 'embodied, feeling human beings in specific historical and social contexts'. Importantly, Held emphasizes the feminist roots of this approach, which pays attention to the neglected experience of women – not only as 'carers', but also as those subject to oppression – through, for example, violence and sexual objectification.[39]

Joan Tronto's highly influential work on care ethics explicitly foregrounds 'the political' in the context of care. Notably, Tronto is critical of Noddings's 'unmediated ideal of care', and her unwillingness to admit any use for institutional or structural types of care.[40] Care, as a private or social virtue, cannot simply be imported into political life, according to Tronto.[41] In a manner reminiscent of the realist political theory discussed above, Tronto is thus critical of what she calls a 'morality first' strategy, which posits care as a moral value that should inform politics.[42] By contrast, she conceptualizes care as a 'practice' and 'political ideal'; as she explains, '[b]ecause the practice of care is also a political idea, I do not face the problem of trying to import a moral concept into a political order'.[43] She holds that the practice of care 'describes the qualities necessary for democratic citizens to live together well in a pluralistic society, and that only in a just, pluralistic, democratic society can care flourish'.[44]

More recent work on care ethics has emphasized the 'ongoing dialogue between the normative and the empirical' and acknowledges the 'interplay of context and value'.[45] Tove Petterson stresses the way that care ethicists have paid particular and careful attention to the 'interface between the normative and the empirical, between philosophy and practice'.[46] She argues that care ethics starts from the way we live our lives, especially, but not exclusively, the practices of care in which we engage – and uses this knowledge as a basis for developing analytical concepts and theories in order to better understand and handle what one empirically faces up to.[47] In this vein, other scholars have emphasized the need to pay attention not simply to the empirical realities of sociopolitical life, broadly understood, but specifically to actual practices of care, understood more conventionally or narrowly. For example, Leget, van Nistelrooij and Visse refer to the importance of 'concrete practices of caring' as the point of departure of any care-ethical reflection. They emphasize that empirical research is needed in order to learn what occurs in everyday practice – for example, nursing on an intensive care unit (ICU) or a hospice. They describe their 'normatively loaded' care-ethical theory that can be used as a theoretical framework and as a hypothesis that is tested and adapted on the basis of empirical research and theoretical reflection. Morally good practices must be (a) meaningful for those engaged in the practice, (b) in accordance with internal standards of that particular practice and (c) in accordance with some form of justice.[48]

Among the newest research on care ethics is work focused on 'decentring' it – in other words, acknowledging the diversity of forms of care, as well as the wide-ranging ways of knowing associated with care ethics.[49] While genealogies of care ethics often trace this thinking back to the work of Carol Gilligan, the broad idea of an ethic of caring has played a significant but often under-recognized role in Black feminist and Indigenous thought. Patricia Hill Collins writes of the way that the emphasis on expressiveness and emotion in African American communities bears marked resemblance to feminist perspectives on the importance of what she calls 'personality' in connected knowing. Here she is referring to the concrete subject, who is unique yet relational, and whose sense of self is achieved in relation to others, thus 'enriching' the whole.[50] Anishinaabe scholar Eva Jewell explains that care is 'at home in Anishinaabe worldviews, and is a vital concept in our onto-epistemologies'.[51] Andrea Smith's influential work demonstrates how Indigenous cosmologies offer new insights into potentially more just forms of governance. As she puts it: 'Whereas nation-states are governed through domination and coercion, indigenous sovereignty and nationhood are predicated on interrelatedness and responsibility. In opposition to nation-states, which are based on control over territory, these visions of indigenous nationhood are based on care and responsibility for the land that all can share.'[52] These perspectives ground their normativity in the concrete – for Black feminists, in the family, the community, the church and for Indigenous feminists, in the land and the more-than-human world. Notably, however, unlike the care ethics of many white and Western feminists, their experience of giving and receiving care cannot be extricated from their experience of oppression and violence. Making sense of this demands an approach to ethics that foregrounds, rather than erases, power and the political in the empirical 'realities' it examines. In order to tease out this idea, I turn now to the work of Margaret Urban Walker, whose work on morality, normativity and power is particularly instructive here.

Walker begins her 1998 book, *Moral Understandings*, with four theses on morality: first, morality itself consists in practices, not theories; second, the practices characteristic of morality are practices of responsibility; third, morality is not socially modular; and fourth, 'moral theorizing and moral epistemology need to be freed from the impoverishing legacies of ideality and purity that make most of most people's moral lives disappear, or render those lives unintelligible'.[53] In fleshing out these arguments, Walker insists that moral practices cannot be 'extricated from other social practices, nor can moral identities from social roles and institutions in particular lifeways'.[54] Morality is therefore not a special cognitive or practical skill or process that we consciously bring to bear when moral dilemmas arise. Thus, when Walker claims that morality is 'not socially modular', she means that morality is not a dimension of reality beyond or separate from shared life or a distinct and detachable set of understandings within it.[55] On the contrary, in our real lives, moral understandings are entwined with social ones and, importantly, moral understandings are 'typically effected *through* social ones'.[56] Seen in this way, our moral lives are distinctly unlike philosophy classrooms, where moral and political philosophers can debate such dilemmas – of shallow ponds, tortured (or not) terrorists, and stolen (or not) drugs. In our real lives, we cannot isolate moral dilemmas from other aspects of our collective lives, and the various demands, responsibilities, hopes and aims that define them.

Walker explains how moral theorizing within what she calls the 'theoretical-juridical approach' typically universalizes and homogenizes 'the' moral point of view or position of 'the' moral agent, and traffics in claims about 'our' concept of responsibility, sense of justice, institutions or obligations.[57] The implications of this, moreover, are not benign. Indeed, the idea of a 'pure and compact core of moral knowledge' permits philosophers to 'bypass the interlacing of moral vocabularies and practices with other historically and culturally embedded beliefs and social practices'.[58] It also 'shields' the 'historical, cultural and social location of the moral philosopher' and, indeed, of moral philosophy itself.[59]

Importantly, Walker emphasizes that if morality is not 'socially modular', as she claims, then understanding morality requires understanding 'how it is seated and reproduced in actual human societies'.[60] In relation to this, she describes the urgent task of what she calls 'critical moral ethnography': 'If it is characteristic of human societies (including our own) that moral standards, statuses, and distributions of responsibility work through social differences, rather than in spite of them, then to understand morality – what it is – is to see how morality works, and works better or worse, in just this way.'[61] For Walker, then, morality works *through* power differentials, not in opposition to them. Her approach to ethics is thus a project of critique which rejects not only the separation of the empirical and the normative, but the dichotomy between knowledge (ideals) and power (the political). When we reject the 'theoretical-juridical' approach, we open up space for a new kind of moral 'theorizing', which can 'directly interrogate some of the most morally troubling aspects of human life: domination, oppression, exclusion, coercion and basic disregard of some people by others'.[62] Indeed, Walker is very clear in her thinking about the role that 'morality' has often played in human relations:

> The fact is that morality as actual human practice has more often supplied understandings that legitimate such human relations than ones that condemn them. If we know such things are deeply wrong, it is because we have found our way to another actual human practice of responsibility that condemns these others. Or at least some of us have found our way to the bare image, or specific fragments, of such a practice. It is the practice in this world we need to know how to defend and make real.[63]

We know, Walker argues,

> that powers of several types ... in various linked dimensions (economic, political, social, discursive and cultural) can allow some people to rig both the arrangements and the perceptions of them, and so to obscure what's really happening to whom and why. It is this fund of knowledge that needs to be enlarged and theoretically articulated in general accounts and specific studies of *different relative moral positions in differentiated social lives*. (emphasis in original)[64]

The implication of these claims is not simply that we must have an awareness of empirical 'context' in order to be able to make moral judgements, but that we must understand the ethical as effected in and through the political – in other words, through relations of power. Those moral judgements – and the resolutions to moral problems – gain their authority not through reference to immutable foundations or principles, but, as Walker puts it, through the 'character of the common life they lead us to'.[65] They will be more or less acceptable depending on how they sustain or alter the integrity of the parties, and the terms of their relationships.[66] An ethics of care that is guided by this critical, political sensibility will not simply espouse the moral value of care as a route to global justice but will provide the critical resources for thinking about the different forms and relations of power that prevent, prohibit and inhibit practices of care. In the final section, I consider this account – which provides the groundwork for a critical, feminist ethic of care – in the context of thinking about global (in)justice.

11.3 RETHINKING GLOBAL ETHICS

The Covid-19 global pandemic brought with it a heightened sense of insecurity and precarity to regions normally insulated from large scale suffering and crisis. This insecurity has deepened as the world has witnessed a proliferation of climate-change-induced weather events, many of which have led to loss of life and the destruction of homes and communities. Violent conflicts rage in many parts of the globe, as the possibility of widespread or even 'world' war no longer seems remote. Humanitarian crises abound, as people flee violence, risking their lives to do so. Income inequality deepens daily, both within and among nation-states. While some may respond by 'doubling down' on principles of rights, justice and just war, others may be struck by the failure of our moral theories to provide the normative basis for ways forward.

It is no accident that abstract moral theories, which fail to connect with the way that we live our everyday lives, seem increasingly irrelevant, or that the concept of care is experiencing what Andreas Chatzidakis et al refer to as 'discursive explosion'.[67] They argue that the Covid crisis has finally foregrounded 'care' as a keyword of our time – one that hitherto had remained largely peripheral in the lexicon of the left, despite the persistent efforts of a long line of feminist theorists.[68] While these scholars are primarily interested in the way that 'care' has crept into the lexicon of media, popular culture, corporations and politicians, I am interested in the ways that ideas related to the normative, empirical and political significance of care have been increasingly used by feminist scholars to conceptualize and understand moral harms in contemporary global politics. Notably, this work foregrounds the moral value of caring practices while grounding these claims in socially differentiated political and economic 'realities', and recognizing and interrogating relations or power at multiple sites and scales. Put differently, we can see the work of these scholars as highlighting both the positive, but often hidden aspects of care and love as responses to violence and harm, as well as the social relations of power that make practices of care dangerous, difficult or impossible. In all cases, what is morally valuable – a normatively good in human lives – is not dissociated from our social lives, or from political and economic relations of power. While no theories or principles of justice are espoused, they take us further towards understanding the nature of injustice, as well as the ethical and political value of our moral-social practices of care.

The first body of work, by feminist scholars of global political economy, focuses on the consequences of the global failure to recognize or account for the contribution of social reproductive labour – sometimes called 'care work' – to national economies. In their 2014 article, authors Shirin Rai, Cathryn Hoskyns and Dania Thomas mobilize the concept of 'depletion', which occurs as the level at which the resource outflows exceed resource inflows in carrying out social reproductive work over a threshold of sustainability, making it harmful for those engaged in this unvalued work.[69] When this occurs, the sustainability of the everyday lives of women and men is undermined, leading to decrease, exhaustion and loss – of the body, the household and community. In their efforts to understand these harms – which they classify as discursive, emotional, they ask:

> what are the axes of class, caste and race, North and South, that mark social reproductive labour and consequent depletion? Are some benefiting from the present regimes of labour and able to trade off depletion with the labour of others? Are some households able to withstand the costs of buying in aspects of social reproduction while others are buffeted by economic crises and go under?[70]

The authors are concerned with bodies here – which, while discrete, are also relational, and while being depleted on an individual basis, must do so within social frameworks that position them in relation to other bodies. But they emphasize the household as the central unit of analysis, where the question of who does what in contributing to social reproduction and with what resources – money, time and health – are of paramount importance.[71]

While Rai, Hoskyns and Thomas do not use the language of ethics and morality, or indeed of care, they point to the 'urgent need' to address the issue of depletion in the context of social reproduction. Furthermore, while social reproduction is not identical to 'care', it includes valuable emotional and affective practices that maintain families and relationships, as well as forms of social provisioning and voluntary work directed and meeting needs in and of the community.[72] The concept of depletion – notably first used by scholars of environmental politics – provides a framework for critical evaluation of these practices, recognizing that the consequences of the depletion of social reproduction will depend on geopolitical, class and gendered positionings.

In their 2022 article 'Taking Love and Care Seriously: An Emergent Research Agenda for Remaking Worlds in the Wake of Violence', Roxani Krystalli and Phillip Schulz explore the practices of love and care that 'sit alongside' experiences of harm in the context of armed conflict. Specifically, they ask, 'how can centring practices of love and care illuminate different pathways for understanding the remaking of worlds in the wake of violence?' Building on interdisciplinary literature, the authors conceptualise love and care as 'practices and potential sites of politics that shape how people survive and make sense of violence as well as imagine and enact lives in its wake'. Drawing from their research in Colombia and Uganda, their argument draws attention to the simultaneity of harms and care, sheds light on the textured meanings of politics and political work, and highlights ethical and narrative dilemmas regarding how to capture these political meanings without reducing their intricacies.[73]

While the feminist global political economy research on depletion addresses familiar sites and practices of care – namely, reproductive labour in the household – Krystalli and Schulz's research focuses on sites where care is assumed to be absent. As they note, scholarly narratives about armed conflicts are typically characterized by a primary, if not exclusive, focus on violence, suffering and harm.[74] Notably, the empirical discussion of Uganda and Columbia is central to their analysis, and is structured around a series of analytic themes, including the relationship of love and care to the political. As such, the authors draw from their interlocutors' narratives to demonstrate not only that care is political work but also that political work requires the work of care. But importantly, and tied to Walker's insights, they also consider how a focus on love and care can risk depoliticizing subjects and relationships.[75] Here, Krystalli and Schulz are reading love and care as both 'pathways for remaking worlds' and potentially, moral discourses and practices that may, through depoliticization, reinforce existing relations of power. As they put it, 'narratives about being motivated by love and care to do their work risk eliding the ways in which the same bureaucracies can simultaneously neglect, cause harm, or reinforce forms of structural and systemic violence against those they purport to serve'.[76] Their work thus ties the normative to the empirical in ways that foreground the value everyday practices of care while refusing idealization and recognizing how the ethical operates in and through the political.

CONCLUSION

In this chapter, I have considered the particular insights that care ethics can bring to conversations about the relationship between the normative and the empirical, especially in relation to questions of global ethics. After briefly tracing the question as it is navigated in political and international political theory, I moved to a consideration of this question in care ethics. This revealed the ways and extent to which care ethics is committed to an 'ongoing dialogue' between the normative and the political.[77] Here, I focused specifically on the insights of feminist moral theorist Margaret Urban Walker, whose analysis of the 'empirical burdens' of moral philosophy focused on the relationship between the moral and the sociopolitical, and the importance of considering relations of power in order to understand the distribution of responsibilities for care in any given context. Finally, I concluded the chapter by considering recent work in feminist IR which addresses the moral importance of practices of care (including 'love' and social reproduction) while focusing on the empirical sociopolitical and economic contexts in which they are immersed. Care ethics cannot provide a theory of global justice, but it can reveal the ubiquitous and life-sustaining nature of quotidian practices of care around the world while emphasizing their embeddedness in social and political life.

NOTES

1. Peter Railton, 'Normative Force and Normative Freedom: Hume and Kant, but not Hume *versus* Kant', *Ratio* 12, no. 4 (1999): 320.
2. Onora O'Neill, 'Applied Ethics: Naturalism, Normativity and Public Policy', *Journal of Applied Philosophy* 26, no. 3 (2009): 221.
3. Ibid.
4. Immanuel Kant, 'Groundwork of the Metaphysics of Morals', in *Practical Philosophy*, ed. and trans. Mary J. Gregor (Cambridge: Cambridge University Press, 1996) [originally published in 1785], 4: 442–3.
5. Kimberly Hutchings, *International Political Theory* (London: Sage, 1999), 23.
6. Richard Price, *Moral Limit and Possibility in World Politics* (Cambridge: Cambridge University Press, 2008), 67.
7. Brooke Ackerly et al., 'Unearthing Grounded Normative Theory: Practices and Commitments of Empirical Research in Political Theory', *Critical Review of International Social and Political Philosophy* 27, no. 2 (2021): 159.
8. Margaret Walker, *Moral Understandings: A Feminist Study in Ethics* (New York: Routledge, 1998), 22.
9. Ibid., 13.
10. See: Fiona Robinson, *Globalizing Care: Ethics, Feminist Theory and International Relations* (Boulder, CO: Westview Press, 1999); and Fiona Robinson, *The Ethics of Care: A Feminist Approach to Human Security* (Philadelphia, PA: Temple University Press, 2011). See also Joan C. Tronto, *Caring Democracy: Markets, Equality and Justice* (New York: New York University Press, 2013); Maurice Hamington, *Embodied Care: Jane Addams, Maurice Merleau-Ponty, and Feminist Ethics* (Champaign: University of Illinois Press, 2004); Daniel Engster, *The Heart of Justice: Care Ethics and Political Theory* (Oxford: Oxford University Press, 2007); and M. FitzGerald, *Care and the Pluriverse: Rethinking Global Ethics* (Bristol: Bristol University Press, 2022).
11. Walker, *Moral Understandings*, 16.
12. Ibid., 27.
13. Simon Caney, 'Global Distributive Justice', in *The Oxford Handbook of International Political Theory*, ed. Chris Brown and Robyn Eckersley Moore (Oxford: Oxford University Press, 2018), 108.
14. Walker, *Moral Understandings*, 16.
15. Tronto, *Caring Democracy*.
16. Alasdair C. MacIntyre, 'Hume on "Is" and "Ought"', *The Philosophical Review* 68, no. 4 (1959): 452.
17. Kimberly Hutchings, *Global Ethics: An Introduction*, 2nd ed. (Cambridge: Polity Press, 2018), 25.
18. Raymond Geuss, *Philosophy and Real Politics* (Princeton, NJ: Princeton University Press, 2008), 9.
19. Geuss, *Philosophy and Real Politics*, 7.
20. Price, *Moral Limit and Possibility in World Politics*, 4.

21. Charles R. Beitz, *Political Theory and International Relations* (Princeton, NJ: Princeton University Press, 1979), 15.
22. Beitz, *Political Theory and International Relations.*
23. Price, *Moral Limit and Possibility in World Politics*, 1.
24. Ibid., 2.
25. Ibid., 6–7.
26. Ibid., 7.
27. Price, *Moral Limit and Possibility in World Politics.*
28. Fiona Robinson, 'Bridging the Real and the Ideal in International Ethics', *International Studies Review* 11, no. 2 (2009): 397.
29. Ackerly et al., 'Unearthing Grounded Normative Theory', 3.
30. Glen Coulthard and Leanne B. Simpson, 'Grounded Normativity/Place-Based Solidarity', *American Quarterly* 68, no. 2 (2016): 254.
31. Ibid., 253.
32. Ibid., 254.
33. Ibid., 251.
34. Carol Gilligan, *In a Different Voice: Psychological Theory and Women's Development* (Cambridge, MA: Harvard University Press, 1982).
35. Nel Noddings, *Caring: A Relational Approach to Ethics and Moral Education*, 2nd ed. (Berkeley and Los Angeles: University of California Press, 2013), 2.
36. Ibid., 3.
37. Ibid., 8.
38. Virginia Held, *The Ethics of Care: Personal, Political, and Global* (New York: Oxford University Press, 2005), 159.
39. Ibid., 160.
40. Joan C. Tronto, *Moral Boundaries: A Political Argument for an Ethic of Care* (New York: Routledge, 1993), 160.
41. Ibid., 161.
42. Ibid., 158.
43. Ibid., 161.
44. Ibid., 161–2.
45. Tove Pettersen, 'The Ethics of Care: Normative Structures and Empirical Implications', *Health Care Analysis* 19 (2011): 61.
46. Ibid.
47. Ibid.
48. Carlo Leget, Inge van Nistelrooij and Merel Visse, 'Beyond Demarcation: Care Ethics as an Interdisciplinary Field of Inquiry', *Nursing Ethics* 26, no. 1 (2019): 17–25.
49. Sophie Bourgault, Maggie FitzGerald and Fiona Robinson, eds, *Decentering Epistemologies and Challenging Privilege: Critical Care Ethics Perspectives* (New Brunswick, NJ: Rutgers University Press, 2024).
50. Patricia H. Collins, 'Toward an Afrocentric Feminist Epistemology', in *Turning Points in Qualitative Research: Tying Knots in a Handkerchief*, ed. Yvonna S. Lincoln and Norman K. Denzin (Lanham, MD: Rowman & Littlefield, 2003), 62.
51. Andrea Doucet, Eva Jewell and Vanessa Watts, 'Indigenous and Feminist Ecological Reflections on Feminist Care Ethics: Encounters of Care, Absence, Punctures, and Offerings', in *Decentering Epistemologies and Challenging Privilege: Critical Care Ethics Perspectives*, ed. Sophie Bourgault, Maggie FitzGerald and Fiona Robinson (New Brunswick, NJ: Rutgers University Press, 2024).

52. Andrea Smith, 'American Studies without America: Native Feminisms and the Nation-State', in 'Forum: Native Feminisms without Apology', ed. Andrea Smith and J. Kēhaulani Kauanui, *American Quarterly* 60, no. 2 (2008): 311–12.
53. Walker, *Moral Understandings*, 14–18.
54. Ibid., 17.
55. Margaret U. Walker, 'Morality in Practice: A Response to Claudia Card and Lorraine Code', *Hypatia* 17, no. 1 (2002): 176.
56. Walker, *Moral Understandings*, 17.
57. Ibid.
58. Ibid., 56.
59. Ibid.
60. Ibid., 211.
61. Ibid.
62. Ibid., 15.
63. Ibid., 15–16.
64. Ibid., 219.
65. Ibid., 68.
66. Ibid., 70.
67. Andreas Chatzidakis et al., 'From Carewashing to Radical Care: The Discursive Explosions of Care during Covid-19', *Feminist Media Studies* 20, no. 6 (2020): 889–95.
68. Ibid., 890.
69. Shirin M. Rai, Catherine Hoskyns and Dania Thomas, 'Depletion: The Cost of Social Reproduction', *International Feminist Journal of Politics* 16, no. 1 (2014): 88–9.
70. Shirin M. Rai, Catherine Hoskyns and Dania Thomas, *Depletion and Social Reproduction* (Coventry: Centre for the Study of Globalisation and Regionalisation, University of Warwick, 2011) [Working Paper No. 274], 7–8.
71. Ibid., 8.
72. Rai, Hoskyns and Thomas, 'Depletion', 87.
73. Roxani Krystalli and Phillip Schulz, 'Taking Love and Care Seriously: An Emergent Research Agenda for Remaking Worlds in the Wake of Violence', *International Studies Review* 24, no. 1 (2022), 1.
74. Ibid.
75. Ibid., 4.
76. Ibid., 16.
77. Pettersen, 'The Ethics of Care'.

BIBLIOGRAPHY

Ackerly, Brooke., Luis Cabrera, Fonna Forman, Genevieve F. Johnson, Chris Tenove and Antje Wiener. 'Unearthing Grounded Normative Theory: Practices and Commitments of Empirical Research in Political Theory', *Critical Review of International Social and Political Philosophy* 27, no. 2 (2021): 156–82.

Bourgault, Sophie, Maggie FitzGerald and Fiona Robinson, eds. *Decentering Epistemologies and Challenging Privilege: Critical Care Ethics Perspectives*. New Brunswick, NJ: Rutgers University Press, 2024.

Beitz, Charles R. *Political Theory and International Relations*. Princeton, NJ: Princeton University Press, 1979.

Caney, Simon. 'Global Distributive Justice,' in *The Oxford Handbook of International Political Theory*, edited by Chris Brown and Robyn Eckersley, 103–17. Oxford: Oxford University Press, 2018.

Chatzidakis, Andreas, Jamie Hakim, Jo Littler, Catherine Rottenberg and Lynne Segal. 'From Carewashing to Radical Care: The Discursive Explosions of Care During Covid-19', *Feminist Media Studies* 20, no. 6 (2020): 889–95.

Collins, Patricia H. 'Toward an Afrocentric Feminist Epistemology', in *Turning Points in Qualitative Research: Tying Knots in a Handkerchief*, edited by Yvonna S. Lincoln and Norman K. Denzin, 47–72. Lanham, MD: Rowman & Littlefield, 2003.

Coulthard, Glen, and Leanne B. Simpson. 'Grounded Normativity/Place-Based Solidarity', *American Quarterly* 68, no. 2 (2016): 249–55.

Doucet, Andrea, Eva Jewell and Vanessa Watts. 'Indigenous and Feminist Ecological Reflections on Feminist Care Ethics: Encounters of Care, Absence, Punctures, and Offerings', in *Decentering Epistemologies and Challenging Privilege: Critical Care Ethics Perspectives*, edited by Sophie Bourgault, Maggie FitzGerald and Fiona Robinson. New Brunswick, NJ: Rutgers University Press, 2024, 15–30.

Engster, Daniel. *The Heart of Justice: Care Ethics and Political Theory*. Oxford: Oxford University Press, 2007.

FitzGerald, Maggie. *Care and the Pluriverse: Rethinking Global Ethics*. Bristol: Bristol University Press, 2022.

Geuss, Raymond. *Philosophy and Real Politics*. Princeton, NJ: Princeton University Press, 2008.

Gilligan, Carol. *In a Different Voice: Psychological Theory and Women's Development*. Cambridge, MA: Harvard University Press, 1982.

Hamington, Maurice. *Embodied Care: Jane Addams, Maurice Merleau-Ponty, and Feminist Ethics*. Champaign: University of Illinois Press, 2004.

Held, Virginia. *The Ethics of Care: Personal, Political, and Global*. New York: Oxford University Press, 2005.

Hutchings, Kimberly. *International Political Theory*. London: Sage, 1999.

Hutchings, Kimberly. *Global Ethics: An Introduction*, 2nd edn. Cambridge: Polity Press, 2018.

Leget, Carlo, Inge van Nistelrooij and Merel Visse. 'Beyond Demarcation: Care Ethics as an Interdisciplinary Field of Inquiry', *Nursing Ethics* 26, no. 1 (2019): 17–25.

Kant, Immanuel. *Groundwork of the Metaphysics of Morals*, in *Practical Philosophy*, edited by Mary J. Gregor, 37–108. Cambridge: Cambridge University Press, 1996 [originally published in 1785].

Krystalli, Roxani and Phillip Schulz. 'Taking Love and Care Seriously: An Emergent Research Agenda for Remaking Worlds in the Wake of Violence', *International Studies Review* 24, no. 1 (2022): 1–23.

MacIntyre, Alasdair C. 'Hume on "Is" and "Ought"', *The Philosophical Review* 68, no. 4 (1959): 451–68.

Noddings, Nel. *Caring: A Relational Approach to Ethics and Moral Education*, 2nd ed. Berkeley and Los Angeles: University of California Press, 2013.

O'Neill, Onora. 'Applied Ethics: Naturalism, Normativity and Public Policy', *Journal of Applied Philosophy* 26, no. 3 (2009): 219–30.

Pettersen, Tove. 'The Ethics of Care: Normative Structures and Empirical Implications', *Health Care Analysis* 19 (2011): 51–64.

Price, Richard. *Moral Limit and Possibility in World Politics*. Cambridge: Cambridge University Press, 2008.

Rai, Shirin M., Catherine Hoskyns and Dania Thomas. *Depletion and Social Reproduction*. Coventry: Centre for the Study of Globalisation and Regionalisation, University of Warwick, 2011. Working Paper No. 274.

Rai, Shirin M., Catherine Hoskyns and Dania Thomas. 'Depletion: The Cost of Social Reproduction', *International Feminist Journal of Politics* 16, no. 1 (2014): 86–105.

Railton, Peter. 'Normative Force and Normative Freedom: Hume and Kant, but not Hume *versus* Kant', *Ratio* 12, no. 4 (1999): 320–53.

Robinson, Fiona. *Globalizing Care: Ethics, Feminist Theory and International Relations*. Boulder, CO: Westview Press, 1999.

Robinson, Fiona. 'Care, Gender and Global Social Justice: Rethinking "Ethical Globalization"', *Journal of Global Ethics* 2, no. 1 (2006): 5–25.

Robinson, Fiona. 'Bridging the Real and the Ideal in International Ethics', *International Studies Review* 11, no. 2 (2009): 396–8.

Robinson, Fiona. *The Ethics of Care: A Feminist Approach to Human Security*. Philadelphia, PA: Temple University Press, 2011.

Smith, Andrea. 'American Studies without America: Native Feminisms and the Nation-State', in *Forum: Native Feminisms without Apology*, edited by Andrea Smith and J. Kēhaulani Kauanui. Special section of *American Quarterly* 60, no. 2 (2008): 309–15.

Tronto, Joan C. *Moral Boundaries: A Political Argument for an Ethic of Care*. New York: Routledge, 1993.

Tronto, Joan C. *Caring Democracy: Markets, Equality and Justice*. New York: New York University Press, 2013.

Walker, Margaret U. *Moral Understandings: A Feminist Study in Ethics*. New York: Routledge, 1998.

Walker, Margaret U. 'Morality in Practice: A Response to Claudia Card and Lorraine Code', *Hypatia* 17, no. 1 (2002): 174–82.

CHAPTER TWELVE

The ethics of care as a transformation in moral philosophy

SANDRA LAUGIER

INTRODUCTION

In recent moral philosophy, the importance of care has come into its own, both in relation to the moral attitudes upon which it draws, such as solicitude, attentiveness and responsiveness, and to the practice of care in attending to the needs of others in everyday contexts. Yet the idea of a 'female morality', central to Carol Gilligan's work and first established in her seminal study, *In a Different Voice*, remains to be fully appreciated.[1] The concept is at once so provocative and so reasonable that we forget it is first and foremost feminist, and that it stakes a claim for an alternative form of morality. In searching for the latter, Gilligan's treatise seeks to capture a different, hitherto neglected yet universally present alternative ethical perspective, one easy to ignore because it relates to women and women's activities. In this respect, Gilligan's approach is not claiming an 'essence' of the female, or a specific female ethics; but it is plainly ordinary, imbued with the perspective of the everyday.[2]

The ethics of care is also a plea for 'realism', in the sense given to it in Cora Diamond's *The Realistic Spirit* to mean the necessity of seeing (or attending to) what lies close at hand.[3] Reflections on care brings ethics back to its proper domain of *everyday practice* – much as Wittgenstein sought to bring language back from the metaphysical level to its everyday use, where words have ordinary meanings grasped by the speakers of the language.

According to this perspective, ethics is not grasped by reference to an enumerable set of pre-existent rules – nor by attending to a metaphysically independent moral realm. Rather, it is grasped in the mere immanence of situations, affects and practices. The ethics of care affirms the importance of care and of paying attention to others; in particular, it concerns those whose life and wellbeing depend on particularized and sustained everyday patterns of care. Moreover, the ethics of care is based on an analysis of the historical conditions that have promoted a division of moral labour in which the activities of care are socially and morally devalorized. The relegation of women to the domestic sphere translates into the demotion of legitimate acts and concerns to the status of mere 'private' sentiments lacking moral and political weight. It is because the work and activities of care have traditionally fallen to women that care is first and foremost a women's issue.

By proposing to valorize moral values such as caring, attention to others and solicitude, the ethics of care has contributed to modifying the dominant conception of ethics in profoundly changing how we understand ethics. Moreover, the ethics of care introduces ethical stakes into politics, by effecting a critique of prominent theories of justice. But, most significantly, it has given due representation to *the ethically ordinary*. The ethic of care draws our attention to what we are unable to see, not because it is hidden or secret but because it is right before our eyes. It is, moreover, an ethics that closely attends to those who are undervalued precisely because they perform unnoticed tasks.

To locate this discussion, observe that the ethics of care, as rooted in the ordinary, adumbrates Wittgenstein's definition of *the ordinary*: 'what we are supplying are really remarks on the natural history of human beings ... observations which no one has doubted, but which have escaped remark only because they are always before our eyes'.[4] Wittgenstein addresses the question of what is 'important' and the fact – concretely substantiated by the ethics of care – that what seems the most important often is not so in the least: 'Where does our investigation get its importance from, since it seems to destroy everything interesting, all that is great and important? What we are destroying is nothing but houses of cards.'[5] This chapter aims to bring together the kind of 'destruction' to which Wittgenstein refers, and the appeal to the ordinary in the ethics of care. It pursues a connection I have built since 2005 between the ethics of care and ordinary language philosophy as represented by Wittgenstein and Cavell.[6]

12.1 A SENSITIVE SUBJECT

The subject of care is sensitive. In a first sense, broadly presented, reflection on care tends to give rise to objections, or even to outright rejection. It is thus a 'sensitive' subject matter. At first encounter, it seems to oppose a 'female' and a 'male' conception of ethics. As discussed by Gilligan and Nel Noddings, feminine ethics is defined by the concepts of attentiveness, concern for others, and a sense of responsibility reflecting close personal ties, while masculine ethics is defined by the concepts of rights, justice and autonomy. Much has been said, especially by Joan Tronto in her influential book *Moral Boundaries: A Political Argument for an Ethic of Care* about the difficulty of opposing a feminine and a masculine ethics as the ethics of care and the ethics of justice, respectively, which incurs the risk of reproducing the very ingrained prejudices that the ethic of care meant to counter. As proposed by Gilligan,[7] one can argue that far from being oppositive concepts, care and justice are in fact complementary perspectives, the choice of which depends on the context of application. In another sense, then, the subject of care is a sensitive subject. Thus, care is fundamentally embedded in a form of life unfolding in a context of relationships.

In addition to forming a new point of departure in philosophy, reflection on care effects a transformation of the very status of ethics. The question of *sensitivity* is indeed at the core of care. It is therefore urgently necessary to understand what is meant by this important concept, and what kind of sensitivity is involved in the ethics of care. Indeed, it is not so much *feeling* – for example, to be contrasted with rationality – as *perception*. Yet it is but an *ordinary* perception, not an 'objectifying' philosophical ersatz. It is here that we must look for the starting point for a modification of the ethical framework.

Gilligan herself, in returning to the antithesis of care and justice perspectives in 1987, starts from the paradigmatic duck–rabbit illustration of perspectival switching, using Wittgenstein's well-known example, first used by psychologist Joseph Jastrow, of an ambiguous image in which a rabbit or a duck can be alternatively seen. Like Wittgenstein, by drawing attention to it she does not aim to introduce a relativism of moral perspectives, but rather to indicate several important observations about 'seeing as'.[8] First, it indicates the possibility of changing viewpoints, even if one viewpoint necessarily dominates the choice. Moreover, it indicates the necessity of attending to only one perspective at any given time (in other words, the impossibility of mastering both at any given instance). In the third place, it indicates the importance of context to the representation of choice. By analogy, ethics is a matter of highlighting, for each moral situation we examine, not only different visual 'orientations', but a *framework* of perception.[9] Gilligan suggests a *Gestalt* approach to ethics, insisting, as did Wittgenstein, on the necessity of choosing aspects of salience against a given background.

Philosopher Cora Diamond defines the specificity of this approach as follows: 'Our *particular* moral conceptions emerge against a more general background of thought and sensibility. We differ in the way we allow (or do not allow) moral concepts to shape our lives and our relationships with others, in the way these concepts structure our accounts of what we have done or experienced.'[10] Such a perceptual approach, which may be seen as an ancestor to the philosophy of care, will be not only situational or dynamic, but also particularistic. It is only through attending to the particular, as opposed to the general, aspects of a situation that we will find the right perspective in ethics – as in aesthetics, for that matter.

Remember that in the *Tractatus*, Wittgenstein took a firm stand against the very existence of moral philosophy, given that the purpose of philosophy is said to be the logical clarification of propositions. Philosophy itself is not a body of doctrine, but an activity, which consists in making our thoughts clear.[11] From this description of the central task of philosophy it follows that there can only be such a thing as 'moral philosophy' if there is a body of propositions such that it is the task of moral philosophy to clarify them. But Wittgenstein also maintained, for reasons beyond the scope of this chapter, that there can be no ethical propositions.[12] And he described the *Tractatus*, which denied the existence of moral philosophy and ethical propositions, as having an ethical aim. In thus maintaining an ethical aim, he did not intend to represent the *Tractatus* as entirely silent on moral philosophy. Rather, the point is that ethics does not arise from theorizing, but from ordinary life. His position was that a work – for example, a novel or a short story – could have a moral purpose even in the absence of any moral teaching or theorizing. Such a work could help us to tackle the tasks of life in the required spirit.

The aim of such thinking is not to reject the idea of morality, nor of moral philosophy understood in a specific sense, but of a systematic moral theory. This is evinced, for example, by John McDowell in his essays on Wittgenstein[13] and Diamond in *The Realistic Spirit*. For example, we seek to determine the nature of the obligation inherent in a rule by relating it to 'something' in reality, rather than by looking at the ordinary way of saying what a rule requires. Thus, an examination of our particular moral practices is more *realistic* (in the sense proposed by Diamond) than the theoretical search for a 'moral reality'. We are dealing here with a moral philosophy inscribed in our ordinary practices and emerging from particular questionings.

12.2 ORDINARY REALISM

In his later works, which converge with Cavell and Diamond's ideas, Hilary Putnam proposed to abandon a certain form of realism in ethics and the possibility of a common ground for ethical discussions: 'Our ethical life cannot be captured by half a dozen words like "ought", "right", "duty", "fairness", "responsibility", "justice", and the ethical problems that concern us cannot be reduced to debates between the metaphysical propositions of the proponents of natural law, utilitarianism, common sense and so on.'[14] Putnam, like Diamond, reflects Iris Murdoch's legacy, which is to *take care* of *what we say*: 'There are ethical propositions which, while being more than descriptions, are also descriptions. One is then "entangled" by descriptive words like "cruel", "impertinent", "inconsiderate".'[15] These *entangled* terms, which are 'both evaluative and descriptive' and *ordinary*, are for Putnam at the heart of our ethical life: the elucidation of their uses is part of moral knowledge, which is a knowledge or ethics without ontology or metaphysics. This is owed to Murdoch's legacy and her reliance on the *vision* and ordinary *texture* of language. In contrast to metaphysics, the ordinary ethical approach should bring us back 'to the roughground of ordinary language'. There is nothing ontological in this realistic approach to ethics: 'logic as well as ethics can be found *there*, in what we do, and something like a fantasy prevents us from seeing it'.[16] The elements of an ethical vocabulary only make sense in the context of our uses, given a particular form of life; they may be said to 'come to life' against the background of a specific *praxis*. Context gives words their meaning – a meaning that is never fixed, always particular. Meaning is defined not only by use or context (as many philosophers have recognized) but is inscribed and perceptible only in the dynamic background of language practice, which is modified *by what we do with it*: '"Beautiful" is linked to a particular game. Similarly in ethics: the meaning of the word "good" is linked to the very act it modifies. We can only establish the meaning of the word "beauty" by considering how we use it.'[17] One might then be tempted to connect ethics with a particularistic ontology, which would put abstract particulars (e.g. from perception) at the centre of a value theory or a realism of particulars. But this would be to lose the meaning of the idea of family resemblance, which is precisely the negation of an ontology, including abstract particulars. Wittgenstein criticizes the craving for generality – the tendency to look for something common to all entities that we standardly subsume under a general term. The idea that a general concept is a property common to its particular cases is related to other primitive and overly simple ideas about the structure of language.[18] What is needed, as Putnam has suggested, is an ethics without ontology rather than an *ontology of the particular*.[19] The philosophical drive for generality is 'contempt for the particular'. By contrast, moral perception is care for the particular. In her important essay 'Vision and Choice in Morality', Murdoch invokes the importance of attention in morality.[20] According to her interpretation, a first way of expressing care is to pay attention to something, that is, to be attentive. The word attention is a possible version of the term *care* – perhaps drawing it a little too much from the perceptual side vs. the agency of caring, but highlighting the anticipatory dynamics of this perception. Murdoch also evokes the differences in morality in terms of differences in Gestalt. She wants to avoid the classical idea of perceiving an object via a concept: 'Moral differences here are less like differences in choice, and more like differences in vision. In other words, a moral concept is less like a movable and expandable ring placed over a certain domain of facts, and more like a *Gestalt* difference.'[21] Here Murdoch operates a critique of the *general* in ethics. There are no univocal moral concepts that can only be applied to reality to delimit objects. Nevertheless, our concepts depend on it through their application relative to a domain of interest – a given narrative or description, and our personal interest and desire to explore these in terms of what is important to us. Here, in the idea of importance, we discover the means for another formulation of the concept of care, as attending to what is important or matters to us: what counts.

12.3 IMPORTANCE OF IMPORTANCE

This relationship of care to *what matters* was highlighted by Harry Frankfurt in *The Importance of What We Care About* (1988). In an analogous spirit, Stanley Cavell discusses cinema and the films that *matter* to us, which are the objects of our attention and care, requiring the education of perception and attentive vision:

> The moral I draw is the following: to answer the question 'what happens to objects when they are filmed and projected?' – as well as 'what happens to particular people, places, subjects and motives, when they are filmed by this or that filmmaker?' – There is only one source of data, namely the appearance and meaning of these objects, these people, which we will in fact find in the sequence of films, or passages of films, that matter to us. ('What happens to things on the screen?')[22]

The importance of cinema lies in the way it brings out visually what matters, in order, as Cavell puts it, 'to magnify the feeling and meaning of a moment'. But: 'it is also his task to go against this tendency and, instead, to recognise this tragic reality of human life: the importance of its moments is not usually given to us with the moments while we are living them, so that it can take a lifetime's work to determine the important crossroads of a life'.[23] It is possible to understand the concept of care in terms of the specific attention to the *unseen* importance of things and moments required by the appreciation of filmic art. 'The inherent concealment of importance' is part of what cinema also teaches us about our ordinary life. Redefining morality on the basis of importance, and its link to the structural vulnerability of experience, produces the necessary elements to constitute the ethics of care. The notion of care is inseparable from a whole cluster of cognate terms, which constitute a language game of the particular. Among these are *attention, concern, importance, significance* and *mattering*. Our capacity for care becomes, according to Murdoch, 'a detached, non-sentimental, non-selfish, objective version of care'. The emergent attention is the result of the development of a perceptual capacity. It is rooted in the ability to see the detachment of detail, of expressive gesture, against a background, without undue ontological reification.

This particularism of attention to detail has also been propounded by Diamond, notably in her important essay 'Getting a Rough Idea of What Moral Philosophy Is', which closes *The Realistic Spirit*.[24] According to her construal, moral philosophy needs to shift its focus from examining general concepts to examining particular visions, the 'configurations' of thought of individuals. Murdoch is again the source here:

> We consider something more elusive which may be called their total view of life, as manifested in the way they speak or remain silent, their choice of words, their ways of appreciating others, their conception of their own lives, what they find attractive or praiseworthy, what they find amusing: in short, the configurations of their thinking which are continually manifested in their reactions and conversations. These things, which may be shown openly and intelligibly or elaborated intimately and guessed at, constitute what may be called a man's texture of being, or the nature of his personal vision.[25]

It is indeed in the use of language, in the choice of words, style of conversation, etc., that the moral vision of a person is openly shown or intimately elaborated, which for Murdoch is not so much a theoretical point of view as a *texture of being* – which is still a Gestalt term, since texture can appear in various modalities: visual, aural and tactile.

This texture has nothing to do with moral choices or ethical argumentation. Rather, it once again pertains to 'what matters' and what makes and expresses the differences between individuals. Diamond expresses this very clearly: 'We cannot see the moral interest of literature unless we recognise gestures, manners, habits, turns of speech, turns of thought, styles of face, as morally expressive – of an individual or a people. The intelligent description of these things is part of the sharp, intelligent description of life, of what *matters*, what makes a difference, in human lives.'[26] It is these differences that are to be the object of 'the intelligent, sharp description of life'. The idea of a human life alludes to the Wittgensteinian form of life, which similarly defines a texture. Texture, then, designates an unstable reality, which cannot be pinned down by concepts, or by particular determined objects, but is nevertheless accessible through the recognition and identification of gestures, manners, styles, etc. The form of life is, from an ethical point of view, defined by perception.

12.4 LIFE FORMS

Wittgenstein speaks of a 'pattern in the tapestry of life and of a "whirl"'; or, as in *Zettel*, of *place* and *connections*: 'pain occupies *such and such a* place in our life, it has *such and such* connections'.[27] As Diamond observes, connections 'in our lives' are not hidden but have their being right before our eyes. Here she alludes to the well-known simile of the 'figure in the carpet' in Henry James's classic short story, 'The Figure in the Carpet'. We perceive through concepts, including moral ones, because our concepts 'grasp' (their referents) in the unfolding of a texture of life, which is dynamic, and where patterns recur and emerge: 'If life were a tapestry, this or that pattern (pretending, for example) would not always be complete and would vary in many ways. But we, in our conceptual world, always see the same thing repeated with variations. This is how our concepts *grasp* (*auffassen*).'[28] The background of the life form is neither causal nor fixed like a set, but living and mobile. Again, we can appeal to *life* forms, instead of *forms of life*. The distinction marked is not a definitive or stable form, but the forms that our life *takes* under the attentive gaze – the 'whirl' of our life lived within a language, of our 'visions', as opposed to a stable body of meanings or social rules.

The term background (*Hintergrund*) appears in Wittgenstein to designate a background of description, which 'brings out' the nature or meaning of actions. It is not intended to *explain* anything. The background cannot have a causal role, for it is language itself in its instability and sensitivity to practice:

> We judge an action by its background in human life ... The background is the train of life; And our concept refers to something in this train.[29]

> How can the human way of acting be described? Only by showing how the actions of the diversity of human beings blend together in a swarm. It is not what an individual does, but the whole swarming whole (*Gewimmel*) that forms the background against which we see the action.[30]

We see the action but we are *caught* in the midst of a life form against which it stands out and becomes sensible and thus important. It is not at all the same to say that the application of the rule is causally *determined* by a background, and to say that it is to be *described in* the background of human actions and connections. This is the difference between a Gestalt and a descriptive conception of ethics and a 'conformist' conception that attempts to provide justification by reference to prior agreement bestowed by the community. The background does not provide or determine ethical meaning, since there is none, but allows for a clearer view of what is important and meaningful to us, in the important moment: the connections in the texture of our lives. Wittgenstein mentions, in *Culture and Value*, 'the background against which what I can express receives meaning'.[31] The 'accepted' or given background does not determine our actions (thus, no causality is involved) but allows us to see them clearly.

The mythology of 'moral theory' lies in the idea of elaborating a number of principles that can produce a 'morally correct answer' to most moral problems *in all circumstances*. The anti-theoretical, 'unorthodox' view, however, rejects the possibility of substantive and general moral principles, or metaethical theories about the nature of moral or normative statements, from which one can develop modes of justification and reasoning that would hold for all situations. Most of the unorthodox moral philosophers (e.g. Anscombe, Baier, Diamond, Lovibond and McDowell) are influenced by Wittgenstein's thinking as the best philosopher to counter 'orthodox' moral philosophy.[32] Certainly, many will agree that there is a duty, for example, to care for one's family and friends – but one does not usually want to be loved out of duty, and this very concern not to be loved out of duty would be a more interesting topic for morality than obligation itself. Similarly, as Diamond notes, there may be something mean-spirited and 'ungenerous' about a perfectly rigorous person who is consumed by the idea of doing what they consider to be their duty.[33] The *unlikability* in the strong sense that taints the character of the dutiful ethicist is something that should be part of moral reflection, rather than consigned to the litter of ethically marginal questions. Annette Baier suggests that one should be interested in a virtue like *kindness*, which can only be treated in both descriptive and normative terms, and 'resists analysis in terms of rules',[34] being an appropriate response to the other according to the circumstances: it requires an experimental attitude, sensitivity to a situation and the ability to improvise, to 'move on' from certain reactions: care. Baier defines moral attitudes such as expectation, patience, or simply waiting to see what happens rather than applying principles. Without these expectation-based attitudes, moral reflection runs the risk of becoming locked into the 'view from sideways on', of losing sight of *what matters* in morality, what it is we care for and about.

Baier criticizes, as did Murdoch, Diamond and Anscombe, the idea that moral philosophy is reducible to questions of obligation and choice – as if a moral problem, by being formulated in these terms, becomes thus treatable.[35]

We may recall the proposition in the *Investigations* where Wittgenstein defines agreement *in* form of life.[36] We may take it that our language usage and practices are given as a set of rules to which we have no choice but to adhere. But another of Wittgenstein's discoveries is that usage is not enough. My agreement with or belonging to *this or that* form of life, whether social or moral, is not given. The background is not *a priori*, but it is modifiable through the practice itself. The acceptance of the form of life as 'a given for us' – which Wittgenstein advocates – is acceptance of a natural given (as Cavell says in *This New Yet Unapproachable America*: 'the fact of being a man, therefore with that (extent or scale of) capacity for work, pleasure, endurance, seduction'[37]). But the form of this acceptance – the 'extent and scale' of our agreement – is not knowable *a priori* 'any more than the extent or scale of a word can be known *a priori*', because the use of moral language is improvised. Thus, one doesn't agree to everything in advance. The moral burden is at all times in '*what* we *should say when*'.[38] The fact that moral language is given to one does not imply that one knows *a priori* how one is going to get along, to agree *in* this language with one's fellow language users, to find the right expressions to respond, etc. What constitutes language agreement and moral agreement is the ever-open possibility of rupture, the threat of scepticism, of the loss of moral voice.[39]

12.5 LOSING CONCEPTS

According to Diamond, many of the statements found in contemporary moral philosophy are, in her own words, 'stupid or *insensitive* or delusional'. She gives as an example a passage in which Peter Singer argues in favour of the defence of animals:

> What I mean by 'stupid or insensitive or delusional' can be made clear by a single word, the word 'even' in the quotation: 'We have seen that the experimenter reveals a bias in favour of his own species when he experiments on a non-human in a case where he would not consider it justified to use a human being, even a retarded human being.'[40]

What is wrong with such an argument is not the argument itself, but the use of the word 'even'. What is wrong is the absence of care. When Diamond says that moral philosophy has become mostly blind and insensitive, she means it has become insensitive to the human specificity of moral questioning, and to ordinary moral life.

What matters in moral perception is not agreement and harmony, but the perception (sometimes violent) of contrasts, distances and differences, and their expression – that moment when, as Diamond says, there is a 'loss of concepts', when it no longer works. Cavell describes this difficulty in terms of scepticism, as a sensation and temptation of inexpressiveness, as our inability to go beyond our natural reactions to know the other – to go beyond the limits of my understanding and concepts, but also of my *experience*.

Our ability to communicate with him depends on his 'natural understanding', his 'natural reaction' to our instructions and gestures. It depends, therefore, on our mutual agreement in judgements. This agreement takes us remarkably far along the path of mutual understanding, but it has its limits – limits which, one might say, are not only those of knowledge, but are also those of experience.[41]

What is important in the ethical situation is not just the agreement, but the disagreement that the sensitivity to words creates: the exposure of the *loss of our concepts*, the difficulty of applying them in new contexts. The important point for Diamond is that there is no opposition between sensibility and understanding, but that sensibility is a form of conceptual life. This explains the 'sensitive' reactions we have to conceptual matters.

Reconnecting with experience and finding a voice for its expression is perhaps the primary perfectionist and political aim of ethics. It remains to articulate this subjective expression with the attention to the particular that is also at the heart of care, and thus to define a *knowledge through* care. The moral knowledge, for example, that literature or film brings to light through the education of sensibility (i.e. the training of the virtue of sensitiveness) is not necessarily fully translatable into rational or moral argumentation, but it *is* nevertheless knowledge. This idea is playfully at work in Nussbaum's ambiguous book title, *Love's Knowledge*. The syntactical play on meanings signals not the knowledge of a general abstract object 'love', but the particular knowledge that the sharpened perception of love grants us through the experience of love itself. As her title suggests, there is no contradiction between sensibility and knowledge, care and rationality.

12.6 ATTENTION TO ATTENTION

Care ethics is an attention to others, and to the way they are caught along with us in connections. The philosophical lines explored so far make it possible to understand a fundamental requirement of the ethics of care. Through a 'loving and attentive' and thus *caring* reading we perceive moral situations differently and actively. This changes our perception of the responsibility of the moral agent and of agency itself. The attention to others both enjoined and creatively explored by literature and the arts does not give us new certainties or the literary or artistic equivalent of theories. Rather, it confronts us with uncertainty and scepticism. By focusing on a narrow conception of ethics and perception, one risks *missing the adventure*, in Diamond's phrasing. That is, one risks missing a dimension of morality, specifically the visible *aspect of* moral thinking, or 'what moral life looks like'.[42] Moreover, it is owing to a lack of care that we manage to miss this all-important aspect of ethics. Conceptual adventure is hence a component of moral perception. There is adventure in any situation that mixes uncertainty, instability and 'the sharp sense of life'. Diamond and Nussbaum refer to a passage from Henry James that beautifully makes explicit this adventurous *form* that moral life takes:

> A human, personal 'adventure' is not an a priori, positive, absolute and inextinguishable thing, but just a matter of relationship and appreciation – in fact, it is a name we give, appropriately, to any passage, any situation that has added the sharp taste of uncertainty to a sharp sense of life. Hence the thing is, quite admirably, a matter of interpretation and of particular conditions; and without a perception of these, the most prodigious adventures may vulgarly count for nothing.[43]

Famous passages in the novel *The Ambassadors* highlight this adventure of perception. The novel's hero, the sensitive, ageing, sheltered Lambert Strether, comes to acquire a new moral attitude and a 'new standard of perception' in the 'great swarm' of Parisian life, which turns out to be difficult, uncertain and dangerous: 'I see it now, I haven't seen it enough before – and now I'm old! Too old for what I see. Oh, but at least I *do* see.'[44] These troubled moments in the novel define caring as seeing, and, conversely, attentive and anticipatory perception as caring. Caring is activity, mobility and improvisation.

Thus, we can see the moral life as an adventure that is both conceptual (one extends one's concepts) and sensitive (one exposes oneself). Put another way, it is both passive (one allows oneself to be transformed, to be touched) and agentive (one seeks 'an active sense of life'). There is no need to separate conceptual life and affection, just as there is no need to separate, in moral experience, thought (spontaneity) and receptivity (vulnerability to reality and to others). James adds that it is necessary that nothing escapes the attention: '*Try to be one of the people on whom nothing is lost.*' With this magisterial Jamesian insight we have reached our final construal of the ethics of care.

In our times, it is arguably in film and television productions that the Wittgensteinian attention to detail proper to care is most strongly evinced. A number of examples drawn from recent cinema describe, through the description and fine narration of caring, what the agential dimension of care is, within the great diversity of forms of care. It is as if cinema, having exhausted the representations and conversations of romance (emblematized in the comedy of remarriage and the melodrama genres of the Golden Age of Hollywood), now describes a wider variety of forms and objects of affection. We might think of the accentuation of care in the disaster or science-fiction film, the plot of which is often centred on the preservation or survival of a family structure. Recent TV series focus on care (*The Leftovers,*[45] *This is Us*[46]) and some present the concrete work of care: *Unbelievable,*[47] *Maid.*[48,49] Film and TV have the capacity to highlight the necessity and importance, for all humans, of this dimension of our lives – and to shape both perception and morality altogether.

12.7 SUBVERTING HIERARCHIES

The radicality of the ethics of care is that it subverts well-established intellectual and social hierarchies and attracts attention to a number of phenomena that are overlooked because they are connected to the female. Gilligan's ethics takes as its starting point the idea that the (moral) sentiments and expressions of women are not inferior forms of morality, but are rather moral resources that have been ignored and, if taken into account, would allow for a profound renewal of moral and social thought. This will only become apparent if we see care not only as a sensibility or affectivity but as an ordinary practice, an ethics defined by the concrete work done for the most part by women, and neglected for that very reason: only, then, if we see care as attention to the ordinary.

To regain our contact with experience and to find a voice for its expression: this is the definition of an ordinary ethics. Care, understood as attention and perception, is to be differentiated from a sort of suffocation of the self by affect or devotion. It confronts us with our own inabilities and inattentions, but, above all, it shows us how these inattentions are then translated into a theory about what matters. 'What we are destroying is nothing but houses of cards.'[50] Wittgenstein's point is also that the importance of the grammatical investigation lies precisely in 'destroying everything great and interesting', displacing our interests, our hierarchies.

12.8 THE ETHICAL IS POLITICAL

Joan Tronto has suggested that the dyadic and affective conception of care to which Gilligan remains attached is too narrow to allow the ensemble of social activities having to do with attentive care for others to be thought of. She holds that the philosophical valorization of care must base itself not so much on a particularistic ethics but rather on an enlargement of the concept of action. This obliges us to give up on one part of the ethics of care, the idea of a specifically feminine ethics. Gilligan's position was indissociable from a gendered ethics; for her, the relationship to self and others as expressed in moral judgement takes opposing directions for men and for women. Tronto, however, proposes an anthropology of human needs in order to found the social dignity of care: not only do certain of our needs call directly for care, but also care defines the (political) space in which listening to needs becomes possible, as a veritable, non-affectivist attention to others. Reflection on care seems to set a feminine and a masculine conception of ethics against one another, the first being defined by attention, care for the other, responsibility and the connections we have to an ensemble of persons; the second by justice and autonomy. There is no need to emphasize the difficulty in contrasting a feminine ethics and a masculine ethics in such terms, opposing care and justice (for who doesn't love justice?), and the risk one would run of reproducing the very prejudices that the ethics of care as a feminist ethics was aimed at combating. One can, as Tronto does, integrate care into a general ethical, social and political approach which would not be reserved for women, but would be an aspiration for all, and would thus allow for an amelioration of the concept of justice. Or one can, as Diamond, Gilligan herself and I have suggested, redefine care and justice together by redefining ethics on the basis of moral perception.

For Tronto, the valorization of care passes through *politicization*. Truly carrying out the ethics of care would imply both including practices linked to care in the agenda of democratic reflection and empowering those concerned – caregivers and care recipients. The recognition of the theoretical pertinence of ethics of care necessarily passes through a practical revalorization of activities linked to care and a concomitant modification of intellectual and political agendas, defining citizenship through bounds of care. There can be no ethics of care, then, without politics: in their political articulation, dominant liberal (masculine) ethics, as well as some feminist philosophy and ethics, may be the product and expression of a social practice that devalorizes the attitude and work of care.

> The world of care, needless to say, has generally been ignored by social and political theorists. The world of care, needless to say, is often inhabited more thoroughly by women, people of lower class and caste status, working people, and other disregarded ethnic, religious, linguistic groups. They are the people most often excluded by politics. Even to bold thinkers who wanted to support the claims for women greater public roles, such as Simone de Beauvoir, the vilification of the 'immanent' life continued.[51]

So the ethics of care is a subversion of intellectual and ethical hierarchies. The perspective of care then leads us to explore the ways in which we – in practice and in theory – treat the demarcation between the spheres of personal relations (familial relations, as well as love, friendship) and the so-called 'impersonal' spheres of public relations, with, of course, a hierarchy involved.

Tronto notes that the care/justice debate has been really 'one-sided', as if it were always the burden of the ethics of care to prove that it is compatible with justice. She aims to integrate care into a general ethical and political approach that would not be reserved for women, but would be an aspiration for all, and would thus allow for an amelioration of the concept of justice. For Tronto it is only in 'passing' from ethics to politics (like a kind of promotion) that ethics of care can be given their critical power. It is quite surprising that Tronto is widely seen as having 'overcome' the different voice by a social theory of care. The question is: how is the kind of new attention that care forces upon us to be separated from women's point of view, and the mere fact that women's voices and activities have been deadened? The focus on moral notions such as duty or choice (a result of the influence of Kant and Rawls) leaves out the essential of ordinary moral questioning. When we get down to the ways in which we actually live our lives, care activities are central and ubiquitous. When we begin to take these activities seriously, 'the world will look different if we place care, and its related values and concerns, closer to the centre of human life'.[52] So the ethics of care is also for Tronto a matter of perception, it draws our attention to the ordinary, to what we are unable to see, although it is right before our eyes. It claims to give voice to humans (mostly women, but all the subaltern and disadvantaged) who are undervalued precisely because they are assigned to activities that have been socially and morally devalorized; denied because we do not want to see, acknowledge, what we depend on. So the ethics of care is political in itself – it provides all the politics we need.

The perspective of the ethics of care calls our attention to a general situation of dependence, and develops an analysis of social relations organized around dependence and vulnerability – blind spots in the ethics of justice. Thus, care-based approaches target the theory of justice as it developed and took the dominant position in political and moral thinking over the second half of the last century. This is not only because, as the controversies between the partisans of care and those of justice illustrate, these approaches call into question the universality of Rawls's conception of justice, but also because they transform the very nature of moral questioning – expressing not merely a negative criticism of justice but rather the positive need for 'more than justice'.[53]

12.9 ESSENTIALISM

Gilligan's recent writings may clear up some misunderstandings about her 'essentialism' by showing that her main concern is in combining theories of justice and care rather than opposing them via a gender dichotomy:

> The potential error in justice reasoning lies in its latent egocentrism, the tendency to confuse one's perspective with an objective standpoint or truth, the temptation to define others in one's own terms by putting oneself in their place. The potential error in care reasoning lies in the tendency to forget that one has terms, creating a tendency to enter into another's perspective and to see oneself as 'selfless,' by defining oneself in other's terms.[54]

It is a matter, then, beyond the justice/care debate, of each individual finding his or her voice, and of hearing and expressing both the voice of justice and that of care, avoiding the following two distortions or deformations: 'the equation of human with male, unjust in its omission of women; and the equation of care with self-sacrifice, uncaring in its failure to represent the activity and the agency of care'.[55]

Care, then, appears as one of the existent paths towards a genuine ethics, one that is concrete, attentive to actual practices and forms of life, and not only normative. It is not a matter of making justice and sensibility compatible, in a sort of moralistic half-measure, nor of introducing a dose of care into the theory of justice. Numerous works in ethics have convincingly argued in favour of this compatibility. It is instead a matter, more radically, of seeing *sensibility,* attention and care as necessary conditions of justice. The centre of gravity of ethics is shifted from the 'just' to the 'important', and again this is done by destroying what seemed to be important. This ethical move is linked to the definition of ethical competence in terms of a refined and active perception, which certainly has not been followed out in all its feminist consequences, and in particular the analysis it provides of differences and inequalities *between* women (some of which are created by care networks and relations). What is at stake in ethics of care ends up epistemological: ethics of care seeks to highlight the connection between our lack of attention to neglected realities and the lack of theorization of these social realities rendered 'invisible', and in this way to understand why ethical, and often philosophical and political, thought is blind to certain ordinary realities, those connected with the domain of the private, the domestic and the female. Thus, we find the continuation of the definition of *the ordinary*, supplied by Wittgenstein himself: 'what we are supplying are really remarks on the natural history of human beings ... observations which no one has doubted, but which have escaped remark only because they are always before our eyes'.[56]

The ethics of care does not aim at installing pity, compassion, solicitude and benevolence as subsidiary values that would soften the hardness of an impartial conception of justice based on the primacy of rights attributed to autonomous, rational individuals. The ethics of care – and its philosophical point – makes it obvious that we depend on others in a world that values autonomy highly in both theory and practice. It even demonstrates that the most autonomous people are actually the most dependent, because of all the help and support they get. It does not aim to enlist compassion and solicitude. Its goal is the acknowledgement of a whole part of life that is systematically ignored in political discourse and moral philosophy. *Care is just what makes ordinary form of life possible.* Tronto and Fisher, in their definition of care, suggest that care should be defined at the most general level as a generic activity including all that we do in order to perpetuate and repair our 'world', so that we can live in it as well as is possible. 'This "world" includes our bodies, our environment, and ourselves.' Ethics, then, is not about how to live better or more virtuous or rational lives, but simply how anyone can live an ordinary life in this world; it is about achieving the ordinary and recovering the human.[57]

Standard ethics and political analysis, when they deal with the social contract, do not enquire into the society in question is made sustainable – thus carefully expelling out of ethics the world of care, and, more generally speaking, all those actions that make ordinary social and moral relations possible and living. Ignoring the issue of care in ethics and politics amounts to ignoring the origin of what allows a moral society to exist and endure.

This can help us see ethics of care not as 'essentialist' but rather as an ethics that gives expression to humans who are undervalued *because* they perform unnoticed, invisible tasks. Ordinary realism in ethics,[58] on this view, consists in *returning to* ordinary language, in examining our words and paying attention to them, in taking care of them (taking care of our words and expressions, and of ordinary others).[59]

The perspectives of care claim a moral dimension that has been overlooked, and question this underestimation. They challenge the liberal ethics of Rawls's theory of justice, confronting a morality centred on equity, impartiality and autonomy, with a morality rooted in the experience, work and voices of women. These voices are not only those of women, but of all disadvantaged, ethnicized and racialized social categories, to whom the tasks of care, which make life possible, have historically been reserved. It is the links to these people that the ethics of care seeks to bring to light.

Care, when understood in its feminist dimension, thus raises the difficulty faced in other terms, a few years after Gilligan, by Carole Pateman. It consists in following through on the critical and democratic idea that was at the root of the *care* ethic: that majority ethics, linked to past and present theories of contract, are the product and expression of a system in which women have no voice, are forgotten. Ethics and politics as they appear in contemporary philosophical reflection, in its various accepted versions, are the translation of a social practice and theory that devalues the attitude and work of care. Considering the social, moral and political importance of care thus obliges us to refer to 'women', one of the categories to which the work of care has been primarily assigned, and to ask what is the nature of a democratic conversation that excludes that which makes it even materially possible. Care draws our attention to our dependencies – what binds us and to whom. The notion of care encompasses both very practical activities and a sensitivity, a sustained attention to others and a sense of responsibility and dependence. It does not aim to situate pity and compassion, solicitude or benevolence as subsidiary virtues softening an unsympathetic conception of social relations, or (another inverted version of the same analysis) to establish domination under the guise of protection. On the contrary, care aims to gain recognition for a whole area of common life and human relationships that are systematically overlooked and devalued in political discourse, analysis and ethics.

The attention that care proposes is an attention to what *ordinarily* constitutes our commonality, a question then no longer metaphysical or principial, but material (the support of life, as a thread and a continuous, albeit weak, link). The ethics of principles, and often political analysis, when they ask themselves the question of the foundation of 'our' society or of the social bond, carefully omit to ask what enables the perpetuation of this society: they put outside ethics the sphere of fundamental care, and, more broadly, all the actions ensuring the maintenance of ordinary social relations and human bonds. Annette Baier shows how the neglect of *care* in ethical and political theory condemns a society to failing to recognize the source of its own perpetuation – and thus to a radical incompleteness of politics, to a problematic heterogeneity between society in its moral dimension and that which perpetuates it. Reflection on *care*, then, opens the way not so much to new approaches to morality as to a transformation of the very status and meaning of ethics.

CONCLUSION

Let's return to our initial question. It's curious that Gilligan's approach was considered 'essentialist'. Gilligan has shown the generality of her approach and has confirmed it in her later work:[60] it makes justice and care two rival tonalities or voices, present in everyone. The voice of care is less quickly stifled in girls than in boys. But Gilligan's point of view is radical: she demonstrates that mainstream ethics shows a remarkable discontinuity with 'ordinary' experiences – those of women, but not exclusively – of all those, the most disadvantaged, who, in the service of others, have no voice in the definition of justice or the common good. The language of the liberal ethic of justice is unfit to capture the experiences and viewpoints of a whole part of humanity, the part that *sustains* others and especially the privileged, as *caregivers* have done everywhere in recent months.

Taking care into account means morally valuing a field that is constantly scorned by philosophy. The challenge of the ethics of care is to create this moral status for the private, domestic domain, and for the activities of caring for people. Care thus transforms politics and calls for a revolution in the way human activities are valued. It's a question of finding the sources of politics in ordinary lives, understood in terms of the bonds and interdependence of vulnerable human beings against the grain of a liberalism that expels from morality all the relationships of proximity and service where ordinary vulnerability is taken care of.

The fragmentation of care in a variety of fields (from hospitals to food and education) renders invisible the foundations of the autonomy of some in the work of others.

The next stage of the argument is the realization that the very definition of ethics is achieved in philosophy *by* excluding an entire field, and a set of people, whose contribution is nonetheless necessary to life; and by denying the mass of work mobilized to guarantee the functioning of the world. Baier shows how the disregard for care leads to the incompleteness of the liberal conception of morality, condemned to posit a problematic heterogeneity between society in its moral dimension and what sustains it.[61] The neglect of care in moral and political theory leads a society to ignore the source of its own survival as a moral society. This is why care is ultimately a matter of democracy, and leads us to ask how we can involve care workers in defining what counts. And how an essential part of reality has escaped both morality and philosophy.

NOTES

1. Carol Gilligan, *In a Different Voice: Psychological Theory and Women's Development* (Cambridge, MA: Harvard University Press, 1982).
2. See: Sandra Laugier, 'From the Ordinary to the Everyday', *Qui Parle* 33, no. 1 (2024): 17–34.
3. Cora Diamond, *The Realistic Spirit: Wittgenstein, Philosophy, and the Mind* (Cambridge, MA: MIT Press, 1991).
4. Ludwig Wittgenstein, *Philosophical Investigations (Philosophische Untersuchungen)*, ed. G. E. M. Anscombe, G. H. von Wright and R. Rhees (Oxford: Blackwell, 1953), § 415.
5. Wittgenstein, *Philosophical Investigations* §118.
6. See: Sandra Laugier, 'The Ethics of Care as a Politics of the Ordinary', *New Literary History* 46 (2015): 217–40; Sandra Laugier, *Politics of the Ordinary: Care, Ethics, and Forms of Life* (Leuven-Pariol: Peeters, 2020).
7. Carol Gilligan, 'Moral Orientation and Development', in *Justice and Care: Essential Readings in Feminist Ethics*, ed. V. Held (Boulder, CO: Westview Press, 1995), 31–46. See also Carol Gilligan, *In a Human Voice* (Medford, MA: Polity, 2023).
8. See: Sandra Laugier, 'The Will to See: Ethics and Moral Perception of Sense', *Graduate Faculty Philosophy Journal* 34, no. 2 (2013): 263–81.
9. Diamond, *The Realistic Spirit*, 32.
10. Cora Diamond, 'Moral Differences and Distances: Some Questions', in *Commonality and Particularity in Ethics*, ed. Lilli Alanen, Sara Heinamaa and Thomas Wallgren (London: Macmillan, 1997), 197–234.
11. Ludwig Wittgenstein, *Tractatus Logico-Philosophicus*, trans. C. K. Ogden and F. P. Ramsey (London: Routledge & Kegan Paul, 1922), 4.112.
12. Wittgenstein, *Tractatus Logico-Philosophicus,* 6.42.
13. See: John McDowell, 'Non-cognitivism and Rule-following', in *Wittgenstein: To Follow a Rule*, ed. Steven H. Holtzman and Christopher M. Leich (Boston, MA: Routledge, 1981), 141–62.
14. Hilary Putnam, 'Conversation with Jacques Bouveresse', *The Monist* 103, no. 4 (2020): 25–70.
15. Ibid.
16. Ibid.
17. Ludwig Wittgenstein, *Bemerkungen über die Grundlagen der Mathematik*, ed. G. E. M. Anscombe, G. von Wright and Rush Rhees (Frankfurt: Suhrkamp, 1954): 35.
18. Ludwig Wittgenstein, *The Blue and Brown Books* (Oxford: Blackwell, 1958), 57–8.
19. See: Hilary Putnam, *Ethics without Ontology* (Cambridge, MA: Harvard University Press, 2004).
20. Iris Murdoch, 'Vision and Choice in Morality', in *Existentialists and Mystics: Writings on Philosophy and Literature*, ed. Iris Murdoch and Peter J. Conradi (London: Chatto and Windus, 1997), 76–98.
21. Ibid.
22. Stanley Cavell, *Themes out of School: Effects and Causes* (Chicago, IL: University of Chicago Press, 1984), 79.
23. Cavell, *Themes out of School.*
24. Diamond, *The Realistic Spirit,* 495–515.
25. Murdoch, 'Vision and Choice in Morality', 80–1.
26. Diamond, *The Realistic Spirit*, 507.

27. Ludwig Wittgenstein, *Zettel*, ed. E. Anscombe and G. von Wright (Oxford: Oxford University Press, 1967), §§532–3.
28. Ludwig Wittgenstein, *Bemerkungen über die Philosophie der Psychologie*, ed. G. E. M. Anscombe and G. von Wright (Oxford: Blackwell, 1980), §672.
29. Ludwig Wittgenstein, *Vermischte Bemerkungen (Culture and Value)*, ed. G. von Wright (Chicago, IL: University of Chicago Press, 1980), §624–5.
30. Wittgenstein, *Vermischte Bemerkungen (Culture and Value)*, §629; Wittgenstein, *Zettel*, §567.
31. Wittgenstein, *Vermischte Bemerkungen (Culture and Value)*, 16.
32. See: Sandra Laugier, 'Care for the Ordinary', in *The Murdochian Mind*, ed. Silvia C. Panizza and Mark Hopwood (London: Routledge, 2022), 223–35.
33. Cora Diamond, 'Ethics, Imagination and the Method of the Tractatus', in *The New Wittgenstein*, ed. Alice Crary and Rupert Read (London: Routledge, 2000), 149–73.
34. Annette Baier, *Postures of the Mind: Essays on Mind and Morals* (Minneapolis: University of Minnesota Press, 1985), 219.
35. Annette Baier, *Moral Prejudices: Essays on Ethics* (Cambridge, MA: Harvard University Press, 1995).
36. Ludwig Wittgenstein, *Philosophical Investigations*, trans. G. E. M. Anscombe (Englewood Cliffs, NJ: Prentice Hall, 2000): §241.
37. Stanley Cavell, *This New Yet Unapproachable America: Lectures after Emerson after Wittgenstein* (Chicago, IL: University of Chicago Press, 1989), 48–9.
38. John L. Austin, *Philosophical Papers* (Oxford: Oxford University Press, 1962).
39. Sandra Laugier, *Why We Need Ordinary Language Philosophy*, trans. D. Ginsburg (Chicago, IL: University of Chicago Press, 2013).
40. Diamond, *The Realistic Spirit*, 33.
41. Stanley Cavell, *The Claim of Reason: Wittgenstein, Skepticism, Morality, and Tragedy* (New York: Oxford University Press, 1979). See: Sandra Laugier, 'Cavell on Feminism and the Ethics of Care', *Conversations: The Journal of Cavellian Studies*, no. 6 (2018): 55–80.
42. Diamond, *The Realistic Spirit*, 36.
43. Henry James, *What Maisie Knew* (London: Penguin Classics, 2010 [1897]).
44. Henry James, *The Ambassadors* (London: Penguin, 1986 [1903]), 615.
45. *The Leftovers,* Damon Lindelof and Tom Perrotta, HBO, 2014–17.
46. *This Is Us,* Dan Fogelman, NBC, 2016–22.
47. *Unbelievable*, Susannah Grant, Ayelet Waldman and Michael Chabon, Netflix, 2019.
48. *Maid,* Molly Smith Metzler, Netflix, 2021.
49. Sandra Laugier, *Nos Vies en Séries: Philosophie et Morale d'une Culture Populaire* (Paris: Climats, 2019). See also: Sandra Laugier, *TV-Philosophy: How TV Series Change Our Thinking* (Exeter: University of Exeter Press, 2023).
50. Wittgenstein, *Philosophical Investigations*, §118.
51. Joan C. Tronto, *Moral Boundaries: A Political Argument for an Ethic of Care* (New York: Routledge, 1993), 15.
52. Tronto, *Moral Boundaries*.
53. Ibid.
54. Gilligan, 'Moral Orientation', 43.
55. Ibid.
56. Wittgenstein, *Philosophical Investigations*, §415.
57. See: Veena Das, *Textures of the Ordinary: Doing Anthropology after Wittgenstein* (New York: Fordham University Press, 2020).

58. Sandra Laugier, 'Ordinary Realism in Ethics', in *The Ethics of Care: The State of the Art*, ed. Frans Vosman, Andries Bart and Jorma Hoffman (Leuven-Pariol: Peeters, 2020), 113–36.
59. Laugier, 'The Ethics of Care as a Politics of the Ordinary', 217–40; Laugier, *Politics of the Ordinary*.
60. Gilligan, *In a Human Voice*.
61. Baier, *Moral Prejudices*.

BIBLIOGRAPHY

Austin, John L. *Philosophical Papers*. Oxford: Oxford University Press, 1962.

Baier, Annette. *Postures of the Mind: Essays on Mind and Morals*. Minneapolis: University of Minnesota Press, 1985.

Baier, Annette. *Moral Prejudices: Essays on Ethics*. Cambridge, MA: Harvard University Press, 1995.

Cavell, Stanley. *The Claim of Reason: Wittgenstein, Skepticism, Morality, and Tragedy*. New York: Oxford University Press, 1979.

Cavell, Stanley. *Themes out of School: Effects and Causes*. Chicago, IL: University of Chicago Press, 1984.

Cavell, Stanley. *This New Yet Unapproachable America: Lectures after Emerson after Wittgenstein*. Chicago, IL: University of Chicago Press, 1989.

Das, Veena. *Textures of the Ordinary: Doing Anthropology after Wittgenstein*. New York: Fordham University Press, 2020.

Diamond, Cora. *The Realistic Spirit: Wittgenstein, Philosophy, and the Mind*. Cambridge, MA: MIT Press, 1991.

Diamond, Cora. 'Moral Differences and Distances: Some Questions', in *Commonality and Particularity in Ethics*, edited by Lilli Alanen, Sara Heinamaa and Thomas Wallgren, 197–234. London: Macmillan, 1997.

Diamond, Cora. 'Ethics, Imagination and the Method of the Tractatus', in *The New Wittgenstein*, edited by Alice Crary and Rupert Read, 149–73. London: Routledge, 2000.

Frankfurt, Harry G. *The Importance of What We Care About: Philosophical Essays*. Cambridge: Cambridge University Press, 1988.

Gilligan, Carol. *In a Different Voice: Psychological Theory and Women's Development*. Cambridge, MA: Harvard University Press, 1982.

Gilligan, Carol. 'Moral Orientation and Development', in *Justice and Care: Essential Readings in Feminist Ethics*, edited by Virginia Held, 31–46. Boulder, CO: Westview Press, 1995.

Gilligan, Carol. *In a Human Voice*. Medford, MA: Polity, 2023.

James, Henry. *The Ambassadors*. London: Penguin, 1986 [1903].

James, Henry. *What Maisie Knew*. London: Penguin Classics, 2010 [1897].

Laugier, Sandra. *Why We Need Ordinary Language Philosophy*. Translated by Danielle Ginsburg. Chicago, IL: University of Chicago Press, 2013.

Laugier, Sandra. 'The Will to See: Ethics and Moral Perception of Sense', *Graduate Faculty Philosophy Journal* 34, no. 2 (2013): 263–81.

Laugier, Sandra. 'The Ethics of Care as a Politics of the Ordinary', *New Literary History* 46 (2015): 217–40.

Laugier, Sandra. 'Cavell on Feminism and the Ethics of Care', *Conversations: The Journal of Cavellian Studies*, no. 6 (2018), 55–80.

Laugier, Sandra. *Nos Vies en Séries: Philosophie et Morale d'une Culture Populaire*. Paris: Climats, 2019.

Laugier, Sandra. 'Ordinary Realism in Ethics', in *The Ethics of Care, the State of the Art*, edited by Frans Vosman, Andries Bart and Jorma Hoffman, 113–36. Leuven-Pariol: Peeters, 2020.

Laugier, Sandra. *Politics of the Ordinary: Care, Ethics, and Forms of Life*. Leuven-Pariol: Peeters, 2020.

Laugier, Sandra. 'Care for the Ordinary', in *The Murdochian Mind*, edited by Silvia C. Panizza and Mark Hopwood, 223–35. London: Routledge, 2022.

Laugier, Sandra. *TV-Philosophy: How TV Series Change Our Thinking*. Exeter: University of Exeter Press, 2023.

Laugier, Sandra. 'From the Ordinary to the Everyday', *Qui Parle* 33, no. 1 (2024): 17–34.

Maid, Molly Smith Metzler, Netflix, 2021.

McDowell, John. 'Non-cognitivism and Rule-following', in *Wittgenstein: To Follow a Rule*, edited by Steven H. Holtzman and Christopher M. Leich, 141–62. Boston, MA: Routledge, 1981.

Murdoch, Iris. 'Vision and Choice in Morality', in *Existentialists and Mystics: Writings on Philosophy and Literature*, edited by Iris Murdoch and Peter J. Conradi, 76–98. London: Chatto and Windus, 1997.

Putnam, Hilary. *Ethics without Ontology*. Cambridge, MA: Harvard University Press, 2004.

Putnam, Hilary. 'Conversation with Jacques Bouveresse', *The Monist* 103, no. 4 (2020): 25–70.

The Leftovers, Damon Lindelof and Tom Perrotta, HBO, 2014–17.

This Is Us, Dan Fogelman, NBC, 2016–22.

Tronto, Joan C. *Moral Boundaries: A Political Argument for an Ethic of Care*. New York: Routledge, 1993.

Unbelievable, Susannah Grant, Ayelet Waldman and Michael Chabon, Netflix, 2019.

Wittgenstein, Ludwig. *Tractatus Logico-Philosophicus*. Translated by C. K. Ogden and F. P. Ramsey. London: Routledge & Kegan Paul, 1922.

Wittgenstein, Ludwig. *Bemerkungen über die Grundlagen der Mathematik*, edited by G. E. M. Anscombe, G. von Wright and Rush Rhees. Frankfurt: Suhrkamp, 1954.

Wittgenstein, Ludwig. *The Blue and Brown Books*. Oxford: Blackwell, 1958.

Wittgenstein, Ludwig. *Zettel*, edited by E. Anscombe and G. Von Wright. Oxford: Oxford University Press, 1967.

Wittgenstein, Ludwig. *Bemerkungen über die Philosophie der Psychologie*, edited by G. E. M. Anscombe and G. von Wright. Oxford: Blackwell, 1980.

Wittgenstein, Ludwig. *Vermischte Bemerkungen (Culture and Value)*, edited by G. Von Wright. Chicago, IL: University of Chicago Press, 1980.

Wittgenstein, Ludwig. *Philosophical Investigations*. Translated by G. E. M. Anscombe. Englewood Cliffs, NJ: Prentice Hall, 2000.

PART TWO

Applying care ethics

CHAPTER THIRTEEN

The importance of enduring and living complex care-ethical inquiry

A plea for intimacy and reciprocity in collaborative care-ethical research

ALISTAIR NIEMEIJER AND GUSTAAF BOS

INTRODUCTION

Whenever Kerry and Jenny couldn't quite figure it out through sign language, they used 'the book': a collection folder with many (fairly small) pictograms (which are learning disability icons or symbols), but also photos of acquaintances and even photos of her favourite TV programmes (or videos on YouTube). Even though she can't talk very much, she communicates a lot, for instance by making a lot of sounds (often accompanied by a whining-like sound) through which she sometimes tries to articulate something in a targeted manner (such as the 'B' for Bobby the dog). What's more, Jenny can indicate via 'the book' exactly who or what she means or wants (Peppa Pig on the iPad, for example). Several times that afternoon Jenny quickly became frustrated when Kerry did not immediately understand her and then she immediately wanted to grab the book or, in this case, retrieve it from the car, but because we were still at the entrance of the school and the book was in the car and the teacher and the mother were also talking to Kerry, this was not possible, so Jenny started stomping in the puddles in protest, with the result that half of her jeans (which continually fell down, and of which Kerry said they lost their belt at school) got wet.

By the time Kerry had finally finished talking and walked to the care to introduce me, Jenny was angry about the fact that there was no name sign for my name and then she immediately wanted to look in the book to see if my name was in it. Remarkably, there were several instances in which Jenny worried about me or felt a certain responsibility. For example, in the video with my son Samuel (who also can't speak due to his learning disability) that I showed (and then had to show a consecutive six more times). I had originally shown her a photo of Samuel with Peppa Pig because, just like Samuel, she was also a fan of Peppa Pig, after which she made the gesture for a video to indicate that she wanted to see a video of Samuel. In the particular video that I showed to her, you see Samuel at school matching pictograms with each other. Meanwhile, his feeding pump also goes off. Jenny immediately made the gesture for food and pump and it turned out that she not only recognized this from a few of her classmates (whom she then also pointed out in the book), but at a certain point she also became a little sad about the fact that Samuel was not given any food (in the video the pump continues to beep for a long time until the nurse finally turns it off). She was worried whether Samuel would still be okay. So we had to reassure her a few times in words and gestures that this was the case. I was really taken by surprise by the fact that this little girl, despite all her vulnerabilities, could care so deeply about how both I and my son Samuel might be feeling.[1]

The above excerpt is from field notes of the first author (for reasons of privacy, all participant names in this chapter have been pseudonymized), who is both an experiential expert, as father to a twelve-year-old son with multiple disabilities, and a care-ethical researcher. Together with the second author, who is also an experienced qualitative and collaborative researcher in the field of long-term care, we are currently the lead researchers on an ongoing research project which aims to investigate what good care for families with a child with complex care needs entails. The project takes families as a starting point and aims to portray the complexity in their everyday lives, including how family members relate to healthcare providers and systems, by conducting long-term, ideographic research. The main purpose of this form of research is to portray the richness and variety of experiences, patterns and interactions of families with a care-intensive child and their mutual relationships, and not to describe general laws (nomothetic).[2] The eight participating families in this project are thus seen and involved as important partners in being able to provide (knowledge about) good care. This joint exploration of and working on sustainable (collaborative) relationships between parents, siblings and healthcare professionals is extra relevant in a context in which good professionals are difficult to find and retain. The knowledge that our project aims to generate can therefore be used to help family members and (care) professionals do more justice to what is important to each of them, which will benefit their relationships – and therefore the overall care.[3]

One of the reasons we focus so specifically on the everyday lived experience of families is because of the inherent complexity that accompanies these lives, not only in care tasks, formal and informal roles but also in relationships between family members and with care professionals and care institutions. To date, the patterns and interactions within families and between families and healthcare systems have not been sufficiently investigated. Because in this research we want to gain more insight into the lived experience of families with complex care needs and analyse those empirical findings through the lens of care ethics, we utilize collaborative, ethnographic and phenomenological methods. Various studies show that the (versatile) quality of life of someone with a disability is strongly related to the quality and social dynamics of family life.[4] We follow this insight with this research project by conceiving quality of life as a phenomenon that relates to the interaction between all people in and around families with a child with complex care needs, including professionals.

However, this chapter does not centre so much around this project or the findings of the project but rather on the (reflective) potential of the chosen design for gaining more insight in reciprocal and intimate exchanges and relationships in complex care practices. Indeed, we will argue that by conducting care-ethical research in the way we do, our responsibilities extend beyond that of adopting a researcher role. In other words: to conceive of care-ethical research, you cannot avoid living and/or enduring some of it yourself. Personal perspectives, feelings and worlds are not often open to immediate investigation, whereby it is important to acknowledge and address the inherent disparities in power dynamics, contextual backgrounds, and positions of authority between those being studied and the researchers themselves. This recognition is not only a fundamental principle within the responsive research tradition but also holds significant relevance within the broader field of anthropology. Understanding and navigating these variations in power and context is central to conducting ethical and meaningful research.

It is also the reason why it takes a long time to 'get to know each other' and therefore inevitably leads to tension between a personal approach and disruption, growing trust and distrust, intimacy, and friendship issues (both an unsolicited friendship and an 'ethics of friendship')[5] between researcher and research participants. Navigating this, as the above excerpt shows, involves relevant 'lived' knowledge and experience, can be demanding and confronting, but can also result in unexpected reciprocity. The aim of this chapter is thus to explore what it means to live and endure everyday care-ethical inquiry, particularly where this relates to complex healthcare practices such as long-term care. Using excerpts from both author's field notes, we will analyse these excerpts and contend that, in line with Virginia Held's notion of care ethics as 'being in development: an ongoing, cooperative project', there is a continuous need for inquiry into existing understandings and values that are leading in practices of care. We argue that this inquiry necessitates an epistemic responsibility to explore different 'modes of understanding', which might be difficult, challenging, out of the ordinary and/or require a truly long-term commitment.

13.1 TO WHAT EXTENT ARE WE DOING UTRECHTIAN CARE ETHICS?

The Utrecht care ethics group of which we are both members has always embraced an unequivocal empirically grounded care ethics, arguing for the validity of a different sort(s) of moral knowledge by employing empirical research in, and stemming from, practices and lived experiences, taking into account, among other things, factual dependency and relationality, emotions, bodiliness and materiality.[6] As care ethics is inherently interdisciplinary, it has always relied heavily on a diversity of methodological and epistemological approaches, including a variety of techniques in knowledge transfer and understanding in order to make assumptions, generalizations and specific statements about the world in which we live.[7]

In Utrecht, care ethics is regarded as an interdisciplinary domain in which the question 'what makes good care?' is central. This is also what we teach our students who participate in the one-year Care Ethics Master's course. Good is understood here in the moral sense of the word. The answer to this question is sought in an empirically grounded, argumentative, normative theory of care and welfare. As a result, normative theories are brought together with: (a) empirically researched insights and experiences from healthcare and welfare practices; and (b) knowledge and insight from policy and organizational sciences in the field of healthcare and welfare. In doing so, our research group aims to make an active contribution to the improvement of healthcare in the Netherlands through scientific research and substantiated vision development, especially in the field of vision and policy development in healthcare and welfare institutions. This approach, however, focuses not only on scientific-ethical reflection on social organizations in the healthcare sector, but also on the praxis-related anchoring of this reflection in the future professional field. Theory and praxis are continuously linked to each other as two dimensions of the same learning process. The multidisciplinary approach offers us as researchers the opportunity to learn to look at the same problem from different scientific perspectives. It also offers us the opportunity to clarify for ourselves where our own preferences lie, especially in terms of meaning or ethics, both scientifically (with a view to writing a publication) and professionally (how do we want to conduct ourselves as researchers, teachers, etc.?).

As stated above, the theoretical framework built around the concept of care is fed by two sources: on the one hand, the interdisciplinary discussions known as care ethics that have run for more than thirty years now, and, on the other hand, various forms of empirical research. Our research group views these two sources, conceptual and empirical research, as dialectically related, as conceptual and theoretical insights are questioned and enriched by empirical research and vice versa. In other words: the 'Utrechtian' approach to care ethics entails departing from a normatively loaded care-ethical theory that is simultaneously used as a theoretical framework and as a hypothesis that is tested and adapted on the basis of empirical research and theoretical reflection. Within the theoretical framework, a number of developed concepts ('critical in sights') are guiding, such as relationality, contextuality, affectivity, practices, vulnerability, corporeality, attention to power and position, and meaning. The empirical research methods that are used by our research group therefore always focus on lived experiences, practices of care, and the way society is organized (the political-ethical dimension). The methodological toolkit, which is used and developed further for this goal, accordingly contains the following methods: phenomenology, narrative analysis, discourse analysis, (institutional and auto-) ethnography, visual data analysis, participatory action research and responsive evaluation. Some of these methods are also trained in the courses that we give to students. To sum up: the theoretical framework, drawing on the above-mentioned 'critical insights', directs the empirical research approaches towards the lived experiences of those who are involved in caring practices, on these practices as such and/or their political context. As a result, insights are gained about the morally good which emerges here.

Nevertheless, in more recent years, and especially since embarking on our long-term and intensive research project with and for families with a child with complex care needs, we have felt an increasing tension between 'saying that from a normative point of view that in order to do care-ethical inquiry one should conduct empirical research' and then actually doing just that in a way which truly does justice to the complexity of whatever care practice you are trying to conduct research in, without any kind of long-term involvement. And then also taking it even a step further in terms of intensity and position. The felt necessity to take it a step further and truly commit to a long-term involvement is linked with established ethnographic insights. Only through such sustained commitment can a researcher become a well-known presence in the studied settings, build relationships of trust with various parties, and learn to distinguish normal and deviating events in all their complexity.[8] This not only entails a constructivist understanding that we gain knowledge about the reality surrounding us by relating to it with our entire being – thus through our physicality, our observations, experiences and thoughts – in action and interaction,[9] but also that it means working collaboratively with those involved. Any research design in this case should therefore be interpreted as being interactive, interpretive and reflexive, where it is crucial to recognize that the process, content and outcomes of this project are highly dependent on a complex interplay of people, views, emotions, situations, positions and relationships. Everyone involved constructs and reconstructs – in interaction with others and material reality – his or her own reality. His, her or their perspective and the (local) dialogue about it is therefore never separate from that of others, the mutual relationships or the context.[10] That is why a joint, dialogic exploration of the interrelated images and meanings of everyday complexity and collaboration can be considered the most suitable research method at case level, especially because the approach is to support the (collaborative) relationships through the research. Categorizing the research that we do simply as 'Utrechtian care-ethical' might therefore feel like a reduction, because our research project was written in consultation with parents of a care-intensive child, siblings, interest groups, representatives of small-scale residential care initiatives and providers involved, care professionals and researchers from various disciplines. There has already been long-term cooperation and shared problem awareness with these parties. From the very start, we have worked intensively together to formulate the background and problem definition of this research. While Utrechtian care ethics would take specific practices as the main source for understanding how the morally good emerges, we took this *collaboration*, rather than a specific practice, as our central starting point. In doing so, we felt it would increase the opportunity to jointly 'learn about', 'learn to retain' and, if necessary, sustainably, to 'learn to improve' relevant themes in the everyday lives of families with a care-intensive child and their relationships with healthcare professionals and systems. Also, we felt that only in this way the research could come close to providing the most varied and richest possible picture of what quality of life means for all individual family members and healthcare professionals, and how their mutual relationships and those with the researchers are given shape and meaning. All those involved in this research recognize the need not to reduce that quality in an attempt to get a grip on it, but to explore it as a layered, subjective experience, through long-term involvement, exchange of personal narratives, open dialogue and reflection on one's own attitude and action.[11] Therefore, a better way to frame this kind of research might be *collaborative* care-ethical research.

13.2 FEELING USEFUL RATHER THAN INTRUSIVE AS A RESEARCHER-COMPANION

We had to cover an hour even though Jenny clearly really wanted to swim as soon as the word was mentioned. So we then drove to a nearby forest where Bobby the dog could be walked briefly (and also poop, it turned out). When we got there, Jenny wanted to stay in the car to watch her iPad and she wanted me to stay too, but Kerry knew Bobby had to be taken out. So Kerry decided to go for a walk with Bobby as long as I stayed behind in the car with Jenny to look after her for about fifteen minutes. Jenny (who was in the back) wanted me to watch the same Peppa Pig film that she was watching. Fortunately, I also have a Netflix account and the app on my phone, so then we started watching it together, each on our own tablet/phone. When Kerry returned with the dog (which settled back in the car boot) we drove back to the school grounds. For me, this moment was very pleasant to experience, because I had the feeling that by being present I was actually useful. I wasn't just a researcher gathering knowledge, but I was actually able to help Kerry to go out alone for a bit, while I looked after Jenny. It was also nice because both Kerry and Jenny felt enough trust for this to be very normal.[12]

Although most qualitative researchers might not explicitly state in their method sections that they aim to be *useful* to the people they are observing in participant observation, it might still be the case implicitly, because of several factors. For example, because of ethical considerations, as being actually useful to participants might be a way to uphold ethical principles in research. Most. if not all, researchers aim to ensure that their work does not harm or exploit the individuals they study. By contributing to the wellbeing or understanding of the participants, researchers have an opportunity to demonstrate their ethical commitment. There might also be a methodological motivation to building a reciprocal relationship of trust, as building trust with research participants might improve the accuracy (i.e. trustworthiness) of the data collection. By being useful, researchers show their commitment to reciprocity. When participants perceive that the research benefits them in some way, they may be more inclined to engage openly and honestly with the researcher. What is more, when participants find value in the research, they are more likely to provide rich and detailed information.[13] This could contribute positively to the validity and depth of the data, which is an important aspect in qualitative research. From a collaborative care-ethical research point of view, being useful might not only enhance the collaborative relationship, making participants active partners in the research process rather than passive subjects, but also might contribute to the fulfilment of research goals: in some cases, the researcher's objectives may include a commitment to social change or the improvement of the conditions of the studied population. Being useful to participants then becomes a means of achieving these broader research goals, while ensuring that the research has real-world applications and contributes positively to the field. And, of course, there might also be personal motivation and values in play that drive researchers to be of assistance to the people they study. This could be a deeply held belief in social responsibility or a desire to make a positive impact on individuals' lives. Overall, collaborative researchers want to be useful to the people they are observing in participant observation as part of their commitment to ethical and empathetic research, as well as to ensure the quality and relevance of their research findings. Being useful not only benefits the participants but also enhances the quality and significance of the research itself.

For us, it was all of these factors. Especially for the first author, who also knew from his own lived experience how much was already demanded of such families in terms of pressure and the level of care required, to enter their intimate daily life as a researcher in a way that would be perceived primarily as an extra burden rather than an immediate added value felt completely wrong. Although many families were intrinsically motivated to participate due to the long-term consequences, namely an improvement in conditions for these families, he, as a father, knew that you are often just trying to get through each day in such a family, and you can only focus on things day by day. You can't really think too much about the long term, or you won't be able to make it. Thus, his own experiences fuelled his intention that any time he were to observe himself, there would be a *direct short-term* benefit. Acting as a kind of research companion was a crucial element of the whole research design, so all the researchers in this project (the first and second author and two other researchers) often acted as either a walking companion, taxi driver, babysitter, cook or psychologist, accompanying families on visits to the hospital, assisting with certain formal applications or procedures in order to procure care services, referring families to other caregivers or services, but also helping out with more mundane things such as moving large furniture, disposing of garden waste and doing dishes.

13.3 AVOIDANCE OF INTIMACY IN QUALITATIVE RESEARCH

The swimming pool was in an outbuilding of the school, which does not belong to the school, but the school does use it for its own students. According to Kerry, this is not a real swimming lesson with 'normal' children, but more therapeutic. What Jenny participates in, therefore falls under regular swimming lessons, and Kerry really likes the fact that Jenny is taking swimming lessons among these children and is actually taking steps and showing progress. We were early, and the swimming teacher Christina, to whom Jenny was clearly attached was not yet there, which made Jenny impatient. The result was that Kerry had to take Bobby the dog with her, but of course, he was not allowed inside. So Bobby patiently waited outside at the table in front of the large window of the swimming pool, in the pouring rain. Not only were we too early, but when we entered the changing room (adjacent to the pool), there appeared to be a technical problem with the surface of the pool, making it unclear whether the swimming lesson could take place at all. That was all very confusing for Jenny, and she became very upset about it, so much so that at one point she sought physical contact with me (she gave me a hug and wanted me to pick her up), much to the apparent satisfaction of Kerry. Although I was initially a bit hesitant whether to pick Jenny up – unsure whether Kerry would approve of this, when she did make approving facial expressions, it personally also felt like a kind of small victory again. I was building a good rapport with this family! While I was having this intimate moment with Jenny, it was striking that all of the other so-called 'regular' children and their parents were apparently used to the fact that there was a child walking around who was slightly different and made a lot of noises (since Jenny comes there regularly), but the parents hardly made any contact with them.[14]

Reflecting on this above excerpt on intimate moments with research participants, the first author was left wondering whether Kerry and him had created a kind of bubble here as both parents of children with complex care needs. He found it perfectly normal that he was cuddling with Jenny and recognized a lot in her behaviour, namely her impatience, her confusion and her need to physically connect when she couldn't find the words, whilst other parents didn't talk to her, and seemed to only partially acknowledge her existence (they seemed to accept the differences but never seemed to seek any further kind of closeness or relationship). The question then is whether you can expect other people to seek any kind of rapprochement with families with children with complex care needs. While, for a researcher in the type of research we embarked on, we felt that intimacy might actually be a requirement. Nevertheless, the avoidance of intimacy in qualitative research is still very pervasive and can stem from several factors, despite the inherently intimate nature of the research approach. For instance, the cultural anthropologist Louisa Lombard states that although the ideals of friendship, solidarity and closeness have become central to fieldwork relationships, maintaining a respectful distance is also essential in these relationships. In her article on fieldwork boundary negotiation, she advocates a heightened focus on boundaries – acknowledging the importance of understanding one another amidst differences and maintaining respectful distance. According to Lombard, emphasizing this boundary work fosters greater honesty about fieldwork relationships as it empowers those deeply involved in these to approach the boundary work without perceiving it as a failure or risk-taking.[15] Her perspective is indicative of the several (legitimate) reasons why researchers may avoid intimacy in qualitative research. They might be concerned about personal boundaries, biases or their own emotional responses, leading them to maintain a more distant and detached approach. In line with this, researchers may worry about crossing ethical boundaries, particularly in cases where research participants are vulnerable or have experienced trauma. Maintaining distance can also be seen as an attempt to balance power dynamics, particularly in situations where participants are in vulnerable positions. Researchers may want to avoid perpetuating power imbalances. Or researchers may be hesitant to disclose too much about themselves or engage deeply with participants due to concerns about personal privacy, potential misinterpretations or the impact on their own wellbeing.

These tendencies to keep a distance, might also be fuelled by the methodological tradition in which certain qualitative researchers were trained. Many research fields and methodologies – e.g. in medicine and long-term care practices – stem from long-established positivist traditions of maintaining a degree of distance and objectivity, as traditional quality criteria like reliability and validity trump personal involvement and subjectivity.[16] Despite the rise of (post-positivist) collaborative and participatory approaches in the domains of health and social wellbeing over the last three decades,[17] researchers may still adhere to these norms as the gold standard, and fear criticism if they deviate from them, as peers or the broader research community might expect them to maintain a certain level of detachment and objectivity. Intimacy could then be seen as unprofessional or unconventional. Or they might feel that any kind of intimacy can lead to forming stronger emotional connections or (subjective) biases towards their participants, potentially weakening the objectivity of the research. Researchers might fear that their personal feelings could cloud their judgement. There might of course also be more mundane reasons, whereby it is simply a matter of time and resources: building intimate relationships with participants can be time-consuming and resource-intensive. Researchers might opt for more efficient data collection methods to cover a broader sample size in a limited time frame.

While there are perhaps certain legitimate reasons for maintaining some level of distance in qualitative research, it's important to recognize that the level of intimacy can vary depending on the research goals, methods and ethical considerations, and that sometimes intimacy might arise unexpectedly, as the following excerpt shows. Ideally, all field researchers are mindful of their approach and its implications, striving for a balance that allows for rich, empathetic data collection while upholding ethical and methodological rigour.

13.4 THE POTENTIAL OF ENGAGING IN UNLIKELY INTIMATE YET EERIE ENCOUNTERS

Hardly 15 minutes after I enter the shared living room of his residential home for the first time, Carl, about 60 years of age, wants to show me his room. He explains this to John, the residence coordinator, then grabs my hand and takes me upstairs. Although he has a loud voice, Carl articulates unclearly to me. 'Room! Room!' he exclaims. I consciously leave the door open and position myself between Carl and the doorway. You never know. I notice a cupboard, a bed, a chair and some photos. Then I look at Carl, who is silently observing me. After about ten long seconds, he walks towards me. He stops when our bodies and faces almost touch each other, looks me straight in the eye, and says: 'Do!', before he inflates his cheeks. I inflate my cheeks. He stares at me, fascinated. After a few seconds, I let go of the oxygen, but he immediately commands: 'Do!' and inflates his cheeks again. I do what he wants, leaving the oxygen inside a little longer now. Carl pats on my inflated left cheek with his finger, and with each tap, I let go of some of the air. He is not pleased with that, and insists: 'Do!', now inflating only his right cheek. What is he up to? I have no idea, but I start to feel a bit euphoric. Once more he proclaims: 'Do!' before he sucks in his cheeks, which results in the appearance of two little holes. I imitate him again. Quietly, Carl sticks his nose in the hole in my right cheek. I stand very still and aware. What is happening, what does he want? We are in contact, that's for sure, but about what? I feel blood rushing through my veins, feel a lot of energy. I want to understand what he is communicating. Carl and I now stand very close to each other, our shoe tips touching. His commands start to come faster and faster. 'Do thick!', he says, or 'Thin!', when he wants me to suck my cheeks in. I keep following his directions. Sometimes, he touches one of my cheeks gently with his hand, but more often with his nose. He shows me how I should transfer oxygen from one inflated cheek to another, followed by: 'Do!' I do as he demonstrated. The whole time, I keep looking at his face. He has pale blue, staring eyes. Again, a new order: Carl puts a finger vertically on his lips, sucks his cheeks in, and says: 'Do!' As I mimic him, he puts his nose gently in my right cheek and sniffs softly. After that, he puts his face almost completely onto mine. Because my right index finger is still covering my lips, his nose and mouth touch the top of my hand. Carl's directions follow each other at an increasing pace, I have to inflate my cheeks, deflate, suck them in, transfer oxygen from one cheek to the other, etc. Also, he shows and tells me how to place the four fingers of my right hand vertically on my chin, the tips touching my lower lip, and then inflate my cheeks again. While I do all this, Carl stands very close to me, he sniffs in my cheeks and neck, blows gently in my face, pushes his nose against my inflated or hollow cheeks, and observes what I am doing. I feel a rapidly growing tension in my stomach, arms, chest and head; don't know what I am doing, what we are doing, what Carl is up to. By following him, I start losing control over myself, my emotions, my body and the situation. Besides euphoria, I feel an increasing fear, confusion and insecurity. All of a sudden, I realize that I start to look at what is happening between us as if I was standing in the doorway. What is happening here? Carl now sticks out his tongue and says: 'Do!'. Now I shake my head. If I would stick out my tongue, I would touch his face with it. Carl repeats his gesture, followed by a coercive: 'DO!' Again, I shake my head. What if someone else would see us? How could I ever explain myself to the support staff? For a moment, my deep confusion evaporates. I feel certain: this is getting too close. I do not want to engage in this. I take Carl's head and neck gently in my hands, around his lower jaw, and say: 'Done'. For a little while, our eyes are locked. His gaze appears bewildered to me. Then I bow his forehead towards mine, while he repeats one more time: 'Do!' I keep holding his jaw and neck, and respond: 'Carl, I don't want to. It's done. Shall we go downstairs?' Carl does not move at all. When I add: 'I am going to have a cup of tea', he takes a step back, turns away to the window and looks outside, from the middle of his room. Our contact is gone. I continue to feel both certain and confused, but also guilty about this sudden end. I try to get Carl to say something about his room, but he keeps looking the other way. Before I go downstairs, I say: 'Thank you for showing me your room.' Not a single response. Uncomfortable and confused, I walk downstairs. Carl follows in silence. From the clock in the shared living room, I infer that we were upstairs for about 15 minutes. What happened between us?[18]

Although this excerpt from the second author comes from a different research project (his PhD research about encounters between people with and without severe intellectual disabilities in neighbourhood settings), it shows the potential for (unlikely) unexpected intimacy when embarking on a collaborative care-ethical research project. Most researchers would try to avoid such a situation, let alone continuing with it, allowing it to happen and then reflecting on it. The second author did just that in this case, resulting in a variety of reflective questions about asymmetry, what to do with discomfort, but also the risk of clinging to simply one perspective or interpretation. It also touched on the boundaries of what is considered acceptable communication between neighbours with and without intellectual disabilities – and the consequences of this for people in positions of dependence. What do you do as a non-professional when a person with an intellectual disability, whose attitude and behaviour you do not understand at all, seeks physical closeness? To what extent can and may those involved in an institutional setting allow uncertainty, doubt and tension in a meeting with a stranger? To what extent do we want to be responsible for what happens in an interaction with an unknown person in the neighbourhood? How much space do we experience to find out what we can mean to each other without (many) words? And based on what criteria do you determine – when it comes to interpersonal relationships and communication in the neighbourhood – 'that it's okay as it is' or that there is no more to it? Many encounters with residents with intellectual disabilities primarily left the second author feeling confused. While, on the one hand, he tried with all his might to learn more about them, his fascination with them was often accompanied by feelings of discomfort, fear, aversion or annoyance on the other hand. As a result, his doubts about their intentions, opinions and perspectives during and after our interactions often increased rather than decreased.

According to German phenomenologist Bernhard Waldenfels, every encounter begins with an uncontrollable 'bodily response' to the otherness of another person. Waldenfels points out that this preconscious focus on the otherness of another is never neutral; on the contrary, we experience this otherness as something alien that has both an attracting and repelling effect on us. This simultaneously stimulating and piercing strangeness confuses us and cannot be precisely and definitively explained (in retrospect), due to its dependence on the observer and the context of perception. Waldenfels argues that we often neglect the 'relational' aspect of what we find strange in others. Instead of pausing to reflect on the limitations and boundaries of our own understanding of humanity and the world when we experience this sense of strangeness, we typically try to explain the otherness of another person based on what is familiar and inherent to us. Viewed through the lens of Waldenfels, during a meeting like the one with Carl, the second author was initially drawn to his (to him) strange otherness: enjoying this unconventional, physical way of communicating with him without reservations. But it didn't take long before the second author consciously tried to make sense of what he was doing: why is Carl blowing in my face, and why does he want me to puff up my cheeks with air? In what way is he looking at me? What is he trying to communicate to me? When he couldn't formulate (satisfactory) answers to these questions quickly, he became worried and started to wonder what Carl's caregivers would think of their interactions, which were unusual and incomprehensible to him. He doubted to what extent he was allowed to let this unknown man do as he pleased in this unfamiliar (and restricted) care setting. When should the second author intervene, for example, by appealing to generally accepted social norms? Viewed through Waldenfels's lens, by then he was already trying to gain control over his intentions and his preconscious fascination with what Carl and he were doing during their interaction. However, when those attempts proved unsuccessful, he tried to suppress his growing confusion and desire to flee for some time. He thought that by temporarily letting go of his own bodily urges, he could get closer to understanding Carl's intentions, opinions and perspectives. Yet, ultimately, the uncontrollable way in which his body reacted to Carl's otherness was decisive for his explicit withdrawal. When he couldn't make any (satisfactory) sense of the unconventional ways in which Carl communicated with him, his initial fascination gave way to rapidly accumulating confusion and uncertainty.

Even in the days following the meeting, the second author was primarily aware of what he had found exciting and unbearable about their communication, rather than gaining more insight into what Carl might have experienced or wanted to achieve. This made him realize that he cannot simply ignore his body's inclinations during an interaction. Paradoxically, the impressive intimate encounter with Carl brought him back to his self: it made him think about why he was both fascinated and frightened by this unconventional, physical approach. He began to doubt everything – not least himself, his communication skills, and the idea that you can better understand others by listening to them without bias, going along with them and not trying to impose your own will on them. Instead of getting to know Carl – and the other people with intellectual disabilities he met during his fieldwork – better, their interactions made him more aware of his own limitations: he realized more than ever before that feelings like impatience, uncertainty, fear, fatigue or annoyance often significantly influence how he responded to others.

Due to the increasing intensity of this confusion, and also because it frequently led him to be unable to interact attentively with other people he encountered in his PhD research, interactions with a growing number of residents with intellectual disabilities became increasingly challenging for him. More than once, he yielded to the tendency to avoid them or end the interaction prematurely. But was he doing right by them in doing so? What do the other parties involved in reverse integration settings consider preferable: trying to understand why meetings like the one with Carl can make us so alert, uncertain, fearful and confused, or trying to prevent such confusing experiences as much as possible?

> *When I discussed this unlikely, intensive, fascinating and unsettling encounter a few weeks later with residence coordinator John, he was very surprised that Carl had related to me in this way. John told me that Carl normally only tried to engage young, female interns in interactions like that. Without hesitation, he declared that this behaviour of Carl was deemed 'very sexual' – and thus forbidden. John told me that the next time I would visit, he would tell Carl that he was not allowed to take me to his room anymore.*[19]

John's (dominant) explanation only boosted new reflections and questions about what had happened: was 'very sexual' the only sensible interpretation of Carl's behaviour? And, if so, was 'forbidden' the only sensible response to this? Did Carl engage with interns like this because they were female and young? Or maybe (also) because in this restricted context they were the only open, naïve people he met; people who did not hold power over him and were unaware of fixed boundaries? In that case, the position of the second author was quite similar to the interns. But how much interactive space was left for Carl (and for the people he would meet), if he could not touch other people at all? If his body was not allowed to get close to theirs? Could we not think of suitable ways for Carl to enjoy and/or explore this kind of intimacy with others? Perhaps the question that was most pervasive and pertinent was: what would have happened, or how would the second author have perceived Carl, if he had heard this 'sexual' interpretation regarding Carl's behaviour – and the restrictive rule attached to it – straightaway, before their unlikely intimate yet eerie encounter? After all, as an outsider within this restrictive context, he probably would have had no other choice than to follow this interpretation. And this would have left very little space wherein Carl and him would be able to interact, to get to know each other in an interpersonal way, not mediated by said dominant (and seemingly unquestionable) institutional logic.

13.5 IN CONCLUSION: COLLABORATIVE CARE-ETHICAL RESEARCH AS BOTH A METHODOLOGICAL MINEFIELD AND A RELATIONAL PASTURE

In collaborative care-ethical research, researchers and participants often interact for long periods of time. It appears that this collaboration and/or exchange regularly involves both strengthening and disruptive emotional and physically intimate experiences.[20] These do not always seem to be sufficiently understood from the dominant frameworks about professionalism and ethics in care and research, which is still strongly focused on notions such as objectivity and impartiality, and views any kind of personal or emotional involvement with strong scepsis as it presumedly could affect the quality and validity of the data. Especially in cases where the research may be sensitive or involve 'vulnerable populations', maintaining distance is often deemed crucial as a means to minimize any harm or distress experienced by participants.

Of course, we are not saying one does not need to think about such issues. However, since care ethics explicitly requires space for relationality, emotions and embodiment in care practices, it does require us to think about implementing this in a (care) ethically responsible manner in collaborative research. To practise what we preach. It appears that this isn't always easy, in fact quite hard as it requires commitment, endurance and indeed a lot of reflexivity. This reflexivity isn't a mere individual undertaking, but in fact a relational, collective effort that fosters self-awareness, open communication and shared decision making. It is a dynamic process that helps researchers navigate the complexities of collaborating together, and ensures that ultimately everyone benefits equally from this mutual companionship.

Collaborative care-ethical research would therefore stand to gain from the collective reconsideration of assumptions and preconceptions, by challenging certain widely held assumptions, such as those regarding intimacy and reciprocity in research, and actually reflecting on how they might influence both the research and the relationships that we develop with those we collaborate with. In the above cases, we as researchers got incredibly close, conducting at times extremely intimate research (e.g. in someone's home, a precarious family situation, in someone's bedroom, very close to someone's skin). Our aim in this chapter was to highlight the significant reflective potential inherent in intimate research of this nature, as it leads to new questions and new knowledge production, which might be relevant for both devising more suitable, care-ethically inspired policies, and contributing to a more comprehensive and nuanced approach to care-ethical data collection and analysis. However, our primary focus will always be on ensuring that its immediate relevance is felt by individuals like Kerry, Jenny, Carl and John.

NOTES

1. Field notes Alistair, 29 January 2021, research project 'Vulnerability and Strength'.
2. See: Oliver C. Robinson, 'The Idiographic/Nomothetic Dichotomy: Tracing Historical Origins of Contemporary Confusions', *History & Philosophy of Psychology* 13 (2011): 32–3.
3. See: Suzanne L. G. Jansen, Annette A. van der Putte and Clara Vlaskamp, 'Parents' Experiences of Collaborating with Professionals in the Support of Their Child with Profound Intellectual and Multiple Disabilities: A Multiple Case Study', *Journal of Intellectual Disabilities* 21, no. 1 (2017): 53–67; United Nations, 'Convention on the Rights of Persons with Disabilities', *Treaty Series* 2515 (December 2006): 3, art. 23.
4. See: Femke Boelsma et al., 'Rethinking FQoL: The Dynamic Interplay Between Individual and Family Quality of Life', *Journal of Policy and Practice in Intellectual Disabilities* 14, no. 1 (2017): 31–8; Jorien Luijkx, *Family Matters: The Experiences and Opinions of Family Members of Persons with Severe or Profound Intellectual Disabilities* (Groningen: RUG, 2016).

5. See: Lisa M. Tillmann-Healy, 'Friendship as Method', *Qualitative Inquiry* 9, no. 5 (2003): 729–49.
6. Carlo Leget, Inge van Nistelrooij and Merel Visse, 'Beyond Demarcation: Care Ethics as an Interdisciplinary Field of Inquiry', *Nursing Ethics* 26, no. 1 (2019): 1–9.
7. Alistair Niemeijer and Merel Visse, 'When Facts Only Go So Far: Decentering What It Means to Know and Understand as a Care-Ethical Researcher in a Polarized, Post-Truth Era', in *Decentering Epistemologies and Challenging Privilege: Critical Care Ethics Perspective*, ed. Sophie Bourgault, Maggie FitzGerald and Fiona Robinson (New Brunswick, NJ: Rutgers University Press, 2024).
8. See: Charlotte A. Davies, *Reflexive Ethnography: A Guide to Researching Selves and Others*, 2nd ed. (Abingdon: Routledge, 2008); Raymond Madden, *Being Ethnographic: A Guide to the Theory and Practice of Ethnography* (Los Angeles, London, New Delhi, Singapore and Washington, DC: Sage, 2010).
9. See: Kenneth J. Gergen, *An Invitation to Social Construction*, 2nd ed. (London and Thousand Oaks, CA, New Delhi and Singapore: Sage, 2009).
10. See: Kathy C. Charmaz, *Constructing Grounded Theory* (Thousand Oaks, CA: Sage, 2006); Theo J. H. Niessen, *Emerging Epistemologies: Making Sense of Teaching Practice* (Diss., Maastricht: Fontys Hogeschool, 2007); Bernhard Waldenfels, 'In Place of the Other', *Continental Philosophy Review* 44 (2011): 151–64.
11. See: Gustaaf F. Bos, *Eindrapport tweeënhalf jaar onderzoek naar 'Dit vind ik ervan!' 2017–2019* (Amsterdam: Amsterdam UMC, 2020); Alistair Niemeijer and Merel Visse, 'Challenging Standard Concepts of "Humane" Care Through Relational Auto-Ethnography', *Social Inclusion* 4, no. 4 (2016): 168–75.
12. Field notes Alistair, 9 December 2021, research project 'Vulnerability and Strength'.
13. See: Karijn Aussems et al., 'Working Together as Scientific and Experiential Experts: How Do Current Ethical PAR-Principles Work in a Research Team with Young Adults with Developmental Language Disorder?', *Educational Action Research* 32, no. 2 (2024): 311–26; Tom Clark, 'On "Being Researched": Why Do People Engage with Qualitative Research?', *Qualitative Research* 10, no. 4 (2010): 399–419.
14. Field notes Alistair, 9 December 2021, research project 'Vulnerability and Strength'.
15. Louisa Lombard, 'The Interpretation of Relationships: Fieldwork as Boundary-Negotiation', *Ethnography* (2022), https://doi.org/10.1177/14661381211069670.
16. For example, see: Egon G. Guba and Yvonna S. Lincoln, 'Competing Paradigms in Qualitative Research', in *Handbook of Qualitative Research*, ed. N. K. Denzin and Y. S. Lincoln (Thousand Oaks, CA: Sage, 1994), 105–17, https://ethnographyworkshop.wordpress.com/wp-content/uploads/2014/11/guba-lincoln-1994-competing-paradigms-in-qualitative-research-handbook-of-qualitative-research.pdf.
17. See: Tineke Abma et al., *Participatory Research for Health and Social Well-Being* (Amsterdam: Springer, 2019); Sarah Banks and Mary Brydon-Miller, eds, *Ethics in Participatory Research for Health and Social Well-Being: Cases and Commentaries* (Abingdon and New York: Routledge, 2019); Hilary Bradbury, ed., *The SAGE Handbook of Action Research* (London, Thousand Oaks, CA, New Delhi and Singpore: Sage, 2015), https://doi.org/10.4135/9781473921290.
18. Gustaaf F. Bos, *Antwoorden op andersheid. Over ontmoetingen tussen mensen met en zonder verstandelijke beperking in omgekeerde-integratiesettingen* (Diss., Amsterdam: Vrije Universiteit University, 2016), 139–40.

19. Unpublished field notes Gustaaf, 4 November 2010, research project 'Sharing Life: Responding to Otherness'.
20. Sebastian von Peter and Gustaaf F. Bos, 'The Necessity of Unsettling Encounters in Collaborative Research – Reflections of Two Researchers Without Experiential Expertise', *Collaborations: A Journal of Community-Based Research and Practice* 5, no. 1 (2022): 4.

BIBLIOGRAPHY

Abma, Tineke A., Sarah Banks, Tina Cook, Sónia Dias, Wendy Madsen, Jane Springett and Michael T. Wright. *Participatory Research for Health and Social Well-Being*. Amsterdam: Springer, 2019.

Aussems, Karijn, Jet Isarin, Alistair Niemeijer and Christine Dedding. 'Working Together as Scientific and Experiential Experts: How Do Current Ethical PAR-Principles Work in a Research Team With Young Adults With Developmental Language Disorder?', *Educational Action Research* 32, no. 2 (2024): 311–26.

Banks, Sarah and Mary Brydon-Miller, eds. *Ethics in Participatory Research for Health and Social Well-Being: Cases and Commentaries*. Abingdon and New York: Routledge, 2019.

Boelsma, Femke, Irebe Caubo-Damen, Alice Schippers, Menco Dane and Tineke A. Abma. 'Rethinking FQoL: The Dynamic Interplay Between Individual and Family Quality of Life', *Journal of Policy and Practice in Intellectual Disabilities* 14, no. 1 (2017): 31–8.

Bos, Gustaaf F. *Antwoorden op andersheid. Over ontmoetingen tussen mensen met en zonder verstandelijke beperking in omgekeerde-integratiesettingen* Dissertation. Amsterdam: Vrije Universiteit University, 2016.

Bos, Gustaaf F. *Eindrapport tweeënhalf jaar onderzoek naar 'Dit vind ik ervan!' 2017–2019*. Amsterdam: Amsterdam UMC, 2020.

Bradbury, Hilary., ed. *The SAGE Handbook of Action Research*. London and Thousand Oaks, CA, New Delhi and Singapore: Sage, 2015. https://doi.org/10.4135/9781473921290.

Charmaz, Kathy C. *Constructing Grounded Theory*. Thousand Oaks, CA: Sage, 2006.

Clark, Tom. 'On "Being Researched": Why Do People Engage with Qualitative Research?', *Qualitative Research* 10, no. 4 (2010): 399–419.

Davies, Charlotte A. *Reflexive Ethnography: A Guide to Researching Selves and Others*. 2nd ed. Abingdon: Routledge, 2008.

Gergen, Kenneth J. *An Invitation to Social Construction*. 2nd ed. London, Thousand Oaks, CA, New Delhi and Singapore: Sage, 2009.

Guba, Egon G. and Yvonna S. Lincoln. 'Competing Paradigms in Qualitative Research', in *Handbook of Qualitative Research*, edited by N. K. Denzin and Y. S. Lincoln, 105–17. Thousand Oaks, CA: Sage, 1994. https://ethnographyworkshop.wordpress.com/wp-content/uploads/2014/11/guba-lincoln-1994-competing-paradigms-in-qualitative-research-handbook-of-qualitative-research.pdf.

Jansen, Suzanne L. G., Annette A. J. van der Putten, and Clara Vlaskamp. 'Parents' Experiences of Collaborating With Professionals in The Support of Their Child with Profound Intellectual and Multiple Disabilities: A Multiple Case Study', *Journal of Intellectual Disabilities* 21, no. 1 (2017): 53–67.

Leget, Carlo, Inge van Nistelrooij and Merel Visse. 'Beyond Demarcation: Care Ethics as an Interdisciplinary Field of Inquiry', *Nursing Ethics* 26, no. 1 (2019): 1–9.

Lombard, Louisa. 'The Interpretation of Relationships: Fieldwork as Boundary-negotiation', *Ethnography* (2022). https://doi.org/10.1177/14661381211069670.

Luijkx, Jorien. *Family Matters: The Experiences and Opinions of Family Members of Persons with Severe or Profound Intellectual Disabilities*. Groningen: RUG, 2016.

Madden, Raymond. *Being Ethnographic: A Guide to the Theory and Practice of Ethnography*. Los Angeles, London, New Delhi, Singapore and Washington, DC: Sage, 2010.

Niemeijer, Alistair and Merel Visse. 'Challenging Standard Concepts of "Humane" Care Through Relational Auto-Ethnography', *Social Inclusion* 4, no. 4 (2016): 168–75.

Niemeijer, Alistair and Merel Visse. 'When Facts Only Go So Far: Decentering What it Means to Know and Understand as a Care-Ethical Researcher in a Polarized, Post-Truth Era', in Sophie Bourgault, Maggie FitzGerald and Fiona Robinson, eds. *Decentering Epistemologies and Challenging Privilege: Critical Care Ethics Perspective*. New Brunswick, NJ: Rutgers University Press, 2024.

Niessen, Theo J. H. *Emerging Epistemologies: Making Sense of Teaching Practice*. Dissertation. Maastricht: Fontys Hogeschool, 2007.

von Peter, Sebastian and Gustaaf F. Bos. 'The Necessity of Unsettling Encounters in Collaborative Research – Reflections of Two Researchers without Experiential Expertise', *Collaborations: A Journal of Community-Based Research and Practice* 5, no. 1 (2022): 4.

Robinson, Oliver C. 'The Idiographic/Nomothetic Dichotomy: Tracing Historical Origins of Contemporary Confusions', *History & Philosophy of Psychology* 13 (2011): 32–3.

Tillmann-Healy, Lisa M. 'Friendship as Method', *Qualitative Inquiry* 9, no. 5 (2003): 729–49.

United Nations. 'Convention on the Rights of Persons with Disabilities', *Treaty Series* 2515 (December 2006): 3.

Waldenfels, Bernhard. 'In Place of the Other', *Continental Philosophy Review* 44 (2011): 151–64.

CHAPTER FOURTEEN

Inquiring into materialized care

Hospital beds as living landscapes of care

MEREL VISSE AND ALISTAIR NIEMEIJER

INTRODUCTION

A wide range of scholars make a convincing case for the need to acknowledge that human practices, like care, are bound to non-human worlds, including materialities.[1] Think about the parent serving their child with a spoon, a room service worker wearing his uniform, a delivery man using a scanner, a nurse working with a computer, inserting an intravenous line or the administrator counting beds. We know of research on the entanglement of wearable technologies and perceptions of identities and relationships with these technologies for elderly people.[2] The Dutch care ethicist Marcel Boonen also examines how care is produced and emerges through various relationships extending beyond human actors to the more-than-humans, like technology.[3] The term 'more-than-humans' was coined, among others, by Karen Barad and Maria Puig de la Bellacasa, post-humanist scholars who developed an 'ethics of entanglements', indicating the responsibilities that come with entanglements of complex relations among people, other species, practices and things.[4] Boonen's research, for example, demonstrates the entanglement of technology and the spatial positions of nurses and patients in hospitals, literally and figuratively. This aligns with the view that humans are *not* separate entities merely observing and interacting with the world around them. Instead of seeing the world and objects as 'out there', independent of human observation, scholars like Barad and Bellacasa propose that the world is not a pre-existing entity; it is co-constituted through intra-actions between various agencies. These agencies include humans, non-human organisms, technologies and the environment.

Translated to care theory, in her pivotal work, Maria Puig de la Bellacasa meticulously unpacks and expands on Joan Tronto and Bernice Fisher's definition of care, emphasizing 'affective, ethical and hands-on agencies of practical and material consequence'.[5] Puig de la Bellacasa also highlights how care ethics is not just about humans, but about their 'thick, impure, involvement in a world', making ethics 'hands-on'.[6] With an increased focus on our non-human world, the things or objects we use and make are perceived as vehicles for care, implicated *in* care. Care ethicists and researchers do not eliminate or blur distinctions between humans and non-humans, but seek, instead, to understand how such distinctions come into being in everyday practices. Haraway invited us long ago to abandon the myth of the isolated human and embrace a more porous view of ourselves, constantly interfacing with the material world and other species. Thus, 'materialities are not merely a backdrop for care interactions but play an active role in constituting relations of care'.[7] How then can we examine and report on these practices in a way that aligns with this approach?

A growing trend in research methods embraces the entanglements of humans, non-humans and the environment, evident in practice-led and new materialist or post-qualitative research. But in the field of care research and ethics, common qualitative research methodologies like grounded theory, case study, phenomenology, narrative research and ethnography still dominate and care research often lags behind in integrating this interconnectedness in research. This omission overlooks the valuable perspective of researchers as inherently entangled participants in the research process: entangled with objects of care and their environment. This stirred our idea for an approach that acknowledges the researcher's own implicated stance to materialities, specifically related objects. It also opened our thinking about how to 'narrate' about materialities in care research.

In this chapter, we therefore propose a view of inquiry that acknowledges our positionality and entanglements with materials and environments. Our focus lies on the 'aesthetic narrativization' of objects of care, where we weave narratives about objects with visual, poetic and analytic expressions. We integrated this in a guide for aesthetic-led inquiry.[8] This approach, of which the groundwork was laid previously and further developed for this chapter, harnesses inquiry as a process of exploring care and materialities of care. It invites readers to connect with entangled objects and experiences that are hard to capture in words. We will clarify what we mean by 'aesthetics' soon, but in short, we refer to experiencing aesthetic qualities.[9] Here, quality is not perceived as good or bad, or beautiful or ugly, but as in the textural, rhythmic and tone colours of a musical piece, for example. We are less concerned with a view of aesthetics as in beautifying or aesthetic judgement. We are especially interested in poetic, existential experiences of these qualities that move beyond language.[10]

We will work with an example from healthcare and focus on one of the most widely used and symbolically charged objects in healthcare, hospital beds. Our contribution challenges the view of objects (such as the hospital bed) as static and detached, and revitalizes objects as aesthetic and sometimes spiritual *landscapes of living*. We invite researchers to *live* questions about relationships with materialities, and how they constitute practices of care (and vice versa). Understanding care objects as aesthetic and experiential landscapes may provide us with alternative, dynamic views of care.

Our interest in the hospital bed as materialized care did not only emerge from our interdisciplinary professional positions as researchers, teachers and faculty members. We have lived these landscapes in various times and circumstances in our lives ourselves and will draw on those experiences later in this chapter when we present vignettes as the point of departure of our inquiry. We began looking into 'beds' and their relation to theories of care and care ethics in 2017, when one of us, Merel, reported on an artistic research project during an artist-in-residency on 'nests'. She developed an exhibition that inquired into the tensions in everyday life from a care ethics perspective, which sees people as embedded, 'nested' in care-based relationships. In that publication, Merel pursued connections between the nest as a secluded and intimate space and the hospital bed: 'my artistic interest in "nests" began with hospital beds as both a secluded and a public space'.[11] In this chapter, we expand on her artistic inquiry, revitalizing hospital beds as aesthetic and even spiritual landscapes of living, referring to Jullien's living with the 'spirit' of the singular 'milieu' of beds as we know them.[12]

14.1 LIVING THE QUESTIONS: AESTHETIC-APOPHATIC INQUIRY

Central to our aesthetic-apophatic inquiry is meandering and examining questions through detour instead of direct access.[13] Apophatic[14] stands for 'indirect' and puts 'living' the care-ethical concerns at the heart of the research. It acknowledges uncertainty, surprises and unpredictability in inquiry, and we hope to contribute to what phenomenologist Linda Finlay called 'seeing afresh'.[15] For this, we need to 'unknow', and that is what apophatic stands for – 'unknowing'. Instead of generating or producing knowledge, this form of inquiry is a way of relating to the world by 'living our questions' through our inquiry.[16] Even though we usually focus on the object of study directly, what would happen if we would connect with our questions differently?

The history of the word 'apophatic' goes back to the Greek apophatikós, which means negation or 'denial'. Instead of capturing objects or phenomena by describing or analysing what they are, in an apophatic approach we might 'meander' around the object, not aiming to capture it by appropriation as much by actively seeking out a relationship with the questions that have arisen, by 'living' them – for example, through poetry or metaphor. Here, Jullien's concept of 'living' refers to an 'involved' and active relationship with the world around us, with emerging 'shadowy knowledge'[17] that remains integrated with a context that is hard to be drawn out of it, and that does not separate the researcher or ethicist from that same world. It cannot be abstracted from a 'landscape'. It defies codification. Jullien gives several examples:

> A child at its mother's bosom or on her lap has practically no other knowledge than that (or in the usual comparison, early cultures are more *conniving*; later cultures more *knowledgeable*). Then, with school, as the written word flattens and equalizes, and knowledge is divided into disciplines, 'objects' take shape and come into isolation; planes are separated that reason must once more bind together. The conniving relation is covered up as soon as a knowledgeable subject wins its autonomy, but it does not vanish. It persists in silence, buried, tacit, like a water table ready to surface. Landscape is that surfacing.[18]

Aesthetic-apophatic inquiry refers to our lived-bodily, sensorial relationships with the world, people and things around us, and to realms we will not be able to know. It also refers to how that relationality is creative. Thus, we do not follow a more Kantian view of aesthetics as referring to beauty or judgement. But we are interested in letting the creative unfold and finding ways to need to not want to jump to unfold it – how to practise an open receptivity or naturalness. Hanging around 'naturalness' is best illustrated by an example of watercolour painters. Philosopher Peimin Ni wrote 'like the motion of the brush to be as natural as water sliding down from a leaking wall or a stick drawing on sand – this kind of stroke has no arbitrary smoothness, and never appears to be running out of energy'.[19] Un-naturalness, or not being receptive to letting this process unfold, would imply that the watercolour would be forced or controlled to work as an oil paint: being without its fluid and transparent properties, or being thick and dense – which it is not.

Aesthetic-apophatic inquiry offers opportunities to inquire into materialities of care and their concerns through more-than-word logic, such as using performative play, poetry, graphic novels, painting, music and dance or movement.[20] These non-verbal approaches provoke questioning and inspiration to sociopolitical concerns. Aesthetics-based inquiry emerged in the field of art education with a shift from product (the artwork) to process and relationality (artistic or studio practice). This approach is related to other approaches such as 'practice-led research', 'performative research' and 'research through creative practice'.[21] They are similar in that the arts and 'processes of making' produce knowledge that can be different from, but complementary to, the knowledge produced by science. However, there may be value in temporarily leaving the goal of knowledge production aside and practising 'unknowing', before returning to *lived* understandings.[22] Previously, in 'The Unsayable in Arts-Based Research',[23] one of us wrote how materials like watercolour paper and pigment can be partners in conversation, and how researchers are phenomenologically involved the materials, resonating with them, receiving them and being transformed by them.[24] We have conceptualized that approach to the 'unsayable' as aesthetic-apophatic inquiry, which honours and presents the more poetic, mysterious and unfathomable aspects of art and research.

To summarize, in this chapter, we de-emphasize the goal of grasping for answers directly, but to decrease the desire to know and control at least temporarily. Instead, we aim to live the questions in a state of receptiveness and connect with what is 'upstream' in life itself. In line with Liora Bresler, this is more than a change of self or a matter of 're-seeing'[25] or 'seeing afresh'.[26] It is about, to use the poet Rainer Maria Rilke's words, living the questions themselves.

In the following sections, we provide an example of living this inquiry to aesthetically narrate our entanglements with objects. This form of inquiry is multimodal and process-oriented and has various movements, also conceptual and experiential. Researchers may work with mediums to their liking. Some feel attracted to writing and documenting, others to collage, watercolour, drawings, photography, reading, music, cooking, observing and reflecting to generate spaces, where experiences are (re-)lived, and where gradually, an experiential and conceptual landscape is sketched. This approach to inquiry connects materialized, temporal experiences with the poetic, the real and the imaginary.

14.2 A GUIDE

The process of aesthetic-apophatic inquiry consists of several movements through alternating, experiential and concept-led phases of writing, making, reflection, and reading, an approach for 'living the questions themselves'. The groundwork for this approach was laid several years ago with various colleagues,[27] and then further developed and published more recently,[28] followed by slight revisions for the purpose of this chapter. We do not frame this a step-by-step method, but as a process guide that needs to be approached in a holistic way. Below, we present movements for others to adapt to their concerns, questions and contexts. We stress that these 'phases' are not to be disentangled, will overlap and sometimes repeat and reverse.

14.2.1 Being perplexed

Pose a 'grand tour' question to enter an experiential space related to your care-ethical concern. For example, 'what is it like to ... ?' Begin with a felt concern or perplexity about a care-related object and problem: this may vary from a societal to a personal challenge you want to learn about. John Dewey's notion of 'being perplexed by' may be helpful: what are you perplexed by? Hence, your focus does not necessarily need to be an object, concept or phenomenon or round-up question, you can also enter a reflexive realm through societal critique. The question or concern needs to be open, ready to change and to be 'lived' throughout the research. For example: do not start with dichotomies or dualities, or by asking a yes or no question. Instead, begin with a question focused on experiences. In the example we present below, we begin with sharing a narrative vignette, leading us to ask questions to hospital beds, their spaces, our experiences and concerns that unfold in the inquiry. So, you can, for example, start with writing an anecdote, expressing a memory, and describing it. In this chapter, we begin writing short narrative vignettes presenting you with initial contexts of questions. This helped us become aware of the unfolding of the questioning.

14.2.2 Choosing a concept

Choose a theoretical concept relating to your lived questions. Instead of deductively 'applying' this concept, establish a relationship with it by reading, making it your own, 'living' it, not abstracted from your process and yourself. You can do this, for example, by drafting a short summary of the concept in your own words, writing a poem about it, making a drawing of one of the related concepts, or having a conversation with someone. This concept will function heuristically while your inquiry unfolds. It helps you move away from what you first see and enter other realms of living. It helps make you more aware of how the concept and related theory may steer your perception and the presuppositions that may need to be put aside. Using a heuristic concept also helps you avoid overload; it helps you choose the mediums and enter the actual making and creative practice of a multimodal approach. In the example below, we chose François Jullien's concepts of 'landscape' and 'scenery', described in the next section.

14.2.3 Reflection through making

Next, engage your questions through another medium – for example, by making something or by recording a podcast or story on your phone or video camera. Relate what unfolds from your concept, again through making. Begin with anything. You can write, or work with a piece of paper, a pen, a canvas, newspaper clippings, or colours. You can also make a performance or write a play or use objects that you find in any context and create a small installation. Make something rather intuitively, let your hands, senses and body guide the making. It doesn't need to be art or craft. Cooking is making too. Gardening, also. Reflect regularly on what unfolds by listening closely. There is no protocol. You could ask: how does what you see, think, hear and sense relate to where you started, your question or concern or object? How does it relate to your theoretical concept(s)? and what is called for, now? What more can you see, hear and sense? What is going on around you, away from your inquiry? Listen with 'attentive being with',[29] with receptiveness, responsiveness and care. Perhaps keep a journal or create a folder where you collect clippings you've gathered. You will not only study why and what is made along the inquiry, but you will also study forms, sensations and meanings by listening and making interpretations about the unfolding work. Another possibility is to look at what unfolds through the 'lens' of your concept as a heuristic 'device'. You can ask questions to the materials. Listen carefully to what unfolds, as if talking to another person. The work carries its own process and form of knowledge. It will speak to you in its own way, demonstrating a kind of agency. Here, agency is not an attribute of something or someone; rather, it is the process of cause and effect in 'enactment'.[30] Translating this view to phase three means you can reflect on how your words, makings and reflections generate newness and make the work grow into something you couldn't envision in advance. Reflect on how the ongoing process of these interactions shapes your practice.

14.2.4 Indirect dwelling

While you work, enjoy the detours and dwell indirectly. Meandering is meaningful, and sometimes, indirect is more direct.[31] This may help you to connect with implicit processes coming to the fore, but it will also help you to be open. Do not focus too directly on what you think should unfold. Imagine balancing precariously on a ball while circling it, keeping your balance. You cannot look down at the ball because you would lose your balance. You need to create an overall sense of perspective while simultaneously connecting with the ball, through your feet remaining balanced. Try to look away, gaze, meander, and notice what happens. This intricate play is at the heart of this aesthetic-apophatic approach.

14.2.5 Reflecting on qualities

During the inquiry, dwell and reflect on qualities that emerge. By 'quality' we do not refer to judgements like good and bad, or beautiful and ugly, but to perceptual awareness of aesthetic qualities such as lines, shapes, textures, colours and hues or tones.[32] People vary in their ability to discriminate among the qualities that constitute their environment. Various studies have shown how some people perceive qualities and relationships as more subtle and complex. Think about wine connoisseurs who can detect subtle characteristics of wine, varying in aroma, flavour and colour. The ability to perceive, compare and contrast qualities is called perceptual differentiation. Different perceptions evoke different feelings. For example, perceiving jagged lines makes some feel edgy, while smooth lines may be soothing. Not everyone perceives the world and its qualities the same way.

14.2.6 Sharing findings

Finally, once your practice seems to be generating results you might consider 'findings', like lived experiences or novel concepts, you can share them with others. How to convey your insights such that they are alive? We align with the Utrecht phenomenological tradition, where Van Manen advocates the inclusion of an artistic dimension to 'stir our pedagogical, psychological or professional sensibilities'.[33] We sometimes take this further to put the creative practice itself at the heart of inquiry, but that is in no way required to do meaningful inquiry. In the example below, we combine descriptions, discursive strategies with visual ones in encounters but there are other forms as well. A multimodal approach may be fruitful, combining narratives, poetic vignettes, images and even peer-reviewed video essays. Reporting on your process should not be a representational act, but a way to share something about the process.

Let us now see how this approach plays out in care ethics inquiry.

14.3 EXAMPLE

14.3.1 Being perplexed – the hospital bed as 'materialized care'

Our perplexity relates to the (under-researched) hospital bed. In the limited research we've found, hospital beds are primarily viewed as functional tools with specific purposes. They're treated as objects we simply interact with through sight, recognition and basic use. For example, we found that hospital bed design from patients' perspectives, despite its importance, is under-researched. And if there is any attention at all, it is usually focused on specific features or performance testing for purposes of fall prevention, bed manoeuvrability, its impact on caregiver workload, and other risks. We found a few studies focusing on complete design processes considering user needs; however, the caregivers, *not* the patients, are defined as the 'users' of the bed.[34]

Our research interest shifted towards the entangled relationships that shape care practices, with the hospital bed as a specific example of how care materializes in the hospital environment. We read various scholarly studies that reported on people in hospitals spending about 60 per cent of their time in bed. In a Swedish qualitative study, for example, sixty adult people were interviewed about their experiences with the hospital bed.[35] Most hospital patients spent around six to eight hours in bed during the night, and four hours or more during the day. The reasons for being in bed varied from experiencing pain to being fatigued, but a significant number of people stayed in bed during the day because they 'have no other place to be/nothing else to do'.[36] Not reported in Petzäll et al.'s study, the hospital can be the last place people are – for example, when receiving palliative care. Alternatively, people may also be too sick to be anywhere else. While in bed, people talk with staff and fellow patients, they have their meals, go to the toilet, read, listen to the radio and talk on the telephone. Some studies report on patients feeling the beds are uncomfortable and the lamp and bedside table do not 'interact' with the bed when they want to undertake certain activities.[37] Others feel their integrity is challenged, having little privacy. The few studies we found report on a myriad other experiences, highlighting issues with beds being too narrow, hard, rigid, too high (from the floor), handles being too heavy or their grip area too small, mattresses being too lumpy, and blankets even giving them static electric shocks.[38] Many patients find the plastic cover around the mattress disturbing: it can be too hot, cause perspiration and make them slip. In most studies we read for this chapter, a minority mentions satisfying properties of the bed.[39] Without framing it as such, we noticed studies bring important materialized qualities of care to light on the experiences of patients[40] with the hospital bed and we wondered if we could reflect on a deeper level by living questions about entanglements in care aesthetically and poetically.

Yes, we read scholarly work, but our perplexity and concern primarily emerged, however, from our personal experiences with hospital beds. This stirred and focused our search for questioning the bed as a potential resource to learn about materialized care. We reconnected to our memories of when we were admitted as patients to the hospital for one or more overnight stays, as we both also have a medical history of being admitted to hospital on several occasions. We wrote two narrative accounts to reconnect with the hospital bed, demonstrating the first step of immersing ourselves, to move 'up the river', and increase our involvement with our inquiry.

A Landscape (Merel)

My bedhead is placed against a window, surrounded by bleach-white walls. The window sheers slice the too-bright light behind my pillow in rectangles. I was hoping they would soften the mood – my mood – but my blanket is losing its yellow and turns into dingy diagonals. Cold sweat covers my body, my mouth is dry from thirst. I try to reach it, but the nightstand with water is too far out. I stretch some more, but my body brusquely calls me back. First with a sharp pinch. Then a more urgent alert. I call the night nurse, I stretch again, dizzy from craving water.

A few hours later, I regain consciousness. I feel someone carelessly pulling the sheets out underneath my bottom, connecting me with the sticky plastic mattress. The sensation propels me back to the gluey steel plate they pushed underneath me on the surgery table. I wonder why there is such haste and urgency in her movements. She turns on the light, and I feel relief. The power of the sneering shades from behind me vanishes, they messed with my head. But the relief is temporary. My eyes blink and cannot register what they see. Before I grasp what's happened, the nurse urges me there is nothing to worry about: 'Your wound opened up, the stitches broke. The doctor will be here any minute.' I am frightened. The sticky plastic, the stained blanket and red confusion. Only after I rose out of bed and years afterward after looking at images of beds, I gained the perspective that allowed me to see this was more than an unsterile calamity area. It was a testimony to hitting rock bottom, because this was my bed.

The Other Landscape (Alistair)

Here again. It smells the same. A familiar, sterile, oddly comforting and simultaneously harrowing smell. The sheets also feel the same. Cool and clean, institutionally formal and distant, and yet also vaguely caring when I wrap them around myself once more. It's a bit too cold in here without pyjama pants, but I've taken them off because I was getting hot. The sheets are somewhat like a luxury hotel bed in that strangely distant and comforting way, only without the luxury or the overall happy feeling of being on holiday or abroad. Very white. Too white. Far too white for the 'accident' that is inevitably going to happen. Maybe they should make brown sheets for gastroenterological patients. But obviously they are also white for a diagnostic reason, sharply reminding me again why I am here.

I hate the confining square footage of this bed. Give me a king-size hospital bed anytime. I can barely twist and turn without either falling off, or feeling way too close to my neighbour. He looks really ill by the way – they've pulled the curtains around his bed – never a good sign. He must be around my age, surely? Maybe I should read something? I'm too tired to sleep. Does that make sense? How many more nights with this too-thin pillow? I should have brought my own pillow with me. I also shouldn't have fidgeted with the electric controls of the bed, because now the head is raised and it is in the middle of the night so I dare not make noise, lest I wake my fellow roomies. This bed makes an enormous noise even during visiting hours, when it can get quite loud. Why is that? I read somewhere that coffee machines make a loud noise on purpose, so that people know when their coffee is ready. Is it the same for electric patient beds?

The blue draw sheet they always place above the white sheets is tucked in too tight, all the way under the mattress. I managed to wiggle the white sheets out, but the blue draw sheet indignantly stays put, as if it's challenging me to a battle. I can't be bothered. So, I make a bundle of them with my feet. Why do they even have these stupid draw sheets, barely anyone here is using them. I wish I could bring my own bed next time.

14.3.2 Choosing a concept – living landscapes

We continue reading, now connecting our personal and scholarly concern with a theoretical concept. As if weaving a theoretical concept with the previous threads above (studies on hospital beds and narrative vignettes) to deepen and expand our inquiry. To step into the stream even more, now combined with conceptual embankment. As if we build an embankment along the bank of the river of inquiry to control a flooding of insights.

We chose 'living landscapes' as a concept. Merel published previously about Jullien's concept of 'living landscapes' and intuited this would be meaningful to our inquiry.[41] In the West,[42] Jullien proposes, paintings usually have one or more fixed vanishing points and perspective establishes a specific point in space to which all other points relate. Space is defined by points, straight lines and planes. Subjects are framed and bounded, and fixed in their positions. In Eastern approaches to landscapes (we acknowledge there are many exceptions but for the sake of the argument continue with this binary), the subjects are drawn with black outlines with tones applied as detail, and landscapes are rhythmical, in constant flux passing between active and passive states. Accurate depiction is not that important, but revealing natural rhythms and the spirit of the subject is essential. In previous work, Merel was especially triggered by the originality of the Chinese in their indifference to any notion of a telos, a final end for things, for they sought to interpret reality solely on the basis of itself, from the perspective of a single logic inherent in the actual processes in motion.[43]

We do not want to grasp experiences with the hospital beds and develop them into knowledge through realism, but we aim to weave our experiences with the passage of time, while staying fully attached to them, thus living Jullien's notion of '*living*' through becoming part of the landscape. Jullien's view of landscape is inspired by the interplay between opposing and at the same time correlating factors. Jullien proposes we speak of landscape 'when the world, through the activity of its correlations, clears out and opens up within itself and compels us to experience it'. Landscape allows us to overcome the separation of the material (physical) and spiritual, and 'spirit issues from the physical'.[44] From this perspective, landscape addresses not the seeing or the 'knowing' of what is seen, but the experiencing and living of sceneries.

Here, landscape stands for a living relationship with the world that is not distanced, but is about an engaged, 'attached' living that 'endlessly and without limit weave[s] together the landscape, the great correlation of "mountains" and "waters"',[45] with which humans are entangled. The landscape becomes like a bow 'which plays on my soul', writes Jullien, quoting Stendhal.[46] The visuals constitute these landscapes that indicate positions and movements of ourselves: the experience continuously unfolds. They are not metaphors, but can be seen rather as materialized care where the symbolic, the real and the imaginary interconnect. Think of a Möbius strip, for example, demonstrating the intertwining of contraries. Contradiction is on one side of the strip, while always being on the other side as well.

This concept and its logic are like that of a possible journey in stages that are lined together. The field of thought is not defined and contained *a priori*; it just unfolds progressively, from one stage to the next, becoming more fertile along the way. Furthermore, the path along which it unfolds does not exclude other possibilities – which may run alongside temporarily or intersect with it. By the end of the journey, an experience has been lived through, a landscape has been sketched in.[47]

14.3.3 Reflection through making

This brings us to the practice of relating to our narrated experiences anew, but through the detour of making. Merel continued the process of making and shared her progress with Alistair. Through poetry and visuals, two 'sceneries' emerged that we used as a stepping stone for further reflection in subsequent phases.

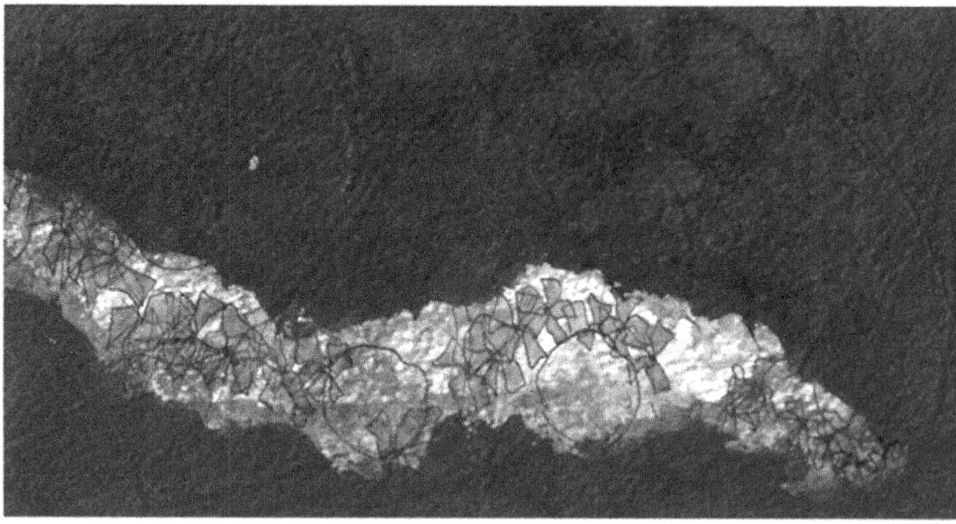

FIGURE 14.1 Scenery 1: Watercolour and ink on paper (Merel).

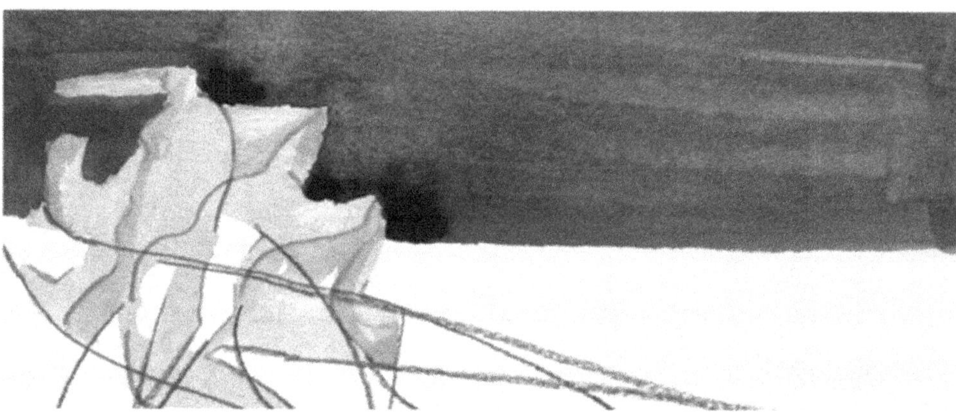

FIGURE 14.2 Scenery 2: Watercolour, ink and charcoal on paper (Alistair).

14.3.4 Indirect dwelling through detours

When we wrote the vignettes and created these visuals, we felt taken 'to the limits of the perceptible'.[48] Something was going on in these narrations and visuals that couldn't be accessed through words or imagery, or colours. For a while, we didn't know how to proceed, and the project stalled for several months. Something felt 'off', which is not uncommon. We 'dwelled' with the imagery and narrations, putting them aside, discussing them with each other, as if we were 'waiting'. In Jullien's terms, our experiences were woven with the passage of time, but it created a sense of having entered 'a void'. An emptiness, but not an abandoned one.

In the meantime, in our own lives, coincidences occurred, such as frequent visits to hospital rooms where loved ones were admitted unexpectedly, offering us a detour from our own experiences with hospital beds, inviting us to meander around others. We were

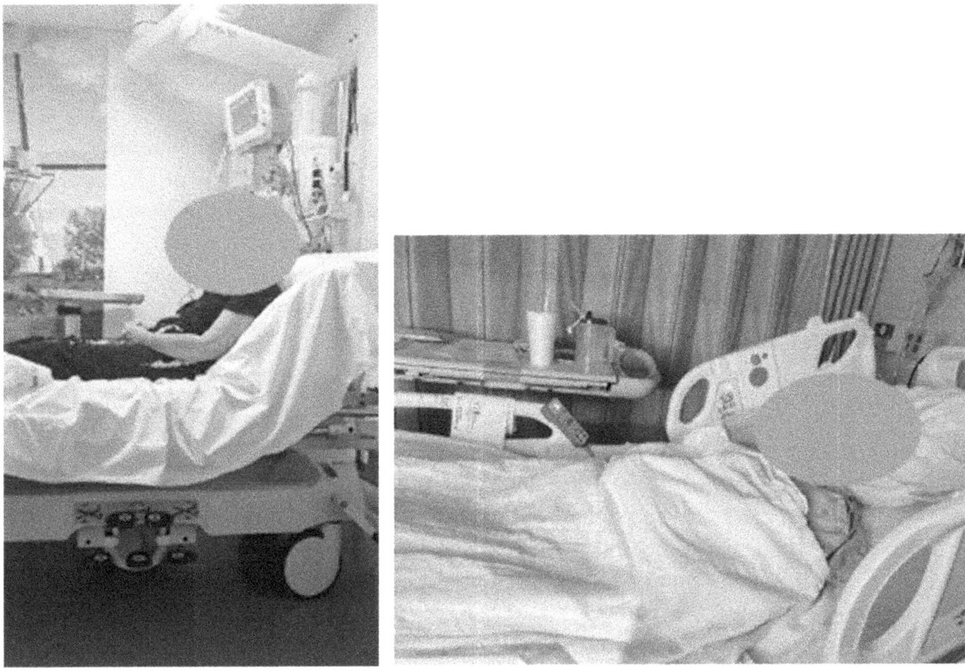

FIGURES 14.3 and 14.4 Sceneries 3 and 4: Unexpected scenery in a Dutch and US hospital, respectively.

'living' the main question of this case example and our orientation to the hospital bed, but through unexpected sceneries.[49] Literally by meandering around the bed of others instead of being bedridden ourselves. Even though we could observe the bed directly, experientially, it was as if we were witnessing the hospital bed indirectly, through secondary experiences (of loved ones). We made some anonymized pictures and will share them here, as these visits and witnessing hospital beds informed further inquiry.

The phenomenologist Finn Hansen proposes that we can gain insights into neglected and unseen aspects by engaging in poetic dwelling. Poetic dwelling can enable us to connect with realms that are not yet apparent to us. Applying this to our inquiry of the hospital bed, we were encouraged to move from perceiving the bed solely as an object (I-It) and perceiving it as a space where lived experiences unfold (I-Thou).

To the people in the photos, the hospital bed meant relief and safety. For them, the bed was a place to rest, sleep, withdraw, even from visitors, nurses, physical therapists or physicians. They 'owned' the bed and their room, as if the bed became them. As if their bodies were unified with the bed, changing into an 'assembled body'.[50] What added to that sense of safety was the technology the bed provided, like an automated function to raise the head or leg support, the call button for the nurse, the phone close by, the colours of the walls and view outside, and the sounds in the hallway all contributed to that lived experience of safety. The perspective of being discharged was quite threatening to them, at least for a while.

Their experience juxtaposed with ours. As if poetically, as Jullien aptly proposes, landscape is like a bow 'which plays on my soul',[51] these two photographs and the related experiences would give us consonant tones that feel peaceful, safe, harmonic, like light, a hopeful violin, while our own experiences with the bed as landscape clearly presented more dissonant, troubling tones. Strangely, these various meanings are unrelated to the gravity of the physical conditions of the bedridden people, as both loved ones were hospitalized because of (temporary) life-threatening conditions, and we were not.

After learning this, we felt a slight shift. The phase of detouring through connecting with others' experiences, of understanding the hospital bed through their eyes, began to give way to a different kind of exploration. Now, we turned to the unique sceneries we carried *within*. We sought not just analysis but an intuitive grasp of the aesthetic qualities the watercolour sceneries embodied: the colours, textures and meanings that whispered their own stories.

14.3.5 Reflecting on qualities

Reflecting on the qualities of the watercolours and our narrative vignettes was helpful. At first, we approached this rather rationally, by analysing their formal qualities, aligning with what Hannes and Siegesmund write in their article on analysing visual images: 'formal qualities are an entry way into tacit experiences that both researchers and participants could tap into to gain a deeper level of analysis'.[52] In this context, roles like researcher and participant collided, providing us an entry into our tacit experiences and the works' agencies. In their article, Hannes and Siegesmund propose three levels of analysis for visual imagery. The first is a form of textual analysis of narratives that the maker of images creates. The second layer of analysis focuses on the meanings given by the viewer of the work. The third layer they propose relates to the meanings the artistically formed object itself is trying to express. This layer recognizes, beyond the maker's intent, the non-human agency of the artistic object.[53]

In our vignettes and visual sceneries, the formative qualities, like the shapes and forms, highlight lines and values affecting our senses. We will simply present the aesthetic qualities we discerned in both the vignettes and our visual sceneries:

> Image 1: aesthetic qualities (line, shape, form, texture, colour, value/tone, spaces): bleach-white walls, sheers, slices, rectangles, flower shapes, yellow, dingy diagonals, sharpness, sticky plastic mattress, gluey steel plate, light, stained, red.
>
> Image 2: aesthetic qualities (line, shape, form, texture, colour, value/tone, space): familiar, sterile, comforting, harrowing smell, white, formal, distance, very white, brightness, brown, square, blue, white, noise, bundle, vanishing.

The first watercolour presents us with something mysterious or uncanny unfolding, despite its warmth of red/orange, possibly by the overwhelming tonal contrast of light and dark, with the small area of light coming through. It demonstrates 'chiaroscuro', the Italian term for clair-obscure, used to create a sense of depth and drama. This image shows relatively sharp edges and blurry see-through shapes behind the reddish flower shapes, also indicating a realm behind the black veil. It is as if we are witnessing a 'tunnel' shape, tightening, and dissolving toward the edges. We are not carrying out a semiotic analysis in this chapter but flowers are often used as symbols of beauty, love and life. In this watercolour, the vibrant flowers and delicate brushstrokes may suggest hope and resilience despite darkness.

The second watercolour, also with a stark contrast of black and white, less mysterious, but evoking another type of tension, invites our eyes to look at a blue bundle, resembling a kind of geometrical, network structure with straight black lines. This bundle – as if it presents us with a perspective – is connected to a vanishing point outside the image. There seems to be a 'stretch' or pull there, but we cannot view who or what is pulling. Also, it is not fully clear if this pull makes the viewer curious or apprehensive. The lines divide the image into two areas: one darker, one lighter, highlighting the contrast, adding tension. This image seems more sterile and icier, possibly because of the blue, and is dominated by more formal and distant meanings, accentuating the coldness or reliability of purity and hygiene. There is less warmth, in contrast to the first watercolour, but more safety, because its starkness leaves less room for doubt or ambiguity.

Image 1: Mysterious, uncanny, chiaroscuro, drama, ambiguity.
Image 2: Sterile, icy, tension, vanishing, purity, clarity.

14.3.6 Sharing findings

In the process of inquiry, we began with the notion of the hospital bed as an object we could tell stories about – a 'narrativized object'. Yet, as we delved deeper, the focus shifted towards visual sceneries – sterile corridors bathed in an icy blue light, the unnerving hum of machinery echoing through empty hallways. These glimpses, analysed and reimagined, led us beyond the physical objects and showed us the lived entanglements, beckoning us towards what lingered beneath the surface. Here, the tangible and intangible collided, and the following elegy took shape, capturing the essence of us, mourning a space both clinical and chilling, familiar yet utterly strange.

I.
Pale walls bleached bare, a canvas stark,
Sheers slice daylight in geometric bark.
Sun spills gold, an unwelcome guest,
On the yellowed wrap, my weary nest.

White walls whisper, aseptic chill,
Sheets like ice, yet comfort still.
Familiar sting, this sterile air,
Echoes of worry, whispered prayer.

Draft chills a body carved by steel,
Throat dry, a desert, unreal.
Thirst claws, limbs protest in vain,
Nightstand taunts, a liquid chain.

II.
Flickering bulb, a beacon's grace,
Banishes browns, their taunting face.
Red haze clears, revealing the scene,
A battlefield where bandages glean.

Nurse's touch, brisk, a hurried pull,
Sticky plastic, sterile and dull.

Memories grip, of cold metal bite,
On that altar where flesh yields to light.

III
This bed, a vessel of chrome and wire,
Enclosed within, my edgy fire.
Hoping for a new-found light,
Not just stains, but my body's might.

14.4 IMPLICATIONS FOR CARE RESEARCH

In this chapter, we ally with an increasing number of scholars interested in care aesthetics[54] and aesthetic narrativization, focusing on the aesthetic narration of objects of care. Our approach may be like a kaleidoscope, challenging the limitations of verbalized accounts of care and instead showing the dynamic vibrancy of colours and textures of care practices including their objects, broadly perceived as 'everything that is done (rather than everything that "we" do) to maintain, continue, and re-pair "the world" so that all (rather than "we") can live in it as well as possible. That world includes ... all that we seek to interweave in a complex, life-sustaining web (modified from Tronto).[55] Here, humans co-exist with non-humans, with materialities and the ecological environment.[56]

We explored where following an aesthetic-apophatic approach would bring us, and aligned with what is so vital to current practices of care and research: life itself. By altering perspectives and observing entanglements and experienced tensions, contrasts and a lack of comprehension previously unnoticed, we may become even more in tune with the objects of care and its practices as 'worlds of becomings', including those who are part of these care webs. The visual sceneries that emerged emphasize these complexities. We return to the sceneries once more to highlight how the first scenery hinted at something uncanny, beyond the indistinctness following the darkness, red, and black webs. In the distance, a glimmer of light suggests an opening. The second visual was more formal in its artistic qualities and invited you to participate by assisting in untangling the strings. It prompted engagement rather than passive viewing or reception, unlike the first. The first visualization beckoned you as a viewer to witness, tune in and contemplate, while the second seemed to encourage action.

In perceiving the visual sceneries and after we detoured through other sceneries, we learned that some of the initial thoughts and ideas we had about the 'hospital bed' changed. For example, in Merel's narrative account, her experience and perception of that experience impacted her presentation accordingly. Her challenging experience was represented (not presented) in dark tones. Only later on, by reflecting on qualities and having travelled various detours, including taking a pause, she learned about the mysterious dimension, also related to the uncanny and ambiguity, but she did not perceive this initially. Perhaps we just cannot see well enough and we need to train perceptive skills. Perhaps we are imagining. In hindsight, though, if we had (only) captured the narrative, analysed it and moved to conclusions without being open to including non-verbal expressions, we would not have encountered something that felt vital and meaningful to her.

In addition, her initial perception could indicate something else. Occasionally, narrative accounts and visuals can interfere with in-depth, qualitative perceptions of *specific* aesthetic qualities in *particular* contexts and times. For example, looking at a man standing in blue light. Although the man standing in blue light appears blue, our knowledge of his 'true' colour interferes with our awareness of the qualities his figure now displays.[57] These hindrances, which emanate from our learned expectations of objects (and phenomena), can – although not necessarily – be related to 'aesthetic constancies'.[58] Aesthetic constancies refer to a gap between what we think we know, what we experience and what we (can) perceive. Aesthetic constancies may interfere with our aesthetic perception of the world and can cause disruption in society as a whole. Aesthetic constancies replace what we think we know (about care) with what we aesthetically perceive and experience. In our chapter, we highlighted this by sharing a 'landscape' of expressions that aligns with the 'apophatic' of the approach: not focusing on the bed as an object that can be perceived and represented through sensory modes alone, but as a coming together of apophatic and aesthetic qualities, including pre-linguistic that reach beyond any expression.

We thus propose a need for recalibration of relationships with subjects and objects of care. In some instances, we may benefit from inquiry that highlights notions of living.[59] We do not reject other forms of research but weave them in, as they are part of the landscape too. Travelling a landscape, immersing ourselves in that landscape, sometimes seeing through a kaleidoscope, does not come easy. We are raised and trained in traditions that need intercultural perspectives to challenge hegemonic categories, repressive languages, and ways of being and doing that may be unproductive or even harmful. With this chapter, we aim to acknowledge the meaning of other ways of relating to objects of care. To live with care objects intimately, to experience objects relationally, we may need to accept new responsibilities. This is our ethico-political commitment to care, including commitment to the neglected or unseen, to that which defies description.[60] We do not deny intellectual, analytical approaches. On the contrary, rather than abandoning critical inquiry, we weave it into the tapestry of our journey, hoping to uncover new questions. We may detour, but we may – paradoxically – find something meaningful.

NOTES

1. See: Karen Barad, 'Posthumanist Performativity: Toward an Understanding of How Matter Comes to Matter', *Signs: Journal of Women in Culture and Society* 28, no. 3 (2003): 801–31; John Law and Annemarie Mol, 'Notes on Materiality and Sociality', *The Sociological Review* 43, no. 2 (1995): 274–94.
2. Michela Cozza, 'Elderliness: The Agential Inseparability of Ageing and Assistive Technologies', in *Socio-Gerontechnology: Interdisciplinary Critical Studies of Ageing and Technology*, ed. Alexander Peine, Barbara Marshall, Wendy Martin and Louis Neven (London: Routledge, 2021), 70–84.
3. Marcel Boonen, *Nurses in Space* (PhD diss., University of Humanistic Studies, Utrecht, 2017).
4. Barad, 'Posthumanist Performativity'.
5. Maria Puig de la Bellacasa, *Matters of Care: Speculative Ethics in More Than Human Worlds* (Minneapolis: University of Minnesota Press, 2017), 4.
6. Ibid., 6.
7. Christina Buse, Daryl Martin and Sarah Nettleton, 'Conceptualising "Materialities of Care": Making Visible Mundane Material Culture in Health and Social Care Contexts', in

Materialities of Care: Encountering Health and Illness Through Artefacts and Architecture (Hoboken, NJ: Wiley-Blackwell, 2018), 1–13.

8. See:Merel Visse, 'Your Thoughts Don't Have Words Every Day', in *Wonder, Silence, and Human Flourishing: Toward a Rehumanization of Health, Education, and Welfare*, ed. Finn Hansen, Solveig Botnen Eide and Carlo Leget (London: Lexington Books, 2023), 97–115; Merel Visse, Finn Hansen and Carlo Leget, 'The Unsayable in Arts-Based Research: On the Praxis of Life Itself', *International Journal of Qualitative Methods* 18 (2019): 1–13.
9. Such as low, high, light, heavy, wet, dry, etc. (see: Karin Hannes and Richard Siegesmund, 'An Analytical Apparatus for Visual Imagery Applied in a Social-Behavioral Research', *International Review of Qualitative Research* 15, no. 2 (2022): 278–302, https://doi.org/10.1177/19408447221097061). By 'aesthetics' we mean this in the broadest sense, not simply restricted to the analytical assessment of (the nature of) beauty as the philosopher Immanuel Kant might have proposed. Instead, having aesthetic ability is a normal capacity of human beings, like walking, cooking, playing, working, learning and nurturing. It is not something only a few of us possess or can cultivate. With this chapter we add to existing views of care closely connected with aesthetic experience as a sensory experience of perception. (See: Maurice Merleau-Ponty, *The Visible and the Invisible* (Chicago, IL: Northwestern University Press, 1968); and James Thompson, *Care Aesthetics: For Artful Care and Careful Art* (New York: Routledge, 2022).)
10. Finn Thorbjørn Hansen, Solveig Botnen Eide and Carlo Leget, eds, *Wonder, Silence and Human Flourishing: Toward a Rehumanization of Health, Education, and Welfare* (London: Lexington Books, 2023); Visse, 'Your Thoughts Don't Have Words Every Day'; Visse, Hansen and Leget, 'The Unsayable in Arts-Based Research'; Merel Visse, Finn Hansen and Carlo Leget, 'Apophatic Inquiry: Living the Questions Themselves', *International Journal of Qualitative Methods* 19 (2020).
11. Merel Visse, 'Nested Tensions in Care', *American Medical Association Journal of Ethics* 19, no. 4 (2017): 399–405, doi: 10.1001/journalofethics.2017.19.4.imhl1-1704.
12. François Jullien, *Living off Landscape or the Unthought-of in Reason*, trans. Pedro Rodriquez (Lanham, MD: Rowman & Littlefield, 2018).
13. Visse, 'Your Thoughts Don't Have Words Every Day'.
14. We have coined this *apophatic inquiry,* based upon the apophatic traditions of philosophers, theologians and artists in Western and Eastern history (see: William Franke, *On What Cannot Be Said: Apophatic Discourses in Philosophy, Religion, Literature and the Arts, Vol. 1: Classic Formulations* (Notre Dame, IN: University of Notre Dame Press, 2007)).
15. Linda Finlay, 'Unfolding the Phenomenological Research Process: Iterative Stages of "Seeing Afresh"', *Journal of Humanistic Psychology* 53, no. 2 (2012): 172–201.
16. See: Visse, 'Your Thoughts Don't Have Words Every Day'; Visse, Hansen and Leget, 'The Unsayable in Arts-Based Research'; Visse, Hansen and Leget, 'Apophatic Inquiry'.
17. Jullien, *Living off Landscape*, 106.
18. Ibid., 107.
19. Peimin Ni, 'Moral and Philosophical Implications of Chinese Calligraphy', *Grand Valley Review* 20, no. 1 (1999): 22.
20. See: Liora Bresler, 'Toward Connectedness: Aesthetically Based Research', *Studies in Art Education* 48, no. 1 (2006): 52–69; Visse, 'Your Thoughts Don't Have Words Every Day'; Visse, Hansen and Leget, 'The Unsayable in Arts-Based Research'; Visse, Hansen and Leget, 'Apophatic Inquiry'.

21. See: Brad Haseman, 'A Manifesto for Performative Research', *Media International Australia* 118, no. 1 (2006): 98–106; Tim Ingold, *Making: Anthropology, Archaeology, Art and Architecture* (London: Routledge, 2013); Erin Manning and Brian Massumi, *Thought in the Act: Passages in the Ecology of Experience* (Minneapolis: University of Minnesota Press, 2014).
22. Visse, Hansen and Leget, 'The Unsayable in Arts-Based Research'.
23. Ibid.
24. See: Ibid., 9; Visse, Hansen and Leget, 'Apophatic Inquiry'.
25. Bresler, 'Toward Connectedness', 57.
26. Finlay, 'Unfolding the Phenomenological Research Process'.
27. Visse, Hansen and Leget, 'The Unsayable in Arts-Based Research'.
28. Visse, 'Your Thoughts Don't Have Words Every Day'.
29. Les Todres, *Embodied Enquiry: Phenomenological Touchstones for Research, Psychotherapy and Spirituality* (Basingstoke: Springer, 2007).
30. Karen Barad, *Meeting the Universe Halfway: Quantum Physics and the Entanglement of Matter and Meaning* (Durham, NC: Duke University Press, 2007), 214.
31. Visse, 'Your Thoughts Don't Have Words Every Day'.
32. See: Rudolf Arnheim, *Art and Visual Perception: The Psychology of the Creative Eye* (Berkeley: University of California Press, 1954); Elliot Eisner, *Educating Artistic Vision* (New York: Macmillan Company, 1972); Hannes and Siegesmund, 'An Analytical Apparatus for Visual Imagery Applied in a Social-Behavioral Research', 282.
33. Max Van Manen, 'Phenomenology of Practice', *Phenomenology & Practice* 1, no. 1 (2007): 25.
34. Davide Bacchin et al., 'Co-Design in Electrical Medical Beds with Caregivers,' *International Journal of Environmental Research and Public Health* 19, no. 23 (2022): 16353, https://doi.org/10.3390/ijerph192316353.
35. Kerstin Petzäll, Barbro Berglund and Christer Lundberg, 'Patients' Opinions and Experiences Regarding the Hospital Bed and the Bedside Equipment: An Interview Study', *Scandinavian Journal of Caring Sciences* 15 (2001): 106–12.
36. Ibid., 108.
37. Calbert H. Douglas and Mary R. Douglas, 'Patient-Friendly Hospital Environments: Exploring the Patients' Perspective', *Health Expectations* 7, no. 1 (2004): 61–73.
38. Petzäll, Berglund and Lundberg, 'Patients' Opinions and Experiences Regarding the Hospital Bed and the Bedside Equipment'.
39. Ibid., 108.
40. We do not report on studies here where caregivers were co-designers of medical beds in hospitals.
41. François Jullien, *From Being to Living: A Euro-Chinese Lexicon of Thought* (London: Sage Publications, 2020).
42. We do not in any way want to evoke the appearance of orientalism by European scholars, but for the sake of this argument we will contrast Western classical landscape paintings with Eastern approaches, acknowledging we should and will simultaneously destabilize this binary after we have made it.
43. Jullien, *From Being to Living*, 17.
44. Ibid., 56.
45. Ibid., 118.
46. Ibid., 68.
47. Ibid., 124.

48. François Jullien, *In Praise of Blandness: Proceeding from Chinese Thought and Aesthetics* (Princeton, NJ: Princeton University Press, 2004), 24–5.
49. Jullien, *Living off Landscape*.
50. Lisa Blackman, *The Body: The Key Concepts* (London: Routledge, 2008).
51. Jullien, *From Being to Living*, 68.
52. Hannes and Siegesmund, 'An Analytical Apparatus for Visual Imagery Applied in a Social-Behavioral Research', 280.
53. This makes us think of Rosi Braidotti and Erin Manning's work on post-human and new materialist theory. In phenomenological inquiry, works of art, and materials in general, have agency too. (See: Rosi Braidotti, 'A Theoretical Framework for the Critical Posthumanities', *Theory, Culture & Society* 36, no. 6 (2019): 31–61; and Erin Manning, 'Ten Propositions for Research-Creation', in *Collaboration in Performance Practice: Premises, Workings and Failures*, ed. Noyale Colin and Stefanie Sachsenmaier (London: Palgrave Macmillan, 2016), 133–41.) The work that emerges in artistic practice is an Ereignis – an event that 'appropriates us' to itself (see: Visse, Hansen and Leget, 'The Unsayable in Arts-Based Research'). Hence, we live in the work; we become part of it, like the sceneries of living, and through the sceneries, we live our questions (see: Visse, Hansen and Leget, 'Apophatic Inquiry').
54. Thompson, *Care Aesthetics*.
55. Joan C. Tronto, 'Care', in *Moral Boundaries: A Political Argument for an Ethic of Care* (New York: Routledge, 1993), 103.
56. Puig de la Bellacasa, *Matters of Care*, 161.
57. Eisner, *Educating Artistic Vision*, 68.
58. Eisner, *Educating Artistic Vision*.
59. Jullien, *Living off Landscape*.
60. Visse, Hansen and Leget, 'The Unsayable in Arts-Based Research'.

BIBLIOGRAPHY

Arnheim, Rudolf. *Art and Visual Perception: The Psychology of the Creative Eye*. Berkeley: University of California Press, 1954.

Bacchin, Davide, Gabriella F. A. Pernice, Leonardo Pierobon, Elena Zanella, Marcello Sardena, Marino Malvestio and Luciano Gamberini. 'Co-Design in Electrical Medical Beds with Caregivers', *International Journal of Environmental Research and Public Health* 19, no. 23 (2022): 16353. https://doi.org/10.3390/ijerph192316353.

Barad, Karen. 'Posthumanist Performativity: Toward an Understanding of How Matter Comes to Matter', *Signs: Journal of Women in Culture and Society* 28, no. 3 (2003): 801–31.

Barad, Karen. *Meeting the Universe Halfway: Quantum Physics and the Entanglement of Matter and Meaning*. Durham, NC: Duke University Press, 2007.

Blackman, Lisa. *The Body: The Key Concepts*. London: Routledge, 2008.

Braidotti, Rosi. 'A Theoretical Framework for the Critical Posthumanities', *Theory, Culture & Society* 36, no. 6 (2019): 31–61.

Bresler, Liora. 'Toward Connectedness: Aesthetically Based Research', *Studies in Art Education* 48, no. 1 (2006): 52–69.

Boonen, Marcel. *Nurses in Space*. PhD thesis, University of Humanistic Studies, Utrecht, 2017.

Buse, Christina, Daryl Martin and Sarah Nettleton. 'Conceptualising "Materialities of Care": Making Visible Mundane Material Culture in Health and Social Care Contexts', in *Materialities of Care: Encountering Health and Illness Through Artefacts and Architecture*, 1–13. Hoboken, NJ: Wiley-Blackwell, 2018.

Cozza, Michela. 'Elderliness: The Agential Inseparability of Ageing and Assistive Technologies', in *Socio-Gerontechnology: Interdisciplinary Critical Studies of Ageing and Technology*, edited by Alexander Peine, Barbara Marshall, Wendy Martin and Louis Neven, 70–84. London: Routledge, 2021.

Douglas, Calbert H. and Mary R. Douglas. 'Patient-Friendly Hospital Environments: Exploring the Patients' Perspective', *Health Expectations* 7, no. 1 (2004): 61–73.

Eisner, Elliot. *Educating Artistic Vision*. New York: Macmillan Company, 1972.

Finlay, Linda. 'Unfolding the Phenomenological Research Process: Iterative Stages of "Seeing Afresh"', *Journal of Humanistic Psychology* 53, no. 2 (2012): 172–201.

Franke, William. *On What Cannot Be Said: Apophatic Discourses in Philosophy, Religion, Literature and the Arts, Vol. 1: Classic Formulations*. Notre Dame, IN: University of Notre Dame Press, 2007.

Hannes, Karin and Richard Siegesmund. 'An Analytical Apparatus for Visual Imagery Applied in a Social-Behavioral Research', *International Review of Qualitative Research* 15, no. 2 (2022): 278–302.

Hansen, Finn Thorbjørn, Solveig Botnen Eide and Carlo Leget, eds. *Wonder, Silence and Human Flourishing: Toward a Rehumanization of Health, Education, and Welfare*. London: Lexington Books, 2023.

Haseman, Brad. 'A Manifesto for Performative Research', *Media International Australia* 118, no. 1 (2006): 98–106.

Ingold, Tim. *Making: Anthropology, Archaeology, Art and Architecture*. London: Routledge, 2013.

Jullien, François. *Living off Landscape or the Unthought-of in Reason*. Translated by Pedro Rodriquez. Lanham, MD: Rowman & Littlefield, 2018.

Jullien, François. *From Being to Living: A Euro-Chinese Lexicon of Thought*. London: Sage Publications, 2020.

Law, John and Annemarie Mol. 'Notes on Materiality and Sociality', *The Sociological Review* 43, no. 2 (1995): 274–94.

Manning, Erin. 'Ten Propositions for Research-Creation', in *Collaboration in Performance Practice: Premises, Workings and Failures*, edited by Noyale Colin and Stefanie Sachsenmaier, 133–41. London: Palgrave Macmillan, 2016.

Manning, Erin and Brian Massumi. *Thought in the Act: Passages in the Ecology of Experience*. Minneapolis: University of Minnesota Press, 2014.

Merleau-Ponty, Maurice. *The Visible and the Invisible*. Chicago, IL: Northwestern University Press, 1968.

Ni, Peimin. 'Moral and Philosophical Implications of Chinese Calligraphy', *Grand Valley Review* 20, no. 1 (1999): 8–18.

Petzäll, Kerstin, Barbro Berglund and Christer Lundberg. 'Patients' Opinions and Experiences Regarding the Hospital Bed and the Bedside Equipment: An Interview Study', *Scandinavian Journal of Caring Sciences* 15 (2001): 106–12.

Puig de la Bellacasa, Maria. *Matters of Care: Speculative Ethics in More Than Human Worlds*. Minneapolis: University of Minnesota Press, 2017.

Thompson, James. *Care Aesthetics: For Artful Care and Careful Art*. New York: Routledge, 2022.

Todres, Les. *Embodied Enquiry: Phenomenological Touchstones for Research, Psychotherapy and Spirituality*. Basingstoke: Springer, 2007.

Tronto, Joan C. 'Care', in *Moral Boundaries: A Political Argument for an Ethic of Care*, 101–24. New York: Routledge, 1993.

Van Manen, Max. 'Phenomenology of Practice', *Phenomenology & Practice* 1, no. 1 (2007): 11–30.

Visse, Merel. 'Nested Tensions in Care', *American Medical Association Journal of Ethics* 19, no. 4 (2017): 399–405. https://doi.org/10.1001/journalofethics.2017.19.4.imhl1-1704.

Visse, Merel. 'Your Thoughts Don't Have Words Every Day', in *Wonder, Silence, and Human Flourishing: Toward a Rehumanization of Health, Education, and Welfare*, edited by Finn Hansen, Solveig Botnen Eide and Carlo Leget, 97–115. London: Lexington Books, 2023.

Visse, Merel, Finn Hansen and Carlo Leget. 'The Unsayable in Arts-Based Research: On the Praxis of Life Itself', *International Journal of Qualitative Methods* 18 (2019): 1609406919851392.

Visse, Merel, Finn Hansen and Carlo Leget. 'Apophatic Inquiry: Living the Questions Themselves', *International Journal of Qualitative Methods* 19 (2020): 1609406920958975.

CHAPTER FIFTEEN

Care ethics and care policies in South Korea

HEE-KANG KIM

INTRODUCTION

Research is currently being conducted on care ethics as a normative basis for public policy.[1] This research criticizes the traditional policy research perspective, which proceeds from an understanding of human beings as independent and rational, impartiality and right-centred principles, policy evaluation based on efficiency and effectiveness, and structure and institutional design based on social contracts. Instead, care ethics focuses on the inevitable dependence and inextricable interdependence of human beings, universal care needs, the public value of care and caring relations, the enhanced status of caregivers, and social responsibility for care. It is presented as a new paradigm in policy research.[2]

In 2004, Olena Hankivsky published a book called *Social Policy and the Ethic of Care*, which examines Canadian social policy from the perspective of care ethics. Hankivsky argues that applying care ethics can lead to greater social justice in social policy, as it offers a new understanding of humans, their social issues and their needs.[3] Maurice Hamington and Dorothy C. Miller's edited book *Socializing Care: Feminist Ethics and Public Issues*[4] also discusses applying care ethics to public issues. They suggest that it breaks down the public/private divide, which underpins existing policy research, and urges changes in entrenched social and cultural norms. They argue that if care ethics is taken seriously in policy and practice, society and the lives of citizens will be more just and inclusive.

More recently, Kari Greenswag has pointed out that the perspective of care ethics as a normative/ethical standard can better explain the issues of power inequality and institutional patterns than the perspective of human rights.[5] She argues that applying care ethics to policy research as a normative/ethical standard is not only a valuable resource that leads to changes in our lives but also can be a catalyst for social change.

The discussions about applying care ethics to social and public fields are not limited to policy research. They are expanding to various areas that require a fundamental transformation of society. This includes criticizing the economic structure and the capitalist system,[6] proposing changes in the labour market time structure,[7] and suggesting changes to the executive bureaucracy system.[8]

The purpose of this chapter is to examine the status and characteristics of care policies in South Korea from the perspective of care ethics. While many of the studies discussing the application of care ethics to public policy target Western countries, this study is meaningful as it applies to the Korean case in the Asian context. In particular, as a third-world country that experienced industrialization and democratization late but has now achieved economic growth in the developed world, it is meaningful to examine Korea's care policy from the perspective of care ethics. In addition, this study can also contribute to finding a more fundamental answer to existing criticisms that 'care' is missing from Korean care policies.[9]

Since the 2000s, the Korean government has begun to recognize care as a national policy issue rather than a personal/private matter, introducing new care policies or significantly expanding existing ones. Behind the expansion of care policies, however, care has been presented and utilized as a means to address other social needs and problems. This chapter aims to examine the expansion of care policies in South Korea within the discourse and policy framework of 'demographic crisis response' and 'economic growth'. It will examine how care is being addressed as part of population policy or economic (labour and industrial) policy. This chapter will argue that this discourse and policy framework has led to the loss of the meaning and value of care and that despite the expansion of care policies over the past two decades, they have not developed into care policies that are in line with care ethics.

15.1 CARE POLICIES SINCE THE 2000S

This section will discuss the expansion of care policies in South Korea since 2000 and explore how this expansion has been framed within the discourse and policy framework of responding to the declining birthrate and ageing population and promoting economic growth. The focus will be on how care policies, such as childcare and elderly care policies, are presented and implemented as solutions to address the crisis at hand and social needs.

15.1.1 Expansion of care policies

South Korea has introduced and expanded many care policies in the last two decades. One of the significant developments in childcare was the institutionalization of national responsibility for the care of preschool children through the Childcare Act in 1991. Universal childcare was introduced in 2004 through a comprehensive revision of the same law. Additionally, in 2013, the partial childcare fee support for low-income children aged 0–5 was expanded to full support for all children aged 0–5. This shift reflects a move from selective childcare, which began with low-income infants and toddlers, to universal childcare for all children. Moreover, it moved from partial to full support, meaning that childcare is now free for all children.[10]

Various policies have been introduced to support families in providing childcare, such as the childcare fee support policy, parental allowance policy, child allowance policy, care service policy, parental leave policy and parental working hours policy. Over time, the scope and content of these policies have gradually expanded. For instance, the childcare allowance, which supports caregivers who care for children at home, was initially provided to low-income families with infants aged 0–1 in 2009. In 2013, it was expanded to all families with children aged 0–5 and is now provided to all preschoolers aged two and older who are not in institutional care. The infant allowance paid to infants aged 0–1 was also expanded and reorganized as a 'parental benefit' in 2023. Parents of infants aged 0–1 are now provided with a parental benefit regardless of income. Starting in 2024, parents of 0-year-old infants will receive one million won, and 1-year-olds will receive 500,000 won monthly. Additionally, the child allowance was expanded from all children aged 0–6 in 2019 to those aged 0–7 in 2022. Concerning parental leave, the paid parental leave system was first introduced for infants aged 0 in 2001, then expanded to children aged 0–5 in 2010 and children aged 0–8 in 2014. Since 2016, a special parental leave system called 'Father's Month' has been in place.[11]

Since 2007, childcare services have been available where childcare workers visit families and provide care. In 2012, the Childcare Support Act was enacted, replacing the pilot operation with the 'Childcare Support Project'. Services for elementary school children have also expanded since the 2000s. In 2004, 'Elementary Care Classrooms' were introduced on a pilot basis for lower grades in elementary school. In 2006, they were provided to dual-income, single parents and underprivileged lower elementary grades. In 2014, the service expanded to all lower elementary grades, and in 2016, it was offered to all grades. Local children's centres were confirmed and institutionalized as government-supported facilities through the revision of the Child Welfare Act in 2003. After-school academies for teenagers began in 2006.[12]

In 2008, a long-term care insurance system was introduced for elderly care, which made it a social insurance. This meant that elderly care, previously only provided to older people without family members or low-income families, was expanded to cover all older adults needing long-term care. The system targets those who are 65 years old or older, as well as those who are 64 years old or younger but have geriatric diseases such as dementia, stroke and Parkinson's disease, regardless of their income level. This approach is geared towards universal welfare and was introduced as a socialization system of care, where the burden of elderly care is shared among the state, society and family.[13]

Since the 2000s, childcare policies have expanded, significantly increasing the number of beneficiaries. Studies estimate that about 50 per cent of preschoolers used daycare centres and kindergartens in 2005. However, the institutionalization rate has continued to increase, with around 90 per cent of preschoolers using these facilities in 2021. For infants aged 0–2 years, the rate of use of daycare centres was only 11.9 per cent in 2002, increasing to 21.4 per cent in 2005 and rapidly increasing to 49.7 per cent in 2010 and 76.2 per cent in 2021. The number of children using care services has also steadily increased from about 50,000 children in 'Elementary Care Classes' and 90,000 children in local childcare centres in 2008 to about 260,000 children and 110,000 children in 2020, respectively. Additionally, the number of childcare organizations has significantly increased. The number of childcare facilities rose from 19,276 in 2000 to 35,352 in 2020, and the number of childcare workers more than tripled from 103,924 in 2001 to 325,669 in 2020, according to the Ministry of Health and Welfare.[14]

Since the introduction of the long-term care insurance system in 2008, the number of its users has continued to increase. As of 2021, around 10.7 per cent of older people, equivalent to 953,511 individuals, are long-term care recipients. This number is more than three times in 2009, only 286,907 people. Moreover, the overall benefit performance of the long-term care insurance system is also increasing. The number of benefit recipients doubled, from 369,587 in 2012 to 899,113 in 2021. The average monthly benefit cost per recipient has risen from 956,986 won in 2012 to 1,322,679 won in 2021.[15]

In South Korea, only 0.8 per cent of the total population receives long-term care, one-third of the average in the Organization for Economic Cooperation and Development (OECD) countries. However, the country is making great strides in improving its infrastructure for long-term care faster than any other OECD nation. For instance, the number of beds in long-term care hospitals and facilities increased by an annual average of 4.5 per cent between 2000 and 2013. As of 2017, South Korea had 54.2 beds per 1,000 people aged 65 or older, higher than the OECD average of 49.7 beds. Nursing facilities also significantly increased, from 8,444 in 2008 to 27,484 in 2022. Furthermore, the number of long-term care workers, mainly caregivers called *yoyangbohosa*, tripled from 182,349 in 2009 to 601,492 in 2022.[16]

15.1.2 Response to the Demographic Crisis

In the early 2000s, the discourse on the crises of low birth rates and population ageing became prominent in Korean society. The total fertility rate dropped below the population replacement level of 2.06 in 1983, and by the early 2000s it had already fallen to the low 1s. Since 2018, it has been below 1.0. At the same time, the ageing of the population in Korean society has been progressing rapidly. The proportion of older people aged 65 or older increased from 7 per cent in 2002 to 10.9 per cent in 2010 and 16.7 per cent in 2021. This means it only took 18 years for the proportion of people aged 65 or older to double from 7 per cent (an ageing society) to 14 per cent (an aged society). This shows that the ageing rate is faster than that of Japan, a super-aged country with more than 20 per cent of the population aged 65 and over. As a result, South Korea is being called 'the first country on Earth to disappear' and 'the fastest aging country in the world' with an 'unprecedented aging rate in history'. It is described as a 'crisis of national existence' and a 'national emergency'.[17]

Care policies were introduced in response to a demographic crisis. The primary reason for low birth rates was identified as the burden of family responsibility for care and, therefore, several childcare policies were proposed to ease the burden on families. Additionally, to address the care burden caused by the ageing population, policies for elderly care were suggested to turn private care into social care.

For example, South Korea has addressed its low birth rate and ageing population crisis since 2005 with the Framework Act on Low Birth Rate in an Ageing Society. It has implemented the Basic Plan for Ageing Society and Population Policy every five years, a medium- to long-term plan. Six Basic Plans have been developed and implemented since 2006, and each has allocated most of the budget to childcare policies. In the First Basic Plan from 2006 to 2010, childcare policies accounted for 87.1 per cent of the total budget, including childcare allowance support, childcare service support and parental leave promotion. In the Second Basic Plan from 2011 to 2015, childcare policies aimed at improving the work–family compatibility system, expanding support for childcare expenses, increasing support for childcare allowances, and expanding support for childcare services accounted for 83.6 per cent of the total budget. While recent Basic Plans have included policies for marriage support, youth employment and housing, close to 50 per cent of the low birth rate policies budget is still allocated and spent on childcare policies.[18]

The Ministry of Health and Welfare, the ministry in charge of childcare policies, has stated that the goal of the performance evaluation of childcare policies, including the internalization of the child allowance system and the expansion of the infrastructure of the all-day care system, is to build a foundation for responding to a declining birth rate and an aging society.[19] In short, the success of childcare policies is measured by how much they contribute to increasing the fertility rate. These policies are intended to relieve the burden of childcare for families, thereby incentivizing them to have more children.

As a response to the ageing crisis, elderly care policies are also being addressed. In Korean society, ageing results in an increase in the number of dependent people, which leads to a decrease in social production and an increase in the social burden of caring for them. This situation has led to the discourse that this is not only a social problem but a social crisis. The long-term care insurance system, a representative elderly care policy, is evaluated as a collective response to social risk through a public social insurance system.[20] The rationale for enacting the Long-Term Care Insurance Act, which is the basis for the long-term care insurance system, also reflects this. The enactment cites the difficulty and increasing cost of caring for older people at home due to the ageing population, the nuclearization of families, and the increasing participation of women in society. This burden is defined as 'a serious social problem that our society urgently needs to address'.

Therefore, it can be said that the long-term care insurance policy has been proposed to respond to the increasing demand for care due to the ageing population and to share the burden on families with society. However, as discussed in the next section, to minimize the burden on national finances for elderly care, the government has established a supply structure that relies on the private market. This market-based care system has ultimately resulted in the marginalization of care.

15.1.3 Means of economic growth

South Korea has implemented a developmental strategy that prioritizes economic growth as the primary goal of the government in a post-colonial global context. In this approach, the state's resources and policies are geared towards achieving economic growth. This also applies to care policies, which are seen as an end to economic growth.[21] Policies related to care are proposed to increase the participation of women in the workforce and create more jobs to boost economic growth.

During the 2000s, South Korea experienced continued growth without an increase in employment. To tackle this issue, the government implemented a significant strategy to utilize women's workforce. However, the female labour force participation rate in South Korea remained lower than the average for OECD countries, and the age-specific employment rate of women exhibits an 'M-curve' due to labour market withdrawal for childbirth and childcare.[22] To address this, the Korean government has proposed care policies to prevent women from leaving the labour market due to childbirth and childcare and to encourage women who have left the labour market to re-enter it. This strategy was to improve national competitiveness by increasing the utilization rate of women in women in the workforce through expanding their employment opportunities.[23]

For example, various care policies such as free childcare, childcare allowances, maternity and paternity leave, and parental leave systems have been introduced and expanded to prevent women from leaving the labour market due to childbirth and childcare. Some people view the parental leave system as a labour policy to prevent workers from leaving the labour market and ensure continuity of employment. In contrast, others view it as a family policy to universally support parents in raising their children. However, many experts believe that South Korea's parental leave system has both objectives but is strongly characterized as a labour policy that provides coverage for workers covered by employment insurance when they are unable to work due to childcare.[24]

Childcare services are an example of a care policy that is part of labour policy. The policy involves childcare workers visiting homes to provide care services to children to promote their safe protection and welfare. Additionally, it aims to support work–family integration by reducing the burden of childcare for working parents and advancing employment for women who take career breaks by training childcare workers. By doing so, the policy aims to link the demand for social services with socio-economic factors such as job creation and the promotion of women's participation in economic activities.[25] The Childcare Support Act of 2012, which the policy is based on, was enacted to 'promote the employment of middle-aged and elderly women with career breaks'. This shows that the policy focuses on women whose careers are interrupted by pregnancy, childbirth and childrearing from the policy design stage.

The South Korean government also identified care policies as a strategic industry for job creation. The goal was to create social service jobs to meet the increasing demand for care. The government emphasized that investment in pre-emptive job creation is essential to tackle the job famine caused by economic growth without employment.[26] In developed countries, the service industry is a significant source of jobs, and the government believed that expanding women's employment in the social service sector would increase national income to $20,000 from $15,000 in 2005.[27]

Below is an excerpt from a 2007 report by the national policy research institute suggesting policy tasks for creating jobs for women in social services. It recommended actively increasing the number of jobs in social services and filling them with women.

> It can be argued that [the increase in women's employment in social services] is because employment creation centered on women-friendly service sectors provides more job opportunities for women wanting to enter the labor market. In addition, the expansion of women's jobs in social services is paving the way for more women to enter the labor market by socially solving care work such as protection, nurturing, and elderly care, which women have mainly performed within the family ... Based on this background, this study aims to propose policy tasks for creating jobs for women in the social service sector as a strategic option for revitalizing women's economic activities.[28]

The case of *yoyangbohosa*, an essential workforce of the long-term care insurance system for older people, was also introduced as a representative social service job. From designing the system in 2006, the Korean government set care as a job development field to actively utilize female workers, including full-time homemakers. It emphasized that *yoyangbohosa* provides suitable employment opportunities for middle-aged and older women.[29] In addition, 'creating jobs and added value' is considered a significant factor in the standards for evaluating the performance of long-term care insurance for older people.[30]

In summary, the Korean government has recognized that social services are in great demand due to the ageing population and has identified and fostered this as an area with great potential for future job creation. The *yoyangbohosa* system, created through long-term care insurance for older people, was also seen as part of the policy to create jobs for women, and bringing the female inactive population into the labour market and utilizing them economically was chosen as the primary strategy for economic growth.

15.2 CARE POLICIES WITHOUT 'CARE'

The previous section examined that behind the expansion of care policies in South Korea since the 2000s, care policies have been used as an immediate response to the demographic crisis of low birthrates and ageing populations and as a means of economic growth to secure the labour force and create jobs. This section will explore where care policies as part of population and economic policies are inconsistent with care ethics by causing and reinforcing the marketization and feminization of care. It will thus show how 'care' is missing from Korea's care policies and how it is marginalized and excluded.

15.2.1 Marketization of care

As mentioned, South Korea has developed a care policy to address the challenges of a declining birth rate and an ageing population. To tackle these issues, the government has adopted a strategy that involves using the private sector to expand care services quickly and efficiently. This approach has essentially turned care provision into a market where private institutions are primarily responsible for providing care services.

Long-term care insurance for older people relies heavily on the private sector. As of 2016, only 1.9 per cent of the 5,295 facilities offering facility benefits were public facilities established and operated by local governments. Similarly, in the case of home-based benefit providers, the public sector accounted for only 0.6 per cent (152) of the 26,375 providers. This is especially true for home-based benefits. Approximately 71.5 per cent and 84.2 per cent of facilities offering facility benefits and home-based benefits, respectively, are operated by small and medium-sized private operators.[31]

Childcare has also become increasingly reliant on the market, with only 16.4 per cent (5,437) of 33,246 childcare facilities being publicly funded as of 2021. The remaining 73.4 per cent (24,494) of childcare facilities comprised private and home daycare centres.[32] Although the government has pledged to increase the public sector's share of childcare centres to 30 per cent, the percentage has decreased in recent years.

The government believed that allowing private organizations to expand care provision through the market would lead to a faster and broader spread of care services to meet social needs. Competition among private providers was also expected to lead to better quality services and increased user choice. This approach was intended to fulfil the public purpose of long-term care insurance for older people.[33] As per the criticism of many experts, however, the government's expectation of marketization of care in a structure where it does not actively participate in providing and operating services has resulted in excessive competition among private institutions. This competition[34] has led to a decline in the quality of care, poor working conditions for care workers, and limited user choice.[35]

The following study by Hee Kyung Choi describes the problems of marketization of care in long-term care for older people.

> The excessive supply of private services has created a competitive service market, and over-competition has led to management difficulties in institutions, creating a vicious circle that ultimately leads to a decline in the quality of long-term care services and the precarious labor of long-term care workers. For home-based service providers, damage to the public interest has continued due to the difficulty of stable operation, such as illegal and unfair methods of securing users and overcharging for services. Although the government provides public financing through the long-term care insurance system … the accountability and guarantee of [the long-term care insurance system's] operation as a social insurance system have been significantly reduced.[36]

Childcare workers, the critical workforce in the childcare sector, also face poor working conditions, including low wages, long hours and no guaranteed breaks. According to a survey, most childcare workers in the private and home daycare centres, who accounted for about 70 per cent of childcare workers as of the end of December 2020, were paid the minimum wage.[37] According to another survey, 94.7 per cent of childcare workers in private and home daycare centres are paid the minimum wage or less, and only 5.3 per cent are paid more than the minimum wage.[38]

Employment instability, low wages, poor working conditions and human rights violations have been consistently reported among caregivers for older people (*yoyanbohosa*). According to the 2015 survey, caregivers working in nursing facilities worked an average of 177 hours per month and earned an average wage of 1.55 million won, while visiting caregivers worked an average of 88.9 hours and earned an average salary of only about 650,000 won.[39] The results of the 2022 survey also reported that their low wages have not improved significantly. The average monthly salary of caregivers is 1.17 million won; by salary type, it is 96.2 million won for visiting caregivers and around 2 million won for facility-based caregivers.[40] In addition to low wages and long hours, caregivers experience problems such as high labour intensity, sick leave and paid leave without career recognition, and blind spots in workers' compensation insurance. In addition, the difficulty of emotional labour involved in caregiving and human rights violations, including sexual misconduct, have led to a significant turnover of caregivers.[41]

As a result, care in the private market has become a for-profit arena for care providers rather than a competition to improve the quality of care. To reduce costs, providers have used downsizing policies to reduce the number of care workers or freeze their labour costs, which is directly related to the poor working conditions of care workers and the decline in the quality[42] of care.[43]

15.2.2 Feminization of care

This study has previously examined how South Korea's care policy has been part of an economic policy aimed at utilizing the women's workforce and creating more jobs. The government's main targets for expanding social service jobs were low-income homemakers in their 40s and older who desired to re-enter the workforce. The objective was to reintroduce women in their 40s and 50s to the labour market by creating social service jobs and utilizing them to provide care at a relatively low social cost. Consequently, the feminization of care has become increasingly prominent, with caregiving jobs primarily concentrated among women: mainly low-income, middle-aged and older women.

Eighty-nine per cent of social welfare workers, such as social workers and childcare workers, are women, and 93.5 per cent of care and health service workers, such as caregivers, nursing caregivers and after-school teachers, who are considered to provide more direct care, are women. Among domestic helpers and babysitters specializing in household chores and childcare, the proportion of women is 99 per cent.[44]

In the case of childcare, 99.5 per cent of childcare workers are female as of 2022, and all babysitters in childcare services are female.[45] In the case of elderly care, the gender imbalance of caregivers for older people, a typical social service job, has been ongoing since the start of long-term care insurance in 2008. Male caregivers accounted for 11.6 per cent of all caregivers in 2009, but the number gradually decreased to 8 per cent in 2012, 6.2 per cent in 2015 and 5.3 per cent in 2019.[46] As of 2022, men accounted for 6.1 per cent of caregivers, while women accounted for 93.9 per cent. By age, those aged 60 and older accounted for 62.9 per cent of all caregivers. Most caregivers (53.6 per cent) are employed on a part-time contract basis, and the proportion of contract workers is relatively higher among women than men as age increases.[47]

This shows that while caregiving has become socially institutionalized outside the home, women still perform it. In other words, while women's labour market re-entry has increased and the creation of social service jobs has been successful, the jobs created are gendered, low-wage, low-skill jobs. Care workers are predominantly female, middle-aged and older, with high rates of temporary work.

Nor did the proliferation of public care reduce the care burden on women at home. The feminization of care continues and intensifies in both public and private settings. The gender gap in total household work hours, including childcare, has not changed significantly even when women are in the workforce. The distribution of domestic work in dual-earner households increased from 3 hours and 20 minutes for women and 36 minutes for men in 2009 to 3 hours and 4 minutes for women and 50 minutes for men in 2019. Even when both men and women are raising children and working simultaneously, women perform more than three times as much household work as men.[48] Between 1999 and 2019, before childcare policies began to expand in earnest, the proportion of men involved in caregiving increased, but women still spent more than twice as much time caring for their children as men.

Therefore, the growth of care policies has led to an increase in care-related jobs. However, this has not necessarily resulted in quality jobs that ensure good care. While the Korean government has shown a keen interest in boosting the number of care jobs to meet the rising demand, little attention has been given to the working conditions of care workers, who they are and how they are treated.

In conclusion, the marketization and feminization of public care have led to an overlooking of the nature and value of care. The market drive for efficiency and profit has overlooked the fact that we are all dependent and interdependent human beings in need of care, with universal care needs. The market dynamics of care have failed to respond proactively to the care needs of vulnerable people and have jeopardized the status of caregivers. The feminization of care has also reinforced traditional public/private dichotomies, ignored the social responsibility of care, and failed to recognize the public value of care and caring relationships.

CONCLUSION: TOWARDS A 'CARING' CARE POLICY

This chapter has examined the quantitative expansion of care policies in South Korea since the 2000s. However, the lack of fundamental consideration of the nature and value of care that underlies the expansion has resulted in care policies being used as an immediate response to the demographic crisis of a declining birth rate and ageing population and as a means of economic growth by securing the labour force and creating social service jobs. It appears that care policies are mainly devoid of efforts to increase the value of care, expand public care, raise the status of care workers and fairly share care responsibilities. Current Korean society shows an irony that care policies devalue care, socially marginalize care workers, and disproportionately distribute care to a certain gender (and class).

In 2024, the future of South Korea's care policy appears to be at a critical point, with both challenges and opportunities. In 2017, the Korean government identified the establishment of a Social Service Agency as a significant policy issue to enhance the state's responsibility and role in care. The agency aimed to improve public care, strengthen the treatment of care workers, and advance care services as a direct provider of public social services created and operated by local governments.

However, as of 2024, the current government has shifted its policy towards the 'marketization of social services' and has removed all support for social service agencies in the 2024 government budget. Even the Seoul Social Service Center, one of the most successful examples of a local government organization, cannot maintain its innovative salary-based wage system for caregivers because it does not receive operating budget support from the Seoul Metropolitan City. The downsizing of the Seoul Social Service Center highlights the precarious state of South Korea's care policies.

In 2023, Gwangju Metropolitan City introduced a public care system called 'Gwangju Community Care', which serves as a core policy. This system is a public care network that allows citizens needing care to apply for and receive care. When citizens use care, they are connected to various service organizations through a '1:1 care manager' in a system that fosters public–private collaboration. The system also features a 'mandatory visit' system, which visits households needing care before they apply. In the same year, Gwangju Community Care was recognized as an exemplary case of urban innovation and won the top prize in the world's most prestigious 'Guangzhou International Urban Innovation Award' by the United Cities and Local Governments (UCLG). This system is seen as a breakthrough in the field of welfare services, as it presents an alternative care system based on caring relationships and solidarity. The mayor of Gwangju explains that 'Gwangju Community Care' enables the practice of caring democracy. Gwangju City's community care policy shows promise in offering a sustainable and inclusive care policy in South Korea.

Policies are inherently based on certain norms and values. Care ethics can offer a unique perspective that can bring about social change that existing approaches have not been able to achieve. In Korean society, it is not enough to have a care policy, but rather a 'caring' care policy rooted in care ethics. A 'caring' care policy can promote better justice and democracy by redefining our understanding of human beings and society.

NOTES

1. See: Maurice Hamington and Dorothy C. Miller, eds, *Socializing Care: Feminist Ethics and Public Issues* (Oxford: Rowman & Littlefield, 2006); Eva Kittay, *Love's Labor: Essays on Women, Equality and Dependency* (New York: Routledge, 1999); Nel Noddings, *Starting at Home: Caring and Social Policy* (Berkeley: University of California Press, 2002); Selma Sevenhuijsen, 'The Place of Care: The Relevance of the Feminist Ethic of Care for Social Policy', *Feminist Theory* 4, no. 2 (2003): 179–97.
2. See: Daniel Engster, 'A Public Ethics of Care for Policy Implementation', *American Journal of Political Science* 64, no. 3 (2020): 621–33; Helena Olofsdotter Stensöta, 'Public Ethics of Care – A General Public Ethics', *Ethics and Social Welfare* 9, no. 2 (2015): 183–200; Kari Greenswag, 'Care Ethics and Public Policy: A Holistic, Transformative Approach', *Politics & Gender* 15, no. 4 (2018): 912–40.
3. Olena Hankivsky, *Social Policy and the Ethic of Care* (Vancouver: University of British Columbia Press, 2004).
4. Hamington and Miller, eds, *Socializing Care*.
5. Greenswag, 'Care Ethics and Public Policy'.
6. Kathleen Lynch, *Care and Capitalism* (Cambridge: Polity Press, 2021).
7. Jennifer Nedelsky and Tom Malleson, *Part-Time for All: A Care Manifesto* (Oxford: Oxford University Press, 2023).
8. Sophie Bourgault, 'Prolegomena to a Caring Bureaucracy', *European Journal of Women's Studies* 24, no. 3 (2017): 202–17.

9. See: Heekyung Choi, 'The Elderly Long-Term Care Insurance System and Care Justice', *Korean Social Policy* 25, no. 3 (2018): 103–30 [in Korean]; Hee-Kang Kim, 'Is the Long-Term Care Insurance in South Korea a Socialising Care Policy?' *Critical Social Policy* 36, no. 4 (2016): 1–19; E-Hae Nam, *A Study of the Characteristics of Korean Care Policies through the Philosophy of Care* (Master's diss., Department of Social Work, Incheon National University Graduate School of Social Work, 2020) [in Korean]; Dayoung Song, 'How is a New Framework of Care Policy Possible? A Critical Review of Care Policy from the Perspective of Care Ethics', *Critical Social Policy* 77 (2022): 197–226 [in Korean].
10. Eunji Kim et al., *A Study on Social Care Reorganization Plan from a Gender Perspective (I): Paradigm Shift in Care Policy in the Age of Personalization* (Korean Women's Development Institute, 2022), 9–10 [in Korean].
11. Yeonkyu Ryu, 'Is a Human-Centered Paradigm Shift in the Low Birthrate Policy Possible? Focusing on Multidimensional Evaluation of Childcare Policies' (paper presented at the 2023 Joint Conference on Social Welfare, 2023), 55–6 [in Korean].
12. Kim et al., *A Study on Social Care Reorganization Plan from a Gender Perspective (I)*, 12.
13. Ibid., 14.
14. Ministry of Health and Welfare, *Childcare Statistics* (2022).
15. Kim et al., *A Study on Social Care Reorganization Plan from a Gender Perspective (I)*, 16–17.
16. *Tomorrow Newspaper*, 'Long-Term Care Recipients Surge, Shortfall of 75,000 Expected by 2027', 10 October 2023.
17. See: *Chosun Ilbo*, 'Korea's First Total Population Decline in History, A National Emergency', 29 July 2022; *Hankyoreh*, 'Steeper "Population Cliff" ... Opportunity for Reversal Within 10 years', 1 August 2022.
18. Yeonkyu Ryu, 'Is a Human-Centered Paradigm Shift in the Low Birthrate Policy Possible? Focusing on Multidimensional Evaluation of Childcare Policies' (paper presented at the 2023 Joint Conference on Social Welfare, 2023), 49–52 [in Korean].
19. See: *Korea Herald*, 'Govt. to lower child-rearing expenses to tackle low birthrate', 7 December 2018, https://www.koreaherald.com/article/1860770.
20. Mijin Lee, 'How to Secure Publicity of the Long-Term Care Insurance System for the Elderly', *Welfare Trends* 8 (2009): 21 [in Korean].
21. Jooha Lee, 'The Development of Welfare Programmes', in *Oxford Handbook of South Korea Politics*, ed. Jeong Hun Han, Romaon Pacheco Pardo and Youngho Cho (Oxford: Oxford University Press, 2021).
22. As of 2022, Korea's female labour force participation rate ranks 31st out of 38 OECD countries (59.9 per cent), below the OECD average of 64.8 per cent.
23. Taehong Kim et al., *Evaluation of Women's Policy in the Last Decade and Future Policy Issues* (Korean Women's Development Institute, 2012) [in Korean].
24. Minjeong Kang, Eunji Kim, Soobum Park, Sooyoung Kwon and Jaeyoung Yoon, *Proposal to Reform the Parental Leave System* (Presidential Committee on Ageing Society and Population Policy & Korean Women's Development Institute, 2019) [in Korean].
25. Nam, *A Study of the Characteristics of Korean Care Policies through the Philosophy of Care*, 34.
26. Eunjin Oh et al., *Policy Tasks for Creating Jobs for Women in the Social Service Sector V: Social Enterprises for Care Workers* (Korean Women's Development Institute, 2011), 4–5 [in Korean].
27. Hyun-Joo Min et al., *Policy Issues for Creating Jobs for Women in Social Services* (Korean Women's Development Institute, 2007), 374 [in Korean].

28. Ibid., iii.
29. Choi, 'The Elderly Long-Term Care Insurance System and Care Justice'.
30. See: Choi, 'The Elderly Long-Term Care Insurance System and Care Justice'; Imryang Ryu, 'Role Construction and Occupational Status of Institutionalized Care Workers: Focusing on the Case of Home Care Workers', *Feminist Studies* 17, no. 2 (2017): 189–231 [in Korean].
31. Seonyoung Seo, *How to Strengthen the Public Nature of Long-Term Care Services* (National Assembly Research Service, 2017), 7 [in Korean].
32. Ministry of Health and Welfare, *Childcare Statistics*.
33. Seo, *How to Strengthen the Public Nature of Long-Term Care Services*.
34. See: Choi, 'The Elderly Long-Term Care Insurance System and Care Justice'; Kim, 'Is the Long-Term Care Insurance in South Korea a Socialising Care Policy?'
35. South Korea's long-term care system is a publicly funded private welfare delivery system that applies market principles. Long-term care insurance is often called 'the privatization of long-term care service provision borrowing from the social insurance model' (Ji 2009, 119).
36. Choi, 'The Elderly Long-Term Care Insurance System and Care Justice'.
37. Young Kim and Soojung Kim, 'Childcare Labor in the Pandemic Era: Old Inequalities and New Risks', *Feminist Studies* 21, no. 2 (2021): 72 [in Korean].
38. *Oh My News*, 'Private and Family Childcare Workers Still "Below Minimum Wage"', 27 April 2022.
39. Keunbok Lee, 'A 10-Year Evaluation of the Long-Term Care Insurance for the Elderly from the Perspective of Caregivers and Needs for Improvement' (presentation at the Grand Debate for the Comprehensive Reform of Long-Term Care Insurance for the Elderly, 2017) [in Korean].
40. Yoonkyung Lee et al., *2022 Long-Term Care Survey* (Ministry of Health and Welfare & Korea Institute for Health and Social Affairs, 2022), 26 [in Korean].
41. A study that analysed care workers' wages over ten years found that the hourly wage of care workers was only 69.1 per cent of the average for employed workers (see: Wonjeong Kim and Yeonkyu Lim, 'The Current Status of Care Work in the Wake of Covid-19: Focusing on Changes in the Scale and Wages of Care Workers 2008–2019', *KWDI Brief* 58 (2020): 1–11 [in Korean]). Another study also found that care workers face a wage disadvantage of about 30 per cent compared to other service occupations, even after controlling for the effects of human capital, such as education and experience. Given care workers' low average hourly wage, their low wages are not due to insufficient hours worked. See: Seonyu Ham and Hyeji Kwon, 'A Study of the Mechanisms of Low Wages of Care Workers', *Industrial Labor Studies* 23, no. 3 (2017): 131–76 [in Korean].
42. Kim, 'Is the Long-Term Care Insurance in South Korea a Socialising Care Policy?'
43. A study notes that, while the wage penalty for care workers is an international phenomenon, the wage gap between care and non-care workers in South Korea is enormous compared to other countries. Using data from the OECD's Programme for the International Assessment of Adult Competencies (PIAAC) to analyse the hourly wage gap between care and non-care jobs, controlling for work experience, training and competency scores, they found that care jobs in the childcare sector in South Korea earned 46.2 per cent less per hour than non-care jobs, compared to 6 per cent in Denmark, 12.9 per cent in France, 19.6 per cent in Japan and 24.8 per cent in the UK (see: Youngmin Shin and Taeil Kim, 'An International Comparative Study of Care Work

Characteristics and Wage Levels', *Journal of Policy Analysis and Evaluation* 32, no. 4: 16 [in Korean]).
44. Kim and Lim, 'The Current Status of Care Work in the Wake of Covid-19'.
45. Ministry of Health and Welfare, *Childcare Statistics*.
46. Nam, *A Study of the Characteristics of Korean Care Policies through the Philosophy of Care*, 101–2.
47. Lee et al., *2022 Long-Term Care Survey*, 26.
48. Kim and Kim, 'Childcare Labor in the Pandemic Era'.

BIBLIOGRAPHY

Bourgault, Sophie. 'Prolegomena to a Caring Bureaucracy', *European Journal of Women's Studies* 24, no. 3 (2017): 202–17.

Choi, Heekyung. 'The Elderly Long-Term Care Insurance System and Care Justice', *Korean Social Policy* 25, no. 3 (2018): 103–30 [in Korean].

Chosun Ilbo. 'Korea's First Total Population Decline in History, A National Emergency', 29 July 2022.

Engster, Daniel. 'A Public Ethics of Care for Policy Implementation', *American Journal of Political Science* 64, no. 3 (2020): 621–33.

Greenswag, Kari. 'Care Ethics and Public Policy: A Holistic, Transformative Approach', *Politics & Gender* 15, no. 4 (2018): 912–40.

Ham, Seonyu. 'Reflections on Care as a Social Right', paper presented at the 2017 Autumn Conference of the Korean Social Welfare Association (2017) [in Korean].

Ham, Seonyu, and Hyeji Kwon. 'A Study of the Mechanisms of Low Wages of Care Workers', *Industrial Labor Studies* 23, no. 3 (2017): 131–76 [in Korean].

Hamington, Maurice, and Dorothy C. Miller, eds. *Socializing Care: Feminist Ethics and Public Issues*. Oxford: Rowman & Littlefield, 2006.

Hankivsky, Olena. *Social Policy and the Ethic of Care*. Vancouver: University of British Columbia Press, 2004.

Hankyoreh. 'Steeper "Population Cliff" … Opportunity for Reversal Within 10 years', 1 August 2022.

Hong, Hyunkyun, and Jeongseung Gong. *Current Status and Prospects of Childcare Services*. Korea Employment Information Centre, 2022 [in Korean].

Ji, Eunkoo. 'Social Welfare Privatization and the Long-Term Care Insurance System for the Elderly', *Korean Social Policy* 15, no. 2 (2009): 99–143 [in Korean].

Kang, Minjeong, Eunji Kim, Soobum Park, Sooyoung Kwon and Jaeyoung Yoon. *Proposal to Reform the Parental Leave System*. Presidential Committee on Ageing Society and Population Policy & Korean Women's Development Institute, 2019 [in Korean].

Kim, Eunji, Kyunghee Ma, Inhee Choi, Yisun Kim, Jinhee Choi, Kyung Sung and Jaeyoung Yoon. *A Study on Social Care Reorganization Plan from a Gender Perspective (I): Paradigm Shift in Care Policy in the Age of Personalization*. Korean Women's Development Institute, 2022 [in Korean].

Kim, Hee-Kang. 'Is the Long-Term Care Insurance in South a Socialising Care Policy?', *Critical Social Policy* 36, no. 4 (2016): 1–19.

Kim, Taehong, Hyekyung Jang, Jungim Hwang and Hojung Bae. *Evaluation of Women's Policy in the Last Decade and Future Policy Issues*. Korean Women's Development Institute, 2012 [in Korean].

Kim, Wonjeong, and Yeonkyu Lim. 'The Current Status of Care Work in the Wake of COVID-19: Focusing on Changes in the Scale and Wages of Care Workers 2008–2019', *KWDI Brief* 58 (2020): 1–11 [in Korean].

Kim, Young, and Soojung Kim. 'Childcare Labor in the Pandemic Era: Old Inequalities and New Risks', *Feminist Studies* 21, no. 2 (2021): 39–88 [in Korean].

Kittay, Eva. *Love's Labor: Essays on Women, Equality and Dependency*. New York: Routledge, 1999.

Lee, Jooha. 'The Development of Welfare Programmes', in *Oxford Handbook of South Korea Politics*, edited by Jeong Hun Han, Romaon Pacheco Pardo and Youngho Cho. Oxford: Oxford University Press, 2021.

Lee, Keunbok. 'A 10-Year Evaluation of the Long-Term Care Insurance for the Elderly from the Perspective of Caregivers and Needs for Improvement', presentation at the Grand Debate for the Comprehensive Reform of Long-Term Care Insurance for the Elderly, 2017 [in Korean].

Lee, Mijin. 'How to Secure Publicity of the Long-Term Care Insurance System for the Elderly', *Welfare Trends* 8 (2009): 21–5 [in Korean].

Lee, Yoonkyung, Sunhee Lee, Eunna Kang, Sejin Kim, Eunha Namgung and Yoojung Choi. *2022 Long-Term Care Survey*. Ministry of Health and Welfare & Korea Institute for Health and Social Affairs, 2022 [in Korean].

Lynch, Kathleen. *Care and Capitalism*. Cambridge: Polity Press, 2021.

Min, Hyun-Joo, Min-Jung Kang, Sangwon Lee, Soonyoung Moon, Sekyung Park, Hyegyu Kang, Hyungyong Kim, Changhak Shim, Kiwook Um and Eunyoung Choi. *Policy Issues for Creating Jobs for Women in Social Services*. Korean Women's Development Institute, 2007 [in Korean].

Ministry of Health and Welfare. *Childcare Statistics*. 2022.

Tomorrow Newspaper. 'Long-Term Care Recipients Surge, Shortfall of 75,000 Expected by 2027', 10 October 2023.

Nam, E-Hae. *A Study of the Characteristics of Korean Care Policies through the Philosophy of Care*. Master's thesis, Department of Social Work, Incheon National University Graduate School of Social Work, 2020 [in Korean].

Nedelsky, Jennifer, and Tom Malleson. *Part-Time for All: A Care Manifesto*. Oxford: Oxford University Press, 2023.

Noddings, Nel. *Starting at Home: Caring and Social Policy*. Berkeley: University of California Press, 2002.

Oh, Eunjin, Nanju Kim and Wonbong Jang. *Policy Tasks for Creating Jobs for Women in the Social Service Sector V: Social Enterprises for Care Workers*. Korean Women's Development Institute, 2011 [in Korean].

Oh My News. 'Private and Family Childcare Workers Still "Below Minimum Wage"', 27 April 2022.

Ryu, Imryang. 'Role Construction and Occupational Status of Institutionalized Care Workers: Focusing on the Case of Home Care Workers', *Feminist Studies* 17, no. 2 (2017): 189–231 [in Korean].

Ryu, Yeonkyu. 'Is A Human-Centered Paradigm Shift in the Low Birthrate Policy Possible? Focusing on Multidimensional Evaluation of Childcare Policies', paper presented at the 2023 Joint Conference on Social Welfare, 2023 [in Korean].

Seo, Seonyoung. *How to Strengthen the Public Nature of Long-Term Care Services*. National Assembly Research Service, 2017 [in Korean].

Sevenhuijsen, Selma. 'The Place of Care: The Relevance of the Feminist Ethic of Care for Social Policy', *Feminist Theory* 4, no. 2 (2003): 179–97.

Song, Dayoung. 'How is a New Framework of Care Policy Possible? A Critical Review of Care Policy from the Perspective of Care Ethics', *Critical Social Policy* 77 (2022): 197–226 [in Korean].

Stensöta, Helena Olofsdotter. 'Public Ethics of Care – A General Public Ethics', *Ethics and Social Welfare* 9, no. 2 (2015): 183–200.

CHAPTER SIXTEEN

Notes from a care network

Lessons from the pandemic

SUNITA GEORGE AND RAYMOND GREENE

INTRODUCTION

Crises lend clarity to our conditions, and provoke our responses. During the peak of the Covid-19 virus pandemic (2020–22), much of the world's attention was focused on the upheavals and disruptions occasioned by the failure of societies to contain the virus's spread. As more people around the world became infected with the Covid-19 virus, *being* careful, or careless, could itself become a matter of life or death. Care, thus, was central to our very existence during this period. The vulnerabilities of living through a global pandemic showed us our mutual interdependence and accentuated the relational and emotional aspects of giving and receiving care and our responsibility for one another. These are concepts which are central to the ethics of care and they became the customary response to the crisis in many spheres of pandemic life.

Was the valorization of care workers, care networks, and caring generally, merely an accommodation to tide us through difficult times, or did it provoke our collective moral imaginations – granting us a clarity to see the world from the perspective of those being cared for? If so, did it enhance our long-term ability to make empathetic, ethically sound choices? There are stories from all over the world of citizen groups, individuals and agencies, taking great risks, making sacrifices and pooling resources, to provide care and comfort to the afflicted. These tales invite the questions: (1) Are people more caring during a crisis? (2) Do *all* crises provoke empathy? (3) Are we selective in our dispensation of care? – what crises are 'deserving' of our care? (4) Are the many instances of caring during the pandemic extendable to 'normal' times? Using these questions as our motive, in this chapter we examine the Food for Chennai network that arose and was developed during the 2020–22 coronavirus global pandemic and lockdown.

Food for Chennai (FFC) was started as an effort by the founder to provide home-cooked food to the elderly parents of her friends who, immobilized by national and international lockdowns, could not reach their elderly or Covid-stricken parents. It soon grew to a network of over 200 volunteers who cooked and delivered meals to patients and their families, free of cost, during the first and second wave of Covid-19 infections in Chennai, India. According to various estimates, the Chennai Metropolitan Area has a population of over 11 million, making it the fifth largest metropolitan area in India, and the city alone has a population of over 4 million people. The city of Chennai is broadly divided into three regions – North Chennai, Central Chennai and South Chennai – and the volunteers of the FFC were geographically dispersed in all three regions of the city. The project to provide food to the sick and incapacitated could not have been implemented without the digital social arrangements that connected people and supported the provisioning of a variety of services. At the hub of these virtual connections were individuals like Latha Dubay, a social activist, marketing, public relations and non-profit consultant, with both a disposition for caring and experience in providing care. She drew supporters to her mission by posting affective stories of the people she had helped and, in doing so, she not only humanized the pandemic/lockdown's suffering but also offered a way for the common citizen to join her in the mission of rendering care. The network of volunteers provided free hot home-cooked meals to over 40,000 people in the city of Chennai during the peak pandemic years, and ebbed as things returned to normal. By examining the FFC network, we hope to learn how the care network, fashioned during the Covid-19 crisis, is sustained during normal times.

Based on interviews with Latha Dubay, who founded FFC, we explore the idea of 'care influencers', people who draw others' attention to a need, who provoke a commitment of action, and who are able to guide individual competencies to achieve broader goals. Care influencers respond to the needs of those for whom they care in ways that Joan Tronto framed as the central elements of the theory of care ethics.[1] We offer the case of FFC, and the founder of FFC in particular, as an example of a care influencer who can effect change by drawing on a network of care that was created during the pandemic.

Drawing from the central elements of care ethics developed in Fisher and Tronto, as well as the latter's solo-authored work, we argue that providing food to the sick and their families during the Covid-19 pandemic differs from other co-extant moral questions, such as the allocation of scarce resources, in several fundamental ways.[2] In the section that follows, we describe the evolution and expansion of the FFC, and consider the engagement practices of FFC volunteers, both with each other and with the households to which they provided food. We then develop the *centrality* of care influencers to the creation of informal networks of care, networks which may lie dormant in non-crisis periods but which can be revivified as the need arises. Social media platforms are full of stories of crowdfunding efforts by individuals and groups for causes that evoke empathy, and invite people to show they care through monetary support. We will outline ways in which 'care influencers' are similar, yet distinct from other influencers on social media. Finally, we posit that the ideation of 'care influencers' allows us to approach caring from the standpoint of informally networked groups that construct solidarity in the face of developing vulnerabilities.

16.1 THE MORPHOLOGY OF 'CARING' DURING THE COVID-19 CRISIS

Covid-19 showed the essential, yet often relegated, realm of care work in capitalist societies, and prompted a societal re-evaluation of the necessity for care in the smooth functioning of society. From shifts in state strategies, to individual responsibilities and collective actions, the pandemic offered, at many scales, opportunities to reimagine a world which 'put responsibilities for caring at the centre of [its] democratic political agenda'.[3] We examine two domains where the ethics and practices of care were central during the crisis period: (a) in providing livelihood support by the state and (b) in taking care of the basic needs of Covid-19 patients by individuals and community-based care networks. We posit that individual acts of care, such as providing food for the ailing during the pandemic, can evolve into community networks of care, where an individual's caring practices can become integrated into societal structures and, thus, individual behaviours more widely.

On 28 March 2020, during the first wave of the Covid-19 crisis, the Prime Minister of India, Mr Narendra Modi tweeted:

> It is my appeal to my fellow Indians, kindly contribute to the PM-CARES Fund.[4] This Fund will also cater to similar distressing situations, if they occur in the times ahead. This link has all important details about the fund.

That the acronym of the trust fund established by the central government of India to fund relief efforts was 'PM-CARES' (and similarly, the economic rescue bill in the United States signed around the same time by President Trump was the CARES Act (for Coronavirus Aid, Relief, and Economic Security Act[5])) tells us of the perceived political need to frame the state's response in an emotive way that could call forth charity in the citizenry. This call to the ordinary citizen to care, and in that caring to aid the state, in the desperate time of a pandemic, inverted the usual power hierarchy in which a parental state provides aid to her citizen children. Care work and its practitioners tend to be marginalized in capitalist societies, where a Ricardian, additive, model of contribution to value – and therefore reward to labour – is accepted. In responding to the dislocations of Covid-19, the Indian state's attempt to 'crowdfund' its rescue mission arguably emphasized how fundamental the work of caring is to the smooth functioning of society, and indeed for how care is vital in effective governance.

Efforts to reduce the devastating impacts of the pandemic on livelihoods were undertaken by governments across the globe, e.g. by enacting social protection measures such as unemployment benefits, cash transfer schemes and direct support for struggling families.[6] These relief measures raised ethical questions about the adequacy of these responses for those most in need of support – the self-employed, undocumented migrants and those in the informal sector. These are the people typically excluded from conventional income-supporting measures. Introducing these relief measures also showed how the unaddressed conditions of societal vulnerability could be, and were, exploited by the Covid-19 virus. The exploitation manifested as both physical and economic dislocations to individuals and societies. Although the rolling out of supportive measures by states had shortcomings, the shifts in states' strategies to care for their citizens – by expanding protective measures, by suspending restrictions on pre-pandemic entitlement policies, by rapidly scaling up social protection measures to meet the greater need, all these shifts allowed us insight into what is possible should states put 'caring at the centre of their democratic political agenda'. Indeed, evidence from the US Census[7] shows that fiscal interventions by the government were instrumental in substantially reducing poverty among key demographic subsets, underscoring therefore the potential of prioritizing care in policymaking.

The Covid-19 period also saw the engagement of non-state actors and individuals who, at great risks to themselves, formed local networks of care for people afflicted by the virus, Many of these local efforts were concerned with tending to the basic needs of vulnerable people, for example, shopping for household supplies and checking on the wellbeing of the elderly, and providing food for the hungry. In the physical delivery of 'basic needs' we saw the care terrain of the pandemic populated with actors, often not reimbursed by the state or other organizations, trying to fill the delivery gap created by the fear of transmission of the Covid-19 virus through physical contact. At the heart of it, the central questions during the pandemic revolved around sustaining life and doing so in an ethically responsible manner. While there was consensus that life needed to be protected and cared for in the most effective ways possible, the practices of caring varied widely from place to place.

The actions of care and the question of *how* to show care are socially constructed and regionally normative. The culturally and geographically varying normative practices of care are less theorized or scrutinized within the larger body of care ethics, yet are central to how care is understood, interpreted and translated to practices of care around the world. In our investigation of the FFC care network, a nuanced picture emerged. Food habits and food taboos are shaped by culture and personal preferences, and in a country like India, where religion and caste widely complicate diets, to accept home-cooked food from strangers is an act of faith on the part of the receiver that the food provider has not violated the faith and cultural traditions of the receiver. Responsiveness, one of the elements of care ethic theory developed by Tronto, addresses this inherently unequal nature of vulnerability. The dependent nature of the sick in this case, and the relative privilege of the network of caregivers who are not ill, and who may be members of higher social-economic groups than the receivers of care, meant that caregivers had to be attentive to the needs and diet specifications of those being cared for, beyond just the action of providing food.[8] However, as Tronto pointed out, responsiveness is not a one-way street where the needs of care receivers take complete precedence over everybody else's needs; rather, she argued for the necessity of a balance between the needs of the care receivers and the needs of the care providers.[9] From its inception, FFC made it its mission to only provide home-cooked vegetarian meals, thus signalling that the food was cooked to meet the basic needs of the broadest group of people. Strategic thinking and attentiveness to the needs of the vulnerable, under cover of utilitarian ethics, seems to have been the broad ethos of this care network.

Beyond sustaining physical life, sharing food builds a community's social cohesion and solidarity. Restrictions on population movement and physical interactions (the lockdown enacted to attempt to slow down the spread of the Covid-19 virus) during the pandemic was particularly hard for elderly people who were not only more susceptible to infection by the virus but were also less capable of performing self-care under infection. Latha Dubay, the founder of FFC, recounted how the project of cooking for the sick started as a response to pleas from friends who were 'locked down' in other cities and countries, to check on their sick parents. She then decided to extend this act of care by offering home-cooked food to strangers who were unable to feed themselves because they were ill. She posted her offer along with her contact details on social media (Facebook), asking that anyone who could help also get in touch. Soon, the number of people asking for help grew dramatically, and the bond between her and the people she helped became stronger. She recalled in a WhatsApp interview how an elderly man battling Covid-19, and who had lost his wife to the virus, called her not to request food but to share his sorrow and his despair. As she recounted to us, 'this is not just about food, it is about the whole person ... we want to feed the soul as well. It is food for the body and soul. We are not just food providers.'[10]

During the pandemic, and perhaps in normal times too, people hunger not just for food, but also for connections. The provisioning of basic needs during the pandemic was not just about the delivery of tangibles, but the delivery of connections, of human bonding, of nursing the spirit. In this regard, the rendering of care through the medium of food embraces two elemental human needs – sustaining the body, and supporting the need for belonging in community – both of which came into sharp relief during the pandemic. The morphology of caring in its myriad forms during the pandemic allowed us to 'rethink our conceptions of human nature to shift from the dilemma of autonomy or dependence to a more sophisticated sense of human interdependence'.[11] The network of care that was developed over a two-year period by the FFC is a system of interdependence, where the efficiency-based division of labour from the pre-pandemic economic systems was adapted to the circumstances of the pandemic-induced realities by harnessing the competencies of many to engage in the practice of care. Can the lessons gleaned from the pandemic help rekindle care networks in 'distressing situations, if they occur in the times ahead'. What if the PM's call to set up emergency funds to tide distressing situations was a clarion call to awaken dormant informal networks of care? Next, we explore the scaling up of this network from one woman's kitchen to the work of many micro-volunteers.

16.2 CAN 'CARING ABOUT' AND 'CARING FOR' BE SCALED UP TO A NETWORK OF CARE?

Before it came to be called Food for Chennai, FFC was the story of one woman who paid attention to a need – the practical difficulties of cooking and feeding oneself (and sometimes a family) when suffering from the Covid-19 virus – and responded to the need by delivering home-cooked meals, free of cost, to those in quarantine. From helping her friends and those in her social circle, she decided to scale up her efforts by communicating to her social circle (on Facebook) her offer to deliver food to strangers in similar situations. This scaling up in practical terms meant that she was cooking up to 40–45 meals in a day, often waking up at 4.00 am to make the meals and deliver them on time. Dubay's story might have gone unknown, as many of the individual works of caring during this time are unknown, and the enterprise would have had a smaller impact had it not been posted to social media. The second crucial scaling up happened when two other denizens of Chennai with extensive connections in the city were drawn to her story and decided to help her. The three of them, possessing a complex of connections, and competencies in public relations, chose the hashtag #foodforchennai, grew the network to more than 200 volunteers and, according to their posts on Instagram and Facebook, at one point delivered food to nearly 40,000 people.

Using social media to encourage acts of charity was commonplace even before the Covid-19 pandemic. However, the pandemic-dominated context in which much of the world lived for nearly two years, meant that there was an abundance of time to focus people's attention on specific issues such as providing food for the sick, thus encouraging commitments of both time and money. The practice of caring during the pandemic, as discussed in the previous section, took varied expressions as caring individuals responded to the needs of the moment according to their individual lights.

The literature on the theory of care ethics argues for the need to consider care not so much as something which some people are disposed to by their circumstances, but as a necessary component of a well-structured society – thus, care must be inculcated in all people and in the structures that uphold society. For example, Sara Ruddick[12] and Joan Tronto both warn that framing care only as a disposition carries the danger of sentimentalizing care, and consigning it to the ambit of individual attributes, rather than recognizing that the systematic, deliberate and practised nature of effective caring places this activity within the purview of a well-functioning society. Further, Tronto writes, 'to think of care solely in dispositional terms allows us to think of care as the possession and province of an individual'.[13] This argument against viewing care as a disposition comes from its long and troubled association with the gendered nature of care, where women are viewed as 'naturally' more caring than men, thereby marginalizing the vital practice of care and undervaluing the social contributions of practitioners of care. Without disputing this position, we assert that dispositional caring, regardless of the gender of the practitioner, can influence others' worldview, and thereby create more engagement with causes that require the practice of care.

Individuals with a caring disposition can use their agency to influence others through the constructions of evocative stories on social media. In our interview with Dubay, she repeatedly stressed her vision of the kind of care she wanted to deliver to the sick – her aversion to mass-produced communal-kitchen-style food,[14] her insistence that emotional connections with the receivers of her caring practices were as important as the food itself[15] – these became the guidance for the volunteers who joined her mission to cook and deliver food. The articulation of a compelling narrative with which to galvanize others' desire to care is a persuasive factor which can be used to scale up caring practices beyond the individual. The evocative power of storytelling makes room for others to see themselves in the narrative, by engaging their own creativity; this was central to the expansion of the FFC's network.

By steering the narrative and drawing attention to a need, we have the potential to shape moral principles in times of disasters such as the Covid-19 pandemic. Drawing from the literature on disasters, Pascoe and Stripling summarize three distinct ways in which calamity can alter the lens of ethics with which the world is regarded. First, calamitous times alter perceptions and challenge established ways of seeing the world; this often requires improvised responses to the new situations. Second, new realities can expedite the adoption of innovative ways of responding to a need, and prompt new ways of thinking. Lastly, disasters often provoke a sense of community and solidarity as denizens of a place come together to deal with situations beyond their normal experience.[16] In the aftermath of the 11 September 2001 attacks on New York City, Solnit described how people from different walks of life and socio-economic classes came together to try to understand, and created a consensus of purpose and communal engagement, of caring and giving.[17] Faced with disaster, people may lean on community and rely less on individualism; in situations which remind us of our mortality, our values, indeed our assessment of the worth of life itself, can be evaluated using different, previously unconsidered, metrics. These 'disaster imaginaries', as Pascoe and Stripling called them, are 'collective narratives that shape our experience of this (Covid-19) disaster and inform what kinds of moral problems we see', and by extension, the solutions we propose.[18] We propose that individuals like Latha Dubay can, through their caring dispositions and social media praxes cajole people into acts of caring, and create spaces for people to see themselves as actors in the macro-narratives of the pandemic. While a caring disposition does not always guarantee engagement in acts of care (caring for), a caring disposition, coupled with acts of care as promoted on social media, can be key to scaling care actions from those of an individual to the fully fledged undertakings of a city-spanning, wide-scope network.

16.2.1 Social media and strategic communication: Can care influencers be used as strategic tools?

When the world was in global and local quarantine, social media platform substituted virtual connections for banned physical interactions. In this substitution such virtualized existence became all too real as people found solace in being able to consolidate purpose by engaging in the micro-activism that was central to many works of care during the peak periods of the pandemic.[19] Even the Indian prime minister's appeal on X (formerly Twitter) was testament to the central role of social media in mounting persuasion campaigns during this period. Social media influencers have emerged as powerful agents of social influence by shaping public perceptions, behaviours and responses during the pandemic.[20] Finland was one of the first countries to harness the potential of social media influencers to disseminate crucial information regarding the pandemic, and created one of the first public communications campaign using this avenue of outreach.[21]

Social influence theory informs us that people's behaviour can be moderated and modulated by the presence and actions of others but can people be persuaded by 'care influencers' to continue to engage in caring actions even beyond times of hardship? As the Covid-19 pandemic threats of scarcity and danger recede, can people who acted beyond their personal needs be persuaded to continue to be their brothers' keepers? Cialdini explored the principles of persuasion, and held that people tend to be persuaded by (1) those whom they like (i.e. those whom they follow on social media) and (2) by figures invested with a public authority (large numbers of followers approximate this authority).[22] Thus, it is that people are guided in their behaviours by 'social proof' that they do not walk alone but are ensconced in a reality beyond themselves, and this is demonstrated by the 'evidence' that their self-thinking also has currency with a large number of others. We propose that this model can be applied to understanding the thought-leading reach of social media influencers who (1) keep their audiences engaged and (2) can shape opinions to comply with the norms which propound.[23] While some social media influencers are content experts, the persuasive appeal of many influencers lies in their personal attributes, such as perceived authenticity,[24] enthusiasm and trustworthiness, and the ability to tell a compelling story, rich in emotions and visuals.[25] With this general understanding of what gives individuals the power to influence, we explore what makes for a care influencer using Fisher and Tronto's[26] and Tronto's[27] elements of care ethics. In particular we try to understand how robust is the nature of social-media-based care influence, and whether it is strong enough to be potent even beyond crisis times, when enhanced social caring is required.

Based on five interviews with Latha Dubay (on WhatsApp, Facebook Messenger and text message exchange) over a three-year period (2021–23), we reflect on her place in the development of the FFC network and its continued evolution in post-Covid-19 'normal times'.

Latha Dubay described herself as a passionate social activist who believes in 'Transforming Lives, Spreading Smiles' (the hashtag of all her social media posts) and, in interviews (2021, 2023) she asserted that she was not interested in being an armchair activist, and that she had been involved in works of care since the 2004 Boxing Day Tsunami in the Indian Deccan that affected people living along the coast of Tamil Nadu state in southern India. She called herself an unflinching optimist with an ability to see 'some good in everything'. In the interviews, Dubay talked about the beginnings of her efforts in 2004, the ethos of her approach to care, the growth of the network, the organizational framework and much more.

Two themes emerged from these interviews. First, the work Latha Dubay was doing appealed to people, so that the seeds she was sowing landed in fertile ground. Second, the rapid growth of her care network was attributable to: (1) her optimistic, non-demanding attitude to problem solving and (2) the fact that, under globalized quarantine, people had plenty of time for existential reflection on the question of a better life. In a bleak time of dire news, with catastrophic loss of life just from pursuing daily activities, optimism was a scarce commodity that was, perhaps, much needed. Those who could shape the 'disaster imaginaries' by instilling a modicum of optimism, and who could persuade her friends and followers to apprehend opportunities for action which would meet the (sometimes vital) needs of others, were well placed to garner or increase social influence. When asked what she thought had been the appeal of her initial Facebook post, the one that persuaded many people to join her efforts to cook and deliver food to the sick, she remarked, 'Most people want to help, they just don't know how. I was able to show them a way.'

Among the four elements of care ethics developed by Tronto, the first and crucial aspect of an ethics of care is attentiveness or paying attention to a need.[28] In order to take responsibility for a problem, we must first give it our attention. While Tronto may have meant this with respect to individuals, we suggest that care influencers use social media to so frame a problem as to draw the attention of a larger group of people. Visual amplification of a problem for which care is needed creates the possibility of a scale-up of reach; in this extended reach lies opportunities for people to integrate their efforts and take responsibility for meeting the problem's needs.

The second ethical dimension of care is that of taking responsibility for those things for which care is needed. Responsibility is multifaceted, as Tronto writes, '[responsibility] is a term that is embedded in a set of implicit cultural practices, rather than in a set of formal rules or series of promises'.[29] Most problems that need to be cared for are multidimensional in nature, and require addressing a series of smaller tasks to fulfil the broader goal of exercising care. As an example of this in the FFC context, the need to get food to the sick necessitates a series of tasks done in a culturally appropriate manner – from shopping for groceries, to cooking and matching the food preparer with the recipient of the food, to delivering the food, to engaging with social media to encourage more volunteers to reach more people. For one person to take responsibility for all these tasks would require an enormous commitment of time and energy. Latha Dubay acknowledged that her initial Facebook post soon attracted people with varying skills, and she credits the widened reach of her mission to the expansion of the network of people who wanted to show their care.

Ultimately, the success of caring can be assessed by whether or not the deficit, whose remediation required others to care, was ameliorated to an acceptable degree. Competency as a moral precept determines the success or failure of the project of caring. Most problems are multifaceted and multiple competencies are required to resolve them competently. The FFC was able to build up the multiple competencies needed to accomplish its mission because people were restricted to their residences by the lockdown imposed by the national government. As Latha Dubay pointed out, because of the pandemic lockdowns, she had access to a virtually free supply of labour with diverse skills and the time to engage with her in the care work of the FFC. This fact was critical to FFC being able to grow its network.

Responsiveness as a moral imperative in care ethics engages the caregiver and care recipient in a process of mutual engagement and reflection. From the standpoint of the caregiver, this involves a shift from being a mere functionary of apparently caring actions, to a reflective practitioner who evaluates the outcome of caring actions from the standpoint of the cared for, such that the goals of caring about and caring for coalesce in the fulfilment of caring actions not as a performance, but rather as an engaged understanding of the needs of the other as they wish to be understood. In his book *Oneself as Another*, Paul Ricœur speaks of the mediating nature of care, and its effect on creating a connection between the giver and the receiver – such that the giver of care is also a receiver of something large, i.e. an ability to see in the care recipient one's own vulnerabilities. It is in this – it is through caring that the 'search for equality in the midst of inequality' and 'the shared admission of fragility' are realized.[30] This view of responsiveness to care as a two-way street reflects the widening of the self and an awakening of the awareness of the human experience. In this connection, several volunteers made social media posts of how satisfying it was to participate in the work of the FFC.

The hub-spoke structure of the FFC network emerged from the needs and circumstances of Latha Dubay's decisions in enacting care in Chennai. At the hub, Latha Dubay could both highlight people in need, and shape the nature of care that could be delivered to those in need. Volunteers acted as spokes/connections to the needy, as vectors of home-cooked meals, for example. As the worst of the pandemic seems to be behind us, and many of the volunteers have already gone back to their regular office jobs, what has become of the network and, fundamentally, can the network persist in normal times given that a particular set of circumstances (lockdowns, tech-savvy workers working from home, the affective nature of social media to provoke empathy and use talents and passions) inspired its creation?

16.3 THE AFTERMATH: WHAT NEXT? LESSON LEARNED?

We wondered if the care network of FFC had been dissolved once the crisis abated or what, if anything, remains of the network? In our conversations, Latha Dubay ruminated on her life's journey of caring about and caring for, a journey that started well before the pandemic. During the pandemic, the use of social media gave her a wider platform to influence others, and the FFC network quickly scaled up the reach of her caring actions. Earlier tragedies which affected Chennai had ignited a desire to care in Latha Dubay. In fact, during the 2015 city-wide flooding, when large swathes of Chennai were inundated, Dubay used public Facebook posts to draw attention to, and seek assistance from, others who were willing to help those affected by the floods. When asked, if she considered herself to be a social media care influencer, she quickly rejected the idea, saying that she had very limited expertise in navigating social media platforms, but she did acknowledge that the success of the FFC was in large part because of the use of social media, particularly WhatsApp, Facebook and Instagram. Dubay also conceded that she had gained more visibility as a result of her role in the FFC efforts, and that a lot more people were now asking for her help.[31] She sees her role as that of a hub in the mission of providing help to those in need.

We can report that the network of FFC volunteers is still connected, and they continue to assist Dubay when she asks their support for smaller needs. Engagement within the group is mostly sporadic, and used to keep the connections alive to make sure that the connections are available should the need for their use arise. The network of volunteers, many of whom were strangers to each other before the pandemic, continue to engage with each other because perhaps, as Ricœur suggested, caring for another transforms the caregiver in fundamental ways.

Our original intention for this chapter was to learn from members of the FFC volunteer network how, if at all, their engagement with FFC had affected them, and whether or not it had altered their ways of engaging in caring practice. In the end this was not possible as the transition to normality after the pandemic meant that most volunteers went back to their office jobs and so could not easily be reached. The resumption of the hurried way of life, as Dubay implied, is the enemy of care. The multitude of cares that compete for our attention, from the individual, to the family and beyond also competes for our time. In this regard, being a part of the loosely formed care network – with Dubay as a hub and a clearinghouse for the needs that need to be cared for – allows the FFC volunteers to still collectively engage in practices of care in normal times. She uses her influence within the network to both seek financial help for individuals in need (recently she sent a request for funds for a student who had lost his parents and was unable to pay for his college tuition) and to request food for the needy.

Dubay, who had been active in supporting palliative care patients even before the pandemic, now uses the old FFC network to seek volunteers who are able and willing to cook meals for cancer patients after chemotherapy and radiation treatments. The FFC volunteer network had expanded throughout the city during the pandemic, and so it was easy to request a volunteer near the person in need of the food to cook a meal or two. Dubay said, 'I am happy to say we have never had to say no to anyone who requested food.' Explaining why this is so, she said, 'most people cook for themselves and their families anyway, asking them to make a little extra does not burden them too much in terms of time or money'. In this regard, the provision of food is quite different from the other care-related work done during the pandemic, much of which was focused on pandemic-specific needs such as providing masks, vaccines or ventilators, but the ubiquitousness of food transcends the pandemic. Where food is concerned, there is a continuity of need even when the context has changed. The fact that food preparation at home can quite easily be scaled up based on the need allows this network to continue beyond the pandemic.

We asked Dubay how she uses social media to manage the varying requests for meal help at different times. She explained that, based on her assessment of perceived need (disasters versus normal times), she engages differently with social media. Typically, when the demand for food is limited, as in normal times, the FFC volunteers communicate with each other to find a volunteer to provide food. However, when there is a greater need for food (as in when there is a broader social crisis situation), her posts to her personal Facebook and Instagram accounts are made public in an effort to reach more people. As the need for help arises, Dubay switches the privacy level of her posts from closed to only her followers on the social media platform, to zero-privacy, public posts so as to reach the greatest number of possible volunteers located as widely across the city as possible. Because the volunteers have varied skills and knowledge backgrounds, it is important to FFC that a range of people be brought on board when the need arises. Depending on what care is sought, a combination of skills within FFC is used to enable care to be delivered to the individual in need. We asked Dubay if she considered formalizing and registering the FFC as an NGO. Her response was nuanced. While the idea of creating an NGO for financial reasons (donations from corporations would facilitate a scaling up of her efforts) was appealing to her, she was hesitant to seek such funds in large part because it would mean the loss of autonomy to practise care as she sees fit.

To keep the FFC network close to the grassroots rather than to establish a formal structure with a depersonalized network has two compelling benefits for Dubay. First, an NGO may dissuade small donors whose time and labour of care are fundamental to the ethos of how Dubay perceives caring should be done. She does not believe that one size fits all when it comes to caring praxes, believing instead that a situationally appropriate approach makes it easier to attract volunteers. Second, having a less rigid organizational approach encourages creative ways to approach care. The immediacy and the uniqueness of a need is best served when there are guiding principles rather than rigid requirements for deciding the best course of action. This aspect of her approach to providing food during the pandemic required improvising and, even in normal times, improvisation is a key feature of her approach. Finally, Latha Dubay, in assessing the success of an action of care, considers the closing of the loop – the response of the care recipient to the caring actions; this psychological aspect of care is as important as the physical delivery of care itself. Ultimately, as Maio said when summarizing the critical role of relationships that frame the essence of care ethics, 'the demand for an adequate perception of the situation, and the prioritising of creative solutions over deductive inference necessitate implicit forms of knowledge such as experiential knowledge, situational knowledge, and relationship knowledge'.[32] In keeping these aspects of care ethics, the continuation of the work of FFC during normal times provides a case study in imagining a framework for the practice of care.

NOTES

1. Joan C. Tronto, *Moral Boundaries: A Political Argument for an Ethics of Care* (London: Routledge, 1993).
2. Berenice Fisher and Joan C. Tronto, 'Toward a Feminist Theory of Caring', in *Circles of Care: Work and Identity in Women's Lives*, ed. Emily K. Abel and Margaret K. Nelson (Albany: SUNY Press, 1990), 36–54.
3. Joan C. Tronto, *Caring Democracy: Markets, Equality, and Justice* (New York: New York University Press, 2013), ix.
4. PM-CARES Fund or the Prime Minister's Citizen Assistance and Relief in Emergency Situations Fund was set up on 27 March 2020 as a Public Charitable Trust whose objectives are 'To undertake and support relief or assistance of any kind relating to a public health emergency or any other kind of emergency, calamity or distress, either man-made or natural, including the creation or upgradation of healthcare or pharmaceutical facilities. To render financial assistance, provide grants of payments of money or take such other steps as may be deemed necessary by the Board of Trustees to the affected population. To undertake any other activity, which is not inconsistent with the above objects.'
5. The CARES Act was an economic stimulus bill signed into law by President Trump on 27 March 2020 to provide assistance to those affected by Covid-19.
6. The OECD's 2020 report '*Supporting Livelihoods During the COVID-19 Crisis: Closing the Gaps in Safety Nets*' provides information about various strategies adopted by governments in countries around the globe in providing quick livelihood assistance to people (see: OECD, 'Supporting Livelihoods during the COVID-19 Crisis: Closing the Gaps in Safety Nets', *OECD ILibrary* (Paris, 20 May 2020), https://www.oecd-ilibrary.org/content/paper/17cbb92d-en).
7. According to the US Census, government assistance lifted 45.4 million people out of poverty in 2021, https://www.census.gov/library/stories/2022/09/government-assistance-lifts-millions-out-of-poverty.html.
8. Tronto, *Moral Boundaries.*
9. Ibid.

10. Sunita George and Raymond Greene, 'Care Ethics in the Time of COVID-19: Are We Our Brother's Keepers? Some Insights from the Efforts of "Food for Chennai," India', *Research in Political Sociology* 29 (May 2022): 127–54.
11. Tronto, *Moral Boundaries,* 101.
12. Sara Ruddick, *Maternal Thinking* (Boston, MA: Beacon Press, 1989).
13. Tronto, *Moral Boundaries*, 118.
14. In a Facebook Messenger interview with us, Dubay remarked, 'Who likes to eat restaurant food when they are sick? You want to eat your mother's *Rasam* and bland food, no?'
15. The care packages delivered to the sick included handwritten notes, handcrafted cards and contact information, in case the recipient of the package needed to connect. In some cases, the sick individuals requested the kind of meals they were craving, and while this was not always realizable, many times the caregivers tried to fulfil their desires.
16. Jordan Pascoe and Mitch Stripling, 'Surging Solidarity: Reorienting Ethics for Pandemics', *Kennedy Institute of Ethics Journal* 30, no. 3–4 (2020): 419–44.
17. Rebecca Solnit, *A Paradise Built in Hell* (New York: Penguin, 2010).
18. Pascoe and Stripling, 'Surging Solidarity', 421.
19. George and Greene, 'Care Ethics in the Time of COVID-19'.
20. Much of the literature emerging from empirical studies during the pandemic highlights the negative impacts on public health by social media influencers who were instrumental in spreading misinformation and conspiracy theories about the dangers of vaccines and fake cures for the virus. (See: Michael A. Gisondi et al., 'A Deadly Infodemic: Social Media and the Power of COVID-19 Misinformation', *Journal of Medical Internet Research* 24, no. 2 (2022): e35552; Eva L. Jenkins et al., 'Strategies to Improve Health Communication: Can Health Professionals Be Heroes?', *Nutrients* 12, no. 6 (2020): 1861; Amy E. Leader et al., 'Understanding the Messages and Motivation of Vaccine Hesitant or Refusing Social Media Influencers', *Vaccine* 39, no. 2 (2020): 350–6.)
21. Essi Pöyry, Hanna Reinikainen and Vilma Luoma-Aho, 'The Role of Social Media Influencers in Public Health Communication: Case COVID-19 Pandemic', *International Journal of Strategic Communication* 16, no. 3 (2022): 469–84.
22. Robert B. Cialdini, *Influence: The Psychology of Persuasion* (Melbourne: Business Library, 1994).
23. Robert Cialdini, in his book *Influence: The Psychology of Persuasion*, explores the principles of influence and persuasion. He identifies six key principles of persuasion – reciprocity, commitment, social proof, authority, liking and scarcity – that are often used in marketing and sales and other arenas to influence decision making. (See: Cialdini, *Influence*.)
24. Pöyry, Reinikainen and Luoma-Aho, 'The Role of Social Media Influencers in Public Health Communication'.
25. Michael T. Lee and Carol Theokary, 'The Superstar Social Media Influencer: Exploiting Linguistic Style and Emotional Contagion over Content?', *Journal of Business Research* 132 (November 2020): 860–71.
26. Fisher and Tronto, 'Toward a Feminist Theory of Caring'.
27. Tronto, *Moral Boundaries*.
28. Ibid.
29. Ibid., 132.
30. Paul Ricœur, *Oneself as Another*, trans. Kathleen Blamey (Chicago, IL: University of Chicago Press, 1994), 192.

31. She was featured as one of India's 100 COVID-19 heroes in a campaign called #Dettolsalutes, a collaborative effort by The Better India and Dettol India to highlight the work of caring done by ordinary citizens during the pandemic. A picture of the heroes along with their story was featured on their limited-edition liquid soap bottles.
32. Giovanni Maio, 'Fundamentals of an Ethics of Care', in *Care in Healthcare: Reflections on Theory and Practice*, ed. Franziska Krause and Joachim Boldt (Cham: Springer International Publishing, 2018), 59.

BIBLIOGRAPHY

Cialdini, Robert B. *Influence: The Psychology of Persuasion*. Melbourne: Business Library, 1994.

Fisher, Berenice and Joan C. Tronto. 'Toward a Feminist Theory of Caring', in *Circles of Care: Work and Identity in Women's Lives*, edited by Emily K. Abel and Margaret K. Nelson, 36–54. Albany: SUNY Press, 1990.

George, Sunita, and Raymond Greene. 'Care Ethics in the Time of COVID-19: Are We Our Brother's Keepers? Some Insights from the Efforts of "Food for Chennai," India', *Research in Political Sociology* 29 (May 2022): 127–54. https://doi.org/10.1108/s0895-993520220000029012.

Gisondi, Michael A., Rachel Barber, Jeremy Samuel Faust, Ali Raja, Matthew C. Strehlow, Lauren M. Westafer and Michael Gottlieb. 'A Deadly Infodemic: Social Media and the Power of COVID-19 Misinformation', *Journal of Medical Internet Research* 24, no. 2 (2022). https://doi.org/10.2196/35552.

Henley, Jon. 'Finland Enlists Social Influencers in Fight against Covid-19', *The Guardian*, 1 April 2020. https://www.theguardian.com/world/2020/apr/01/finland-enlists-social-influencers-in-fight-against-covid-19.

Jenkins, Eva L., Jasmina Ilicic, Annika Molenaar, Shinyi Chin and Tracy A. McCaffrey. 'Strategies to Improve Health Communication: Can Health Professionals Be Heroes?', *Nutrients* 12, no. 6 (2020): 1861. https://doi.org/10.3390/nu12061861.

Krause, Franziska, and Joachim Boldt. *Care in Healthcare: Reflections on Theory and Practice*. Cham: Springer International Publishing, 2018.

Leader, Amy E., Amelia Burke-Garcia, Philip M. Massey and Jill B. Roark. 'Understanding the Messages and Motivation of Vaccine Hesitant or Refusing Social Media Influencers', *Vaccine* 39, no. 2 (2020). https://doi.org/10.1016/j.vaccine.2020.11.058.

Lee, Michael T., and Carol Theokary. 'The Superstar Social Media Influencer: Exploiting Linguistic Style and Emotional Contagion over Content?', *Journal of Business Research* 132 (November 2020): 860–971. https://doi.org/10.1016/j.jbusres.2020.11.014.

Maio, Giovanni. 'Fundamentals of an Ethics of Care', in *Care in Healthcare: Reflections on Theory and Practice*, 51–63. Cham: Springer International Publishing, 2018.

OECD. 'Supporting Livelihoods during the COVID-19 Crisis: Closing the Gaps in Safety Nets', *OECD ILibrary*. Paris, 20 May 2020. https://www.oecd-ilibrary.org/content/paper/17cbb92d-en.

Pascoe, Jordan, and Mitch Stripling. 'Surging Solidarity: Reorienting Ethics for Pandemics', *Kennedy Institute of Ethics Journal* 30, no. 3–4 (2020): 419–44. https://doi.org/10.1353/ken.2020.0022.

Pöyry, Essi, Hanna Reinikainen and Vilma Luoma-Aho. 'The Role of Social Media Influencers in Public Health Communication: Case COVID-19 Pandemic', *International Journal of Strategic Communication* 16, no. 3 (2022): 469–84. https://doi.org/10.1080/1553118x.2022.2042694.

Ricœur, Paul. *Oneself as Another*. Translated by Kathleen Blamey. Chicago, IL: University of Chicago Press, 1994.

Ruddick, Sara. *Maternal Thinking*. Boston, MA: Beacon Press, 1989.

Solnit, Rebecca. *A Paradise Built in Hell*. New York: Penguin, 2010.

Tronto, Joan C. *Moral Boundaries: A Political Argument for an Ethics of Care*. London: Routledge, 1993.

Tronto, Joan C. *Caring Democracy: Markets, Equality, and Justice*. New York: NYU Press, 2013.

CHAPTER SEVENTEEN

Queer care and pleasure activism

AMY MCKIERNAN

INTRODUCTION: THE MOMENTS BEFORE

In 'Your Emergency Contact Has Experienced An Emergency', Chen Chen dedicates the poem 'Elegy While Listening to a Song I Can't Help But Start to Move to' to Pulse, the gay nightclub where forty-nine people were murdered on 12 June 2016 in Orlando, Florida, almost all of whom were Latinx.[1] Chen begins, 'what breaks me is their giddy, their swaying,/ moments before' and asks, 'how does a body forget all danger & become song, swoon?'[2] There is much to learn from how LGBTQIA+ community members care for each other while grieving and expressing righteous anger in contexts of homophobic and transphobic violence.[3] With Chen, though, I also think about the moments before the violence, not to avoid looking directly at this violence, but to remember the joyful anticipation, storytelling on the way to the club, smiling from across the room, and experiences of delight that risk getting overshadowed by focusing only on the violence and its aftermath. The poem ends, 'their laughter. I keep hearing their laughter, moments before.'[4]

In an interview about this poem, J.A. Dela Cruz-Smith says to Chen, 'I really appreciate how you close that poem with their laughter. It was such a wonderful way to honor their lives, to honor their fun, to honor their dancing.'[5] Chen responds:

> What I feel most moved by is not pain or suffering. What I'm moved by, is people trying to go through the world and find connection and kindness despite it all, despite how unjust and cruel so much of the world can be. They're still seeking it or longing for it, or trying to build it, to connect with more people and better.[6]

It is true that those who fear expressions of queer and trans flourishing have tried to eradicate it. They have attempted to straighten out, convert, and explain us away as unfortunate (at best) anomalies. These attempts at eradication take many forms: shame, surveillance, incarceration, humiliation, silencing, mistrust, abuse and neglect, grief denied, healthcare denied, employment denied, self-expression denied, family denied, boundaries policed and conformity rewarded.

This chapter considers how, 'despite it all', we still aim 'to connect with more people and better'.[7] I argue for the value of engaging with what adrienne maree brown calls 'pleasure activism' when theorizing and practising care ethics. I understand this as an accountability practice aimed at making sure care ethicists do not mostly focus on the meaning of care ethics in relation to queer and trans suffering and death. Queer and trans theorists and activists have considered the danger of overemphasizing violence and death in relation to queer and trans care. For example, in *Trans Care*, Hil Malatino[8] writes, 'Aftercare is a concept that might move us beyond a focus on death, and in particular the spectacular homicides that continue to be enacted upon trans women of color, characterized by a form of violence that Eric Stanley has termed "overkill".'[9] Making explicit connections between care ethics and pleasure activism serves as a reminder of the importance of considering, not only the survival-based needs of queer and trans members of our communities, but also the desires and the pleasures that contribute to queer and trans flourishing.

In this chapter, I begin by defining pleasure activism. Then, I devote one section to each of the five features of the ethics of care identified by Virginia Held in *The Ethics of Care: Personal, Political, and Global*. In these sections, I explain the feature and demonstrate how attention to pleasure activism can hold care ethicists accountable for affirming queer and trans flourishing, not merely attending to harms against queer and trans community members. Based on this analysis, I think it is important to advance an ethics of care attuned to, at least, these three aims: those theorizing and practising care ethics should (1) seek liberation from oppressive social norms and expectations for all people; (2) not remain complacent in ways that trade the pleasurable comfort of conformity for the further isolation, shame, and suffering of marginalized others; and (3) make an effort to emphasize the creative ways queer and trans people are building communities of care anchored in radical ways of loving ourselves and each other, including emphasizing models of care that rethink the dominance of the traditional nuclear family.

There is no one-size-fits-all way to attend to these aims (and this is good). I do not assume the acronym LGBTQIA+ represents a monolithic group and by writing about 'queer and trans' experiences, I mean for this phrase to be inclusive of important differences. In the introduction to *Pleasure Activism*, brown writes, 'trust is a crucial part of the intimacy that yields pleasure for ourselves and others. Most likely you don't know me, so whatever trust can exist between us will come from how well I can share and how much you can open yourself to what I share.'[10] Most likely you don't know me, so I, too, will briefly share. I write as a queer, cis, white woman. I am neurodivergent, love living alone and do not plan to get married, and am happily partnered. I connect deeply with animals, know the grief of watching my father die when I was a child, and the PTSD that followed. I love to swim and hike in the Pennsylvania woods. My friends are my 'other significant others', and I have a supportive family, including an almost two-year-old, to whom I am so proud to be an aunt.[11] I know the growth and harm that can come from placing trust in religious institutions. I regularly practise internal family systems therapy, though going to therapy and taking medication made me feel ashamed when I was younger. I love to play dungeons and dragons; I am a theatre kid at heart.[12]

Throughout this chapter, I do my best to include a wide range of perspectives while resisting co-optation, tokenism and exploitation. As relational selves situated in multiple groups, we may find ourselves oppressed by virtue of one part of our identity, while privileged due to another part. On this point, Iris Marion Young explains:

> This view of group differentiation as multiple, cross-cutting, fluid, and shifting implies another critique of the model of the autonomous, unified self. In complex, highly differentiated societies like our own, all persons have multiple group identifications. The culture, perspective, and relations of privilege and oppression of these various

> groups, moreover, may not cohere. Thus individual persons, as constituted partly by their group affinities and relations, cannot be unified, themselves are heterogeneous and not necessarily coherent.[13]

With these important differences in mind, I suggest that care ethicists use the three aforementioned aims as helpful reminders when developing accounts of what constitutes morally good care, especially given how often queer and trans people have experienced paternalistic bad care in the name of what is 'for their own good' or 'best for them'.

Finally, by way of introduction, I want to say that before beginning work on an effort called 'Care Ethics Otherwise', with Sarah Clark Miller and Hil Malatino, I thought of myself as something like 'care curious'. I sometimes struggled to connect with care ethics. I endorsed so much of what care ethicists said, especially about the importance of valuing emotions in our moral lives and rethinking the influence of traditional, patriarchal public and private divisions in moral theory. Yet, as I continued to grow into the person and ethicist who I am today, I needed some alternative ways to reconsider (1) the meaning of the 'maternal' in care ethics and (2) the focus on the child as the paradigmatic figure representing the cared-for in a carer/ cared-for dyad.[14]

When offered the opportunity to serve as co-editors for a special issue of *Essays in Philosophy* focused on care ethics, Hil, Sarah, and I issued a call to 'the margins, to the underground, to unconventional domains' to queer care ethics in generative ways. This special issue led to a conference by the same name in June 2023 at Penn State University, an interdisciplinary gathering devoted to theorizing care ethics and care theory in new directions. I owe a lot to the folks who have come together to explore 'caring otherwise' because of the plentiful examples of diverse and radical care they have offered this community.

It is my hope that this chapter creates space within this anthology for readers to consider how queer and trans care affirms, challenges and expands previously developed accounts of care ethics. As far as moral theories go, these are early days for care ethics. Dismantling homophobia, transphobia, racism, classism, misogyny, ableism and other forms of oppression will require ongoing critical and creative engagement with care ethics. As Maggie Nelson says, 'if we want to do more than claw our way into repressive structures, we have our work cut out for us'.[15] As we theorize and practise care with the aim of dismantling oppression, we would do well to keep in mind Audre Lorde's call for us to move beyond mere necessity and convenience, to move beyond 'the shoddy, the conventionally expected', to connect with the erotic in ourselves and each other:

> For the erotic is not a question only of what we do; it is a question of how acutely and fully we can feel in the doing. Once we know the extent to which we are capable of feeling that sense of satisfaction and completion, we can then observe which of our various life endeavors bring us closer to that fullness.[16]

17.1 WHAT IS PLEASURE ACTIVISM?

In *Pleasure Activism: The Politics of Feeling Good*, readers are quickly made aware that the 'pleasure' in 'pleasure activism' is not merely a pursuit of individual preferences. Much like Virginia Held explains 'we need an *ethics* of care, not just care itself',[17] pleasure activism is not merely committed to advancing pleasure in and of itself.[18] brown explains, 'I have seen, over and over, the connection between tuning into what brings aliveness into our systems and being able to access personal, relational, and communal power.'[19] Tuning into what feels good can illuminate the ways we are already embedded in our relationships to self, others, ancestors, social institutions and shared ecosystems. This serves as a fruitful entry point for thinking about the breadth and depth of our interconnectedness, a core component of care ethics.

While it may be tempting to think about pleasure as a luxury aimed at individual satisfaction, brown's pleasure activism is deeply concerned with questions of care and justice:

> Pleasure activism is the work we do to reclaim our whole, happy, and satisfiable selves from the impacts, delusions, and limitations of oppression and/or supremacy. Pleasure activism asserts that we all need and deserve pleasure and that our social structures must reflect this. In this moment, we must prioritize the pleasure of those most impacted by oppression. Pleasure activists seek to understand and learn from the politics and power dynamics inside of everything that makes us feel good. … Pleasure activism includes work and life lived in the realms of satisfaction, joy, and erotic aliveness that bring about social and political change. Ultimately, pleasure activism is us learning to make justice and liberation the most pleasurable experiences we can have on this planet.[20]

In direct conversation with Audre Lorde's 'Uses of the Erotic: The Erotic as Power', brown asks, 'How do we learn to harness the power and wisdom of pleasure, rather than trying to erase the body, the erotic, the connective tissue from society?'[21] Lorde's influence runs through *Pleasure Activism*, motivating a commitment to exploring pleasures and desires in the face of domination and oppression. brown explains why she shifts from 'erotic' to 'pleasure' in her work, 'I am aware that Lorde uses the language of the erotic, which specifies the pleasures and aliveness associated with sex. I love the erotic, and it's all over this book, but I also wanted to broaden the scope to all the experiences that bring us happiness, aliveness, transcendence – which is why this is *pleasure* activism and not *erotic* activism.'[22]

brown recounts first reading and hearing 'Uses of the Erotic' when she was in college. I also discovered Lorde's collection *Sister Outsider* in my early twenties. I still have the coffee-stained copy of the book from the campus women's centre where I worked. I vividly remember my first time with this text. Reading 'Uses of the Erotic' floored me. I emailed my dear friend who had recently moved to New York City to tell her to go find the book and read 'Uses of the Erotic' as soon as she could. I remember the urgency, the buzz, the feeling of needing to share this sacred text about creativity, excellence and the erotic. She called me later to tell me that when she asked the bookstore clerk where she could find Lorde, they directed her to the 'Gay and Lesbian' section. We marvelled at how taboo and dangerous that felt to two young women who attended Catholic school from grade school through college.

Twenty years later, I'm still floored. Lorde's words knock me back, wake me up, and remind me, if and when I can, to get in touch with erotic power. I have desires that stretch far beyond mere survival towards freedom and pleasure. I'll spend my whole life feeling grateful for and accountable to Lorde's work. I say this wanting to honour Lorde as 'Black lesbian feminist'.[23] Additionally, *Pleasure Activism*, brown explains, 'includes a few voices that are not Black or woman-identified but that I trust in the human experience of finding pleasure beyond oppression'.[24] I aim to join in this chorus of voices led by Black queer women helping to spread the word about pleasure activism such that we might explicitly incorporate this wisdom into theorizing and practising care ethics.

One might wonder, isn't it a privilege to focus on pleasure when there is so much harm we ought to attend to if we take our caring responsibilities seriously? Isn't this especially true in the context of the violence queer and trans people face every day across the world? These are good questions. In their most recent book, *The Future is Disabled: Prophecies, Love Notes, and Mourning Songs*, author of the influential *Care Work: Dreaming Disability Justice*, Leah Lakshmi Piepzna-Samarasinha addresses this concern:

> 'Pleasure activism,' the term coined by writer and activist adrienne maree brown to mean a politic that uplifts joy and pleasure in activism and radical life, is both a beloved and controversial concept among people I know. I have a piece about the pleasures of giving and receiving care in brown's book *Pleasure Activism*. I appreciate a focus on joy and sensuality in activism and the lives we make, as a form of healing, prefiguratively making the lives and communities we want in the Good Future to happen now, and also just helping us withstand the struggle. I also have had friends make reasonable critiques of how they see some people using the term 'pleasure activism' to lift up individual self-care and hedonism as the world burns, without a class analysis of who gets to afford certain pleasures and how we define pleasure with regards to what things cost.[25]

Piepzna-Samarasinha notes that, while they appreciate the fair criticisms of some uses of terms like 'pleasure activism' and 'rest is radical', it is important to remember that '[a] s disabled people, particularly disabled BIPOC, wild disability joy and disabled forms of pleasure – including kinds that are not legible to abled and neurotypical people, or that they are repelled by – are a core part of our resistance'[26] and 'disabled people are the best people I know at prioritizing pleasure in our lives'.[27]

One might also worry that pleasure activism amounts to 'rainbow capitalism' or 'pink washing'. I am writing this in June 2024 in the United States. I am surrounded by corporate celebrations of all things 'equality', 'love' and 'respect' – that is, until the rainbow products are replaced with the 'freedom', 'liberty' and flag-themed items in time for Independence Day on 4 July. Rest assured I am not suggesting that care ethicists should buy into some corporate attempt to paint smiles and rainbows over violence. Suggesting that we bring brown's pleasure activism into more deliberate contact with care ethics does not mean that we should neglect homophobic and transphobic oppression in favour of this shallow corporate window dressing. As will become clear, pleasure activism includes evaluating how our desires and capacities to experience pleasure have been shaped by oppressive social, political and economic forces.[28]

Having addressed some initial worries about a focus on pleasure activism in care ethics, including the worry that we should focus on suffering instead and the worry that pleasure activism amounts to corporate co-optation, I now turn to the exciting potential I see for bridging care ethics and pleasure activism in more explicit ways. For the purpose of this chapter, I rely on the five features of the ethics of care developed by Virginia Held in *The Ethics of Care: Personal, Political, and Global*. I welcome readers to make additional connections between aspects of care ethics and pleasure activism that I do not cover here.

17.2 FOCUS ON DEPENDENCY AND VULNERABILITY

Held begins: 'care is both value and practice'.[29] When I teach this chapter in my 'Practical Ethics' course, I ask students what they think Held means by this. Students offer insightful examples of how a diverse range of needs and practices might get lost if we generalize or idealize too much about care. So, we spend some time thinking about what is universal in care ethics given these important differences. We tend to arrive at our mortality and our interdependence. Held explains that most care ethicists understand our shared dependency as a feature that unites members of the moral community:

> First, the central focus of the ethics of care is on the compelling moral salience of attending to and meeting the needs of the particular others for whom we take responsibility. Caring for one's child, for instance, may well and defensibly be at the forefront of a person's moral concerns. The ethics of care recognizes that human beings are dependent for many years of their lives, that the moral claim of those dependent on us for the care they need is pressing, and that there are highly important moral aspects in developing the relations of caring that enable human beings to live and progress.[30]

Key here is Held's claim that there is 'moral salience' in our experiences of giving and receiving care throughout our lives. We are interdependent creatures deeply invested in each other's lives, even when this investment does not carry the urgency of my immediate need for you to keep me alive. As Held notes, 'there are highly important moral aspects in developing the relations of caring that enable human beings to live and progress'.[31] I am interested in reminding us not to forget the 'progress' part of this claim as we work to identify and meet basic needs. Flourishing is, I think, the point of ethics. Or, Lorde might say, 'The aim of each thing which we do is to make our lives and the lives of our children richer and more possible.'[32]

Here, I see potential for pleasure activism to remind us that when we speak of features of care ethics like dependency, need, vulnerability and precarity, it is helpful to draw distinctions between these terms. This way, we have a strong vocabulary through which we can differentiate between basic needs for survival and the desires and pleasures involved in aiming for flourishing. To this end, in 'From Vulnerability to Precariousness: Examining the Moral Foundations of Care Ethics', Sarah Clark Miller offers the following helpful distinctions: 'need suggests an absence. Vulnerability expresses an openness to some form of reception. Dependence calls to mind a leaning on another, while precariousness implies a teetering perch from which one could well fall. Care, for its part, signifies a response to all four circumstances.'[33] Miller's discussion of vulnerability is well positioned to shed light on a fruitful connection between care ethics and pleasure activism. She clarifies:

> Vulnerability represents a manner of openness to the world and other people – for example, corporeal, psychological, or emotional openness – over which we have limited control. Initially, scholars tended to understand vulnerability as exposure to types of harm … More recently, however, philosophers have emphasized that vulnerability should be understood not solely or even primarily in the negative sense of susceptibility to harm. The receptivity that our vulnerability signifies means we are open to a whole host of experiences – positive, negative, and many in between – and, therefore, is a concept that should not be understood merely in terms of potential injury of some kind. Instead, there are forms of vulnerability that we should value.[34]

As we consider queer and trans experiences and expressions of care, we need not only think of vulnerability in 'the negative sense of susceptibility to harm'.[35] Instead, vulnerability offers a point of entry for care ethicists to get curious about how embracing the moral salience of our shared dependency and vulnerability offers opportunities for growth and expansion. brown says, 'pleasure activists believe that by tapping into the potential goodness in each of us we can generate justice and liberation, growing a healing abundance where we have been socialized to believe only scarcity exists'.[36] So, when it comes to the first feature Held describes, pleasure activism offers pathways by which we can get curious about how our shared dependency and vulnerability can facilitate openness to flourishing beyond harm reduction.

17.3 CARE ETHICS VALUES EMOTIONS

Held introduces a second feature common to most articulations of care ethics. Emotions are not dismissed as corrupting or distracting forces in our moral lives. Emotions can direct our attention to who and what we care about. Held quickly anticipates the following objection and responds, 'this is not to say that raw emotion can be a guide to morality; feelings need to be reflected on and educated. But from the care perspective, moral inquiries that rely entirely on reason and rationalistic deductions or calculations are seen as deficient.'[37] She explains that emotions also have the power to fuel domination and facilitate harm, so, the emotions that accompany 'various aspects and expressions of care and caring relations need to be subjected to moral scrutiny and evaluated, not just observed and described'.[38]

This careful attention to the role that emotions play in our moral lives works well with the critical thinking and curiosity involved in pleasure activism. Pleasure activism is not about generating *excessive* pleasure. brown writes,

> sometimes when I bring up this work to people, I can see a bacchanalia unfold in their eyes, and it makes me feel tender. I think because most of us are so repressed, our fantasies go to extremes to counterbalance all that contained longing. Pleasure activism is about learning what it means to be satisfiable, to generate, from within and from between us, an abundance from which we can all have enough.[39]

Further, when we consider how to create the conditions where queer and trans joy can thrive, we may find ourselves interrogating so many of our assumptions about what constitutes 'a good life'. We may find ourselves critically examining our desires as we become curious about what full-bodied flourishing would feel like. Pleasure activism includes getting curious about so-called 'negative' emotions like anger, shame, envy and grief. For example, I smiled when I read the following in Amia Srinivasan's *The Right to Sex*: 'what if the envy you feel for another woman's body, her face, her charm, her ease, her brilliance, were not envy at all – but desire?'[40] I remember when this dawned on me about some of my own desires. I recall wishing I looked more like other girls, then, as I aged, like other women. Over time, I experienced the transformation of this envy into pleasurable desire. Sometimes erotic desire; sometimes other kinds of admiration, especially as I learned more about my sexuality. I let myself be vulnerable to this experience, and I am so glad I did. Our emotions and desires can be sites of critical thinking and personal transformation about what we feel and why. However, without the space to do this while feeling safe enough and free enough to transform, it will be difficult to engage with our emotions in the ways that Held describes as valuable for our moral lives.[41]

On this point, in a chapter of *Pleasure Activism* called 'Confessions of a Queer Sex Goddess', brown writes:

> One of the most important areas of pleasure activism is to acknowledge and unlearn the regressive beliefs inside our own pursuit of pleasure. I have been on my own journey of decolonization in the work of crafting these pages. It is embarrassing to name, but one key area of this kind of unlearning in my life has been around sex with partners of the same sex. It's taken me most of my life to have this particular aha, that 'gay sex' is not abnormal or subpar or missing something or evil or even gay. It's just dope.[42]

Here, we see the kind of scrutiny and evaluation of emotions that Held describes as crucial if emotions are to be considered valuable for our moral lives. I know the feelings of embarrassment, shame and fear that can accompany queer desires. If I took these feelings at face value as if they merely *revealed* something about the moral dimensions of my desires, I would (and did) think of myself as sinful or broken. Care ethics and pleasure activism stress the importance of feeling our emotions, and interrogating these feelings with the aim of unlearning internalized oppression and 'regressive beliefs'.

17.4 CARE ETHICS VALUES RELATIONSHIPS WITH PARTICULAR OTHERS

The third feature Held discusses deals with care ethics and partiality. For so long, I assumed partiality was a bad word in moral theory and practice. Yet, Held clarifies that care ethics 'rejects the view of the dominant moral theories that the more abstract the reasoning about a moral problem the better because the more likely to avoid bias and arbitrariness, the more nearly to achieve impartiality. The ethics of care respects rather than removes itself from the claims of particular others with whom we share actual relationships.'[43] As a moral theory, the ethics of care does not require us to take an objective or impartial stance towards significant others like friends and family. When a moral question or conflict emerges with loved ones, we need not bracket the commitments that come along with our love and shut down our vulnerability in order to engage in moral deliberation. This is not to say that there are not some domains of ethics where attempting impartiality makes sense. Held elaborates:

> The ethics of care may seek to limit the applicability of universal rules to certain domains where they are more appropriate, like the domain of law, and resist their extension to other domains. Such rules may simply be inappropriate in, for instance, the contexts of family and friendship, yet relations in these domains should certainly be evaluated, not merely described, hence morality should not be limited to abstract rules. We should be able to give moral guidance concerning actual relations that are trusting, considerate, and caring and concerning those that are not.[44]

Held makes it clear that care ethicists can and should have something to say about how to engage in moral inquiry without stripping away the richness, depth and partiality that come from loving our significant others.

Here, I want to flag the fact that care ethicists are not immune from what we might call objectivity drift (or creep). Bracketing the kinds of complex commitments that constitute caring relationships can make theorizing more straightforward. Zena Sharman focuses on her experiences with care ethics inside and outside of academia. Sharman shares her frustration with some academic writing that sanitizes care by neglecting experiences of giving and receiving care in real time and practice:

> I feel a sense of detachment when I read more conventionally academic accounts of care ethics where care is held at a distance like an object to be turned over and examined, or conceptualized as a scarce resource to be distributed. Care recipients are positioned as dependent subjects who deserve better and ought to be protected from the ravages of neoliberalism. There are flashes of passion and glimmers of lived experiences in these writings and what I perceive to be deeply-felt desires for societal transformation, yet they often feel hemmed in by the conventions of discipline and the strictures of academic voice. I poked curiously at my feelings of frustration as I put the used wet wipes in the garbage can, flushed my kid's poop down the toilet, and washed my hands. What was it about these experiences of reading that felt so irritating to me? I found my answer in the very act of butt-wiping: that is, a yearning for theorizing about care and more care-full futures that engages with the messy, embodied, durational, and relational aspects of care work and the everyday/night solidarities, interdependencies, and survival strategies it's embedded in.[45]

brown's pleasure activism is filled with interviews, stories and rich descriptions of pleasure practices. brown says:

> In these pages, I am intentionally bringing academics into conversation with experiential experts, to show the patterns of aligned interest and learning happening across the language barriers that exist between us. I am bringing together a lot of different styles of expression in order to weave this tale. I asked contributors to share themselves as whole people, in the spirit of the Combahee River Collective, who taught me that 'from the personal, the striving toward wholeness individually and within the community, comes the political, the struggle against those forces that render individuals and communities unwhole. The personal is political, especially for Black women.' Each person in this text is whole, complex, and brave in how they are shaping the world around them.[46]

As a philosopher, I experience the temptation to bracket where I should 'be able to give moral guidance concerning actual relations that are trusting, considerate, and caring and concerning those that are not'.[47] As care ethics continues to develop as a moral theory and gets taken seriously by more academic philosophers, we should be wary of *why* it is being taken seriously. We should be careful of the kind of sanitizing to fit convention that Sharman describes. Engaging with pleasure activism keeps me honest on this front. Further, when thinking about queer and trans care, the intentional bringing together of academics *and* experiential experts is especially important to avoid making assumptions about what it means to be 'whole, complex, and brave' for members of such a diverse community. This focus on the personal as political leads well into the fourth characteristic of the ethics of care.[48]

17.5 CARE ETHICS VALUES RETHINKING THE PUBLIC AND PRIVATE

It is not uncommon to hear queer and trans folks talk about 'chosen family' or 'queer kinship'. This family can be created over and against a family of origin that has neglected, rejected, or been violent towards a person because of their sexual orientation and/or gender identity. If we assume that this treatment falls outside the scope of ethics because it is 'private' or 'a family affair', we risk failing to attend to serious moral harms experienced by queer and trans members of our community. Held explains that insofar as the ethics of care is a feminist ethical theory, it is committed to a thorough rethinking of the public and private domains:

> Feminists have shown how the greater social, political, economic, and cultural power of men has structured this 'private' sphere to the disadvantage of women and children, rendering them vulnerable to domestic violence without outside interference, often leaving women economically dependent on men and subject to a highly inequitable division of labor in the family. The law has not hesitated to intervene into women's private decisions concerning reproduction but has been highly reluctant to intrude on men's exercise of coercive power within the 'castles' of their homes. Dominant moral theories have seen 'public' life as relevant to morality while missing the moral significance of the 'private' domains of family and friendship. Thus the dominant theories have assumed that morality should be sought for unrelated, independent, and mutually indifferent individuals assumed to be equal.[49]

Importantly, as we rethink the public and private in bringing care ethics together with queer and trans experiences, we should consider that some queer and trans people may only be deemed 'socially acceptable' if they 'appropriately' reproduce dominant public and private dynamics. In *The Care Manifesto: The Politics of Interdependence,* the Care Collective warns against maintaining a strong social commitment to the traditional nuclear family:

> The traditional nuclear family still provides the prototype for care and for contemporary notions of kinship, all stemming from the mythic ramifications of the first 'maternal bond.' This remains true even as queer people have been increasingly incorporated into the mainstream – on the condition that they reproduce the traditional nuclear-family model. Our circles of care have not broadened out but have, in fact, become painfully narrow. These caring arrangements are unreliable and unjust. The nuclear family cannot be the assumed basic unit of care, nor can market outsourcing be the solution to the gender inequality of current care expectations or practices.[50]

This passage from *The Care Collective* calls to mind brown's chapter in *Pleasure Activism* titled 'Love as Political Resistance'. Here, she writes, 'We don't learn to love in a linear path, from self to family to friends to spouse, as we might have been taught. We learn to love by loving. We practice with each other, on ourselves, in all kinds of relationships.'[51] Insights from pleasure activism can assist in imagining what broadening these 'painfully narrow' circles of care might look like. For example, on 14 February 2017, ALOK posted this on their webpage. I appreciate how they demonstrate how we can rethink the public and private, including the dominance of the traditional nuclear family. ALOK imagines:

> i want a world where friendship is appreciated as a form of romance. i want a world where when people ask if we are seeing anyone we can list the names of all of our best friends and no one will bat an eyelid. i want monuments and holidays and certificates and ceremonies to commemorate friendship. i want a world that doesn't require us to be in a sexual/romantic partnership to be seen as mature (let alone complete). i want a movement that fights for all forms of relationships, not just the sexual ones.

> i want thousands of songs and movies and poems about the intimacy between friends. i want a world where our worth isn't linked to our desireability, our security to our monogamy, our family to our biology.[52]

As we move to rethink the public and private in care ethics, it is important to stay curious about how we can expand our vocabulary and practices to include more possibilities for honouring relationships with significant others that are both personal and political, through and through.

17.6 CARE ETHICS VALUES A RELATIONAL CONCEPTION OF THE SELF

The final feature Held discusses as common across approaches to care ethics is a shift away from individualism towards an understanding of the self as relational. Care ethics posits that '[e]very person starts out as a child dependent on those providing us care, and we remain interdependent with others in thoroughly fundamental ways throughout our lives. That we can think and act as if we were independent depends on a network of social relations making it possible for us to do so.'[53] This focus on the self as relational and interdependent invites us to think critically about accounts of moral agency that seem to position the moral agent as radically self-sufficient. We need others to survive, and our actions can harm or nurture people at the level of *who* they are and who they feel free enough to become.

When I first read *Pleasure Activism*, I thought so much about how brown models what it can look like to take seriously the claim that the self is relational without suggesting that there is no 'self' or the 'self' is an illusion. In the introduction, she invites readers to get to know her by sharing 'a bit about my identity, contradictions, practices, and desires as they relate to pleasure'.[54] The section immediately following the introduction is called, 'Who Taught You To Feel Good?' In this section, brown constructs the lineage of those who instructed her on the path to becoming a pleasure activist. At the conclusion of this section, she encourages readers to do the same: 'Write up *your* pleasure activism lineage! Who awakened your senses? Who politicized your experiences of body, identity, sensation, feeling good?'[55] The book itself is a whole made up of autobiographical contributions, interviews, standalone essays by others, and invitations to readers. Because the self is relational and interdependent, we have so much to offer each other as 'part of a natural world that is constantly changing, and we need to learn to adapt together and stay in relationship if we hope to survive as a species'.[56] The text reflects this commitment in content and form.

CONCLUSION: TO 'CONNECT WITH MORE PEOPLE AND BETTER'

In December 2021, I logged in to 'The Revolution Is My Personfriend: Dismantling the Romance Myth', a Zoom lecture with Dean Spade, sponsored by The Poetry Project. Zoom felt like second nature in the context of the global pandemic and I had long loved Dean Spade's work. When I first read the following in 'For Lovers and Fighters', it felt like taking a deep breath:

> One of my goals in thinking about redefining the way we view relationships is to try to treat the people I date more like I treat my friends to be respectful and thoughtful

> and have boundaries and reasonable expectations – and to try to treat my friends more like my dates – to give them special attention, honor my commitments to them, be consistent, and invest deeply in our futures together.[57]

The nearly 100 participants contributed to the chat when prompted to share examples of how the romance myth takes hold from a young age. This myth, Spade argues, is one we 'have been immersed in all our lives', supported by the 'corporate media, diet and beauty industries, and the legal marriage system that determines things like who has healthcare, housing, and immigration status'. An hour in, Spade shared a slide titled 'The Truth About Romance':

> The idea that there is scarcity of partners, or only one right person, is harmful. Many of the needs we are encouraged to meet through romantic and sexual connections like sexual gratification, physical affection, affirmation about our appearance, play, intellectual stimulation, feeling seen, companionship, sharing our stories, caring labor, sharing holidays, sharing meals and cohabitation, can be met through friendships, family and/or though our relationship with ourselves.[58]

Spade went on to explain that one of the best things to happen to him was learning to ask, 'Who do I want to do that with?'

When I started to imagine this chapter, I looked at my bookshelf and thought, 'Who do I want to do this with?' Some texts nearly jumped off the shelf; others showed themselves over time. In the 'Outro' of *Pleasure Activism*, brown writes, 'pulling the essays and interviews [in the book] together has been medicinal for me, and I hope that something in here helps with your own liberation'.[59] I hope this is true of this chapter. Care ethics is well-positioned to insist on the importance of affirming the depth of thinking and feeling that can come from learning how 'to connect with more people and better'.[60] In Chen's use of 'better', I hear a commitment to what Lorde called 'the erotic' and what brown calls 'pleasure activism'.

Weaving together Held's work on the ethics of care with pleasure activism leads me to think it is important to advance an ethics of care attuned to, at least, the three aims I included in the introduction: those theorizing and practising care ethics should (1) seek liberation from oppressive social norms and expectations for *all* people; (2) not remain complacent in ways that trade the pleasurable comfort of conformity for the further isolation, shame, and suffering of marginalized others; and (3) make an effort to emphasize the creative ways queer and trans people are building communities of care anchored in radical ways of loving ourselves and each other, including emphasizing models of care that rethink the dominance of the traditional nuclear family. As brown reminds us, 'Pleasure is the point. Feeling good is not frivolous, it is freedom. We can gift it to each other in a million ways: with authentic presence, abundant care, and honesty.'[61]

NOTES

1. John Paul Brammer, 'Why It Matters That It Was Latin Night at Pulse', *Slate*, 16 June 2016, https://slate.com/human-interest/2016/06/it-was-latin-night-at-pulse-heres-why-that-matters.html (accessed 24 July 2024).
2. Chen Chen, *Your Emergency Contact Has Experienced An Emergency* (Rochester, NY: BOA Editions, 2022), 40.

3. For the purpose of this chapter, LGBTQIA+ stands for 'Lesbian, Gay, Bisexual, Trans, Queer, Intersex, Asexual/Aromantic/Ace' and the '+' signifies openness to and inclusion of additional identities and relationship orientations, e.g. poly, pan, gender non-conforming (GNC), and two-spirit (2S). In the chapter, I use 'queer and trans' to refer to these identities, experiences and relationship orientations. I welcome readers to revise and remain open to how these identities may shift based on time, culture and context.
4. Chen, *Your Emergency Contact Has Experienced An Emergency*, 52.
5. J.A. Dela Cruz-Smith, 'The School of Chen Chen, Hottie Poet Extraordinaire', *Joy Sauce*, https://joysauce.com/chen-chen/ (accessed 24 July 2024).
6. Cruz-Smith, 'The School of Chen Chen, Hottie Poet Extraordinaire'.
7. Chen, *Your Emergency Contact Has Experienced An Emergency*.
8. Hil Malatino, *Trans Care* (Minneapolis, MN: University of Minnesota Press, 2020), 3–4.
9. Consider also Trans Day of Visibility as an important complement to Trans Day of Remembrance: 'The International Transgender Day of Visibility (TDOV) is an annual day of recognition, celebrated around the world on March 31st, which is dedicated to celebrating the accomplishments and victories of transgender and gender-expansive people, while simultaneously raising awareness of the work that is still needed to combat discrimination and violence. TDOV was founded in 2009 by US-based transgender activist Rachel Crandall, a licensed psychotherapist and the Executive Director of Transgender Michigan, both in reaction to the lack of LGBTQ+ days of recognition for the successes achieved by trans people, as well as the frustration that the only well-known transgender-centered day of recognition was the Transgender Day of Remembrance (TDOR). TDOV is a much-needed day of empowerment, celebrating the lives and achievements of our transgender and gender-expansive loved ones.' (See: PFLAG, 'Transgender Day of Visibility', PFLAG, https://pflag.org/transgender-day-of-visibility/, last modified 8 July 2024.)
10. adrienne maree brown, *Pleasure Activism: The Politics of Feeling Good* (Chico, CA: AK Press, 2019), 4.
11. See: Rhaina Cohen, *The Other Significant Others: Reimagining Life with Friendship at the Center* (New York: St. Martin's Press, 2024).
12. For examples of how previously white, cis, male D&D spaces have expanded to include iterations of D&D that queer and trans folks find pleasurable, exciting and empowering, see: Rowan Zeoli, 'Queer Dungeons & Transgender Dragons: Exploring Gender Through Imagined Worlds', *Autostraddle*, https://www.autostraddle.com/queer-trans-dungeons-and-dragons/ (accessed 24 July 2024); and Rowan Zeoli, 'Dimension 20's Dungeons and Drag Queens is a Cultural Reset for Queer Nerds', Polygon, https://www.polygon.com/23797617/dimension-20-dungeons-and-drag-queens-cast-review-where-to-watch, last modified 19 July 2023.
13. Iris Marion Young, *Justice and the Politics of Difference* (Princeton, NJ: Princeton University Press, 1990), 48.
14. Hil Malatino offers an example of this by explaining that what Sara Ruddick called 'maternal thinking' does not only describe the experiences of cis women who have biological children: 'Sara Ruddick, in *Maternal Thinking* – a groundbreaking work in feminist care ethics – frames preservative love as one of the central acts of mothering, which is the relational position from which she derives an entire epistemology of care. It's important to note, as well, that Ruddick understands "mothering" to be a practice taken up by persons of any gender; rather, anyone who commits themselves "to responding to children's demands, and makes the work of response a considerable part of her or his life,

is a mother". Preservative love is shorthand for all of those acts that keep a being alive and intact, and it is characterized by a specific response to the vulnerability of an other' (see: Malatino, *Trans Care,* 67). For an account that 'resist[s] the heteronormative standards of "good" mothering and, in doing so, provide[s] a model for queering motherhood', see also: Shelley M. Park, *Mothering Queerly, Queering Motherhood: Resisting Monomaternalism in Adoptive, Lesbian, Blended, and Polygamous Families* (New York: State University of New York Press, 2014), 2.

15. Maggie Nelson, *The Argonauts* (Minneapolis, MN: Graywolf Press, 2015), 26.
16. Audre Lorde, *Sister Outsider: Essays and Speeches* (Trumansburg, NY: The Crossing Press, 1984), 55–67.
17. Virginia Held, *The Ethics of Care: Personal, Political, and Global* (New York: Oxford University Press, 2006), 11.
18. Similarly, in 'Creating Caring Institutions: Politics, Plurality, and Purpose', Joan Tronto differentiates between *good* and *bad* institutional care, including seven assumptions that are likely to generate bad care because these lack 'adequate accounts of power, purpose, and plurality'. (See: Joan Tronto, 'Creating Caring Institutions: Politics, Plurality, and Purpose', *Ethics and Social Welfare* 4, no. 2 (2010): 163–6.)
19. brown, *Pleasure Activism,* 6.
20. Ibid., 13.
21. Ibid., 23.
22. Ibid., 22.
23. Lorde, *Sister Outsider*, 59.
24. brown, *Pleasure Activism*, 5.
25. Leah Lakshmi Piepzna-Samarasinha, *The Future Is Disabled: Prophecies, Love Notes and Mourning Songs* (Vancouver, BC: Arsenal Pulp Press, 2022), 305–6.
26. Ibid., 307.
27. Ibid., 308.
28. In 'An anatomy of carewashing: Corporate branding and the commodification of care during Covid-19', Andreas Chatzidakis and Jo Littler demonstrate how 'care' too has been co-opted by corporations claiming to support social justice. In a section on the genealogies of carewashing, they explain: 'Carewashing can be understood as a mutation or adaptation of other types of corporate attempt to wash themselves "clean" from the stain of unethical behaviour. The term "carewashing" itself is an adaptation of "whitewashing", the older term used for glossing over or covering up vices or crimes. Originally referring to the cheap paint used to give a quick uniform clean appearance, "whitewashing" has been used for over two centuries in the context of cover-ups in a political and corporate context. More recent variants on the term have included the well-established term "greenwashing", in which corporations (and sometimes governments) flamboyantly present their actions as environmentally friendly, while marginalising the fact that they are, to a significant degree, ecologically damaging. "Pinkwashing" has likewise been used to refer to both the cause-related marketing of companies selling pink products and giving a small percentage of the proceeds to breast cancer charities, while they continue to produce products containing carcinogens and to the promotion of LGBT issues in a positive light in order to distract attention from negative actions.' (See: Andreas Chatzidakis and Jo Littler, 'An Anatomy of Carewashing: Corporate Branding and the Commodification of Care During Covid-19', *International Journal of Cultural Studies* 25, no. 3–4 (2022): 271.)

29. Held, *The Ethics of Care,* 9.
30. Ibid., 10.
31. Ibid.
32. Lorde, *Sister Outsider,* 55.
33. Sarah Clark Miller, 'From Vulnerability to Precariousness: Examining the Moral Foundations of Care Ethics', *International Journal of Philosophical Studies* 28, no. 5 (2020): 645.
34. Ibid., 646.
35. Ibid.
36. brown, *Pleasure Activism,* 13.
37. Held, *The Ethics of Care*, 10.
38. Ibid., 11.
39. brown, *Pleasure Activism,* 15.
40. Amia Srinivasan, *The Right to Sex: Feminism In the Twenty-First Century* (New York: Bloomsbury Publishing, 2021), 97.
41. This treatment of care, desire and emotion deserves far more attention than I give it here, as does this account of personal transformation. I hope to continue to work on making distinctions between these terms in care ethics in my future work and I am grateful to the editor for the opportunity to begin this work here.
42. brown, *Pleasure Activism,* 151.
43. Held, *The Ethics of Care*, 11.
44. Ibid., 11–12.
45. Zena Sharman, 'Imagining More Care-Full Futures: Care Work as Prefigurative Praxis', *Essays in Philosophy* 24, no. 1–2 (2023): 15–16.
46. brown, *Pleasure Activism,* 12.
47. Held, *The Ethics of Care*, 11–12.
48. I am grateful to my dear friend Sarah Gorman for pointing out that the language of 'wholeness' may mean something different to those who are disabled, given how often this language is paired with ableist notions of 'health' and 'wellness'.
49. Held, *The Ethics of Care*, 12–13.
50. The Care Collective, *The Care Manifesto* (New York: Verso Books, 2020), 17.
51. brown, *Pleasure Activism,* 59.
52. Alok, 'Friendship Is Romance', https://www.alokvmenon.com/blog/2017/2/15/friendship-is-romance, last modified 15 February 2017 (accessed 24 July 2024).
53. Held, *The Ethics of Care*, 13–14.
54. brown, *Pleasure Activism,* 4.
55. Ibid., 25.
56. Ibid., 10.
57. Dean Spade, 'For Lovers and Fighters', in *We Don't Need Another Wave: Dispatches from the Next Generation of Feminists*, ed. Melody Berger (New York: Seal Press, 2006), 31.
58. Dean Spade, 'The Revolution Is My Personfriend: Dismantling the Romance Myth with Dean Spade', *The Poetry Project*, https://www.youtube.com/watch?v=5WPDUIk4VW0 (accessed 24 July 2024).
59. brown, *Pleasure Activism,* 438.
60. Chen, *Your Emergency Contact Has Experienced An Emergency*
61. brown, *Pleasure Activism*, 441.

BIBLIOGRAPHY

ALOK. 'Friendship Is Romance'. https://www.alokvmenon.com/blog/2017/2/15/friendship-is-romance. Last modified 15 February 2017 (accessed 24 July 2024).

Brammer, John Paul. 'Why It Matters That It Was Latin Night at Pulse', *Slate*, 16 June 2016. https://slate.com/human-interest/2016/06/it-was-latin-night-at-pulse-heres-why-that-matters.html (accessed 24 July 2024).

brown, adrienne maree. *Pleasure Activism: The Politics of Feeling Good*. Chico, CA: AK Press, 2019.

Chatzidakis, Andreas, and Jo Littler. 'An Anatomy of Carewashing: Corporate Branding and the Commodification of Care During Covid-19', *International Journal of Cultural Studies* 25, no. 3–4 (2022): 268–86.

Chen, Chen. *Your Emergency Contact Has Experienced An Emergency*. Rochester, NY: BOA Editions, 2022.

Cohen, Rhaina. *The Other Significant Others: Reimagining Life with Friendship at the Center*. New York: St. Martin's Press, 2024.

Dela Cruz-Smith, J.A. 'The School of Chen Chen, Hottie Poet Extraordinaire', *Joy Sauce*. https://joysauce.com/chen-chen/ (accessed 24 July 2024).

Held, Virginia. *The Ethics of Care: Personal, Political, and Global*. New York: Oxford University Press, 2006.

Lorde, Audre. *Sister Outsider: Essays and Speeches*. Trumansburg, NY: The Crossing Press, 1984.

Malatino, Hil. *Trans Care*. Minneapolis: University of Minnesota Press, 2020.

Miller, Sarah Clark. 'From Vulnerability to Precariousness: Examining the Moral Foundations of Care Ethics', *International Journal of Philosophical Studies* 28, no. 5 (2020): 644–61.

Nelson, Maggie. *The Argonauts*. Minneapolis, MN: Graywolf Press, 2015.

Park, Shelley M. *Mothering Queerly, Queering Motherhood: Resisting Monomaternalism in Adoptive, Lesbian, Blended, and Polygamous Families*. New York: State University of New York Press, 2014.

PFLAG. 'Transgender Day of Visibility'. https://pflag.org/transgender-day-of-visibility/. Last modified 8 July 2024.

Piepzna-Samarasinha, Leah Lakshmi. *The Future Is Disabled: Prophecies, Love Notes and Mourning Songs*. Vancouver, BC: Arsenal Pulp Press, 2022.

Sharman, Zena. 'Imagining More Care-Full Futures: Care Work as Prefigurative Praxis', *Essays in Philosophy* 24, no. 1–2 (2023): 11–25.

Spade, Dean. 'For Lovers and Fighters', in *We Don't Need Another Wave: Dispatches from the Next Generation of Feminists*, edited by Melody Berger, 66–75. New York: Seal Press, 2006.

Spade, Dean. 'The Revolution Is My Personfriend: Dismantling the Romance Myth with Dean Spade', *The Poetry Project*. https://www.youtube.com/watch?v=5WPDUIk4VW0 (accessed 24 July 2024).

Srinivasan, Amia. *The Right to Sex: Feminism In the Twenty-First Century*. New York: Bloomsbury Publishing, 2021.

The Care Collective. *The Care Manifesto*. New York: Verso Books, 2020.

Tronto, Joan. 'Creating Caring Institutions: Politics, Plurality, and Purpose', *Ethics and Social Welfare* 4, no. 2 (2010): 158–71.

Young, Iris Marion. *Justice and the Politics of Difference*. Princeton, NJ: Princeton University Press, 1990.

Zeoli, Rowan. 'Dimension 20's Dungeons and Drag Queens is a Cultural Reset for Queer Nerds', Polygon. https://www.polygon.com/23797617/dimension-20-dungeons-and-drag-queens-cast-review-where-to-watch. Last modified 19 July 2023.

Zeoli, Rowan. 'Queer Dungeons & Transgender Dragons: Exploring Gender Through Imagined Worlds', *Autostraddle*. https://www.autostraddle.com/queer-trans-dungeons-and-dragons/ (accessed 24 July 2024).

CHAPTER EIGHTEEN

Imagining care ethics

Disability, violence and caring spaces – Trudy's mothering story

CHRISSIE ROGERS

INTRODUCTION

> *People talk about care in the community, care in society, it doesn't bloody exist! It's some utopia that doesn't exist* (Trudy, 2016). *Because my son is now being treated in a hospital that cares for him as a person. I can relax now, knowing he's being taken care of, and it now gives me time to have cancer! I relaxed* (Trudy, 2017).

> *He has totally come back to me. During the time he was in the hospital, he had a very good named nurse. Eventually she facilitated a meeting where my son apologized to me. But I got very emotional then, even though he was very unwell at the time it happened (the violent attacks). But by the time we had the session, it remarkably happened in an unremarkable way. He apologized and I accepted it* (Trudy, 2020).

Who is Trudy? What is Mother? Lalvani describes, '*Mother* is often understood in dominant discourse as a person without further identity, or as existing without context; however, motherhood is a relational identity' (emphasis in original).[1] In 2016, England, UK, I met Trudy, a 63-year-old mother, when she responded to my call for research participants about disability and criminal justice. We met again in 2017 for a follow-up, and then remotely via telephone and email in 2020, 2023 and 2024. She had a lot to say, as her autistic son Mathais had been so violent towards her, she was hospitalized on more than one occasion. The final time she was attacked, Mathais was arrested, charged and imprisoned. I discovered on listening to her story she will always be Mother and will always be caring.

Mathais was in his thirties when Trudy first responded to me. She told me, although he displayed some aggressive behaviour as a young child, he became increasingly violent, withdrawn and paranoid as he entered his twenties. Trudy, over the years had been to her local general practitioner to log bruises, but never officially went to the police to press charges for these attacks – he was her son. She cared for and about him. As Trudy recalled, it was in 2013 when her neighbours witnessed a life changing attack on her, and Mathais was arrested and charged. He then spent almost 8 months *on remand*, in prison, and was subsequently sentenced under section 37/41 and was transferred to hospital (secure services).[2] Seven years after his arrest, in 2020, Mathais was released from hospital, to supported housing, some distance from Trudy. When I had an update from Trudy in 2023, she told me, Mathais now lives 'independently', in his own flat, in their hometown. As we hear about the caring story of Trudy in more detail below, we can only imagine her life, her caring spaces, both care-less and care-full, as disability, mothering, violence, and care practices are woven throughout her narrative.

This chapter is about Trudy, The Mother – the one caring – about disability and violence, and about the micro-politics of everyday life. Significant to this story are care ethics in relation to mothering, responsibility and neurodivergence, as well as mental health and criminal justice processes. None of these can be fully understood without contemplating history, biography and social structure – that is, personal troubles, and the public issues of society,[3] and what it means to care relationally.

18.1 CARE ETHICS OF DISABILITY AND CARING SPHERES

In my research, sons who have been physically or emotionally abusive towards their mothers are over the age of 18, but due to being neurodivergent and 'disabled', extended mothering and therefore caring work is apparent, whether their son lives at home or elsewhere in the community. Furthermore, whilst abuse is both seen and unseen, and physical and emotional, evident is interdependent caring, love and support. When it comes to mothering adult children, some consider their 'job' is such that they must take care of their son/daughter whatever the circumstances and consequences, and however damaging.[4] The small number of researchers who have carried out qualitative studies with prisoners' families do offer insight into everyday life,[5] yet remarkably there is limited research that engages with the caring and the emotional health of mothers with criminalized disabled sons.[6]

When reflecting upon mothering, disability, and what it means to be human, I previously developed a care ethics (model) of disability.[7] Largely because although the social model of disability has had a transformative impact for disabled people, it is not wholly satisfactory when it comes to understanding interdependency, relationality and care, especially for disabled people with additional impairment effects, such as learning difficulties.[8] In my research, I propose three spheres of caring: the emotional caring sphere, where love and care are psychosocially experienced; the practical caring sphere, where day-to-day care is carried out; and the sociopolitical caring sphere, where social intolerance and aversion to difficult differences are played out. It is within these spheres of caring we find people inhabit care-less and care-full spaces (and perhaps something in-between). Specifically, a care ethics of disability is about trust and webs of relationships, and the focus is on both the receiver and the giver of care, within an interdependent relationship.

Understanding interdependence, disability and caring is pertinent when considering Trudy's story, as a mother who has an adult autistic son who has been violent towards her. Namely because Trudy has experienced exclusion and discrimination, directly and vicariously,[9] via the caring spheres – emotionally (her mental health), practically (her daily care practices for and about Mathais), and sociopolitically (external responses to her experiences). Notable is the fact that prisoners' families are cumulatively deprived of support.[10] Indeed, in the UK, the Prison Reform Trust and Partners of Prisoners (POPS) found that for those caught up in the criminal justice system (CJS), desisting from crime 'can be a long, difficult and complex process, and that strong family relationships can help to reduce the likelihood of reoffending'.[11]

In addressing care ethics *and* socio-legal structures, therefore, if we shift how we comprehend autonomy, as people are interdependent and 'vulnerability' is considered part of the human condition,[12] perhaps we can contemplate changes in the way we understand families, violence, caring and disability practices, particularly, in this case, Trudy's. What can a care ethics of disability do here? Arguably, it can help us to identify care-less and care-full spaces, via the emotional, practical and sociopolitical caring spheres, and offer understanding – particularly as people 'need to be cared for and nurtured throughout their lives by other people, at times more urgently and more completely than at other times'.[13]

For Trudy's caring story, I would suggest, feminist care ethics critiques established ways of thinking about care, ethics, justice, morality, security and vulnerability,[14] and a care ethics of disability interrogates caring, just, political and relational implications for disabled people and their families.[15] Significantly, for Trudy, a feminist care ethics prioritizes relationality, as Held asserts, 'moralities built on the image of the independent, autonomous, rational individual largely overlook the reality of human dependence and the morality for which it calls'.[16] Moreover, an 'ethics of care that is political and critical must be grounded in the concrete activities of real people in the context of social relations'[17] and this is key in the telling of Trudy's story.

18.2 RESEARCH AND STORYTELLING WITH CARE

18.2.1 Care-full storytelling and the sociologist

Research, according to Brannelly and Barnes,[18] 'leaves a legacy that extends beyond that of which we are aware', and that once 'you have embraced feminist care ethics it feels like you have tried to live it throughout your life'. Furthermore, when it comes to storytelling, Baglieri suggests, 'memory work is slippery work' and that 'stories are shaped in the moments of their remembering, imagining, and telling, as much as they are formed in relation to events originally ordered in space and time'.[19] Also in her work, Baglieri creatively weaves mothering in the panopticon, and as others have done before her, suggests, 'we are always in the moment of becoming' as each moment in life, comes into play as a combination of the past and present.[20] These recollections, in that instant when talking, mould the way we perform, respond to, and merge our experiences into the stories we tell, 'the narratives we construct to give order to our lives'. Trudy, in the opening of this chapter, Brannelly and Barnes[21] and Baglieri,[22] are all talking about care, relationality and stories, explicitly or not. Remembering, recalling, listening, and researching with care, are part of doing feminist care ethics: are all part of being feminist.

I try to do research with care. Perhaps I am not always successful, but I present stories that are told to me through a caring lens, and via a sociological imagination to make meaning of social life. It is pertinent moreover, to see the difference in stories and narratives, as they are not quite the same.[23] 'All stories are narratives, but not all narratives are stories. Power features in both.'[24] Apposite in my research is how Plummer discusses narrative power. He suggests that '*stories* direct us to *what* is told, while *narratives* tell us *how* stories are told. I take stories to be the skeleton of "who, what, where, when and why" of *what* we tell and narratives to be the underlying ways we tell and communicate *how* a story is deeply fashioned by apparatus of telling' (emphasis in original).[25] My research explores life stories with criminalized disabled people, particularly those who are neurodivergent and/or learning disabled, mothers who have a criminalized disabled son, and those who work within education or the CJS.[26] Stories I tell are viewed and told through a particular narrative, and like narrative criminologists Presser and Sandberg,[27] I do not view 'offender's narratives as accurately – or inaccurately – describing events'. Furthermore, and in response to Sykes and Matza's neutralization, I too recognize, unlike 'narratives, neutralisations attend only to the offense, not to a lifetime of criminal and non-criminal actions'.[28] It is the lifetime I am interested in, despite the fact that, for Trudy, the offence that led to Mathais's imprisonment is obvious.

Critically, all the stories I tell, and specifically in this chapter for Trudy, are personal and traumatic. Yet more often the story is rooted in broader sociopolitical structural and systemic violence, and always with a history, personal or otherwise.[29] In total I carried out over forty life-story interviews with fifteen criminalized 'disabled' adults, five mothers with criminalized disabled sons, and ten professionals who work in education with disabled young people or in the community with criminalized disabled adults.[30] All interviews lasted between one and a half to two and a half hours. This chapter is based on one part of one story alone – Trudy – this is her story.

18.2.2 Ethics

In the UK, social science research generally requires ethical approval when involving human participants.[31] In the case of this research regarding ethics, I asked,

- What claims can be made in addressing ethics for the purpose of exploring 'new' knowledge around the diverse lives of these families and individuals?

As I understand, I cannot make 'truth' claims, as my participants are not a homogenous group. Yet, it is important to understand from the beginning of research into such areas of injustice, crime, disability, inequalities and social life, that doing, or at least attempting to do, ethical and care-full research is vital.[32] I needed to be flexible, empathetic, caring and responsive as I listened to stories. I gained university ethical approval to carry out the research in 2016, and as I changed institutions, and continued to maintain research connections, I further gained ethical approval via subsequent amendments in 2018 and 2020. All participants had the capacity to consent, but it was a negotiated and ongoing process. No real names are used in any work I present.

18.2.3 Data analysis and the story

In my research, I amassed qualitative data that included field notes (handwritten, voice-recorded and typed), voice-recorded face-to-face life-story interviews, letters to and from prison, and photographs. I write in more detail about my data gathering elsewhere and especially life stories and field notes as they 'expose a range of emotional and practical responses to a chaotic data collection process, and more often a moment in time, a moment that perhaps is continuous and bound up with the micro-politics of a domestic environment and embedded in the sociopolitical sphere of the criminal justice system'.[33] Evidently, data collection and analysis are interwoven and identify a feminist and reflexive process that is often fraught with 'ethical dilemmas and personal costs, where moral judgements are conceivably suspended'.[34] Moreover, I would like to think, as a feminist, that in all troubled stories there ought to be hope.[35] The stories I tell and the relationality between the participant (Trudy) and the researcher (me) are no exception.

18.3 EXTREME VIOLENCE, EXTREME CARING

18.3.1 Introduction

Thinking broadly about violence against parents, Condry and Miles caution us not to get caught up in the criminalization and blaming of young people and particular families but say it 'is important to understand family violence in all its forms and how these forms may be interconnected.[36] Family violence is relational and requires a different understanding to individual isolated incidents of violence between strangers.' They also highlight that in March 2015, the Serious Crime Act introduced a new criminal offence of 'coercive or controlling behaviour in an intimate or family relationship'.[37] This is important, not least because it can be applied to anyone over the age of criminal responsibility (10 years old) and could lead to the 'prosecution of adolescents who are abusive towards their parents'.[38] However, prisoners' families generally, and specifically Trudy, are cumulatively deprived of support due to familial/mother–son relationships and caring practices.

For this chapter, the strength of care ethics is 'its capacity to address everyday lives, politics and policymaking as well as offering a perspective on specific care practices'.[39] The potency of a care ethics of disability builds upon this, and facilitates the interrogation of caring spheres – emotionally, practically and sociopolitically, whilst identifying care-less and care-full spaces. As I have said, I interviewed and communicated with Trudy a number of times between 2016 and 2024. In 2020, Trudy said to me in our third interview about Mathais: 'Well, as a parent you are always, always affected by what's going on with your "child", aren't you? I am not a victim; I am a survivor. The difference between surviving and not surviving is about finding what it is to survive.' This becomes even more pertinent as we hear Trudy's story that speaks about lifelong caring for and about, in the context of violence and resolve. Below, we see just where Trudy had been, and what she has survived. We explore how Trudy has negotiated a darker side of life: physically and emotionally, and her responses to it. Not all mothers with criminalized disabled sons experience physical violence, abuse or emotional trauma, but it is an area that warrants discussion due to caring practices, care-full and care-less implications for the carer, social processes and everyday support needs.

Caring and love are evident within Trudy's story as she vividly describes and reflects upon two episodes of violence she experienced at the hands of her son, but critically, those bits beyond the violence. Her story gives us a glimpse not only into the physical violence, but also how Trudy acknowledges Mathais's autism and then her own maternal role, during and after his arrest and incarceration. The first excerpt of violence is an incident when she did not press charges, despite the police becoming involved. The second, in the subsequent section, shows the violence she experienced which led to the arrest and incarceration of Mathais. As we move through her story, we uncover the sheer caring and care-full work involved in the first stages of Mathais's arrest, charging and imprisonment. Not least the toll it takes on her, but also perhaps how Mathais is, sometimes unknowingly, being held, being cared for and about, emotionally and practically, so much so, that by 2023, after years of institutionalization, he lives independently in his hometown; still cared for and about, by his mother, Trudy.

18.3.2 Caring for and about the self and (an)other – 'I wasn't prepared to risk him going to prison'

When I first met Trudy, she told me about her life, her upbringing and how she lost her husband, Mathais's father, when he was only young. Later in the interview she moved on to reflect upon Mathais, and said that in his early 20s he had managed to get his own place to live, not too far from the family home, and she had helped secure a care coordinator to support with his mental health, but said, 'I don't think she (the support worker) understood mental health, she certainly didn't know anything about autism.' Trudy, at that point in her life, was becoming more concerned about Mathais; as she said, he was 'just sitting on his sofa, just looking, looking really weird'. She said that he seemed to have a problem with electricity, and she assumed it was something to do with 'being psychotic', as 'he wasn't using the heating, he wasn't cooking anything. He wasn't in a fit state to know whether it was night or day, to be honest' and basically told me Mathais was not managing everyday life terribly well.

Wanting to tell me about the first 'significant' attack, Trudy recalled that the weather had turned cold, and because Mathais was not using the fire or other electrical gadgets, 'he wasn't making hot drinks as that involved using the kettle'. Trudy would therefore visit often, taking him cooked meals daily, and said, 'he accepted me going round', but revealingly she told me that taking food round was a useful way to gain access to his flat. This was her way of caring – of making sure other aspects of his life were managed without being overly intrusive – and she said, for example, 'I was trying to keep an eye on what letters he had, and if he had any outstanding bills.' This seemingly mundane caring work was crucial, because if Trudy were not to visit and support domestic life for Mathais, it could have led to minor criminalization, or at the very least a loss of fuel to the house, and a build-up of further anxiety and financial chaos if bills were left unpaid. Arguably, in considering caring spheres, Trudy was in a care-less space, for several reasons, not least as she was spending significant parts of her day managing her adult son's affairs, yet Mathais was in a care-full space, as he experienced displays of practical and emotional caring work.

Over a short period of time, it got to a point where Trudy was scared to visit Mathais. She told me, 'I would come away from his flat, close the front door and take a deep breath. It was almost like I was holding my breath in there. Because it was getting quite scary.' Then, on the occasion described below, we begin to understand why, as Trudy had visited within the usual routine and was washing up, and said,

> I was at the sink. He was rolling a cigarette ready to go out and I was just thinking 'I'm making too much noise here, I better just leave this, till after', and I don't quite know what happened next as he lashed out because of the noise. I was knocked unconscious, I fell into the kitchen door, and my head was impaled on the glass in the kitchen door, and as my head hit the glass, I became conscious again and the rest of my body followed, and in a split second I slumped down on the kitchen floor and bruised all my coccyx and laying there on the floor with my head impaled in the glass, and my son said, 'and don't make that noise again', and got his coat on and went for a walk! And I felt very vulnerable laying there, and I wrenched my head from the glass and there was blood and I dialled 999, there was blood pouring out, there was cuts just above my ears, where that had severed, and eventually an ambulance came and they stitched and stuck my scalp back together, and I had 14 stitches in one place on its own. They kept me in overnight, um, discharged me the following day.

Trudy went on to tell me the police did arrest Mathais because of this violent attack, but there were no witnesses, and she would not press charges, because she was 'terrified of him ending up in prison'. She paused at this point in the interview, as she recalled such a harrowing memory, and then emphasized, *'I wasn't prepared to risk him going to prison.'*

Trudy's injuries and her relationship with her son display vulnerability. Yet regardless of police and health professionals' involvement in this attack, no systematic (legal, health or otherwise) follow-up occurred in response to the violence against Trudy and her unmistakably volatile position. Critically, as Trudy said, she did not want to press charges, as she assumed this would mean Mathais was criminalized, and therefore go to prison. However, simply because she did not want to press charges, it did not follow that she was free from fear, indeed safe or without need for support, care and intervention. Or, that Mathais was not in need of further support from the care coordinator or other health professionals. The concern with asserting the relevance of care to issues of justice is one that is fitting in feminist care ethics and political philosophy. Robinson has articulated it in terms of 'human security'. Broadly speaking, she refers to a '"freedom from want" and "freedom from fear"'.[40] Robinson is dissatisfied with the way human security has been developed broadly within scholarship, as everybody would want to feel secure but very few people understand what it means.[41]

In the context of Trudy's mothering, I asked, 'Did you live in fear?' Trudy's response was twofold, as it included fear from Mathais, but also fear of him going to prison, as she said, 'I was very cautious after that! But that's an autistic person's response to emotion; it's always about them [*sic*] and I had upset him, by making that noise.' Trudy's reaction to this event was about Mathais, their relationship and how she needed to better deal with, or indeed manage his behaviour. But then she said to me about *not* pressing charges and fear: 'it is the fear of what could happen … and not being able to protect him'. For Trudy, the fear of not being able to protect Mathais if he were arrested and imprisoned was greater than the fear of her own safety. Despite Trudy living in fear, I agree with Robinson in her approach to an ethics of care, as she makes an ontological shift, 'one that allows us to see moral subjects as relational and to recognize ethics as fulfilling responsibilities through practices of care'.[42]

The deeper into Trudy's narrative, the more complicated, relational and blurred care-less and care-full spaces become. Not least because she cares for and about her son yet requires care and safety herself. Clearly recognizing and accepting relational vulnerabilities is key, and as Bridgeman suggests with regard to law, '[u]nless our relational vulnerabilities are articulated we cannot identify ways in which the law can foster and support those partnered with family members in the provision of care to respect their caring relationship. Or the ways in which causing relational harm may be remedied.'[43] By focusing on stories such as Trudy's, change making, for social and legal, local and global care practices, must be identified – by, for example, listening to mothers or carers, without judgement and with care. Through this, we can recognize how the legal processes respond to safeguarding against distress and suffering, and then ascertain how to realize care-*full* spaces and practices. We can also contemplate, methodologically the 'importance of hearing histories and experiences of trauma in human-to-human connection that breaks down the barriers of the "researched" versus the researcher'.[44]

18.3.3 Beyond Caring – 'I had to survive as there were things I needed to do'

Care-fullness (safeguarding) and therefore keeping Trudy free from danger did not adequately happen, as she went on to tell me about a subsequent violent attack. Again, Trudy was visiting Mathais, and told me she had taken his 'tea round', which he ate, and he then asked, 'if they could go to the coast soon'. Trudy positively responded to his request, but said Mathais just walked over to her, as if to give the tray back and said, 'he started punching me full in the face and he was shouting questions at me about up the coast, and I didn't have a clue what he was on about'. She went on to describe, 'I think he did say how many punches he had to give me. I think he had a set number in mind.'

The storytelling was intense, as Trudy's description was graphic, and she said, 'at one point his thumbnail got my skin ... and, and you can see there' and she pointed to a scar and continued, 'so, every time he punched me, his fists, were coming into contact with this blood spurting out'. Trudy managed to get to the kitchen, but then,

> Every time he hit me it [blood] went over the ceiling, over the tiles in the kitchen, it was across the cupboards, it was puddled on the floor, because it was pouring out. It was everywhere. And then, he hit me again, and looked at his fist, and he shook his head, opened the door and motioned for me to go out and I was thinking 'don't let your legs crumple, you can walk', and he motioned for me to go outside and he told the police officer after, I was making too much mess, in his kitchen, with my blood, and that's why he had to get me outside. And so, I went down the stairs, there were imprints of blooded hands down the stairs.

Trudy went on to say, 'I got outside, and he hit me again and I had screamed to alert the neighbours, and they came, and they restrained him.' She said she crawled underneath a trampoline that was in the front garden, 'like a wounded animal, just working on instinct, thinking I'd be safer'. Her storytelling continued as she said, 'I can remember looking back and seeing him screaming at me, and I thought "why can't I hear anything?"'. Trudy recalled then, the neighbours lifted the trampoline, and they told her the police and ambulance were on their way. However, still thinking about and caring for Mathais, she said they arrested him, and exclaimed 'apparently, he told the policewoman he was an inside-out jumper!' Trudy went on to say: 'I was in hospital overnight with suspected concussion, and my face swelled up so much I couldn't see out of my eye. ... so, I was lying there thinking I was going blind. He went to court, and from there went on remand. They said for my safety he had to go to prison until it was sorted out.' Trudy did say, on thinking about Mathais and the situation, 'I knew it was a mental health problem and not a domestic violence one.' She was saying that Mathais was ill, and not that he had a problem with her.

At this point, as a researcher, and a human, I was in a bit of shock over what I was hearing, and blurted out, 'I'm just trying to get my head around what sort of emotion one goes through when ... ', especially as doing caring research 'involves emotion work for ourselves and others we involve in this process. Sometimes the emotions generated are unexpected',[45] but Trudy wanted to continue with her story, and despite being in intensive care at that point in her narrative, interrupted me, emphatically saying,

> *I had to survive*. In order to protect us both. I had to survive as there were things I needed to do. So, they arrested my son, because the neighbours had called the police, and they took him off to the police station. ... I just wanted to protect him. As his mother, I just wanted to put my arms around him and say nobody's going to hurt you.

Significant is that, in October 2020, when I interviewed Trudy for the third time, as I said earlier, but worth repeating, she said, 'I am not a victim; I am a survivor. I have faced danger before. The difference between surviving and not surviving is about finding what it is to survive.' In this violent attack above, Trudy was reflecting upon this, in our first interview in 2016, but again, repeats the survivor narrative a few years later.

Trudy, in our early interviews, continued to talk about the lack of care and responsibility from Mathais's care team, rather than his violent behaviour as the problem, as we hear below, even after such an horrific event that left Trudy hospitalized and scarred, physically and emotionally. This caring work carried out by Trudy is astonishing, as is clear here, when she told me that while she was waiting for the ambulance, a policewoman arrived, and 'I gave her my mobile and I said, "Can you phone Mathais's care co-coordinator and tell her what's happened?"'. Trudy assumed that the care coordinator would come and visit. Despite the police officer passing on this information, the care coordinator 'didn't even tell anybody, she took the phone call, put the phone down, and four days later, the supervisor got in contact and said what on earth has happened to you?' Trudy told me that no one had passed on the information beyond the care coordinator, because 'she said, "ooh, I've not bumped into her this week!"'. Trudy's words evidence violence, caring, and a care lack. I did ask, at this point, if she broke down at all, in the hospital, when her brother came to visit, and her retort was, 'no, no I had things to do', and then laughed. Despite Trudy's humour, she revealed, on discharge from hospital, 'my brother stayed that night coz every time there was a noise, I jumped thinking somehow, Mathais got out from the police station, and he was coming back to finish me off', and went on, 'I've still got a certain amount of post-traumatic stress disorder.' When we spoke in 2020, Trudy revealed she was still having counselling for her post-traumatic stress, and that it was incredibly useful, especially during Mathais's transfer in 2020, from secure hospital, into supported living.

After hearing about such attacks from Trudy when we spoke in 2016, I did venture this question, 'but did you ever feel anything but love?' and Trudy responded with: 'I was very shaky, and I didn't want to see him. I needed to put space between us, so I could sort my head out really, and after that, it was more concern about the situation he was in rather than the one I was in, and so that took over.' Glimpses of Trudy's story show us that she inhabits care-less, frightening spaces, inside *and* outside the home, but too that her caring for and about Mathais is palpable. As in these moments, we hear that she was on the receiving end of significant violence, but she did not stop caring. It is relational. It also highlights, rightly or wrongly, or something in-between, that 'acceptance of responsibility',[46] as care-fullness within a care ethics of disability *does not necessarily* compel us to love or be affectionate, but it does commit us to care-full practices and policies. Leaving aside the care lack from the professional bodies expected to care, it seems that as a mother, Trudy, might love and fear her 'child' at the same time. Trudy sensed danger at times, yet felt obliged to care *for* her son, still always caring *about* him.

Trudy, along with other mothers of disabled adult children,[47] are arguably obliged to care, but the battle between 'I must do something' (caring for) and 'something must be done' (caring about) is perhaps critical in attempting to understand a complicated relationship.[48] 'I must' carries with it obligation';[49] *I must* is different from *I want*. It could be suggested that some of Trudy's motivations and narrative are driven by 'I must' and others by 'I want', yet they seem care-full. Furthermore, relationships can be open to abuse, and are not without power inequalities. The inequalities here between a mother and her son are complicated. There are, embroiled in these narratives, legal and social responses to caring relationships, and, Herring suggests, not all are the same nor reducible to a 'single set of principles'.[50] He suggests that we are all 'ignorant, vulnerable, interdependent individuals, whose strength and reality is not our autonomy, but our relationships with others'.[51] However, this is not wholly satisfactory to the extent that the violence described by Trudy is also bound up with extended mothering and care-full and care-less spaces that are difficult to unravel, because of this interdependent relationship and lack of external sociopolitical caring.

18.3.4 Creative and pragmatic caring practices – 'I wasn't allowed to go and see him or to have contact with him'

For Trudy, mothering is beyond demanding. This is due to several factors that include expectations around mothering and additional practical and emotional care labour, staying alive and care for herself, as well as a lack of care from other external sources. Clearly, in her case, Trudy felt the pressure to take care of her adult son as she said, 'I had to survive in order to protect us both' and 'I just wanted to put my arms around him and say nobody's going to hurt you.' Evidently, Trudy was not going to stop caring *for* and *about* her son, even after his arrest and imprisonment, despite being unable to visit while he was on remand for eight months because she was the victim, and said, 'because I was a victim I wasn't allowed to go and see him or to have contact with him, but as his mother I was desperately worried about him. This is where the law just doesn't allow for this type of situation. I was not allowed to visit him or have any contact with him.' The socio-legal system and the law were a care-less space, as Trudy straddled a complicated mother/victim position. For Trudy, it took a lot of thought and planning to work around some of these legal and procedural barriers to 'display' to her son she was there for him – caring. Some of these barriers were because she was the victim, as well as being a family member, and said, 'I had no right to be involved in his case.' Mathais spent eight months on remand in prison, so this caring work went on for some time.

Listening to Trudy, there were multiple ways of caring – she was indeed incredibly 'creative' and pragmatic. For example, Trudy said she would meet the police van when going to court. She got to know the registration plates of the vans that took Mathais to court and told me she 'would contrive to be there when the vans came in' and would say 'hi and wave to him' so he would notice her. But she said she would also be very careful not to say too much and told me 'as far as they (the officers escorting Mathais) were concerned, I was just a relative who happened to see him on the way in'. This was her way of monitoring, of caring, similar to when she was visiting his home, and keeping an eye on his domestic affairs. She went on to say there were many court appearances. Each time, 'I go to the Crown Court and see Mathais in the dock and assess him and see if he looked like he was being beaten up or abused in prison.' I asked if she thought this was the case, and Trudy said she did not think he was, yet said 'he was very vulnerable, because he wasn't receiving any treatment while he was in there'. To compound this position, Trudy said, 'it seemed the details that the probation officer and others supplied on his state of mind and health, didn't get through'. This is pertinent for several reasons, but not least because as Mathais's mother, she knew him and how he would respond in certain situations. More important even, she was adamant Mathais would not fully understand why he was imprisoned, and told me, 'he didn't think he had done anything bad'. Trudy's caring was not simply to survey the situation with her son, but also to display to him that he is cared for and about. She did this by turning up to the court wearing 'the same jumper every time, so he was aware and had some sense of continuity and he'd know I'd be there' and she would also send cards from other family members to let him know he was cared about. Her caring and care-full performativity, as far as she was concerned, was crucial for Mathais, yet she also gained a sense of relief from doing the caring work.

Mothering and caring work, in this case, is not only extended and creative, but also all-consuming and deeply care-full – emotionally and practically. As we have learned, Mathais was on remand in prison for months and, as Trudy told me, 'It was only the last two weeks that the in-reach team knew of his existence', and work on how Mathais 'would be managed began'. Trudy revealed that some judges *did* understand autism and neurodivergence. She said she had 'written a letter outlining the struggles Mathais had with mental health, and I wanted him to get treatment, and they took a copy and handed it over to the defence and the judge read the letter in court. And I think that helped', as Mathais was eventually 'given a section 37/41, which meant effectively he went to hospital rather than prison'. However, Trudy also said, about the solicitors and probation officers, that 'every step of the way I had to teach them about autism'. It was in 2013 and Trudy was talking about how, if one was injured, a person would have immediate medical intervention, yet, she said her son was 'held in prison without any treatment', and continued, 'but because it's mental health it doesn't matter. So, Mathais was getting worse, to the point he was almost mute, being unable to communicate, so locked into his psychosis.' Trudy told me that, although Mathais was referred and admitted to a secure hospital, after being in an adult prison for eight months, it was two and a half years before he was 'transferred to a hospital nearer to where we live', taking its toll on both Trudy and Mathais. He was then finally transferred into supported living in 2020 about an hour's round trip away, which was better for Trudy.

As we have heard from Trudy, family and caring support can be crucial for a healthy life for anyone released from prison or secure hospital.[52] Remarkably, Trudy, after years of caring, still has the tenacity, cultural capital and caring capacity to advocate for her son, as I continued to hear in 2020, when she was very much involved in Mathais's transfer into the community. For Trudy, throughout her caring work, there was clearly a lack of systematic and caring support and intervention that caused mental health decline as she existed within care-less spaces. Trudy, however, was incredibly stoical and focused on Mathais during our interviews. Yet by the time Trudy and I had our follow-up interview in 2017, she did reveal to me she was going to 'the mental health group' but caveated that with 'but it's one for generic carers'. By the time we met up in 2020, she was having one-to-one post-traumatic stress counselling. Trudy has had experiences of violence and caring and has managed some of her journey via 'doing' tasks, as well as being a vehement advocate for her son. Her caring work is palpable. The inhabitation of caring spheres, both care-less and care-full is obvious.

CONCLUDING REMARKS

Shifts toward family responsibility, autonomy and agency have gripped the social and political landscape, whereas dependency and care (need), particularly on the state, is stigmatized and abhorred,[53] and vulnerable others are repeatedly positioned as victims.[54] Certain groups are seen as 'vulnerable', such as learning-disabled and/or neurodivergent adults, and considered to sometimes lack responsibility. According to Diduck, 'it is as though the vulnerable subject embodies a different subjectivity from the autonomous subject'.[55] In telling Trudy's story, and in the context of caring work, and caring spheres, discourses around vulnerability, responsibility and obligation are pertinent. Trudy cares for and about Mathais, who was violent towards her, criminalized and incarcerated. She straddles careless and care-full spaces, within the emotional, practical and sociopolitical caring spheres. Her experiences of the criminal justice process, health and social care are largely care-less, yet they are also complex, as she did not want to press charges against her son.

Trudy's story tells us about resolve and caring work, but sometimes at the cost of her mental and physical health. She wants to be heard, to be supported, to be cared about, to be informed: she wants social justice. As Brannelly and Barnes say about telling stories, it is important to have a critical lens, because there are normative research processes that are a better fit for some groups and communities, and it is not a surprise that 'dominant communities are better served'.[56] It is important to acknowledge Trudy's caring story, as she gives a *care-full* portrait of love that is unknowable, inconceivable even for the recipient of that care and love – Mathais – and doubtless Trudy, shows that mothering in certain circumstances can cause suffering. The suffering, disquiet and reflection talked about manifests in emotional and physical cruelty and systemic violence and is sociopolitically based on care-less and inhumane legal and moral positions, but Trudy too is clear in her own relationality with Mathais and her decision making around care practices, that do not always take care of herself. It might be Mathais as an incarcerated disabled adult was/is vulnerable and therefore unable to necessarily care for himself. Nevertheless, the mother, Trudy, is also vulnerable during her maternal journey. Bureaucratic processes, and in particular how violence is managed in or by the CJS or health and social care, do not mitigate this suffering, indeed they are care-less, and it is a socio-political matter where health, social care and the CJS are reconceptualized by, in this case recognizing the mother – Trudy – as an interdependent relationship that necessitates care as part of broader care-full practice, because maternal resolve is evident, but is not enough.

Care-full-ness, resolve and survival are obvious in hearing Trudy's story. Caring and care-full-ness ought to be privileged and positioned as not simply about the practical day-to-day aspects of caring (although these are important) but about how practical caring and emotional caring co-exist within the socio-political sphere and through our sociological imagination and care-full storytelling. It is hard to hear how someone experiencing physical and emotional pain can continue to care for and about, and so deeply. Yet beyond Trudy's personal troubles, this story tells us about the bigger picture. A dominant story of care is one that we want to hear, one that we are comfortable with; however, it often works to exclude. As Plummer suggests about narrative exclusion, symbolic violence is committed as we displace, stigmatize and scapegoat certain groups.[57] Human beings – in this case, Trudy and Mathais – are only autonomous *and* interdependent if they are safe and in beneficial relations of care. Fundamentally, as Noddings said thirty years ago, '[i]f caring is to be maintained, clearly, the one-caring must be maintained'.[58] This is certainly the case for Trudy, as ethical caring is nuanced, and care-full practices ought to involve everyone via relational and interdependent responsibility.

NOTES

1. Priya Lalvani, ed., *Constructing the (M)other: Narratives of Disability, Motherhood, and the Politics of Normal*. Disability Studies in Education (Lausanne: Peter Lang, 2019), 2.
2. Section 37 is a hospital order. Section 41 can only be added via the Crown Court and places restrictions on freedom, if it is thought necessary for the protection of the public from serious harm.

3. See: Chrissie Rogers, 'Missing Data: The Sociological Imagination Beyond the Crime', in *The Palgrave Macmillan Handbook of Auto/Biography*, ed. Julie Parsons and Anne Chappell (Basingstoke: Palgrave, 2020), 609–31; C. Wright Mills, *The Sociological Imagination* (New York: Oxford University Press, 1959).
4. Marguerite Bouvard, ed., *Mothers of Adult Children* (New York: Lexington Press, 2013).
5. See: Helen Codd, *In the Shadow of Prison: Families, Imprisonment and Criminal Justice* (London: Routledge, 2008); Megan Comfort, *Doing Time Together: Love and Family in the Shadow of the Prison* (Chicago, IL: University of Chicago Press, 2008).
6. Jenny Talbot, with Rebecca Cheung and Sam O'Sullivan, *Relative Justice: The Experiences and Views of Family Members of People with Particular Needs in Contact with Criminal Justice and Liaison and Diversion Services* (London: Prison Reform Trust and Partners of Prisoners and Family Support Group [POPS], 2015).
7. I have called it a care ethics model of disability in my previous work (see: Chrissie Rogers, *Intellectual Disability and Being Human: A Care Ethics Model* (London: Routledge, 2016)), but as I reflect, I do not consider 'model' to be helpful, or indeed see it as a model. More is that I think of it as a care ethics of disability.
8. Michael Oliver and Colin Barnes, *The New Politics of Disablement* (Basingstoke: Palgrave Macmillan, 2012).
9. See: Comfort, *Doing Time Together*; Rachel Condry, *Families Shamed: The Consequences of Crime for Relatives of Serious Offenders* (Cullompton: Willan Publishing, 2007).
10. Rachel Condry, Anna Kotova and Shona Minson, 'Social Injustice and Collateral Damage: The Families and Children of Prisoners', in *Handbook on Prisons*, 2nd ed., ed. Yvonne Jewkes, Jamie Bennett and Ben Crewe (London: Routledge, 2016), 622–40.
11. Talbot, with Cheung and O'Sullivan, *Relative Justice*, 3.
12. See: Erinn C. Gilson, *The Ethics of Vulnerability: A Feminist Analysis of Social Life and Practice* (London: Routledge, 2014); Catriona Mackenzie, Wendy Rogers and Susan Dodds, eds, *Vulnerability: New Essays in Ethics and Feminist Philosophy* (New York: Oxford University Press, 2014).
13. Eva F. Kittay, 'Dependency, Difference and the Global Ethic of Care', *Journal of Political Philosophy* 13, no. 4 (2005): 443–69.
14. See: Virginia Held, *The Ethics of Care: Personal, Political and Global* (Oxford: Oxford University Press, 2006); Mackenzie, Rogers and Dodds, eds, *Vulnerability*; Fiona Robinson, *The Ethics of Care: A Feminist Approach to Human Security* (Philadelphia, PA: Temple University Press, 2011); Joan C. Tronto, *Moral Boundaries: A Political Argument for an Ethic of Care* (London: Routledge, 1993).
15. Rogers, *Intellectual Disability and Being Human*.
16. Held, *The Ethics of Care*, 10.
17. Rianne Mahon and Fiona Robinson, eds, *Feminist Ethics and Social Policy: Towards a New Global Political Economy of Care* (Vancouver: University of British Columbia Press, 2011).
18. Tula Brannelly and Marian Barnes, *Researching with Care: Applying Feminist Care Ethics to Research Practice* (Bristol: Bristol University Press, 2022), 149.
19. Susan Baglieri, 'Mothering in the Panopticon', in *Constructing the (M)other: Narratives of Disability, Motherhood, and the Politics of Normal*, ed. Priya Lalvani (New York: Peter Lang Publishing, 2019), 167.
20. Ibid.
21. Brannelly and Barnes, *Researching with Care*.
22. Baglieri, 'Mothering in the Panopticon'.

23. Mills, *The Sociological Imagination.*
24. Ken Plummer, *Narrative Power* (Cambridge: Polity Press, 2019), 5.
25. Ibid., 4–5.
26. See: Chrissie Rogers, 'Rape and Sexual Assault: Criminalised and Disabled', *Deviant Behavior* (2024), https://doi.org/10.1080/01639625.2024.2338885; Chrissie Rogers, *Criminalised and Disabled: A Sociological Criminology Beyond the Crime* (Bristol: Bristol University Press, forthcoming).
27. Louis Presser and Sveinung Sandberg, eds, *Narrative Criminology: Understanding Stories of Crime* (New York: New York University Press, 2015), 1–2.
28. Ibid., 6.
29. See: Brian Schiff, Kaylee Altimore and Genevieve Bougher, 'The Hermeneutics of Darkness: Interpreting Perpetrators on Their Crimes', in *The Use and Abuse of Stories: New Directions in Narrative Hermeneutics*, ed. Hanna Meretoja and Mark Freeman (Oxford: Oxford University Press, 2023), 224–43. Mills, *The Sociological Imagination.*
30. See: Chrissie Rogers, 'Life Stories, Criminal Justice and Caring Research', in *Oxford Research Encyclopaedia of Education*, ed. George Noblit (New York: Oxford University Press, 2018), https://doi.org/10.1093/acrefore/9780190264093.013.326;Chrissie Rogers, 'Necessary Connections: "Feelings Photographs" in Criminal Justice Research and Doing Visual Methods', in *Special Issue: Collaborations in Research, Methodological Innovations*, ed. Gayle Letherby and Julie Parsons (2020): 1–13.
31. British Sociological Association, *Statement of Ethical Practice for the British Sociological Association* (British Sociological Association, 2017).
32. See: Brannelly and Barnes, *Researching with Care*; Chrissie Rogers and Geeta Ludhra, 'Research Ethics: Participation, Social Difference and Informed Consent', in *Research and Research Methods for Youth Practitioners*, ed. Simon Bradford and Fin Cullen (London: Routledge, 2012).
33. Rogers, 'Life Stories, Criminal Justice and Caring Research', 4.
34. Rogers, 'Life Stories, Criminal Justice and Caring Research'.
35. Martha Nussbaum, *Citadels of Pride: Sexual Assault, Accountability and Reconciliation* (London: W. W. Norton & Company, 2021).
36. Rachel Condry and Caroline Miles, 'Adolescent to Parent Violence: Framing and Mapping a Hidden Problem', *Criminology and Criminal Justice* 14, no. 3 (2014): 270.
37. Caroline Miles and Rachel Condry, 'Responding to Adolescent to Parent Violence: Challenges for Policy and Practice', *British Journal of Criminology* 55 (2015): 1077.
38. See also: Miles and Condry, 'Responding to Adolescent to Parent Violence'; Amanda Holt, *Adolescent-to-Parent Abuse: Current Understandings in Research, Policy and Practice* (Bristol: Policy Press, 2013).
39. Marion Barnes, 'Contesting and Transforming Care: An Introduction to a Critical Ethics of Care', in *Theorising Feminist Ethics of Care in Early Childhood Practice*, ed. Rachel Langford (New York: Bloomsbury Publishing, 2019), 27.
40. Robinson, *The Ethics of Care*, 47.
41. Robinson, *The Ethics of Care.*
42. Ibid., 28.
43. Jo Bridgeman, 'Relational Vulnerability, Care and Dependency', in *Vulnerabilities, Care and Family Law*, ed. Julie Wallbank and Jonathan Herring (London: Routledge, 2014), 214.
44. Brannelly and Barnes, *Researching with Care*, 117.
45. Ibid., 121.
46. Jonathan Herring, *Caring and the Law* (Oxford: Hart Publishing Ltd., 2013), 25.

47. See: Anna Kingston, 'Mothering Adult Children with Special Needs: Handing in the Uniform', in *Mothers of Adult Children*, ed. Marguerite Bouvard (New York: Lexington Press, 2013); Rogers, *Criminalised and Disabled*; Chrissie Rogers, 'Intellectual Disability and Mothering: An Engagement with Ethics of Care and Emotional Work', in *Critical Approaches to Care: Understanding Caring Relations, Identities and Cultures*, ed. Chrissie Rogers and Susie Weller (London: Routledge, 2013), 132–43.
48. Nel Noddings, 'Caring', in *Justice and Care: Essential Readings in Feminist Ethics*, ed. Virginia Held (Boulder, CO: Westview Press, 1995), 11.
49. Ibid.
50. Herring, *Caring and the Law*, 26.
51. Ibid., 46.
52. See also:Michael Farmer, *The Importance of Strengthening Prisoners' Family Ties to Prevent Reoffending and Reduce Intergenerational Crime* (London: Ministry of Justice, 2017); Talbot, with Cheung and O'Sullivan, *Relative Justice*; Lynn Saunders, 'The Transition from Prison to the Community of People Convicted of Sexual Offences: Policy and Practice Recommendations', *Prison Service Journal*251 (2020): 11–18.
53. Jonathan Herring, *Vulnerable Adults and the Law* (Oxford: Oxford University Press, 2016).
54. Alison Diduck, 'Autonomy and Vulnerability in Family Law: The Missing Link', in *Vulnerabilities, Care and Family Law*, ed. Julie Wallbank and Jonathan Herring (London: Routledge, 2014), 95–114.
55. Ibid., 98.
56. Brannelly and Barnes, *Researching with Care*, 109.
57. Plummer, *Narrative Power*.
58. Noddings, 'Caring', 26.

BIBLIOGRAPHY

Baglieri, Susan. 'Mothering in the Panopticon', in *Constructing the (M)other: Narratives of Disability, Motherhood, and the Politics of Normal*, edited by Priya Lalvani, 167–78. New York: Peter Lang Publishing, 2019.

Barnes, Marian. 'Contesting and Transforming Care: An Introduction to a Critical Ethics of Care', in *Theorising Feminist Ethics of Care in Early Childhood Practice*, edited by Rachel Langford, 17–36. New York: Bloomsbury Publishing, 2019.

Bouvard, Marguerite, ed. *Mothers of Adult Children*. New York: Lexington Press, 2013.

Brannelly, Tula, and Marian Barnes. *Researching with Care: Applying Feminist Care Ethics to Research Practice*. Bristol: Bristol University Press, 2022.

Bridgeman, Jo. 'Relational Vulnerability, Care and Dependency', in *Vulnerabilities, Care and Family Law*, edited by Julie Wallbank and Jonathan Herring, 199–215. London: Routledge, 2014.

British Sociological Association. *Statement of Ethical Practice for the British Sociological Association*. British Sociological Association, 2017.

Codd, Helen. *In the Shadow of Prison: Families, Imprisonment and Criminal Justice*. London: Routledge, 2008.

Comfort, Megan. *Doing Time Together: Love and Family in the Shadow of the Prison*. Chicago, IL: University of Chicago Press, 2008.

Condry, Rachel. *Families Shamed: The Consequences of Crime for Relatives of Serious Offenders*. Cullompton: Willan Publishing, 2007.

Condry, Rachel, and Caroline Miles. 'Adolescent to Parent Violence: Framing and Mapping a Hidden Problem', *Criminology and Criminal Justice* 14, no. 3 (2014): 257–75.

Condry, Rachel, Anna Kotova and Shona Minson. 'Social Injustice and Collateral Damage: The Families and Children of Prisoners', in *Handbook on Prisons*, 2nd edition, edited by Yvonne Jewkes, Jamie Bennett and Ben Crewe, 622–40. London: Routledge, 2016.

Diduck, Alison. 'Autonomy and Vulnerability in Family Law: The Missing Link', in *Vulnerabilities, Care and Family Law*, edited by Julie Wallbank and Jonathan Herring, 95–114. London: Routledge, 2014.

Farmer, Michael. *The Importance of Strengthening Prisoners' Family Ties to Prevent Reoffending and Reduce Intergenerational Crime*. London: Ministry of Justice, 2017.

Gilson, Erinn C. *The Ethics of Vulnerability: A Feminist Analysis of Social Life and Practice*. London: Routledge, 2014.

Herring, Jonathan. *Caring and the Law*. Oxford: Hart Publishing, 2013.

Herring, Jonathan. *Vulnerable Adults and the Law*. Oxford: Oxford University Press, 2016.

Held, Virginia. *The Ethics of Care: Personal, Political and Global*. Oxford: Oxford University Press, 2006.

Holt, Amanda. *Adolescent-to-Parent Abuse: Current Understandings in Research, Policy and Practice*. Bristol: Policy Press, 2013.

Kingston, Anna. 'Mothering Adult Children with Special Needs: Handing in the Uniform', in *Mothers of Adult Children*, edited by Marguerite Bouvard, 75–84. New York: Lexington Press, 2013.

Kittay, Eva. F. 'Dependency, Difference and the Global Ethic of Care', *Journal of Political Philosophy* 13, no. 4 (2005): 443–69.

Lalvani, Priya, ed. *Constructing the (M)other: Narratives of Disability, Motherhood, and the Politics of Normal*. Disability Studies in Education. Lausanne: Peter Lang, 2019.

Mackenzie, Catriona, Wendy Rogers and Susan Dodds, eds. *Vulnerability: New Essays in Ethics and Feminist Philosophy*. New York: Oxford University Press, 2014.

Mahon, Rianne, and Fiona Robinson, eds. *Feminist Ethics and Social Policy: Towards a New Global Political Economy of Care*. Vancouver: University of British Columbia Press, 2011.

Miles, Caroline, and Rachel Condry. 'Responding to Adolescent to Parent Violence: Challenges for Policy and Practice', *British Journal of Criminology* 55 (2015): 1076–95.

Noddings, Nel. 'Caring', in *Justice and Care: Essential Readings in Feminist Ethics*, edited by Virginia Held, 7–30. Boulder, CO: Westview Press, 1995.

Nussbaum, Martha. *Citadels of Pride: Sexual Assault, Accountability and Reconciliation*. London: W. W. Norton & Company, 2021.

Oliver, Michael, and Colin Barnes. *The New Politics of Disablement*. Basingstoke: Palgrave Macmillan, 2012.

Plummer, Ken. *Narrative Power*. Cambridge: Polity Press, 2019.

Presser, Louis, and Sveinung Sandberg, eds. *Narrative Criminology: Understanding Stories of Crime*. New York: New York University Press, 2015.

Robinson, Fiona. *The Ethics of Care: A Feminist Approach to Human Security*. Philadelphia, PA: Temple University Press, 2011.

Rogers, Chrissie. 'Intellectual Disability and Mothering: An Engagement with Ethics of Care and Emotional Work', in *Critical Approaches to Care: Understanding Caring Relations, Identities and Cultures*, edited by Chrissie Rogers and Susie Weller, 132–43. London: Routledge, 2013.

Rogers, Chrissie. *Intellectual Disability and Being Human: A Care Ethics Model*. London: Routledge, 2016.

Rogers, Chrissie. 'Life Stories, Criminal Justice and Caring Research', in *Oxford Research Encyclopaedia of Education*, edited by George Noblit. New York: Oxford University Press, 2018.

Rogers, Chrissie. 'Missing Data: The Sociological Imagination Beyond the Crime', in *The Palgrave Macmillan Handbook of Auto/Biography*, edited by Julie Parsons and Anne Chappell, 609–31. Basingstoke: Palgrave, 2020.

Rogers, Chrissie. 'Necessary Connections: "Feelings Photographs" in Criminal Justice Research and Doing Visual Methods', in *Special Issue: Collaborations in Research, Methodological Innovations* 13, no. 2 (2020).

Rogers, Chrissie. 'Rape and Sexual Assault: Criminalised and Disabled', *Deviant Behavior* (2024). https://doi.org/10.1080/01639625.2024.2338885.

Rogers, Chrissie. *Criminalised and Disabled: A Sociological Criminology Beyond the Crime.* Bristol: Bristol University Press, forthcoming.

Rogers, Chrissie, and Geeta Ludhra. 'Research Ethics: Participation, Social Difference and Informed Consent', in *Research and Research Methods for Youth Practitioners*, edited by Simon Bradford and Fin Cullen. London: Routledge, 2012.

Saunders, Lynn. 'The Transition from Prison to the Community of People Convicted of Sexual Offences: Policy and Practice Recommendations', *Prison Service Journal* 251 (2020): 11–18.

Schiff, Brian, Kaylee Altimore and Genevieve Bougher. 'The Hermeneutics of Darkness: Interpreting Perpetrators on Their Crimes', in *The Use and Abuse of Stories: New Directions in Narrative Hermeneutics*, edited by Hanna Meretoja and Mark Freeman, 224–43. Oxford: Oxford University Press, 2023.

Talbot, Jenny, with Rebecca Cheung and Sam O'Sullivan. *Relative Justice: The Experiences and Views of Family Members of People with Particular Needs in Contact with Criminal Justice and Liaison and Diversion Services*. London: Prison Reform Trust and Partners of Prisoners and Family Support Group (POPS), 2015.

Tronto, Joan C. *Moral Boundaries: A Political Argument for an Ethic of Care*. London: Routledge, 1993.

Wright Mills, C. *The Sociological Imagination*. New York: Oxford University Press, 1959.

CHAPTER NINETEEN

Care in unexpected places

Punishment and forensic detention

HELEN BROWN COVERDALE

INTRODUCTION

This chapter explores the presence of care in unexpected places – primarily practices of criminal punishment. Our initial expectations of punishment – especially that it is undesired, unpleasant and burdensome, as in the case of criminal punishment – seem to run counter to the aims of caring, especially when we frame penal practices in terms of suffering and hardship. Care is not the only thing that happens in punishment. But care is essential for safe and effective penal regimes. We are comforted to imagine that only 'monsters', not people like us, could perpetrate the worst kinds of crimes. This is not true. There are no monsters in our prisons, only human beings.[1] Wherever there are human beings, there must be care; since fragile human bodies and minds cannot flourish without opportunities to give and receive care, and ultimately cannot survive without it. I argue that there is care in these places, and that the insights of care ethics can help us to better understand, and therefore better design, these practices. If our penal aims include reducing recidivism, and enabling people with convictions to build their capabilities to meet their own needs and contribute to our shared communities, then looking at the overlap between caring and penal practices and employing the insights of care ethics will be important for penal policymakers and practitioners. Here I consider the overlap between a range of penal practices with care ethics (I have written elsewhere in more detail on the overlap between the prison and caring, and some of the implications for philosophy and policy),[2] and finish with a borderline case of compulsory detention and treatment for people who are mentally unwell.

19.1 CONCEPTUAL PRELIMINARIES

19.1.1 What is care ethics?

Care ethics is an alternative mode of moral reasoning, distinct from the traditional western mainstream individualist way of thinking, that begins from individuals and their rights, and works outwards to the correlative duties of others. Care and relational ethics more broadly begin from our connection to others and our interdependence.[3] Care ethics has its roots in the everyday practices of giving and receiving care and is heavily tied to the particular. Care gives us three linked key insights, following from the importance of relationships in human lives, the vulnerability of human bodies and minds, which together result in our interdependence. First, good human lives have valuable relationships. Not all of those relationships are chosen – for example, within the family – but all relationships bring responsibilities towards others. As well as other-regarding responsibilities, as social creatures we also rely on one another for our basic needs much more often than an archetypal Classical Millian liberal individualism leads us to believe. Second, we must survive periods of extreme dependence on others[4] because we are variably vulnerable. Accident, illness, disabling conditions, maternity, and age-related dependence are not unusual, and it is in such periods of increased dependency that our reliance on others becomes more visible. In this way, care ethics normalizes dependence and need. Hence, third we are interdependent on and with each other, as needy people who need each other.

Former British Prime Minister Margaret Thatcher famously asserted that there is no such thing as society, only a collection of individuals. On the contrary, there is no such thing as the independent individual, unless a social collective cooperates to provide the conditions for care that the particular individual needs. How the labour of care provision is shared, and how caring is valued, are social and political decisions.[5] Care ethics demonstrates that both caregivers and care receivers require support services, so that the former are not overwhelmed, and the latter are able to meet their needs and develop their capabilities as far as possible, permitting us all to flourish.[6]

19.1.2 What is caring?

The practice of caring is central to care ethics, but because these practices are context-dependent, there are disagreements as to what is to count as care. Core exemplar cases are nursing care and childcare, and helping someone to do things they could not do,[7] or would struggle to do, alone. Daniel Engster offers us a helpful definition: caring work is that which builds capabilities, meets needs, or avoids unwanted harm.[8] This reflects Tronto's phases of caring practice:[9] noticing needs in others (a moral requirement for Tronto);[10] making arrangements for practical assistance to address the need; the provision of caring work, whatever form that practical assistance takes; and a response from the care receiver, which helps to refine care provided to better address a developing need going forwards. Taking these practice elements together as a cyclical process reflects the ongoing collaborative nature of caring between caregiver and care receiver. Even though almost all caring reflects a power imbalance, as one party helps another to achieve something they would find challenging alone, care is helpfully thought of as a practice of solidarity, of caring-with rather than for. This explains the wrongness of abusing that power imbalance to exploit a care receiver, or why engaging in care provision contrary to a care receiver's wishes, cannot count as good care. Moreover, while care work is work, care is more than just work. Engster summarizes the 'attentive, responsive, respectful'[11] attitude necessary for good care, that is open to engaging with the other,[12] in solidarity.[13] Tronto also details the values of care to reflect her practice phases. These ethical elements are: awareness of the needs of the other; taking responsibility for seeing that needs are met; meeting needs competently – and seeking specialized help when needed; and the responsiveness needed to engage openly and care-with in solidarity.[14]

19.1.3 Relationships, trust and time

Trust is needed for care provision, and the ability to build, maintain and restore trust is needed to sustain lasting relationships. Alison Leibling has written on the essential role of trust between staff and residents for maintaining order in British prisons.[15] It is hard to give or receive care from another we do not trust. If my trust is misplaced, I am open to abuse because of the power imbalances inherent in most instances of care provision. But the power to harm, is also the power to help. Both trust and relationships are built and deepen over time, supported by the right conditions.

It is tempting to view care as a snapshot: a discrete moment where one cares for and another receives. Yet Joan Tronto helpfully observes that good care cannot be compartmentalized in time: good care happens when it is needed and simply takes as long as is needed.[16] Good care changes over time, as situations and individuals change and needs develop. The type of caring-with in solidarity that it is possible to do with very young children is limited by their as-yet underdeveloped capacity to reason and choose, but it does not mean that children cannot be respectfully engaged and supported in making choices, in order to build and develop their capabilities. Moreover, individuals whose capabilities will not improve and may decline can also be respectfully engaged and supported in making choices.[17] Respectful engagement includes being mindful of the current ability of the other to engage and to respond; and pitching the interaction appropriately, so that it is inclusive and supportive of building capabilities and meeting needs, rather than imposing additional responsibilities and onerous burdens.

It can also be challenging to separate care out into discrete acts. For example, a nurse might administer medications, comfort a patient, advocate for the patient with a prescribing physician, and support family members. All of these acts are care, but it might be hard to say where one task ends – comforting and medicating, medicating and advocating – and another begins. It is further tempting to view caring relations as one-way: one cares for, another receives. But this misses the mutual interdependence, and the acts of care, however small, that often flow in the opposite direction when the roles are reversed. In reality, caring is a continuous process, and care flows both ways between the parties, even when one party is objectively more dependent. Even young children attempt to care for their parents.[18] It is also the case that a caregiver in one moment might be a care receiver later on from another party. Consider the parent who makes a child's breakfast, packs their lunch and drops them at school, before attending an appointment to receive dental care.

19.2 CARE IN CRIMINAL JUSTICE

19.2.1 Restorative justice practice

Restorative justice is the obvious place to begin when looking for care in responses to crime. Restorative justice aims to repair relationships between those responsible for harm and victims, where possible, rather than a retributive response to wrong.[19] Restorative justice recognizes criminal wrongs as breaches of trust between individuals, that damage relationships both between them, but also the relationships between the community and the individual responsible. Both parties are members of the same community. The community must go on living together, even if the parties themselves choose no further contact.

John Braithwaite proposes a set of standards for restorative justice, which resonate with care ethics values. Braithwaite's minimum standards include empowerment, respectful listening and equal concern.[20] This reflects the respectful, responsive listening Engster and Kittay identify. Whereas mainstream proceedings seek to respond to the offence proportionally to the harm caused, restorative practices seek to repair the harm.[21] These broadly align with Engster's aims of care as meeting needs, developing capabilities and avoiding (or repairing) harm, and reflect Tronto's requirements for awareness of needs and responsiveness to the other.[22]

Following Walker,[23] I do not mean to claim that what is 'really' happening in restorative justice – or any other penal practice – is wholly described by care ethics. Rather, what appears to be central to the practice may be effectively understood as care. Insofar as penal practices reflect care, they can be strengthened and potentially improved by recognizing them as caring practices, and by applying caring values to evaluate the practices and provide direction for improvements.

19.2.2 Fines

The most common form of criminal sentence in England and Wales is a fine.[24] There is nothing especially restorative about fines, but they can be applied in more and less supportive ways. In England and Wales, fines are calculated first relative to the offence, and second relative to the individual's ability to pay, considering income and essential financial obligations regarding dependents. Douglas Husak similarly suggests that day fines, set relative to an individual's capacity to pay, provide an equivalent amount of punishment to rich and poor people, even if the former pay objectively more.[25] Payment might also be ordered in instalments, spreading the cost. Supporting individuals towards compliance with their order is desirable if we have additional aims of punishments. For example, that the punishment should not further alienate the individual from the community, so that it allows the person punished to feel fairly treated, and which may in turn be more effective at reducing recidivism.

19.2.3 Probation

The most common form of sentence in US jurisdictions is probation.[26] The federal probation service's mission is to assist the courts in the fair administration of justice, to protect the community, and to bring about long-term positive change for those under supervision through proactive intervention. Similar roles exist at state and local levels, with some variations in name. Probation officers, parole officers and community supervisors are all community correction professionals. In all cases, this is a dual role: part law enforcement, and part social work. Officers monitor conduct, but they also refer individuals for treatment, education and employment, with the aim of supporting the person towards a crime-free life.[27]

Probation services in England and Wales began as specialized social work, with an ethos of 'advise, assist and befriend' towards individuals in community punishment. Gregory, a probation officer turned scholar, argues that 'an ethics of care underpinned practice'.[28] However, a move towards a 'punitive managerialist' approach followed from a specialized probation diploma, moving away from social work.[29] Gregory argues that her 2003 study still evidenced the use of the moral reasoning of care ethics. As late as 2011, the House of Commons Justice Committee found that 'staff continue to emphasize the original values of probation'.[30]

Advising, assisting and befriending are sympathetic to caring values, since these demand some level of open engagement with recipients, with supportive, enabling attitudes. Moreover, to either 'advise, assist and befriend' or 'rehabilitate' or refer for support through proactive intervention for long-term change, requires an awareness of individuals' personal challenges. This must in part at least be gained through respectful and responsive discussion with service users. Probation officers must take and share responsibility for providing support, with colleagues from other agencies, such as specialist psychologists and addiction workers.

In England and Wales, and many other jurisdictions, most community punishments include probation supervision. While this may be of variable quality and duration, it offers some opportunity to officers to engage with individuals and begin to build trusting relationships. 'McNeill and Robinson ... argue that the supervisory relationship is central to and crucial for development of legitimacy in probation practice; they warn that this legitimacy, in the eyes of the supervisee, "is hard-won, easily lost, and almost impossible to recover"'.[31] Moreover, Dominey and Canton note that empirical evidence indicates the importance of 'good supervisory relationships for probation outcomes including compliance and legitimacy'.[32]

Wherever officers can make time to hear individuals and to respond to their concerns, there is space and time for care. This reflects awareness and taking and sharing responsibility within our capability, seeking specialist support where needed, reflecting Tronto's ethics elements of care. Yet, Dominey and Canton identify several recent features indicating the commodification of probation, restricting the ability of officers to take time, to engage with and respond to, individuals. Moreover, they argue that recent transforming rehabilitation reforms in probation in England and Wales actively discourage departing from standardized procedures to accommodate real people and real lives.[33]

19.2.4 Unpaid work

A common element of community punishment is unpaid work. This work is intended as punitive rather than rehabilitative; however, several scholars[34] note the rehabilitative potential in bringing people in punishment together with others with different personal challenges or greater needs than their own. This opportunity for individuals to connect and understand how their unpaid work helps others is reflected in an individual's comment about their experience of unpaid work as punishment on a social housing estate in Liverpool. Mair and Mililngs quote one worker in punishment as saying:

> *We were on this estate painting these fences and these people said to the probation guy that some of the fences weren't any good ... and you thought why do they care about it but once it was done good they thanked us and you could see it was useful for them.*
> (offender respondent 55)[35]

The Residents' Association of a Liverpool social housing estate benefiting from unpaid work undertaken as punishment echoed similar experiences. While residents were initially apprehensive, things improved once they met and developed relationships with those labouring on their estate. The work demonstrated to residents that those undergoing punishment were ordinary people, and not as bad as media portrayals. Residents offered tea to the workers, and those working went above and beyond to help elderly residents with small chores they could not do alone, such as moving heavy garden furniture. These relationships sometimes outlasted the community orders, with previous workers coming back to visit residents. The work and these experiences helped to give those in punishment some pride in their local area and themselves.[36]

19.2.5 Alternative jurisprudence

The Liverpool examples are drawn from a now-ended experiment in problem-solving justice, based on the highly successful programme at the Red Hook Community Justice Center in New York. Community-based punishments are used here for two reasons: to help keep individuals out of jail, and to address the harms of offending behaviour that have a high impact on local people's lives. In mainstream criminal justice, an order that is inevitably breached leads to a short prison sentence as punishment for the breach, further disrupting already chaotic lives with criminogenic effects.

In problem-solving jurisprudence, punishment practices are tailored to community need, but also to supporting the person in punishment towards complying with an order that may initially have been out of their reach, in light of their context or situation (for example, we cannot simply order individuals with longstanding addiction problems to quit substance misuse and expect them to succeed alone). Support or treatment requirements are provided to the individual, through the co-location and cooperation of local support services with criminal justice, and continual judicial involvement – varying the support provided and conduct expected by gradually amending the order through ongoing collaborative work with the person being punished as their needs change. Unpaid work requirements, centred on improving local public spaces in response to local needs, as in the Liverpool example above, often accompany the support provided. Sentences can be successfully completed, achieving the same ends a mainstream sentence would have ordered (that would most likely have been breached without support), while community facilities are improved, community relationships repaired, and individuals helped to get back on their feet.

A related practice is Therapeutic Jurisprudence, which theorizes ongoing judicial engagement as therapeutic of itself. This practice, championed by Winick and Wexler,[37] requires judicial engagement over a sustained period, again with continually modified achievable goals, and expects judges to use motivational interviewing skills – helping individuals to see how court ordered support to address the issues underlying their offending behaviour, is ultimately also in line with their own personal goals. These practices are not without criticism, but they do evidence individually tailored, responsive, iterative processes, that at least aim to be respectful and inclusive of the person at their centre – the person being punished for an offence – and hence, this reflects the values and practices of care.

19.2.6 Prison

Care is not the first thing that springs to mind when we think about the prison, yet I have argued that caring can be found in present prison practices, even if only as woefully bad caring.[38] Moreover, failing to recognize the presence and practice (however poor) of care in prisons is also a failure to recognize the reach and diversity of care. If we fail to notice care here, we should also consider what other blind spots we have about care provision where needs go unconsidered and unmet. I have argued elsewhere with Bill Wringe that the hyperfocus of penal philosophy on the criminal punishment, by states, of competent adults, through imprisonment, is a disservice to penal thought more broadly understood.

It restricts the way we think about punishment. It also restricts the way we think about prisons.[39] Thinking about prisons in terms of care and caring at once illuminates the presence of care, where these practices fail – and then how policies might be designed to improve the essential care.

The United Nations Standard Minimum Rules for the Treatment of Prisoners (the Nelson Mandela Rules) expect that people in prisons should receive individualized (i.e. responsive) treatment (Rule 89), as members of the community (Rule 88), that fosters their self-respect.[40] The European Prison Rules expect the duties of prison officers to go beyond those 'required of mere guards', facilitating 'the reintegration of prisoners into society ... through a programme of positive care and assistance'.[41] Even Prison Rules in England and Wales have long specified the purpose of a prison sentence as 'training and treatment ... to encourage and assist [people punished by imprisonment] to lead a good and useful life'.[42]

Indeed, care is part of the job description in England and Wales. Prison officers, as key workers, provided one-to-one support. The House of Commons Justice Committee characterized this wide-ranging support with anything from sentence planning to food requirements to bereavements.[43] This reflects Engster's characterization of care, since these examples meet needs (dietary requirements), build capabilities (especially if sentence planning involves rehabilitative skill-building, substance misuse or mental health support, or education), and avoid harm (facilitating bereavement support). In the case of facilitating access to a specialist (perhaps an appropriately trained bereavement counsellor) or signposting a person on to more specialized services, officers also demonstrate competence and responsibility in their caring, by not attempting to care beyond their capability when expert help is on hand. While there are no guarantees, this at least creates space for good care – that is attentive, responsive and respectful – that works in solidarity with the one receiving care, and seeks to avoid poor care by acknowledging the limits of the carer's abilities, and when better help is available elsewhere. Undoubtedly, time and resource constraints will limit officers' abilities to care well. Nevertheless, practices and values central to caring – understanding individuals' needs[44] and responding to meet them – are central to officers' duties.[45] Of course, these examples are cherry-picked, but my purpose is to highlight the essential and intended presence of care.

But basic needs meeting is not the only care in prisons. Chaplaincy workers discuss personal and emotional problems, a practice identified as care even on narrow definitions of care work.[46] Education – building skills and capabilities – ranging from basic literacy to Open University programmes is available in prisons in England and Wales, as is healthcare, addiction treatment and mental health support. Undoubtedly these services suffer from problems with access, resourcing, and issues created by the transfer of individuals between prisons in an overcrowded system.

Peer-to-peer support among people living in prisons is particularly significant. The Samaritans, a charity aiming to prevent suicides, train and support volunteers to listen confidentially to others experiencing distress, despair or contemplating suicide, using the same guidelines as for their community-based volunteers. Listeners across prisons in England and Wales organize themselves so that there is always someone available to listen, usually in private, to a person in distress.[47] Around the edges, care creeps back in, even where it is unplanned, unthought and even apparently undesired. Because those who live and work in prisons are first and foremost human beings, and human beings need – and need to give – care.

19.2.7 Supporting People in Punishment

Supporting people in punishment need not frustrate penal aims or run contrary to the needs of communities for reduced crime. On the contrary, it can help to address those ends. The desistance paradigm for understanding how it is that some people turn away from offending frames non-recidivism as following from an individual's choice, and as a process of new identity building. This requires time, effort, and importantly acceptance by others, and success is most likely with supportive families, communities and state agents, who positively reinforce an individual's project to recast their identity as a non-offender.[48]

Research suggests that the social connectedness and feelings of self-worth of formerly imprisoned US women was enhanced when they were permitted to support other desisting individuals. Acting as role models and mentors for more recently released prisoners, the women drew on shared experiences to help their mentees avoid mistakes. These caregiving mentors supported their mentee's desistance, while simultaneously improving their own community reintegration, and planning careers to give back to the community.[49] This suggests that opportunities to practise caregiving with their mentees and community giveback, facilitated individuals' own desistance, in turn making engagement with others and broader social flourishing possible.

I've suggested three practical reasons for taking care in punishment practices more seriously. First, supporting people in prisons in particular in addressing their own needs reduces the burden on the taxpayer: it helps individuals to be in a position at the end of their punishment where they are ready and able to continue meeting many of their own needs, rather than relying on welfare. Moreover, this amplifies the effects of welfare spending, since this better equips people in and leaving punishment to meet the needs of their dependents as well as their own needs. Second, since caring is a learned behaviour, showing care to people in punishment offers an opportunity to learn about care provision. This may be particularly valuable since most of the people we punish by imprisonment are already heavily socio-economically disadvantaged and excluded. We may be better to consider rehabilitative measures to be habilitative,[50] since they may provide a first opportunity to learn skills – such as how to give and to receive care – that those in punishment have never previously been afforded. Teachers recognize that not all students are able or ready to learn at the first opportunity, so even where these opportunities have been provided and have not previously helped a person to develop the skills, there is no reason to presume further attempts will fail. There are of course good pedagogical reasons to expect better results in a more supportive environment than most modern prisons. But this is where care standards begin to suggest better ways of achieving these ends. So supporting people in punishment better equips them to meet their own needs where they can, and to support others, particularly those they have immediate relationships with and caring responsibilities for. Third, being better equipped to engage in needs meeting facilitates further social contribution to our communities, as neighbours, as employees and as engaged citizens.

Receiving care can be essential for our survival. Kimberley Brownlee[51] has further identified the good of being able to give as well as to receive social connection as so essential to our mental wellbeing as to ground a right against unwanted social deprivation. She argues forcefully that we may not ignore the friendly social advances of others who are vulnerable and have limited other opportunities for social engagement. There seems a clear resonance between Brownlee's right against social deprivation and the findings of desistance research: individuals in the process of desisting from past criminal behaviour are vulnerable, and need support and acceptance. But they also need opportunities to provide support to others, and opportunities to demonstrate their trustworthiness – even though desistance, like recovery from addiction, is a cyclical process and relapses will occur. Although it is not her approach, I have suggested that one way to fulfil Brownlee's right against social deprivation, and to provide supported opportunities to give as well as to receive social connection, might be through employing care ethics as a guide to localized practice.[52] Brownlee identifies isolated groups such as those in residential institutions, including prisons, secure hospitals, hospitals, care homes, and some residential schools as examples of groups of people with limited avenues for social contribution whose advances we have a duty to accept.

19.3 CARE IN FORENSIC DETENTION

Forensic detention is the area where the law and mental health intersect.[53] Compulsory mental health detention for individuals, due to the risk they pose or have evidenced, to others or themselves, takes place in different ways in different jurisdictions. In some states, compulsory mental health detention occurs primarily or only under the criminal law. In others this may be practised only in medical, treatment-oriented settings. In still others, such as England and Wales, either criminal or non-criminal practices and settings may be used in compulsory mental health detention.

Clinical staff working with people who pose risks in secure settings have a dual role[54] – between the care and treatment of individuals resident in the institution; and the safety and security of the institution for staff and residents, and public protection. Tensions arise because decisions about the suitability of less secure conditions or small privileges that may be of great importance to the individual, can conflict with caring. This issue is equally problematic for prison officers, but for clinical staff in particular, this can actively undermine the trust-building essential for forensic care.

Forensic detention shares the locks and physical barriers of a prison environment, although some design differences may hint at the differences in intended regime focus between a medical treatment environment, and a penal detention environment. Yet, even for security-focused prison officers,[55] recognizing the essential presence of care and seeking to improve service delivery as care can contribute to meeting security aims. Care can support desistance from crime through building capabilities to avoid recidivism in the long term, and more immediately protect the health and safety of people living in prisons by meeting needs.[56] So while forensic practice focuses on the treatment and support of patients, both roles are dual roles, and the practices can converge.

Austin et al. recommend a particularized, relational ethics approach for forensic practitioners focusing on what is right for a particular patient, in their particular context, and working with individuals in ways that reflect the solidarity of care ethics. They argue that clinicians must hold separate and minimize neither the individual's crimes, nor the patient's humanity.[57] Providing respectful engagement will always be challenging when an individual is detained involuntarily. But an honest relationship between the healthcare provider and patient requires an acknowledgement of the disapproval of previous criminal conduct, while nevertheless accepting the person in treatment as valuable and worthy of care and respect.

Hannah Pickard, a moral philosopher with clinical experience, has argued that it is possible to decouple the negative attitudes we commonly associate with placing blame, from holding a person causally responsible for their actions. Since the negative attitudes following blame are emotions, it is possible that we can be mistaken about them. Pickard explains this in relation to fear, which can easily be misplaced: we can experience very real fear for no good reason. Pickard suggests negative attitudes following blame are similarly unreliable, and frustrate treatment processes that require practitioner and patient to believe that change is possible.[58] A more detached approach to blame on the part of the care provider allows space for holding responsible, and for consequences – such as forensic detention and treatment – to follow from the conduct without stigmatization. Crucially, this approach also recognizes that the person at the centre still has the capability to learn to respond differently with patient treatment. Pickard has, with Nicola Lacey, argued for bringing this detached form of blaming out of the treatment room,[59] and into the criminal justice process more broadly. Some research suggests that practices supporting individual-led personal change offer better prospects for more rehabilitative success, facilitate desistance from offending, and permit more dignified and humane practices and relationships during punishment. So, while the care-led practices of forensic medicine demand and sometimes conflict with security concerns, even the security-focused features of prisons require care. There is perhaps much that practices can learn from each other about managing this tension, if penal practices can do better at recognizing the essential role of care in punishment.

CONCLUSION

Early care ethics research contrasted an archetypal relational-focused 'care' approach with an archetypal rights-focused 'justice' approach. Everyday caring labour is often undertaken by less privileged groups in society – women, migrants, people of colour.[60] For large parts of human history, these less privileged groups have been excluded from citizenship – we had societies which practised care (since care is essential for human life) but without just inclusion.[61] Justice without care is equally problematic.[62] We need to ensure that people in prison receive justice with care and support, and that people in forensic detention receive care with just inclusion. Care ethics provides one way of thinking differently about detention practices, particularly prison, that highlights the essential presence of caring, and may offer principles to support and guide policymakers and practitioners.

I've identified the care that is essential to penal practice and that occurs in the most unlikely, perhaps the most hopeless, of settings: places and practices of punishment and involuntary confinement. I've shown where we can find care sometimes despite our expectations, in the supportive practices of staff who treat prison or hospital residents with dignity and respect, taking the time to build trusting relationships, and to slowly support individuals in meeting their needs and developing their capabilities. People who are punished are first and foremost people. All humans need care, and to give and receive social connection. Moreover, if we seek to reduce recidivism, a case can be made that supportive practices assist individual desistance, amplify state resources by facilitating individuals in meeting both their own needs and the needs of their dependents, and contribute positively to the community both by reducing crime and by fostering good citizenship in the place of prior offending. Thinking about punishment from the perspective of care then can help us recognize the caring elements of punishment that too often go unthought, untheorized, deprioritized in practice. By doing so, we can use the standards and expectations of care to assess, guide and design improvements to our practices, where they overlap with care provision. I hope I've shown this overlap is greater than we might have first thought.

ACKNOWLEDGEMENTS

This chapter develops and extends some discussion from my PhD thesis *Punishing with care: treating offenders as equal persons in criminal punishment*, available at https://etheses.lse.ac.uk/1080/. I am also grateful for feedback on a more recent version of this paper to organizers and participants at the 4th International Conference of SAFI (Societas Feminarum Apertia in Iuris Theoria), Paris 1, October 2023; and to co-organizers and participants at *Therapeutic Spaces Behind Bars: Eco-psychosocially Supportive Prisons and Forensic Psychiatric Wards*, a British Academy/Wellcome Trust funded conference held in London in February 2024.

NOTES

1. Deborah Drake, *Prisons, Punishment and the Pursuit of Security* (London: Palgrave Macmillan, 2012), 8.
2. Helen Brown Coverdale, 'Caring and the Prison in Philosophy, Policy and Practice: Under Lock and Key', *Journal of Applied Philosophy* 38, no. 3 (2021): 415–30, https://doi.org/10.1111/japp.12415.
3. Jennifer J. Llewellyn, 'Restorative Justice: Thinking Relationally about Justice', in *Being Relational: Reflections on Relational Theory and Health Law*, ed. Jennifer J. Llewellyn and Jocelyn Grant Downie (Vancouver: University of British Columbia Press, 2012), 89–108.
4. Eva Feder Kittay, *Love's Labor: Essays on Women, Equality and Dependency* (New York: Routledge, 1999).
5. Fiona Robinson, *Globalizing Care: Ethics, Feminist Theory, and International Relations* (Boulder, CO: Westview Press, 1999), 33.
6. Daniel Engster, *The Heart of Justice: Care Ethics and Political Theory* (Oxford: Oxford University Press, 2007), 29.
7. Diemut Elisabet Bubeck, *Care, Gender and Justice* (Oxford: Clarendon Press, 1995), 129.
8. Engster, *The Heart of Justice*, 29.
9. Joan C. Tronto, *Moral Boundaries: A Political Argument for an Ethic of Care* (New York: Routledge, 1993), 106–8.
10. Ibid., 127.
11. Engster, *The Heart of Justice*, 31.
12. Eva Feder Kittay, 'When Caring Is Just and Justice Is Caring', in *The Subject of Care: Feminist Perspectives on Dependency*, ed. Eva Feder Kittay and Ellen K. Feder (Lanham, MD: Littlefield Publishers, 2002), 259.
13. Selma Sevenhuijsen, *Citizenship and the Ethics of Care: Feminist Considerations on Justice, Morality, and Politics* (London: Routledge, 1998).
14. See: Tronto, *Moral Boundaries*, 127–37; Joan C. Tronto, *Caring Democracy: Markets, Equality, and Justice* (New York: New York University Press, 2013), 34–5.
15. Alison Liebling, 'Penal Legitimacy, Well-Being, and Trust: The Role of Empirical Research in "Morally Serious" Work', in *Crime, Justice, and Social Order*, ed. Alison Liebling,

Joanna Shapland, Richard Sparks and Justice Tankebe (Oxford: Oxford University Press, 2022), 299, https://doi.org/10.1093/oso/9780192859600.003.0012.

16. Joan C. Tronto, 'Time's Place', *Feminist Theory* 4, no. 2 (2003): 119–38, https://doi.org/10.1177/14647001030042002.
17. Kasim Khorasanee and Matilda Carter, 'Supported Voting: A How-To Guide', *Journal of Applied Philosophy* 38, no. 4 (2021): 674–85, https://doi.org/10.1111/japp.12505.
18. Wendy Hollway, *The Capacity to Care: Gender and Ethical Subjectivity* (London; New York: Routledge, 2006), 43, 60.
19. See: Margaret Urban Walker, 'The Curious Case of Care and Restorative Justice in the U.S. Context', in *Socializing Care: Feminist Ethics and Public Issues*, ed. Maurice Hamington and Dorothy C. Miller (Lanham, MD: Rowman & Littlefield, 2006), 145–62; Tyler G. Okimoto, Michael Wenzel and N. T. Feather, 'Beyond Retribution: Conceptualizing Restorative Justice and Exploring its Determinants', *Social Justice Research* 22, no. 1 (2009): 157.
20. John Braithwaite, 'Setting Standards for Restorative Justice', *British Journal of Criminology* 42, no. 3 (2002): 569, https://doi.org/10.1093/bjc/42.3.563.
21. Howard Zehr and Harry Mika, 'Fundamental Concepts of Restorative Justice', in *Restorative Justice: Critical Issues*, ed. Eugene McLaughlin, Ross Fergusson, Gordon Hughes and Louise Westmarland (London: Sage, in association with The Open University, 2003), 43.
22. Tronto, *Moral Boundaries*, 127–36.
23. Walker, 'The Curious Case of Care and Restorative Justice in the U.S. Context', 154.
24. Office for National Statistics, *Criminal Justice Statistics Quarterly, England and Wales, October 2019 to September 2020* (2021), 1, https://assets.publishing.service.gov.uk/government/uploads/system/uploads/attachment_data/file/962357/criminal-justice-statistics-quarterly-sept-2020.pdf.
25. Douglas Husak, 'The Metric of Punishment Severity: A Puzzle about the Principle of Proportionality', in *Of One-Eyed and Toothless Miscreants* (New York: Oxford University Press, 2019), 111, https://doi.org/10.1093/oso/9780190070595.003.0005.
26. Michelle S. Phelps, 'Mass Probation: Toward a More Robust Theory of State Variation in Punishment', *Punishment & Society* 19, no. 1 (2017): 53–73, https://doi.org/10.1177/1462474516649174.
27. US Courts, Probation and Pretrial Services, 'Probation and Pretrial Services – Mission | United States Courts', December 2023, https://www.uscourts.gov/services-forms/probation-and-pretrial-services/probation-and-pretrial-services-mission.
28. Marilyn J. Gregory, 'Practical Wisdom and the Ethic of Care in Probation Practice', *European Journal of Probation* 3, no. 3 (2011): 63.
29. See: Gregory, 'Practical Wisdom and the Ethic of Care in Probation Practice', 61 (citing: Michael Cavadino, Iain Crow and James Dignan, *Criminal Justice 2000: Strategies for a New Century* (Winchester: Waterside Press, 1999), 54); Marilyn J. Gregory, 'Reflection and Resistance: Probation Practice and the Ethic of Care', *British Journal of Social Work* 40, no. 7 (2010): 2274–90, https://doi.org/10.1093/bjsw/bcq028.
30. House of Commons Justice Committee, *The Role of the Probation Service Volume 1* (London: HMSO, 2011), 13.
31. Jane Dominey and Rob Canton, 'Probation and the Ethics of Care', *Probation Journal* 69, no. 4 (2022): 424 (citing: Fergus McNeill and Gwen Robinson, 'Liquid Legitimacy and Community Sanctions', in *Legitimacy and Compliance in Criminal Justice*, ed. Adam Crawford and Anthea Hucklesby (Abingdon: Routledge, 2012), https://eprints.gla.ac.uk/43317/, 133).

32. See: Dominey and Canton, 'Probation and the Ethics of Care', 424 (citing: Fergus McNeill and Gwen Robinson, 'The Dynamics of Compliance with Offender Supervision', in *Offender Supervision*, ed. Fergus McNeill, Peter Raynor and Chris Trotter (London: Willan Publishing, 2010)); Pamela Ugwudike, 'Compliance with Community Penalties: The Importance of Interactional Dynamics', in *Offender Supervision*, ed. Fergus McNeill, Peter Raynor and Chris Trotter (London: Willan Publishing, 2010).
33. Dominey and Canton, 'Probation and the Ethics of Care', 428.
34. George Mair, Noel Cross and Stuart Taylor, *The Use and Impact of the Community Order and the Suspended Sentence Order* (London: Centre for Crime and Justice Studies, King's College London, 2007), 20.
35. George Mair and Matthew Millings, *Doing Justice Locally: The North Liverpool Community Justice Centre* (London: Centre for Crime and Justice Studies, funded by The Bowlands Trust, 2011), 78.
36. Rt Rev James Jones, 'BBC Radio 4 Programmes', *The Bishop and the Prisoner*, Episode 3 (2012), http://www.bbc.co.uk/programmes/b019h3xs, at 15:43.
37. Bruce J. Winick and David B. Wexler, 'Therapeutic Jurisprudence', in *Principles of Addiction Medicine*, ed. Richard K. Ries, Shannon Miller, David A. Fiellin and Richard Saitz, 4th ed. (Philadelphia, PA: Lippincott Williams and Wilkins, 2009), 1519–20.
38. Coverdale, 'Caring and the Prison in Philosophy, Policy and Practice'.
39. Helen Brown Coverdale and Bill Wringe, 'Non-Paradigmatic Punishments', *Philosophy Compass* 17, no. 5 (2022): e12824, https://doi.org/10.1111/phc3.12824.
40. United Nations, *United Nations Standard Minimum Rules for the Treatment of Prisoners (the Nelson Mandela Rules)* (2015), https://undocs.org/A/RES/70/175.
41. Council of Europe, *European Prison Rules*, Rec(2006)2 (2006), https://search.coe.int/cm/Pages/result_details.aspx?ObjectID=09000016805d8d25#P6_138.
42. Parliament, Great Britain, *The Prison Rules 1999: Prison Rules Consolidated January 2010* (2010), r3, http://www.legislation.gov.uk/uksi/1999/728/contents/made.
43. House of Commons Justice Committee, *Role of the Prison Officer: Twelfth Report of Session 2008-09: Report, Together with Formal Minutes, Oral and Written Evidence* (London: The Stationery Office, 2009), 50, https://publications.parliament.uk/pa/cm200809/cmselect/cmjust/361/361.pdf.
44. *The Woolf Report: A Summary of the Main Findings and Recommendations of the Inquiry into Prison Disturbances* (London: Prison Reform Trust, 1991), 30, https://prisonreformtrust.org.uk/wp-content/uploads/1991/02/Woolf-report-summary-of-findings.pdf.
45. HMPS, 'Prison Officer' (2013), http://www.justice.gov.uk/jobs/prisons/on-offer/prison-officer/job-description.
46. Bubeck, *Care, Gender and Justice*, 129.
47. Samaritans. 'The Listener Scheme', 2013, http://www.samaritans.org/your-community/our-work-prisons/listener-scheme.
48. Fergus McNeill et al., *How and Why People Stop Offending: Discovering Desistance* (Glasgow: Institute for Research and Innovation in Social Services, 2012), 2.
49. G. Heidemann et al., 'Wounded Healers: How Formerly Incarcerated Women Help Themselves by Helping Others', *Punishment & Society* 18, no. 1 (2016): 9, 22, https://doi.org/10.1177/1462474515623101.
50. See: Braithwaite, 'Setting Standards for Restorative Justice', 98; Pat Carlen, 'Against Rehabilitation; for Reparative Justice', in *Crime, Justice and Social Democracy: International Perspectives*, ed. Kerry Carrington (Basingstoke: Palgrave Macmillan, 2013), 89–104; Lawrence Jablecki, 'Changing the Lives of Prisoners: A New Agenda', *The Humanist* (2005): 32.

51. See: Kimberley Brownlee, 'Freedom of Association: It's Not What You Think', *Oxford Journal of Legal Studies* 35, no. 2 (2015): 267–82, https://doi.org/10.1093/ojls/gqu018; Kimberley Brownlee, 'I – The Lonely Heart Breaks: On the Right to Be a Social Contributor', *Aristotelian Society Supplementary Volume* 90, no. 1 (2016): 27–48, https://doi.org/10.1093/arisup/akw008; Kimberley Brownlee, *Being Sure of Each Other: An Essay on Social Rights and Freedoms* (Oxford: Oxford University Press, 2020), https://doi.org/10.1093/oso/9780198714064.001.0001.
52. Helen Brown Coverdale, 'Social Connection, Interdependence and Being Sure of Ourselves', *Analysis*, July 2022, https://doi.org/10.1093/analys/anac041.
53. John Gunn, 'Introduction: What Is Forensic Psychiatry?', *Criminal Behaviour and Mental Health* 14, no. S1 (2004): S1–5, https://doi.org/10.1002/cbm.601.
54. See: Wendy Austin, Erika Goble and Julija Kelecevic, 'The Ethics of Forensic Psychiatry: Moving beyond Principles to a Relational Ethics Approach', *The Journal of Forensic Psychiatry & Psychology* 20, no. 6 (2009): 835–50, https://doi.org/10.1080/14789940903174147; Dave Holmes, 'Governing the Captives: Forensic Psychiatric Nursing in Corrections', *Perspectives in Psychiatric Care* 41, no. 1 (2005): 4, https://doi.org/10.1111/j.0031-5990.2005.00007.x; Charlotte Pollak et al., '"It Had Only Been a Matter of Time Before I Had Relapsed Into Crime": Aspects of Care and Personal Recovery in Forensic Mental Health', *Journal of Forensic Nursing* 14, no. 4 (2018): 231, https://doi.org/10.1097/JFN.0000000000000210.
55. Coverdale, 'Caring and the Prison in Philosophy, Policy and Practice'.
56. Helen Brown Coverdale, 'Punishment and Welfare: Defending Offender's Inclusion as Subjects of State Care', *Ethics and Social Welfare* 12, no. 2 (2018): 117–32, https://doi.org/10.1080/17496535.2017.1364398.
57. Austin, Goble and Kelecevic, 'The Ethics of Forensic Psychiatry', 844–5.
58. Hanna Pickard, 'Responsibility Without Blame: Empathy and the Effective Treatment of Personality Disorder', *Philosophy, Psychiatry, & Psychology* 18, no. 3 (2011): 209–24, https://doi.org/10.1353/ppp.2011.0032.
59. Nicola Lacey and Hanna Pickard, 'From the Consulting Room to the Court Room? Taking the Clinical Model of Responsibility without Blame into the Legal Realm', *Oxford Journal of Legal Studies* 33, no. 1 (2013): 1–29, https://doi.org/10.1093/ojls/gqs028.
60. Tronto, *Moral Boundaries*, 113.
61. Virginia Held, *The Ethics of Care: Personal, Political, and Global* (Oxford/New York: Oxford University Press, 2006), 17.
62. Jonathan Herring, *Caring and the Law* (Oxford: Hart Publishing, 2013), 67.

BIBLIOGRAPHY

Austin, Wendy, Erika Goble and Julija Kelecevic. 'The Ethics of Forensic Psychiatry: Moving beyond Principles to a Relational Ethics Approach', *The Journal of Forensic Psychiatry & Psychology* 20, no. 6 (2009): 835–50. https://doi.org/10.1080/14789940903174147.

Braithwaite, John. 'Setting Standards for Restorative Justice', *British Journal of Criminology* 42, no. 3 (2002): 563–77. https://doi.org/10.1093/bjc/42.3.563.

Brownlee, Kimberley. 'Freedom of Association: It's Not What You Think', *Oxford Journal of Legal Studies* 35, no. 2 (2015): 267–82. https://doi.org/10.1093/ojls/gqu018.

Brownlee, Kimberley. 'I – The Lonely Heart Breaks: On the Right to Be a Social Contributor', *Aristotelian Society Supplementary Volume* 90, no. 1 (2016): 27–48. https://doi.org/10.1093/arisup/akw008.

Brownlee, Kimberley. *Being Sure of Each Other: An Essay on Social Rights and Freedoms*. Oxford: Oxford University Press, 2020. https://doi.org/10.1093/oso/9780198714064.001.0001.

Bubeck, Diemut Elisabet. *Care, Gender and Justice*. Oxford: Clarendon Press, 1995.

Carlen, Pat. 'Against Rehabilitation; for Reparative Justice', in *Crime, Justice and Social Democracy: International Perspectives*, edited by Kerry Carrington, 89–104. Basingstoke: Palgrave Macmillan, 2013.

Cavadino, Michael, Iain Crow and James Dignan. *Criminal Justice 2000: Strategies for a New Century*. Winchester: Waterside Press, 1999.

Council of Europe. *European Prison Rules*, Rec(2006)2. 2006. https://search.coe.int/cm/Pages/result_details.aspx?ObjectID=09000016805d8d25#P6_138.

Coverdale, Helen Brown. 'Punishment and Welfare: Defending Offender's Inclusion as Subjects of State Care', *Ethics and Social Welfare* 12, no. 2 (2018): 117–32. https://doi.org/10.1080/17496535.2017.1364398.

Coverdale, Helen Brown. 'Caring and the Prison in Philosophy, Policy and Practice: Under Lock and Key', *Journal of Applied Philosophy* 38, no. 3 (2021): 415–30. https://doi.org/10.1111/japp.12415.

Coverdale, Helen Brown. 'Social Connection, Interdependence and Being Sure of Ourselves', *Analysis*, July 2022. https://doi.org/10.1093/analys/anac041.

Coverdale, Helen Brown, and Bill Wringe. 'Non-Paradigmatic Punishments', *Philosophy Compass* 17, no. 5 (2022): e12824. https://doi.org/10.1111/phc3.12824.

Dominey, Jane, and Rob Canton. 'Probation and the Ethics of Care', *Probation Journal* 69, no. 4 (2022): 417–33. https://doi.org/10.1177/02645505221105401.

Drake, Deborah. *Prisons, Punishment and the Pursuit of Security*. London: Palgrave Macmillan, 2012.

Engster, Daniel. *The Heart of Justice: Care Ethics and Political Theory*. Oxford: Oxford University Press, 2007.

Gregory, Marilyn J. 'Reflection and Resistance: Probation Practice and the Ethic of Care', *British Journal of Social Work* 40, no. 7 (2010): 2274–90. https://doi.org/10.1093/bjsw/bcq028.

Gregory, Marilyn J. 'Practical Wisdom and the Ethic of Care in Probation Practice', *European Journal of Probation* 3, no. 3 (2011): 60–77.

Gunn, John. 'Introduction: What Is Forensic Psychiatry?' *Criminal Behaviour and Mental Health* 14, no. S1 (2004): S1–5. https://doi.org/10.1002/cbm.601.

Heidemann, G., J. A. Cederbaum, S. Martinez and T. P. LeBel. 'Wounded Healers: How Formerly Incarcerated Women Help Themselves by Helping Others', *Punishment & Society* 18, no. 1 (2016): 3–26. https://doi.org/10.1177/1462474515623101.

Held, Virginia. *The Ethics of Care: Personal, Political, and Global*. Oxford/New York: Oxford University Press, 2006.

Herring, Jonathan. *Caring and the Law*. Oxford: Hart Publishing, 2013.

HMPS. 'Prison Officer', 2013. http://www.justice.gov.uk/jobs/prisons/on-offer/prison-officer/job-description.

Hollway, Wendy. *The Capacity to Care: Gender and Ethical Subjectivity*. London/New York: Routledge, 2006.

Holmes, Dave. 'Governing the Captives: Forensic Psychiatric Nursing in Corrections', *Perspectives in Psychiatric Care* 41, no. 1 (2005): 3–13. https://doi.org/10.1111/j.0031-5990.2005.00007.x.

House of Commons Justice Committee. *Role of the Prison Officer: Twelfth Report of Session 2008–09: Report, Together with Formal Minutes, Oral and Written Evidence*. London: The Stationery Office, 2009. https://publications.parliament.uk/pa/cm200809/cmselect/cmjust/361/361.pdf.

House of Commons Justice Committee. *The Role of the Probation Service Volume 1*. London: HMSO, 2011.

Husak, Douglas. 'The Metric of Punishment Severity: A Puzzle about the Principle of Proportionality', in *Of One-Eyed and Toothless Miscreants*. New York: Oxford University Press, 2019. https://doi.org/10.1093/oso/9780190070595.003.0005.

Jablecki, Lawrence. 'Changing the Lives of Prisoners: A New Agenda', *The Humanist*, 2005.

Jones, Rt Revd James. *The Bishop and the Prisoner*, Episode 3. BBC Radio 4 Programmes, 2012. http://www.bbc.co.uk/programmes/b019h3xs.

Khorasanee, Kasim, and Matilda Carter. 'Supported Voting: A How-To Guide', *Journal of Applied Philosophy* 38, no. 4 (2021): 674–85. https://doi.org/10.1111/japp.12505.

Kittay, Eva Feder. *Love's Labor: Essays on Women, Equality and Dependency*. Thinking Gender. New York: Routledge, 1999.

Kittay, Eva Feder. 'When Caring Is Just and Justice Is Caring', in *The Subject of Care: Feminist Perspectives on Dependency*, edited by Eva Feder Kittay and Ellen K. Feder, 257–76. Feminist Constructions. Lanham, MD: Rowman & Littlefield, 2002.

Lacey, Nicola, and Hanna Pickard. 'From the Consulting Room to the Court Room? Taking the Clinical Model of Responsibility without Blame into the Legal Realm', *Oxford Journal of Legal Studies* 33, no. 1 (2013): 1–29. https://doi.org/10.1093/ojls/gqs028.

Liebling, Alison. 'Penal Legitimacy, Well-Being, and Trust: The Role of Empirical Research in "Morally Serious" Work', in *Crime, Justice, and Social Order*, edited by Alison Liebling, Joanna Shapland, Richard Sparks and Justice Tankebe. Oxford University Press: Oxford, 2022. https://doi.org/10.1093/oso/9780192859600.003.0012.

Llewellyn, Jennifer J. 'Restorative Justice: Thinking Relationally about Justice', in *Being Relational: Reflections on Relational Theory and Health Law*, edited by Jennifer J. Llewellyn and Jocelyn Grant Downie, 89–108. Vancouver: University of British Columbia Press, 2012.

Mair, George, Noel Cross and Stuart Taylor. *The Use and Impact of the Community Order and the Suspended Sentence Order*. London: Centre for Crime and Justice Studies, King's College London, 2007.

Mair, George, and Matthew Millings. *Doing Justice Locally: The North Liverpool Community Justice Centre*. London: Centre for Crime and Justice Studies, funded by The Bowlands Trust, 2011.

McNeill, Fergus, and Gwen Robinson. 'The Dynamics of Compliance with Offender Supervision', in *Offender Supervision* edited by Fergus McNeill, Peter Raynor and Chris Trotter. London: Willan Publishing, 2010.

McNeill, Fergus, and Gwen Robinson. 'Liquid Legitimacy and Community Sanctions', in *Legitimacy and Compliance in Criminal Justice*, edited by Adam Crawford and Anthea Hucklesby. Abingdon: Routledge, 2012. https://eprints.gla.ac.uk/43317/.

McNeill, Fergus, Stephen Farrall, Claire Lightowler and Shadd Maruna. *How and Why People Stop Offending: Discovering Desistance*. Glasgow: Institute for Research and Innovation in Social Services, 2012.

Office for National Statistics. *Criminal Justice Statistics Quarterly, England and Wales, October 2019 to September 2020*. 2021. https://assets.publishing.service.gov.uk/government/uploads/system/uploads/attachment_data/file/962357/criminal-justice-statistics-quarterly-sept-2020.pdf.

Okimoto, Tyler G., Michael Wenzel and N. T. Feather. 'Beyond Retribution: Conceptualizing Restorative Justice and Exploring its Determinants', *Social Justice Research* 22, no. 1 (2009): 156–80. https://doi.org/10.1007/s11211-009-0092-5.

Parliament, Great Britain. *The Prison Rules 1999: Prison Rules Consolidated January 2010*. 2010. http://www.legislation.gov.uk/uksi/1999/728/contents/made.

Phelps, Michelle S. 'Mass Probation: Toward a More Robust Theory of State Variation in Punishment', *Punishment & Society* 19, no. 1 (2017): 53–73. https://doi.org/10.1177/1462474516649174.

Pickard, Hanna. 'Responsibility Without Blame: Empathy and the Effective Treatment of Personality Disorder', *Philosophy, Psychiatry, & Psychology* 18, no. 3 (2011): 209–24. https://doi.org/10.1353/ppp.2011.0032.

Pollak, Charlotte, Tom Palmstierna, Magnus Kald and Per Ekstrand. '"It Had Only Been a Matter of Time Before I Had Relapsed Into Crime": Aspects of Care and Personal Recovery in Forensic Mental Health', *Journal of Forensic Nursing* 14, no. 4 (2018): 230–7. https://doi.org/10.1097/JFN.0000000000000210.

Robinson, Fiona. *Globalizing Care: Ethics, Feminist Theory, and International Relations*. Feminist Theory and Politics. Boulder, CO: Westview Press, 1999.

Samaritans. 'The Listener Scheme', 2013. http://www.samaritans.org/your-community/our-work-prisons/listener-scheme.

Sevenhuijsen, Selma. *Citizenship and the Ethics of Care: Feminist Considerations on Justice, Morality, and Politics*. London: Routledge, 1998.

Tronto, Joan C. *Moral Boundaries: A Political Argument for an Ethic of Care*. New York: Routledge, 1993.

Tronto, Joan C. 'Time's Place', *Feminist Theory* 4, no. 2 (2003): 119–38. https://doi.org/10.1177/14647001030042002.

Tronto, Joan C. *Caring Democracy: Markets, Equality, and Justice*. New York: New York University Press, 2013.

Ugwudike, Pamela. 'Compliance with Community Penalties: The Importance of Interactional Dynamics', in *Offender Supervision*, edited by Fergus McNeill, Peter Raynor and Chris Trotter. London: Willan Publishing, 2010.

United Nations. *United Nations Standard Minimum Rules for the Treatment of Prisoners (the Nelson Mandela Rules)*. 2015. https://undocs.org/A/RES/70/175.

US Courts, Probation and Pretrial Services. 'Probation and Pretrial Services – Mission | United States Courts', December 2023. https://www.uscourts.gov/services-forms/probation-and-pretrial-services/probation-and-pretrial-services-mission.

Walker, Margaret Urban. 'The Curious Case of Care and Restorative Justice in the U.S. Context', in *Socializing Care: Feminist Ethics and Public Issues*, edited by Maurice Hamington and Dorothy C Miller, 145–62. Lanham, MD: Rowman & Littlefield, 2006.

Winick, Bruce J., and David B. Wexler. 'Therapeutic Jurisprudence', in *Principles of Addiction Medicine*, 4th edition, edited by Richard K. Ries, Shannon Miller, David A. Fiellin and Richard Saitz, 1519–20. Philadelphia, PA: Lippincott Williams & Wilkins, 2009.

Woolf, Lord Justice. *The Woolf Report: A Summary of the Main Findings and Recommendations of the Inquiry into Prison Disturbances*. London: Prison Reform Trust, 1991. https://prisonreformtrust.org.uk/wp-content/uploads/1991/02/Woolf-report-summary-of-findings.pdf.

Zehr, Howard, and Harry Mika. 'Fundamental Concepts of Restorative Justice,' in *Restorative Justice: Critical Issues*, edited by Eugene McLaughlin, Ross Fergusson, Gordon Hughes and Louise Westmarland, 40–3. London: Sage, in association with The Open University, 2003.

CHAPTER TWENTY

Care ethics and public administration

An overview of the field and a look forward

PETR URBAN

INTRODUCTION

The social and political dimension of care was a focus of care ethics from the outset and it received the explicit attention of care ethicists as early as about the mid-1980s.[1] Tronto famously demonstrated how the traditional boundary between private institutions (the family, the household) and public institutions (the market, the state) has for centuries served as the main vehicle of marginalizing and devaluing care.[2] Over the long history of the West, care was relegated to the domain of intimate personal relationships in the family and the household, was excluded from political discussions and deliberations, and was gendered as a primary activity of women. To see care as a crucial element in the life of all individuals and communities thus means to challenge the current institutional arrangements of caring and propose alternative ways of organizing care in our societies and polities. Over the last four decades, care theorists have been rethinking the role and responsibility of larger social and political structures, such as the state and its institutions, in securing care as a public value. They formulated the idea of a 'public ethic of care'[3] which served as a starting point for both the criticism of the neoliberal policies of market-oriented care arrangements and the paternalistic modes of the welfare state care provision.[4]

Besides the primary interest in a critical analysis of policies of states in various geographical, cultural and economic contexts, care ethicists gradually started to pay attention to the ways in which the state governs the public sector and implements its laws and policies through public administration. Engster recently offered a compelling argument for the importance of a care-ethical perspective on legal and policy implementation. He points out that public administrators play a seminal role in determining whether citizens perceive the state's policies as just, since they often have to make decisions about whether and how a rule applies to a particular situation and individual.[5] If they use their discretionary powers in inappropriate ways, citizens may experience the interaction with the state and its policies as unjust, regardless of the content and nature of those policies. Engster finds care ethics particularly suitable to develop a procedural theory for guiding how public administrators ought to relate to individuals and communities, and concludes that care ethics offers a new public ethics which is needed 'for the proper exercise of discretion in liberal-democratic states'[6] and which therefore helps both liberal and republican governance 'to live up to its ideals at the very point where the state most directly interacts with citizens'.[7]

In this chapter, I will provide an overview of the formation of the idea of a care-centred public administration[8] in care ethics literature. I will also zoom in on three new areas in which the research on care-centred public administration entered only recently and which open possibilities for further investigation. The chapter is divided into three sections. In the first section, I reconstruct the birth and formation of the idea of care-centred public administration in the works of DeLysa Burnier, Helena Stensöta and Sophie Bourgault. The second section discusses different views of the relationship between care and justice perspectives in public administration, and particularly explores the role of these different perspectives in everyday practice of public administrators. In the third section, I take a closer look at some current debates that apply a care ethics perspective to three newly established areas of public administration: a) crisis management, b) governance for environmental sustainability and c) digitalizing public administration.

20.1 CARE-CENTRED PUBLIC ADMINISTRATION

Drawing on the classical account proposed by Carol Gilligan, an ethic of care can be characterized as a distinctive style of moral judging and constructing moral problems.[9] It centres around responsibility for human relationships, builds moral judgement on concrete knowledge of a particular situation and context, emphasizes the priority of connection and starts from the insight that there is no contradiction in acting responsibly towards oneself and others. An ethic of care foregrounds the ideal of non-dominating relationships based on responsibility, respect, understanding, cooperation, sensitivity to the needs of the other, compassion and tolerance. According to Fisher and Tronto's influential definition, care is 'a species activity that includes everything we do to maintain, continue, and repair our "world" so that we can live in it as well as possible'.[10] Fisher and Tronto famously distinguish four phases of the process of caring: *caring about* (attentiveness) – paying attention to something with a focus on continuity, maintenance and repair; *taking care of* (responsibility) – taking responsibility for activities responding to the facts noticed in caring about; *caregiving* (competency) – the concrete tasks and the hands-on care work; and *care receiving* (responsiveness) – the response of those towards whom caring is directed.[11] Fisher and Tronto conceive of good caring in terms of the integrity of the caring process where the four phases fit together into a whole. Deficient caring, on the contrary, consists in the alienation of and fragmentation in the caring process (e.g. when care receivers have little control over how their needs are defined). Tronto shows that the patterns of fragmentation of caring are mainly created by deficient social and political arrangements. She further argues that 'only in a just, pluralistic, democratic society can care flourish'.[12] Yet, the goal of non-dominating relationships does not imply that a politically formulated ethics of care should aim to eliminate power in caring relations. Instead, it should provide an understanding that helps to differentiate between power and domination, by making power recognizable and manageable.[13]

Building on the normative foundations of a moral and political theory of care laid by Gilligan, Fisher and Tronto, Sevenhuijsen and others, the American care theorist and administrative scientist DeLysa Burnier was the first to propose and systematically develop an idea of a *care-centred public administration*.[14] Burnier identifies the core assumption of a care-centred public administration in the belief that administering is a situational and relational practice which seeks to improve the lives of all individuals and communities.[15] If care ethics 'gives precedence to contextual, concrete knowledge and to values such as attentiveness, responsibility, competence and responsiveness',[16] applying it to public administration has a number of normative implications. Burnier identifies the following four: (1) good administrative processes and outcomes should reflect not only expert judgement but a collaborative work that takes into account different viewpoints and lived experiences; (2) good administrators should use their discretionary authority not to accumulate more power but to reach out to the public and invite them to join a dialogue; (3) good administrative knowledge should be situated in experience and dialogical reflection; and (4) good administrators should be critically reflexive, willing to question and challenge their own values, assumptions and professional judgements.[17] In other words, care-centred public administrators would take into account the circumstances of citizens and seek their input when implementing policies. They would become collaborators with citizens in applying policies according to their situations. Power would be applied in ways that track citizens' interests and the administrators would avoid dominating citizens at the implementation stage.[18]

It is worth noting that Burnier arrives at the characteristics of a care-centred public administration not only through a theoretical normative reflection, but also through an analysis of real-life examples of administrative practice (both past and present). Drawing on Stivers, Burnier examines the organizational efforts and activities of the American 'settlement women' from the turn of the twentieth century and finds them driven by an 'alternative ethos for governance and administrative practice'[19] which emphasizes relationality, viewing situations from multiple perspectives, concern for others, cooperative problem solving, care and compassion. She argues that though this alternative construction of administrative reality has never become public administration's dominant construction – Stivers speaks of 'public administration's buried heritage'[20] – neither has it completely disappeared. Burnier observes that 'for many public administrators, especially those working at the street and agency levels, care-centered administration is already at the core of what they do'.[21] If we carefully listen to the everyday talk of government employees and administrators, Burnier argues, a fresh discourse emerges that illuminates 'how care as a value and practice is inextricably tied to everyday judgments that clients, citizens, and administrators make about what it means to do a job well or what it means to be a "good" administrator'.[22]

Burnier also considers a set of practical measures that could help public administration become more care-centred, such as changing the organizational structure and culture, deploying 'relational leadership', introducing formal recognition and compensation for care work and emotional labour in the public sector or teaching, and training public officials aimed at acquiring knowledge and skills needed for individuals to become caring administrators. As regards the behaviour of administrative leaders and managers, Burnier emphasizes a transformative potential of 'relational leadership'.[23] The relational leader practises facilitating and reciprocal power as 'power with' rather than 'power over'. Such a leader promotes collaboration, caring, courage and vision within an organization and remains open to the perspectives of others. The relational leader should 'communicate that care is an organizational value to be embraced and practiced by individuals throughout the organization'.[24] The emotional labour and care work of relational leaders as well as other employees go often unrecognized in public sector agencies. It is a marginalized and devalued practice, although it can substantially contribute to creating better working conditions in an organization and enhancing the wellbeing of its clients. Thus, Burnier argues, we need to introduce measures of formal recognition and compensation for emotional labour and care work in organizations, such as alternative modes of evaluation, incorporating this work in job descriptions or audits.[25] Finally, governments and public agencies should bear responsibility for providing public administrators with quality education and training aimed at acquiring knowledge and skills needed for individuals to exercise good administrative discretion.

Independently of Burnier, the Swedish care ethicist and political theorist Helena Stensöta proposed the idea of a *public ethics of care* which is 'directed to assist in policy formation and implementation'[26] and aims 'to provide a guideline for employees in their handling of relevant cases in relation to citizens'.[27] Like Burnier, Stensöta stresses context sensitivity and responsiveness as fundamental tenets of a public ethics of care[28] due to which a care-oriented policy implementation can contribute to diminishing the danger of paternalistic public administration.[29] To achieve the goal of a flexible and trustful attitude towards citizens, administrative institutions are advised to implement 'an organizational form that puts the client in the center in a contextualized way'.[30] One of the ways to achieve this goal may consist in promoting diversity in the institution 'in order to increase the diversity of experiences represented, with which asset one thinks that the organization will be able to handle a broader range of tasks in a qualitatively good manner'.[31] The Canadian care ethicist and political philosopher Sophie Bourgault offers a more detailed analysis of what creating a caring administrative institution entails. Bourgault argues that the institution should ensure that it has administrators with solid listening and communicative skills (personal attentiveness) and puts in place extensive institutional consultation processes that enable reflective ways of defining and addressing the needs of all affected groups (institutional attentiveness).[32] A caring institution should place good administrative discretion at its centre. Yet, this is a complex issue. On the one hand, administrators should be encouraged to exercise discretion. On the other hand, some measures must be in place to ensure that discretion is exercised without falling into illegitimate arbitrariness. Bourgault makes the case that these measures do not need to be reduced to adopting more institutional rules and stronger control mechanisms. In her view, it is possible to facilitate good discretion by hiring and promoting administrators with good communicative and listening skills, providing administrators with adequate training and support in acquiring needed cognitive and emotional skills combined with professional expertise and developing an organizational culture that recognizes and values good discretion.[33] If an institution seeks to create such a culture it must also pay adequate attention to the issue of time, for bad discretion often occurs under the circumstances of a lack of time.[34]

Good communicative and listening skills on the part of public officials and administrators are clearly central to a care-centred public administration. This does not apply solely to the relationships between street-level bureaucrats and their clients, but also to the level of government's communication with the wider public. Dong and Morenhouse recently explored how 'care ethics can help government practitioners navigate relational challenges by shifting the focus of government–public relationships (GPRs) from an organization-centric, goal-oriented managerial function to the process of relationship nurturing and building between communicator and publics'.[35] In particular, Dong and Morenhouse examined government communicators' conceptualization of care-based communication strategies by interviewing thirty-two public relations practitioners working at county government agencies in the United States. Their data reveal a number of facets of care in GPRs that seem crucial for creating a care-centred public administration.

(1) The communicators described how they proactively initiate communication with their publics 'to understand publics' evolving needs, issues, concerns, and expectations of the government organization'.[36] For this purpose, they use various tactics in proactive outreach such as inviting participants to town hall meetings and community outreach meetings, reaching out to the publics via radio stations and social media platforms, or informally reaching out to the publics through casual conversations in neutral locations.

(2) The communicators emphasized the role of empathic listening which offers them 'an opportunity to put themselves in the shoes of publics and understand the rationale behind publics' confusion, anger, or fear'.[37]

(3) The participants stressed that care means 'recognizing the diversity in demographics, education, media literary, information accessibility and cultural backgrounds' which sometimes involves a strategic use of plain language, enabling translations and multilingual options or cooperating with community advisers to engage with local residents.[38]

(4) Referring to care as a way of recognizing and protecting human vulnerabilities, the participants contended that government communicators' responsibilities include 'safeguarding publics' information, privacy, security, online political participation, and freedom of speech'.[39]

(5) The participants conveyed a view that care entails 'understanding their limitations as communicators and constantly striving to overcome and improve those limitations'.[40] These empirical findings clearly illustrate the strong link between a care-centred public administration and care-based government–public relations and how these relations can be developed through care-based cultivation strategies, going beyond the classical communication strategies of openness and access.

Looking back at the two decades of the development of the idea of a care-centred public administration, it seems justified to claim that a care ethics perspective helped to ground and establish a distinct approach to policy implementation which foregrounds the importance of attentiveness, responsiveness, sensitivity to context, good communicative/listening skills and democratic needs interpretation. Since its first formulation in the work of DeLysa Burnier, the idea of a care-centred public administration has undergone a detailed elaboration with respect to concrete institutional and organizational measures that are instrumental to achieving the goal of a care-centred administrative practice and policy implementation. Yet, one could easily raise the question of whether such a view of public administration challenges the traditional normative foundation of administrative ethics, given the fact that a traditional pillar of administrative ethics is the Weberian ideal-type bureaucracy based on the values of justice, impartiality, rule-following and accountability. The relationship between care and justice has been a matter of lively discussion in moral and political theory for decades. In the next section, I will explore different views of how the relationship between care and justice might be conceptualized in the context of administrative practice and how these views rhyme with the idea of a care-centred public administration.

20.2 CARE, JUSTICE AND EFFICIENCY IN PUBLIC ADMINISTRATION

Engster points out that to the extent that mainstream political theorists (both liberal and republican) have studied policy implementation, their favoured model was 'a legal-rational organization arranged hierarchically with a division of offices, specialized tasks, fixed rules, paid professionals, and … an impersonal and rule-bound ethics' where 'bureaucratic discretion should be sharply constrained, oriented around fixed rules, and exercised impersonally for maintaining limited and responsive government in the implementation of laws and policies'.[41] The traditional emphasis on the importance of impartially applying rules and decisions based on merit has made the justice perspective an especially relevant moral framework for public administrators. It is therefore no surprise that 'the justice perspective has long been regarded as more appropriate to the public sphere of our lives, where, as citizens or as public employees, one must weigh the rights of others and dispassionately apply laws that bind all citizens alike'.[42] However, there seem to be a good reason for thinking that an exclusive reliance on the justice perspective in the administrative context is 'seriously deficient'.[43] This is mainly due to the importance of flexible and responsive discretion for the just implementation of laws and policies. The need for a flexible and responsive discretion in the administrative context is an old idea expressed already by Aristotle who argued that 'equity must be applied to the law when, in particular cases, enforcing the universal rule would result in an outcome contrary to the law's intended aims'.[44] Engster seeks to make the case that a public ethics of care, with its emphasis on flexible and responsive discretion, does not only comply with the principle that like cases should be treated alike, but 'might actually better fulfil the principle of treating like cases alike than a Weberian ethics of rule'. He maintains that by taking into account the differences between individual cases and their unique contexts 'a public ethics of care can achieve a kind of equality and consistency in the implementation of laws and policies that Weberian bureaucratic ethics cannot'.[45] Since a flexible and responsive exercise of discretion which a care-centred public administration promotes seems to be essential also for 'avoiding state domination' and protecting citizens against the exposure to 'an alien coercive power in the application of laws and policies',[46] Engster concludes that 'a public ethics of care provides a better public ethics'[47] than the Weberian bureaucratic ethics; thus, 'if street-level bureaucrats are to align the exercise of their discretion with liberal and republican principles … they should adopt a public ethics of care … as their guide'.[48]

While Engster seems to view care ethics as 'the proper or best public ethics' for legal and policy implementation,[49] Jos and Hines propose a comparatively more moderate and balanced view of the relationship between the care and justice perspectives in public administration. By their account,

> an examination of the care and justice perspectives shows that both are relevant to the administrative task and that it is unwise to employ either perspective to the exclusion of the other. … The public employee who becomes preoccupied with procedural fairness and client rights and neglects to understand and care for particular clients with particular needs is less likely to recognize harms done in the name of abstract ideals.[50]

Jos and Hines particularly argue that without the relationship to particular individuals and their needs it is difficult to evaluate whether one is adequately serving the public, since 'it is through caring for real individuals that we can gain perspective on the moral adequacy of rules and procedures'.[51] On the other hand, because an exclusive reliance on one's relationship to particular clients might lead to biased and unfair decisions, 'an appeal to rules and individual rights of all clients can serve to check the tendency towards bias and paternalism as well, just as sensitivity and compassion are required to avoid the complacency that results from turning clients into cases and the public interest into an abstraction'.[52] Thus, Jos and Hines conclude, 'an ethics of justice is a necessary but not sufficient basis for public administration ethics and political ethics more generally'[53] and the care perspective serves to remind us that the 'public administrator must serve the public in both generalized fashion (impartial, rule-oriented administration of nomothetic law) and in a specific way[54] (engaged, particularistic, and idiographic service to persons)'.[55]

Engster eventually voices some sympathy with respect to this more balanced view, as he considers 'a total overhaul of Weberian bureaucracy' as unnecessary[56] and argues that even in a care-centred public administration 'bureaucratic discretion would still exist under the law and be oriented toward agency aims'.[57] He admits that 'a public ethics of care must be practiced within laws and agency goals that set some limits to what street-level bureaucrats can legitimately do'.[58] Similarly, when Burnier talks about the need for 'a care transformation of the public sector' which 'values care, makes care work visible, and places care values and practices at the center of public administration scholarship and practice',[59] she does not suggest that care should replace the values of bureaucracy and the market, but rather that public administration should take care as seriously as it has taken bureaucracy and markets.

The complex relationship between care and justice in public administration raises the question: how do the care and justice perspective relate in the everyday practice of public administrators? Jos and Hines contend that a good public administrator seeks to connect, balance and reconcile the different perspectives of care and justice in their everyday practice. Although public administrators may experience conflicts between bureaucratic requirements of neutrality and objectivity and care requirements of cooperative and contextual problem solutions, good administrators would take into consideration both as they inevitably work under multiple ethical contexts.[60] At the same time, the good public administrator, characterized by the ability to combine and accommodate both perspectives, can hardly avoid the ambiguity and uncertainty of 'how to weigh considerations of care and justice in a particular situation'.[61] Bourgault – in accordance with a bulk of recent research on public institutions[62] – speaks in this context of a dissonance which public administrators often experience.[63] It is a tension between the principles that guide administrative practice but, at the same time, pull in different directions, that is, towards greater neutrality and impartiality on the one hand, and towards more attentiveness and responsiveness on the other hand.[64]

The tension between justice and care perspectives, however, is not the only tension that public administrators experience. The New Public Management (NPM) reforms of the 1990s challenged the Weberian ideal-type bureaucracy with its emphasis on impartial delivery of public goods and services. The value of efficiency took over the role of the normative foundation of public administration and the governmental delivery of goods and services to citizens was, to a considerable extent, transformed into a market transaction where private providers of services compete for customers seeking to maximize their choices. Despite the criticism which the NPM reforms faced,[65] the principle of maximizing productivity has become a widely accepted normative pilar of current administrative practice. In the view of Jos and Hines it is possible to reduce the tension between the values of care and efficiency in public administration 'by directing attention to how the web of relationships among particular people contributes to organizational productivity', since 'the ethic of care is not at all inconsistent with attaining organizational goals and should not be dismissed as the kind of personal caring and concern that necessarily leads to indulging employees at the expense of the public treasury'.[66] Most public administration theorists, however, seem to contend that the values of care, fairness and efficiency represent competing normative demands which pull the public administrator in different directions and create dissonance.[67] Burnier's moderate proposal that care should not replace the values of fairness and efficiency, but rather be taken as seriously as bureaucracy and markets, seems a realistic and pragmatic suggestion in the context of a post-NPM public administration.

The aim of this section has been to demonstrate that the idea of a care-centred public administration can be fruitfully incorporated in the complex picture of the real-life administrative practice which is characterized by a nontrivial relationship between diverse normative frameworks. Thus, care ethics not only provides a viable distinct perspective on public administration and policy implementation, but also contributes to a more complex and nuanced understanding of the everyday practice of public administrators and administrative institutions. In the next section, I want to zoom in on three newly established areas of public administration which gained in urgency over the last decade, but were so far only provisionally discussed from a care ethics perspective: (1) crisis management, (2) leadership for environmental sustainability and (3) digitalizing public administration in the era of new technologies. The aim of this concluding section is to exemplify the applicability of a care ethics perspective to concrete areas of current administrative practice as well as to point out some possible future directions of research in care ethics and public administration.

20.3 CRISIS MANAGEMENT, SUSTAINABILITY AND DIGITALIZED PUBLIC ADMINISTRATION

The twenty-first century has been marked by a number of crises, which include the climate crisis, financial crisis, crisis of democracy, geopolitical crises and the Covid-19 crisis. The concurrence of these crises made many scholars and journalists start to talk about the 'age of the polycrisis'.[68] With respect to the recent global developments, 'crisis management [has] become the subject of a growing and increasingly prominent strand of management and practice'.[69] How a crisis is managed has considerable material and societal consequences, hence it is an important task to explore different ways of crisis management and their expected effects. Branicki observes that the current mainstream approaches to crisis management are based on a set of rationalist and masculinist assumptions. When dealing with the Covid-19 crisis, for instance, leaders and politicians often invoked the language of the battlefield or war-like metaphors.[70] Branicki points out that the classical discourse of crisis management 'emphasizes the calculation of impacts in financial, legal and human terms, and … inherent to crisis management is a philosophy of crises being "manageable"'.[71] The objective of rationalist crisis management is a return to 'normal' and 'the emphasis is on coordination via a specialist managerial function'.[72] During the Covid-19 pandemic, the evidence began to emerge that the mainstream management approaches to the crisis caused that 'people from already structurally disadvantaged groups were being disproportionately impacted by both Covid-19 and the measures put in place to control its spread'.[73] Similar evidence exists with respect to the climate crisis, the global financial crises and many others. Branicki suggests that the negative consequences of classical crisis management demonstrate the inappropriateness of the approach and the need for 'a new theorization of crisis management that is grounded in feminist ethics to provide a care-based concern for all crisis affected people'.[74] The feminist alternative to rational crisis management, which Branicki advocates, is centred on the values of non-violent conflict resolution, contextual and narrative understanding, the activity of care, and networks of relationships and responsibilities. It entails 'a heightened appreciation of reciprocal care and relational needs and capacities'.[75] Instead of a return to 'normal', the objective of feminist crisis management is individual and social transformation, and the resolution is based on webs of connections produced by interpersonal relationships. Feminist crisis management also entails a different temporality. It sees crises as 'enduring and overlapping phenomena that are enmeshed and embedded within each other to a significant extent. Crises compound and confound each other within webs of relationships informed by care.'[76]

The relational logic invoked in feminist crisis management plays also a crucial role in Nicholson and Kurucz's idea of 'relational leadership for sustainability'.[77] Sustainability is a complex notion which refers to a set of urgent social, economic and environmental issues. Leadership for sustainability became a prominent notion in recent literature on business management and public administration. Yet, Nicholson and Kurucz argue that the current debate on leadership for sustainability is based on 'the fundamental assumption about effective leadership as an individual pursuit'.[78] They suggest that it is possible to develop a more effective approach to leadership for sustainability, an approach which 'emphasises the importance of co-creation within the complexity of multiple, often conflicting, perspectives, rather than the more prevalent view of leadership as an individual rallying around a common, though often leader-generated, vision'.[79] Nicholson and Kurucz coin the term 'relational leadership for sustainability' which they conceive as 'an ongoing process of meaning making and reflection within a nested system of the biosphere and society that enables this integration (of principles, strategies, and actions) to take place ... Much of this meaning making involves value-laden decisions and questions about "who wins and who loses" in the process of integrating environmental, social, and economic concerns.'[80] The ethics of care perspective is helpful in this context, since it refocuses our attention on the role of caring in leadership practice and puts emphasis on 'encouraging the collaborative capacity of the organization, in order to strengthen the stakeholder network as a whole. Leadership efforts from this perspective are primarily aimed at fostering this collaboration.'[81] In the relational approach to leadership for sustainability 'the meaning of "value" includes the contribution to present and future well-being, considering an integrative view of economic, societal, and environmental flourishing'.[82] Care ethics' sensitivity to context, whether organizational or cultural, makes it also 'particularly useful as an ethical framework for leadership for sustainability which requires coordination of local and global actions to address issues of the commons that transcend national and cultural boundaries'.[83]

Both Branicki and Nicholson and Kurucz deploy the care ethics perspective to propose an alternative to the mainstream approaches to crisis management and leadership for sustainability. They formulate the alternative relational approaches primarily with respect to organizational management and business leadership. However, both crisis management and leadership for sustainability are of utmost importance in public administration too, as the cases of the mismanaged Covid-19 crisis and poorly tackled climate crisis on the governmental level clearly demonstrate. This reveals a gap in the existing literature on care-based public administration which needs to be filled by exploring the potential of 'feminist crisis management' and 'relational leadership for sustainability' in the context of public administration and governance. A good start might consist in establishing a dialogue between the current research in crisis management and the body of literature on care-centred public administration which was discussed in the previous sections of this chapter. Moreover, while Nicholson and Kurucz operate with a human-centred notion of sustainability, referring to 'human development within the limits of the biosphere ... with the ultimate goal of individual and societal flourishing',[84] future research on relational leadership for sustainability in public administration would better draw from more progressive care-ethical approaches to environmental sustainability that seek to overcome the humanist and anthropocentric positions.[85]

Another area which has attracted growing attention from administration scholars is the digital transformation of management and administration, both in the private and public sector. Over the last two decades, we have witnessed 'the massive entry of digital tools in institutions, including those that some scholars thought were immune to algorithms or disembodied technology (that is, social work, education and health)'.[86] Administration theorists noticed that 'pushing digitalization as an efficiency tool *does* something to public space as well as to private life and it has practical, political and ethical consequences'.[87] Studies have shown that digitalization of public administration in particular is far from being just about injecting digital and information technologies into the public sector, rather it implies a process in which 'we also get reconfigured citizen roles, new ways of understanding the bureaucratic profession and changed bureaucratic practices, in which the public and private spheres are activated and blended in new ways'.[88] The techno-optimistic images of digital technologies as a neutral upgrade of the state, introduced with the aim of creating more efficient welfare provision, often tend to overlook 'how adjustments of practice might have intrusive effects on the way governance is performed' and how the unintended effects of new roles for both citizens and bureaucrats can lead to 'intrusive reconfigurations of the time and space of the bureaucratic encounter'.[89]

Bourgault offers a critical view of the digital transformation of public administration from a care ethics perspective. On the one hand, the usage of digital technologies in state–citizen interaction clearly helps to diminish social marginalization and increase fairness in service provision through anonymization of files and removing the particular biases of imperfect civil servants at the street-level bureaucracy. On the other hand, Bourgault argues, 'what is sacrificed when resorting to anonymisation and digital citizen-government encounters is the consideration of particulars that may appear at first glance irrelevant for decision making but are, in fact, critical'.[90] By removing the bodily presence and veiling the particular traits of individual citizens, digital technologies can contribute to avoiding prejudicial treatment in public administration. However,

> the bodily absence entailed in the institutional recourse to digital service delivery might, paradoxically, lead to the loss of significant means to undercut negative prejudice in the long term. ... To give up on the human capacity to correct for some of our hermeneutic/epistemic difficulties by resorting to more reliable/impartial 'technological' means or to anonymising measures of various sorts, might, in the long run, increase some of our discursive and epistemic failures.[91]

The main concern here is that digital rigidity of algorithms used in public sector compromises the responsiveness and attentiveness of public services. Moreover, Bourgault also notices that 'the losses entailed in "going digital"/veiling are significant not only for citizens, but also for the public employees themselves, who can derive satisfaction from face-to-face encounters and the exercise of discretion'.[92] Bourgault does not conclude that we ought to completely put aside digital technologies in public administration; however, she does present 'a concerned reminder, voiced from a care perspective, about the ethical and political importance of face-to-face contact'[93] and argues that 'the path of anonymisation, which tends to compromise attentiveness, is at odds with what care ethics celebrates'.[94]

Bourgault's concerned view of the growing recourse to digital service delivery in the public sector begs a question whether a care ethics perspective motivates an overall negative stance with respect to introducing digital technologies in public administration. It is important to note that Bourgault's focus is primarily on citizen–state encounters at the street level and the issue of replacing street-level bureaucrats by digital tools of public service provision. Thus, her 'concerned reminder' relates to the ethical and political implications of the losses of face-to-face encounters between street-level civil servants and their clients. Bourgault does not reflect on the ethical and political implication of the usage of digital technologies at higher (central governmental) levels of institutional decision making which involve no bodily presence of citizens even in the traditional pre-digital public administration.[95] In her account, Bourgault also leaves aside the question of designing and developing technologies to be used in public administration, or, to be more precise, she touches on it only in passing in her critical remark about discretionary power moving 'into the hands of system designers' who now have discretion over the very 'drafting and composing of the rules themselves'.[96] In the remaining part of this section, we shall explore the question whether it plausible to think of a reconciliation between a care ethics perspective and the ongoing process of digitalizing public administration in particular by taking these two areas into account.

In a recent paper, Villegas-Galaviz and Martin zoom in on the introduction of digital technologies, in particular AI, into administrative decision making and propose the ethics of care as a moral framework to analyse the moral implications of AI-based decision making. In a similar way as Bourgault, Villegas-Galaviz and Martin contend that the use of digital technologies can contribute to creating a 'moral distance' which 'abstracts those who are impacted by the decision and leads to less ethical decisions'.[97] According to Villegas-Galaviz and Martin, the moral distance can be created both in the development and deployment of AI and other digital tools. They propose to distinguish between two types of moral distancing: (1) *proximity distance* which relates to 'the elimination of face-to-face interactions (creating a distance of space, time, and culture)' and (2) *bureaucratic distance* which is 'derived from hierarchy, complex processes, and principlism'.[98] Proximity distance entails not only special distance or absence of face-to-face interactions, but also temporal distance which can be created by the change of algorithms over time with the introduction of new data.[99] Another important aspect of moral distancing is linked to cultural differences, e.g. with respect to culturally different privacy expectations and norms, or culturally different ways of evaluation at educational institutions. Villegas-Galaviz and Martin point out that 'AI exacerbates the cultural distance issue by automating ethical decision-making and the fact that the same model may be deployed in different cultures'.[100] Bureaucratic distance, in turn, typically entails issues such as algorithmic opacity ('we do no longer know how it [an algorithm] works, what it does, and indeed what we are doing'),[101] and formal rationality, a type of moral distance created by 'a blind attachment to guidelines and principles'.[102]

Villegas-Galaviz and Martin point to concrete examples to illustrate the issue of the moral distance created by the use of AI in administrative decision making. For example,

Amazon has deployed an automated system for firing delivery drivers, where the whole process, from rating to firing, is controlled by AI. Villegas-Galaviz and Martin argue that, in such cases, 'where decision reduces to data, ignores circumstances, vulnerabilities, and the specific harm that can be done to that individual – the firm misses the moral implications of the decision for which it is responsible. The firm is blinded to the impact of its decisions behind the veil of AI while also being responsible for those decisions.'[103] In other cases, where digital technologies are deployed in areas such as university acceptance programmes or companies' decision about granting a loan or insurance, 'automating that decision could have a great impact in the future with the marginalization of … entire societies, leaving them with no possibility of prospering'.[104]

In contrast to Bourgault, Villegas-Galaviz and Martin suggest using care ethics as a 'bridge for moral distance in AI'[105] and a moral framework to 'ameliorate the downsides of moral distancing from the use of AI'.[106] In particular, drawing on the shared understanding in care ethics that 'ethical decision making should consider interdependent relationships, context and circumstances, attend to particular vulnerabilities, and also should respond to different points of view, and hear different voices', Villegas-Galaviz and Martin contend that these notions should guide 'the critical thinking of those who design, develop, and deploy AI'.[107] In terms of more concrete recommendations, Villegas-Galaviz and Martin argue that those who develop and deploy digital technologies are 'responsible for ensuring that algorithms do not eliminate variables such as context (like space and time), circumstances, or historical-cultural background'.[108] To apply a care ethics perspective to AI requires that

> those who develop and deploy AI could certify that algorithms do not prevent the possibility of fostering the needs of protected classes, people at risk of social exclusion, or marginalized stakeholders. Also, those working with AI could guarantee that the data used does not imply exploiting the vulnerabilities of those affected by the algorithm and that vulnerabilities are not used as variables to prevent their future enhancement.[109]

The care-ethical emphasis on listening to different voices and giving space to voicing marginalized points of view translates into the recommendation that 'in the try to give voice to every affected part, those working on AI are considering the implications of the passage of time, the interest of those who are not present (whom they cannot see or who may never have a physical approach), and the needs and values according to different cultures'.[110] In sum, care ethics 'brings to the forefront circumstances and context, interdependence, and vulnerability in analyzing algorithmic decision making'[111] and as such has a potential to become 'a complementary and integrative proposal to augment existing work in AI Ethics'.[112]

Villegas-Galaviz and Martin's proposal for a care-based perspective on the development and use of digital technologies in administrative decision making represents an important step towards a more constructive and realistic approach to a care-sensitive public administration in the area of growing digitization. However, it is important to note two limitations of their account. First, Villegas-Galaviz and Martin operate with a rather narrow understanding of care ethics, derived primarily from the work of Nel Noddings who emphasizes the values of helping the other and bridging the distance between me and the other. Further research is needed to explore the potential of the political and institutional theory of care[113] for the reflection on the digitalization of political and institutional decision making. Second, Villegas-Galaviz and Martin focus mainly on the introduction of AI into decision making of companies and business organizations. The conclusions reached with respect to this area do not necessarily apply to public administration and governmental agencies. Thus, further research is needed to investigate what it entails to develop and deploy digital technologies in the context of public administration in ways which pay attention to the values and practices promoted by the moral and political theory of care.[114]

CONCLUSION

This chapter aimed to show that a care ethics perspective has inspired a distinct approach to public administration which foregrounds the importance of attentiveness, responsiveness, sensitivity to context, good communicative skills and democratic needs interpretation. It has argued that the idea of a care-centred public administration can be fruitfully applied to the complexity of administrative practice which is characterized by a nontrivial relationship between diverse normative demands. Thus, care ethics not only provides a distinct normative perspective on public administration, but also contributes to a better and more nuanced understanding of the everyday practices of administrators and public institutions. Care ethics also has a clear potential to enrich the current discussions about crisis management, sustainability governance and the digital transformation of public administration, but more work in these domains is needed.

NOTES

1. See: Petr Urban and Lizzie Ward, 'Introducing the Contexts of a Moral and Political Theory of Care', in *Care Ethics, Democratic Citizenship and the State*, ed. Petr Urban and Lizzie Ward (Basingstoke: Palgrave Macmillan, 2020), 1–27.
2. Joan C. Tronto, *Moral Boundaries. A Political Argument for an Ethic of Care* (London: Routledge, 1993).
3. See: Grace Clement, *Care, Autonomy, and Justice: Feminism and the Ethic of Care* (Boulder, CO: Westview Press, 1996); Nel Noddings, *Starting at Home: Caring and Social Policy* (Berkeley: University of California Press, 2002); Helena Olofsdotter Stensöta, 'Public Ethics of Care – A General Public Ethics', *Ethics and Social Welfare* 9, no. 2 (2015): 183–200.
4. See: Marian Barnes, *Caring and Social Justice* (Basingstoke: Palgrave Macmillan, 2006); Marian Barnes, *Care in Everyday Life. An Ethic of Care in Practice* (Bristol: Policy Press, 2012); Daniel Engster, *Justice, Care, and the Welfare State* (Oxford: Oxford University Press, 2015); Olena Hankivsky, *Social Policy and the Ethic of Care* (Vancouver: University of British Columbia Press, 2004); Virginia Held, *The Ethics of Care. Personal, Political, and Global* (New York: Oxford University Press, 2006); Joan Tronto, 'Who Cares? Public and Private Caring and the Rethinking of Citizenship', in *Women and Welfare: Theory and Practice in the United States and Europe*, ed. Nancy J. Hirschmann and Ulrike Liebert (New Brunswick, NJ: Rutgers University Press, 2001), 65–83; Eva Feder Kittay, *Love's Labor: Essays on Women, Equality, and Dependency* (London: Routledge, 1999); Joan C. Tronto, *Caring Democracy: Markets, Equality, and Justice* (New York: New York University Press, 2013); Anne Julie White, *Democracy, Justice, and the Welfare State. Reconstructing Public Care* (University Park: Pennsylvania State University Press, 2000).

5. Daniel Engster, 'A Public Ethics of Care for Policy Implementation', *American Journal of Political Science* 64, no. 3 (2020): 1–13.
6. Ibid., 6.
7. Ibid., 1.
8. Public administration can be defined as a cooperative group effort in a public setting that comprises those activities that are involved in implementing the policies and programmes of governments but also have a role in the formulation of public policy. Theoretically, public administration is an interdisciplinary field of study that examines the structure and workings of institutions that are charged with the administration of governmental functions, and studies the behaviour of officials responsible for the conduct of these functions.
9. Carol Gilligan, *In a Different Voice. Psychological Theory and Women's Development* (Cambridge, MA: Harvard University Press, 1982).
10. Berenice Fisher and Joan C. Tronto, 'Toward a Feminist Theory of Caring', in *Circles of Care: Work and Identity in Women's Lives*, ed. Emily K. Abel and Margaret K. Nelson (Albany: SUNY Press, 1990), 40.
11. Fisher and Tronto, 'Toward a Feminist Theory of Caring', 40.
12. Tronto, *Moral Boundaries,* 162.
13. Selma Sevenhuijsen, *Citizenship and the Ethics of Care. Feminist Considerations on Justice, Morality and Politics*, trans. Liz Savage (London: Routledge, 1998).
14. Engster contends that 'Stensöta, in particular, has led the way in showing how care ethics can provide the basis for a public administrative ethics' (see: Engster, 'A Public Ethics of Care for Policy Implementation', 8). Though it is fully appropriate to credit Stensöta for her original contribution to the development of a care-oriented public administrative ethics, Burnier's research on a care-centred public administration predates Stensöta's work almost by a decade and should therefore be considered foundational. Other pioneering works on a care-centred public administration that often get overlooked in care ethics literature include: Lynn G. Beck, 'Meeting the Challenge of the Future: The Place of a Caring Ethic in Educational Administration', *American Journal of Education* 100 (1992): 454–95; Philip H. Jos and Samuel M. Hines Jr, 'Care, Justice, and Public Administration', *Administration & Society* 25, no. 3 (1993): 373–92; and Anneka Davidson, 'Gender Differences in Administrative Ethics', in *Handbook of Administrative Ethics*, ed. Terry L. Cooper (New York: Marcel Dekker, 1994), 415–33.
15. DeLysa Burnier, 'Other Voices/Other Rooms: Towards a Care-centered Public Administration', *Administrative Theory and Praxis* 25, no. 4 (2003): 529–44.
16. DeLysa Burnier, 'The Long Road of Administrative Memory: Jane Addams, Frances Perkins and Care-Centered Administration', in *Handbook on Gender and Public Administration*, ed. Patricia M. Shields and Nicole M. Elias (Northampton, MA: Edward Elgar, 2022), 63.
17. Burnier, 'Other Voices/Other Rooms'.
18. See also: Engster, 'A Public Ethics of Care for Policy Implementation', 8.
19. DeLysa Burnier, 'The Shock of Recognition: Reflections on Bureau Men, Settlement Women', *Administrative Theory and Praxis* 31, no. 4 (2009b): 586–9. See also: DeLysa Burnier, 'Jane Addams: Care-Centered Leadership and the Democratic Community', in *The Oxford Handbook of Jane Addams*, ed. Patricia M. Shields, Maurice Hamington and Joseph Soeters (Oxford: Oxford University Press, 2023), 75–92.
20. Camilla Stivers, *Bureau Men, Settlement Women: Constructing Public Administration in the Progressive Era* (Lawrence: University Press of Kansas, 2000), 49.

21. DeLysa Burnier, 'Markets No More: Toward a Care-centered Public Administration', *Administrative Theory and Praxis* 31, no. 3 (2009): 396.
22. Burnier, 'Other Voices/Other Rooms', 541. See also: DeLysa Burnier, 'Embracing Others with "Sympathetic Understanding" and "Affectionate Interpretation:" Creating a Relational Care-centered Public Administration', *Administrative Theory & Praxis* 43, no. 1 (2021): 42–57.
23. See also: Jessica Nicholson and Elizabeth Kurucz, 'Relational Leadership for Sustainability: Building an Ethical Framework from the Moral Theory of "Ethics of Care"', *Journal of Business Ethics* 156, no. 1 (2019): 25–43;Helen B. Regan and Gwen H. Brooks, *Out of Women's Experience: Creating Relational Leadership* (Thousand Oaks, CA: Corwin Press, 1995); Kathleen Sernak, *School Leadership: Balancing Power with Caring* (New York: Teachers College Press, 1998).
24. Burnier, 'Other Voices/Other Rooms', 538.
25. Burnier, 'Markets No More: Toward a Care-centered Public Administration'.
26. Stensöta, 'Public Ethics of Care – A General Public Ethics', 184.
27. Helena Olofsdotter Stensöta, 'A Public Ethics of Care for Public Administration and Implementation' (paper presented at the Western Political Science Conference, San Antonio, Texas, 2011), 4.
28. Stensöta, 'Public Ethics of Care – A General Public Ethics', 191.
29. Stensöta, 'A Public Ethics of Care for Public Administration and Implementation', 10.
30. Ibid., 11.
31. Ibid., 12.
32. Sophie Bourgault, 'Prolegomena to a Caring Bureaucracy', *European Journal of Women's Studies* 24, no. 3 (2017): 202–17.
33. Bourgault, 'Prolegomena to a Caring Bureaucracy'.
34. Sophie Bourgault, 'Epistemic Injustice, Face-to-Face Encounters and Caring Institutions', *International Journal of Care and Caring* 4, no. 1 (2020): 91–107.
35. Chuqing Dong and Jordan Morehouse, 'Toward a Caring Government: Advancing Ethical Government Public Relations with a Care-based Relationship Cultivation Model', *Journal of Public Relations Research* 34, no. 5 (2022): 179–207.
36. Ibid., 180.
37. Ibid., 187.
38. Ibid., 188.
39. Ibid., 195.
40. Ibid., 189.
41. Engster, 'A Public Ethics of Care for Policy Implementation', 1–2.
42. Jos and Hines Jr, 'Care, Justice, and Public Administration', 380.
43. Ibid.
44. Engster, 'A Public Ethics of Care for Policy Implementation', 6.
45. Ibid., 10.
46. Ibid., 6.
47. Ibid., 12.
48. Ibid., 9.
49. Ibid., 8.
50. Jos and Hines Jr, 'Care, Justice, and Public Administration', 386–7.
51. Ibid., 385–6.
52. Ibid., 386.
53. Ibid.

54. Ibid.
55. The balanced view of the relationship between care and justice in public administration seems to resonate with the perspective advocated by Gilligan, who – despite numerous harsh contrasts in her exposition of an ethic of care and an ethic of justice – ultimately contends that the two views of morality 'are complementary rather than sequential or opposed' (see: Gilligan, *In a Different Voice*, 33). She argues that 'to understand how the tension between responsibilities and rights sustains the dialectic of human development is to see the integrity of two disparate modes of experiences that are in the end connected' (see: Gilligan, *In a Different Voice*, 174). Tronto points out in a similar way that 'only when care is assessed in its relative importance to other values can it begin to serve as a critical standpoint from which to evaluate public life' (see: Joan C. Tronto, 'Beyond Gender Difference to a Theory of Care', *Signs: Journal for Women in Culture and Society* 12, no. 4 (1987): 656).
56. Engster, 'A Public Ethics of Care for Policy Implementation', 12.
57. Ibid., 8.
58. Ibid.
59. Burnier, 'Markets No More: Toward a Care-centered Public Administration', 396.
60. Burnier, 'Other Voices/Other Rooms'.
61. Jos and Hines Jr, 'Care, Justice, and Public Administration', 388.
62. See: Vincent Dubois, *The Bureaucrat and the Poor: Encounters in French Welfare Offices*, trans. J.-Y. Bart (Farnham: Ashgate, 2010); Paul Hoggett, 'A Service to the Public: The Containment of Ethical and Moral Conflicts', in *The Values of Bureaucracy*, ed. Paul du Gay (Oxford: Oxford University Press, 2005), 165–190; Bernardo Zacka, *When the State Meets the Street: Public Service and Moral Agency* (Cambridge, MA: Harvard University Press, 2017).
63. Bourgault, 'Prolegomena to a Caring Bureaucracy'.
64. Bourgault contends that the dissonance in everyday practice of public administrators is healthy rather than dangerous and can make their work even more interesting. See: Bourgault, 'Prolegomena to a Caring Bureaucracy'.
65. See: Paul Hirst, *From Statism to Pluralism: Democracy, Civil Society and Global Politics* (London: Routledge, 1997); Hoggett, 'A Service to the Public'.
66. Jos and Hines Jr, 'Care, Justice, and Public Administration', 383–4.
67. See: Bourgault, 'Prolegomena to a Caring Bureaucracy'; Zacka, *When the State Meets the Street*.
68. Jeremy Allouche, Steve Metcalfe, Megan Schmidt-Sane and Shilpi Srivastava, 'Are We in the Age of the Polycrisis?', https://www.ids.ac.uk/opinions/are-we-in-the-age-of-the-polycrisis/, last modified 2023 (accessed 4 February 2024).
69. Layla J. Branicki, 'COVID-19, Ethics of Care and Feminist Crisis Management', *Gender, Work & Organisation* 27, no. 5 (2020): 875.
70. Branicki, 'COVID-19, Ethics of Care and Feminist Crisis Management'.
71. Ibid., 875.
72. Ibid., 876.
73. Ibid., 874.
74. Ibid., 872.
75. Ibid., 873.
76. Ibid., 880.
77. Nicholson and Kurucz, 'Relational Leadership for Sustainability'.
78. Ibid., 27.

79. Ibid.
80. Ibid., 26.
81. Ibid., 31.
82. Ibid., 33.
83. Ibid., 40.
84. Ibid., 25.
85. See: Michael Flower and Maurice Hamington, 'Care Ethics, Bruno Latour, and the Anthropocene', *Philosophies* 7, no. 2 (2022): 31, https://www.mdpi.com/2409-9287/7/2/31; Sandra Laugier, 'Care, the Environment, and Global Ethics', *Cahier du genre* 59, no. 2 (2015): 127–52; Elena Pulcini, *Care of the World: Fear, Responsibility and Justice in the Global Age*, trans. Karen Whittle (Dordrecht: Springer, 2013); Kyle Whyte and J. Chris Cuomo, 'Ethics of Caring in Environmental Ethics: Indigenous and Feminist Philosophies', in *The Oxford Handbook of Environmental Ethics*, ed. Stephen M. Gardiner and Allen Thompson (Oxford: Oxford University Press, 2016), 234–47.
86. Bourgault, 'Epistemic Injustice, Face-to-Face Encounters and Caring Institutions', 104.
87. Anja Svejgaard Pors and Eva Pallesen, 'The Reorganization of the Bureaucratic Encounter in a Digitized Public Administration', *Ephemera: Theory & Politics in Organisation* 21, no. 3 (2021): 34.
88. Ibid., 33.
89. Ibid., 34.
90. Bourgault, 'Epistemic Injustice, Face-to-Face Encounters and Caring Institutions', 100.
91. Ibid., 103.
92. Ibid., 101.
93. Ibid., 104.
94. Ibid., 100.
95. See: Petr Urban, 'Organizing the Caring Society: Toward a Care Ethical Perspective on Institutions', in *Care Ethics, Democratic Citizenship and the State*, ed. Petr Urban and Lizzie Ward (Basingstoke: Palgrave Macmillan, 2020), 296.
96. Bourgault, 'Epistemic Injustice, Face-to-Face Encounters and Caring Institutions', 99.
97. Carolina Villegas-Galaviz and Kirsten Martin, 'Moral Distance, AI, and the Ethics of Care', *AI & Society*, 1, https://link.springer.com/article/10.1007/s00146-023-01642-z, last modified 2023.
98. Ibid., 2.
99. Ibid., 4.
100. Ibid., 5.
101. Mark Coeckelbergh, 'Drones, Information Technology, and Distance: Mapping the Moral Epistemology of Remote Fighting', *Ethics and Information Technology* 15 (2013): 87–98.
102. Villegas-Galaviz and Martin, 'Moral Distance, AI, and the Ethics of Care', 6.
103. Ibid., 1.
104. Ibid., 5.
105. Ibid., 7.
106. Ibid., 2.
107. Ibid., 8.
108. Ibid., 9.
109. Ibid.
110. Ibid., 10.
111. Ibid., 1.

112. Ibid., 2.
113. For example: Tronto, *Caring Democracy*.
114. I am very grateful to Maurice Hamington, Daniel Engster and Lysa Burnier for their insightful suggestions and comments which I received on a previous version of this chapter. My big thanks go also to Matilda Carter, the editor of this volume, for her helpful feedback and patient support. The work on this chapter greatly benefited from my conversations with a number of fellow care ethicists, including Sophie Bourgault, Joan Tronto, Lizzie Ward, Helena Stensöta, Brunella Casalini, Elena Pulcini, Fiona Robinson, Carlo Leget, Andries Baart, Frans Vosman, Virginia Held and many others. I am indebted to all of them.

BIBLIOGRAPHY

Allouche, Jeremy, Steve Metcalfe, Megan Schmidt-Sane and Shilpi Srivastava. 'Are We in the Age of the Polycrisis?' https://www.ids.ac.uk/opinions/are-we-in-the-age-of-the-polycrisis/. Last modified 2023 (accessed 4 February 2024).

Barnes, Marian. *Caring and Social Justice*. Basingstoke: Palgrave Macmillan, 2006.

Barnes, Marian. *Care in Everyday Life. An Ethic of Care in Practice*. Bristol: Policy Press, 2012.

Beck, Lynn G. 'Meeting the Challenge of the Future: The Place of a Caring Ethic in Educational Administration', *American Journal of Education* 100 (1992): 454–95.

Bourgault, Sophie. 'Prolegomena to a Caring Bureaucracy', *European Journal of Women's Studies* 24, no. 3 (2017): 202–17.

Bourgault, Sophie. 'Epistemic Injustice, Face-to-Face Encounters and Caring Institutions', *International Journal of Care and Caring* 4, no. 1 (2020): 91–107.

Branicki, Layla J. 'COVID-19, Ethics of Care and Feminist Crisis Management', *Gender, Work & Organisation* 27, no. 5 (2020): 872–83.

Burnier, DeLysa. 'Other Voices/Other Rooms: Towards a Care-centered Public Administration', *Administrative Theory and Praxis* 25, no. 4 (2003): 529–44.

Burnier, DeLysa. 'Markets No More: Toward a Care-centered Public Administration', *Administrative Theory and Praxis* 31, no. 3 (2009): 396–402.

Burnier, DeLysa. 'The Shock of Recognition: Reflections on Bureau Men, Settlement Women', *Administrative Theory and Praxis* 31, no. 4 (2009): 586–9.

Burnier, DeLysa. 'Embracing Others with "Sympathetic Understanding" and "Affectionate Interpretation:" Creating a Relational Care-centered Public Administration', *Administrative Theory & Praxis* 43, no. 1 (2021): 42–57.

Burnier, DeLysa. 'The Long Road of Administrative Memory: Jane Addams, Frances Perkins and Care-Centered Administration', in *Handbook on Gender and Public Administration*, edited by Patricia M. Shields and Nicole M. Elias, 53–67. Northampton, MA: Edward Elgar, 2022.

Burnier, DeLysa. 'Jane Addams: Care-Centered Leadership and the Democratic Community', in *The Oxford Handbook of Jane Addams*, edited by Patricia M. Shields, Maurice Hamington and Joseph Soeters, 75–92. Oxford: Oxford University Press, 2023.

Clement, Grace. *Care, Autonomy, and Justice: Feminism and the Ethic of Care*. Boulder, CO: Westview Press, 1996.

Coeckelbergh, Mark. 'Drones, Information Technology, and Distance: Mapping the Moral Epistemology of Remote Fighting', *Ethics and Information Technology* 15 (2013): 87–98.

Davidson, Anneka. 'Gender Differences in Administrative Ethics', in *Handbook of Administrative Ethics*, edited by Terry L. Cooper, 415–33. New York: Marcel Dekker, 1994.

Dong, Chuqing, and Jordan Morehouse. 'Toward a Caring Government: Advancing Ethical Government Public Relations with a Care-based Relationship Cultivation Model', *Journal of Public Relations Research* 34, no. 5 (2022): 179–207.

Dubois, Vincent. *The Bureaucrat and the Poor: Encounters in French Welfare Offices*. Translated by J.-Y. Bart. Farnham: Ashgate, 2010.

Engster, Daniel. *Justice, Care, and the Welfare State*. Oxford: Oxford University Press, 2015.

Engster, Daniel. 'A Public Ethics of Care for Policy Implementation', *American Journal of Political Science* 64, no. 3 (2020): 1–13.

Fisher, Berenice, and Joan C. Tronto. 'Toward a Feminist Theory of Caring', in *Circles of Care: Work and Identity in Women's Lives*, edited by Emily K. Abel and Margaret K. Nelson, 35–62. Albany: SUNY Press, 1990.

Flower, Michael, and Maurice Hamington. 'Care Ethics, Bruno Latour, and the Anthropocene', *Philosophies* 7, no. 2 (2022): 31. https://www.mdpi.com/2409-9287/7/2/31.

Gilligan, Carol. *In a Different Voice. Psychological Theory and Women's Development*. Cambridge, MA: Harvard University Press, 1982.

Hankivsky, Olena. *Social Policy and the Ethic of Care*. Vancouver: University of British Columbia Press, 2004.

Held, Virginia. *The Ethics of Care. Personal, Political, and Global*. New York: Oxford University Press, 2006.

Hirst, Paul. *From Statism to Pluralism: Democracy, Civil Society and Global Politics*. London: Routledge, 1997.

Hoggett, Paul. 'A Service to the Public: The Containment of Ethical and Moral Conflicts', in *The Values of Bureaucracy*, edited by Paul du Gay, 165–90. Oxford: Oxford University Press, 2005.

Jos, Philip H. and Samuel M. Hines Jr. 'Care, Justice, and Public Administration', *Administration & Society* 25, no. 3 (1993): 373–92.

Kittay, Eva Feder. *Love's Labor: Essays on Women, Equality, and Dependency*. London: Routledge, 1999.

Laugier, Sandra. 'Care, the Environment, and Global Ethics', *Cahier du genre* 59, no. 2 (2015): 127–52.

Nicholson, Jessica, and Elizabeth Kurucz. 'Relational Leadership for Sustainability: Building an Ethical Framework from the Moral Theory of "Ethics of Care"', *Journal of Business Ethics* 156, no. 1 (2019): 25–43.

Noddings, Nel. *Starting at Home: Caring and Social Policy*. Berkeley: University of California Press, 2002.

Pors, Anja Svejgaard, and Eva Pallesen. 'The Reorganization of the Bureaucratic Encounter in a Digitized Public Administration', *Ephemera: Theory & Politics in Organisation* 21, no. 3 (2021): 17–41.

Pulcini, Elena. *Care of the World: Fear, Responsibility and Justice in the Global Age*. Translated by Karen Whittle. Dordrecht: Springer, 2013.

Regan, Helen B., and Gwen H. Brooks. *Out of Women's Experience: Creating Relational Leadership*. Thousand Oaks, CA: Corwin Press, 1995.

Sevenhuijsen, Selma. *Citizenship and the Ethics of Care. Feminist Considerations on Justice, Morality and Politics*. Translated by Liz Savage. London: Routledge, 1998.

Sernak, Kathleen. *School Leadership: Balancing Power with Caring*. New York: Teachers College Press, 1998.

Stensöta, Helena Olofsdotter. 'A Public Ethics of Care for Public Administration and Implementation', paper presented at the Western Political Science Conference, San Antonio, Texas, 2011.

Stensöta, Helena Olofsdotter. 'Public Ethics of Care – A General Public Ethics', *Ethics and Social Welfare* 9, no. 2 (2015): 183–200.

Stivers, Camilla. *Bureau Men, Settlement Women: Constructing Public Administration in the Progressive Era*. Lawrence: University Press of Kansas, 2000.

Tronto, Joan C. 'Beyond Gender Difference to a Theory of Care', *Signs: Journal for Women in Culture and Society* 12, no. 4 (1987): 644–63.

Tronto, Joan C. *Moral Boundaries. A Political Argument for an Ethic of Care*. London: Routledge, 1993.

Tronto, Joan C. 'Who Cares? Public and Private Caring and the Rethinking of Citizenship', in *Women and Welfare: Theory and Practice in the United States and Europe*, edited by Nancy J. Hirschmann and Ulrike Liebert, 65–83. New Brunswick, NJ: Rutgers University Press, 2001.

Tronto, Joan C. *Caring Democracy: Markets, Equality, and Justice*. New York: New York University Press, 2013.

Urban, Petr. 'Organizing the Caring Society: Toward a Care Ethical Perspective on Institutions', in *Care Ethics, Democratic Citizenship and the State*, edited by Petr Urban and Lizzie Ward, 277–306. Basingstoke: Palgrave Macmillan, 2020.

Urban, Petr, and Lizzie Ward. 'Introducing the Contexts of a Moral and Political Theory of Care', in *Care Ethics, Democratic Citizenship and the State*, edited by Petr Urban and Lizzie Ward, 1–27. Basingstoke: Palgrave Macmillan, 2020.

Villegas-Galaviz, Carolina, and Kirsten Martin. 'Moral Distance, AI, and the Ethics of Care', *AI & Society*. https://link.springer.com/article/10.1007/s00146-023-01642-z. Last modified 2023.

White, Anne Julie. *Democracy, Justice, and the Welfare State. Reconstructing Public Care*. University Park: Pennsylvania State University Press, 2000.

Whyte, Kyle, and J. Chris Cuomo. 'Ethics of Caring in the Environmental Ethics: Indigenous and Feminist Philosophies', in *The Oxford Handbook of Environmental Ethics*, edited by Stephen M. Gardiner and Allen Thompson, 234–47. Oxford: Oxford University Press, 2016.

Zacka, Bernardo. *When the State Meets the Street: Public Service and Moral Agency*. Cambridge, MA: Harvard University Press, 2017.

CHAPTER TWENTY-ONE

Care ethics, maternity and reproductive justice

INGE VAN NISTELROOIJ AND RODANTE VAN DER WAAL

INTRODUCTION

In feminist scholarship in the second feminist wave, inquiry into the position of women and practices of mothering and care went hand in hand. Particularly groundbreaking was the work of two scholars, Ruddick and Gilligan, who can be considered as the pioneers of care ethics. Following the first feminist wave, with its primary focus upon women's voting rights, the second wave (between the 1960s and 1980s) engaged in discussions on a broader range of issues, including sexuality and reproductive rights, and the power relations in the family, the household and the workplace. A rich number of bestsellers on 'mothering' were published, illustrating the need of many to reflect upon these experiences and the structures that had silenced or neglected them until then. It may be telling that Nancy Chodorow's *The Reproduction of Mothering* was an international bestseller, and its Dutch translation (in its hip 1970s' Dutch spelling with 'k's replacing 'c's, for instance) has been sitting on many bookcases, including our own, for decades as a 'must-have' for any feminist, next to Simone de Beauvoir's *The Second Sex*.[1] It seemed that understanding 'mothering' and women's 'secondary place' were deeply intertwined. Chodorow's work addresses the sociological and structural context of what many considered to be biological, and what in psychoanalysis is usually considered to be personal: mothering and how it comes to be reproduced in every generation. Adrienne Rich wrote *Of Woman Born*, analysing the personal experience of mothering in the patriarchal institution of motherhood.[2] Ruddick's groundbreaking article 'Maternal Thinking' was published in 1980, Gilligan's *In a Different Voice* in 1982. And the list could continue.[3]

This contribution focuses on the analyses of practices of mothering in which care ethics originates, and their moral and political relevance for current questions of reproductive justice. It does so by first sketching the original context and development of care theory. After that, we will centre the works of two pioneering theorists: Sara Ruddick and Margaret Urban Walker. We present Ruddick's work and argue why it is relevant to draw upon embodied practices for moral understandings, and why this is particularly the case regarding experiences and practices of pregnancy, birthing and child-rearing. We also show how Ruddick herself responded to criticisms, how her work was supported in care theory[4] – for example, by Tronto[5] and by other thinkers[6] – as well as criticized.[7] Subsequently, we present the expressive-collaborative model of moral understandings and elaborate upon the idea of 'forced identities', developed by Walker.[8] These insights help to understand the structural pitfalls of connecting the pregnant, birthing and child-rearing body to 'care'. This is particularly true for bodies in which inequalities of gender and race intersect. Power is all too often exercised over those bodies, to their detriment, and creates an 'epistemic firewall' for their knowledge, through processes of *naturalizing, privatizing and normalizing* the ways in which they are treated as people without knowledge.[9] We exemplify the processes described by Urban Walker by turning to our research in reproductive justice, particularly to obstetric violence in obstetric and midwifery practices. We then return to Ruddick's work to underpin the idea of 'midwifery thinking'. We argue that even though the processes that create the epistemic firewall are present in those practices, we can only overcome this firewall by drawing upon the practical forms of thinking that arise within those practices. Our aim is to show what is at stake, what care theory could bring, and what new care theory should be developed.

21.1 THE ORIGINS AND DEVELOPMENT OF CARE ETHICS

Gilligan's *In a Different Voice* had an impact that can hardly be overestimated. This book was acclaimed to have started a revolution leading to the development of the field of the 'ethics of care'. Moreover, *Ms.* magazine made her the 1984 Woman of the Year, and *Time* magazine counted her among the twenty-five most influential people in the United States in 1996. The 'different voice' (as is also described in other contributions to this book) concerns her research findings of a different, rather than a less developed, moral voice that was primarily expressed by girls and women. The idea that their moral development lagged behind when compared to boys and men, as moral development researcher Lawrence Kohlberg had found, was rooted in his biased model of moral development. Kohlberg had based it upon research among only boys and men and created a model of moral development (which is still common knowledge in studies of pedagogy nowadays). Gilligan found that women and girls scored structurally as less developed morally when his model was applied, leading to them being assessed as 'morally less developed' or 'morally immature' (which is – needless to say – quite a staggering judgement). Gilligan, understandably, turned her critique to the model: rather than women and girls failing to develop morally, the way their development was measured was biased. Based upon her research among boys *and* girls, she developed two models of moral development (primarily, but not strictly, distinct according to lines of gender). Whereas Kohlberg's model focused upon the development of an 'ethic of justice', her alternative model described the development of an 'ethic of care', not as 'less moral', but as 'different'. Hence women (and others embedded in practices of care) were not 'less developed' in the moral sense; rather, they expressed a 'different morality'.[10] To sum up, Gilligan's work was rooted in the second feminist wave's critique of scientific knowledge's one-sidedness: if one inquires into issues only among boys and men and subsequently builds a model based upon these findings and pretends that this model has universal validity, one has a biased model and should not be surprised if others then 'fail' or lag behind in comparison to the persons who formed the foundation of the model. A long history of male-biased science and humanities can be viewed similarly, and still requires an uphill battle for women (and other minorities), unfortunately.

Central to Kohlberg's and Gilligan's research was the famous Heinz dilemma. Another part of Gilligan's work has received less attention comparatively. It consists of her research into the experiences of pregnant people who were considering abortion during the obligatory waiting time after their first doctor's visit, in which the wish to end a pregnancy was discussed. Van Nistelrooij and Leget describe how, particularly in this part of her analysis, key insights into the role of 'relationality, affectivity, contextuality, and practice-based morality' come to the fore. And with relationality, 'ambiguities, ambivalences, tensions, and conflicts' come in, rather than 'classic categories that create separation or opposition, like egoism versus altruism, self versus other, professional versus personal, self-sacrifice versus self-realization'.[11] These findings led Gilligan to develop a view of an 'ethic of care' in which a continuous weighing of relational goods rather than dichotomies between mutually excluding obligations are central. Applied to the case of abortion, then, moral deliberation consists of questioning one's ability to have a child within their specific situation, rather than more traditional moral reasoning regarding the question of whether one can morally defend to end a pregnancy. Interestingly, a recent analysis by literary scholar Clair Wills shows that in novels and poetry on abortion, abortion is almost never made out to be a moral dilemma in the traditional understanding, but always a practical, contextual and relational consideration.[12]

Following Gilligan's bestseller, Noddings was the first scholar to develop a thorough 'ethic of caring' that[13] – quite naturally, considering the context as sketched above – draws upon the dyadic model of mothering care for the child.[14] Although Gilligan has rejected the accusation of essentialism in her 'Letter to the Readers' in the 1993 edition of her book,[15] and Ruddick had put aside accounts of gender difference or maternal nature and defined 'maternal' as a social category and not a biological one,[16] Noddings unequivocally embraces essentialism:

> An ethic built on caring is, I think, characteristically and *essentially* feminine – which is not to say, of course, that it cannot be shared by men, any more than we should care to say that traditional moral systems cannot be embraced by women. But an ethic of caring arises, I believe, out of our experience as women, just as the traditional logical approach to ethical problems arises more obviously from masculine experience. (emphasis added)[17]

The fierce and dichotomized debate that followed these early days of care ethics – the Kohlberg–Gilligan – or justice–care – debate was only overcome in the 1990s with the publication of Tronto's *Moral Boundaries*. She addresses the unsuccessful strategy of care theory until that point of claiming feminine essentialist specificity in the public realm and care to be worthy of moral and political impact. She argues for more inclusiveness of care theory by aiming for advancement of equality not only between sexes, but also classes, races and ethnic minorities. She explicitly considers the first care ethicists' work on mothering practices (particularly Noddings) as failing to acknowledge 'the political setting of their moral arguments at their peril',[18] and as following a politically naïve and ineffective strategy.[19] Tronto transcends the dichotomies characteristic of care theory up till that moment by developing a broad political and moral theory of care, which proved to be an invaluable new impetus for care ethics.[20] Moving away from the dichotomized debates in which care theory was stuck, revaluing caring as a moral and political practice, developing care as a valuable analytical tool to dissect power inequalities related to care responsibilities,[21] has proven to be a recognizable and applicable political theory worldwide.

Leading the focus away from mothering was therefore an effective strategy for care theory. Nevertheless, Ruddick's work continued to inspire others, leading to the development of a distinct body of knowledge, 'maternal theory', no longer much related to or embedded in care theory. In particular, sociologist Andrea O'Reilly is considered as the pathbreaking scholar for a 'matricentric feminism' that addresses motherhood as 'the unfinished business of feminism'.[22] We argue, however, that pregnancy, birth and parenting practices are also the 'unfinished business of care theory'. Considering, for instance, the ongoing problems we have with regards to issues of reproductive justice,[23] such as the criminalization of abortion,[24] obstetric violence,[25] obstetric racism,[26] questions around surrogacy and quickly developing technology in reproduction,[27] the ableist assumptions of motherhood,[28] and the global lack of midwives,[29] we think that care theory has much to offer to those questions that arise in embodied care practices of people doing reproductive labour. For in these diverse, global practices and experiences, many forms of inequality and violence continue to harm people involved in care, at both the giving and the receiving end, as well as when this distinction cannot be made – for instance, in pregnancy and labour, where a person both requires and gives care.[30]

Returning to the idea that these questions of pregnancy, birth and parenting are 'the unfinished business of care theory', we now return to two main and pioneering thinkers for addressing them.

21.2 THE RELEVANCE OF RUDDICK'S 'MOTHERING' FOR MORAL UNDERSTANDINGS OF CARE

Before Gilligan published her groundbreaking bestseller *In a Different Voice* there was another groundbreaking text: Ruddick's 'Maternal Thinking'. Sometimes this text, rather than Gilligan's, has been acknowledged as the origin of care ethics.[31] Students reading this text in the 2020s have remarked that this text requires some 'time-travelling'. It is as relevant for practices and persons today in discussing oppression and patriarchy, as it is embedded in a time when certain philosophical categories central to present-day philosophical debates were considered profoundly different or simply lacking, like gender diversity, intersectionality, generalisability and Western supremacy.

It remains worthwhile, however, to consider Ruddick's (1935–2011) work from which both care ethics and maternal theory scholars received much inspiration. Like Robinson, we consider her book as 'wonderful and widely misunderstood',[32] as will become clear below. The misunderstandings concerning her work can already be identified in the debate that followed Gilligan's publication, a debate that failed to take notice of some insights that Ruddick had developed. We therefore take a close look at how Ruddick's work – much like care theory – centres on the aim to reverse philosophy's Reason (she capitalizes the word), with political implications.

In her 1989 book, Ruddick describes her research concern. Loyal to feminist epistemology, her research is rooted in her biography. Trained as a philosopher in the 1960s, she writes, she discovered the uselessness of academic thinking for her post-academic experiences as it was 'philosophy's Reason [itself] that abetted my desire to free myself from the fate of wife-and-mother with its messy, fleshly children and dull duties'.[33] Finding herself, post-academically, married and mothering, she increasingly became conscious of a divide between academic rational thinking and the thinking required by practices to which the majority of women dedicated their lives.[34] Underneath this divide, she discovered a 'pervasive disrespect for women's minds and lives'[35] and writes: 'in my generation, women's attempts to reason were typically met with contempt, still wounding even when too subtle to name'.[36] She therefore wondered if she could serve her great love, Reason, by reversing it: 'Reason was failing me – as a lover, mother, and citizen. As Western philosophers had idealised it, Reason was meant to be detached and impersonal, at best irrelevant to particular affections and loyalties. ... Would it be possible to reverse this judgment, finding fault not in women but in the ideals?'[37]

Ruddick's reversal of 'Reason' has become one of the basic insights for care ethics.[38] This point also shows how profoundly academics in the second wave of the women's movement had to revise the foundations of knowledge.[39] In a later reflection upon her work in 1995, Ruddick reflects upon the utter strangeness at the time of the very idea of 'maternal thinking', as all that was assigned to 'mothers' stood in absolute opposition to what was considered the heart of philosophy: 'rationality'. Mothers contrasted in every way with this, Ruddick contends, in their 'particularity, passionate attachment, and bodily engagement'.[40] She explains how she had to develop a new kind of philosophy, writing:

> A feminist critique of dominant ideals of rationality was entirely absent from my graduate training [as a philosopher] and from my own early sense of the philosophy I taught. Divisions between mind and mother, reason and female/woman, now so discredited, had not been named let alone contested. Today feminists are creating ever more nuanced critiques of reason and clearer accounts of alternative ideals of rationality. By contrast, when I first began to write I felt as if I had to invent a conceptual framework to justify the mere idea of maternal thinking.
>
> Before the recent burgeoning of feminist philosophy, I drew on Wittgenstein and Habermas for two ideas: there are distinctive, though not sharply bounded, kinds of thinking; these kinds of thinking, whether scientific, historical, psychoanalytic, religious ... or *maternal*, arise out of distinctive practices. This 'practicalist conception of reason,' as I label it in Chapter I, provided a space in which to represent mothers as reasoners. The idea of practice-based ways of reasoning, uniting as it does thinking and action, still seems to me one useful way of understanding thinking in general as well as the idea of maternal thinking.
>
> But since writing [the book] *Maternal Thinking* I have not been nearly as interested in the practicalist (or any other) account of reason as in the prior idea of mothering as a practice or work. According to this idea, mothers are not identified by fixed biological or legal relationships to children but by the work they set out to do. In my more particularized conception, mothers are people who see children as 'demanding' protection, nurturance, and training; they attempt to respond to children's demands with care and respect rather than indifference or assault.
>
> This conception of mothering as a kind of caring labor undermines the myth that mothers are 'naturally' loving. (emphasis in original).[41]

This long quotation serves several goals. The first is to show that from the 1970s and 1980s scholars have been working on a framework that is capable of justifying alternative ideas of rationality; a framework that is not separating and dividing, but *uniting thinking and action and is suited to mothering and caring*. With a backlog of centuries or even millennia, this struggle for an adequate conceptual framework of caring practices which require much time, commitment and energy, started just then, and the struggle continues to this day. It is good to keep in mind that this body of knowledge is relatively young, fights an uphill battle, and is met with the same resistance still. Second, this quote shows an *epistemological continuity* between 'maternal thinking' and 'care theory', for which Ruddick co-constructed the groundworks: practice-based ways of reasoning. Care theory has continued this epistemology in the works of Gilligan,[42] Noddings,[43]

Tronto,[44] Walker,[45] and others. The third goal is to show that Ruddick started to *fight against essentialist accounts of gender difference* or maternal nature and instead centred on '*thought*' of those of all genders who were substantially involved in caring for their child – thought which according to her[46] consists of intellectual capacities, judgements, metaphysical attitudes, values that are required in these social practices of childcare. And a fourth goal is to show that Ruddick's work is the opposite of what it is taken for: as focused upon private practices. On the contrary, her work is *highly political*: in its practicalism, anti-essentialism, feminism, reversed epistemology, and in its deriving of insights on 'peace' from those caring practices.[47]

But what *is* maternal thinking? To answer this question, we need to start with practices, for that is where this thinking emerges. Ruddick's idea can be put quite briefly: mothering is work that consists of 'responding to children's demands', and mothers are all those who '[make] the work of response a considerable part of her or his life'.[48] So, when one is engaged in the practice of mothering, one cannot escape the demands that children present and which require a response[49]: preservation, growth and social acceptability.[50] In other words, all children demand that m/others perform the activities of protection and preservation (so that they can survive), nurturance (so that they can flourish), and training for social acceptability (so that they can live with others).[51] Preservation is a universal demand of maternal practice, nurturance and training for social acceptability are historically and culturally different. Typically, however, maternal practice is attuned to the particular demands of each unique child. Conflicts are often part of the practice, both within these demands and between them. Conflicts arise for instance between the demand to protect and the demand to develop the capacity to take care of themselves, but also between social norms and a mother's own ideas about adapting or resisting them.[52] Mothering is – like caring – a responsive practice, that is characterized by particularity and variety, and by conflicting interests. In practices of mothering, a balance is sought between 'too much' and 'too little'. And for these practices, 'good humour and humility' are important as well as acceptance of uncontrollability and change, cheerfulness, and reflection upon dominant values. Finally, they require the capacity of attention and the virtue of love.[53]

Finding oneself in this practice with these activities, conflicts and requirements, leads mothers to *think*[54] and from this thinking a 'distinctive discipline emerges', that is 'maternal thinking'.[55] This discipline, 'like other disciplines, establishes criteria for determining failure and success, sets priorities, and identifies virtues that the discipline requires'.[56] Considering the above characteristics of maternal practice, it is typical of maternal *thinking* that it is strategic and conflict managing, searching for meaning, balancing the importance of goals, identifies 'mothering virtues', and also that knowledge does not automatically lead to a perfect practice.[57]

Her developing work of a new kind of 'reason' was aptly summed up by LaChance Adams:

> Maternal thinking involves the use of seemingly opposed faculties: reason, passion, and love, challenging the idea that reason is detached and impersonal. Reason is not there simply to dominate and control emotion. Emotion can be thought provoking, but it is also thoughtful and reflective in itself. The practical nature of motherhood's ends encourages concrete thought over abstraction. Dilemmas, conflicts, and struggles do not detract from this process, but rather they prompt the need for further thought.[58]

Others have highlighted insights similar to Ruddick's work, of which we name a few: Tronto describes caring as a practice[59] of which conflicts are part,[60] as universal in some respects and particular in other,[61] oriented towards 'concerns and needs of the other'[62] and 'taking the other's needs as the starting point for what must be done'.[63] Bourgault finds that at the heart of the ideals of care ethics is 'attentive listening'.[64] Hamington underscores the potential of Ruddick's characterization of 'care as labour' in removing care theory from traditional ideas of care as instinctual, essentially feminine, and revealing care as a process, as 'the sheer amount of work necessary in many caring relationships'.[65] Baraitser emphasizes the practical ethics that mothers engage with and contrasts it with Emmanuel Levinas's ethical subjectivity that is 'discovered' in the son by the father. She follows Ruddick in stating that '[t]he mother ... attains an ethical subjectivity through her ability to deal with the uncertainty and conflict inherent in child-rearing with grace, humour and good will'.[66]

Ruddick also engages extensively with the critiques that her work received. In her 1980 article she positions herself within these limits: 'the institutions of motherhood in middle-class, white, Protestant, capitalist, patriarchal America as these have expressed themselves in the heterosexual nuclear family in which I mother and was mothered'.[67] She acknowledges her limits and particularity as well as her dependence upon others to correct and translate her ideas across cultures.[68] In her preface of 1995 to the reprinted book *Maternal Thinking* she extensively engages with what she calls 'its deficiencies'.[69] She acknowledges criticisms regarding her emphasis on 'work' while underestimating the temporal dimension and diversity of relationships as well as the differences among children. Her disconnection of birth and mothering was not recognized by many mothers, including adoptive mothers; and fathers did not recognize themselves as 'mothering', a terminology which she aimed to be reformist, but failed. Further, the perspectives of mothers in distinct contexts lead to different kinds of 'demands' of mothering. She refers to anthropological research among impoverished mothers in Brazil whose circumstances lead them 'to select some [of their children] but not others for life or death'. While caring for those with good health, and expecting that not all children will survive, diseases of other children may cause the mothers' neglect of their demands. She names the failure to acknowledge the implicit assumption of children as 'intact' when assuming their growth, development and social acceptability, which is often different for children with impairments. Also the implicit assumption of 'whiteness' leads to a neglect of Black children and children of colour, who demand other things of mothers (we return to this below). These kinds of assumptions run the risk of stigmatization. Ruddick acknowledges her failure of being inclusive and, at worst, exacerbating 'the particular struggles of their mothers'.[70]

Others too have responded to her work in critical ways. For instance, Mullin points out that pregnancy is often ignored, even by feminist thinkers 'who concentrate on the elaboration of maternal thinking', who 'turn to discussions of birth, rather than pregnancy, when they wish to acknowledge the role played by biological mothers'.[71] She blames Ruddick,[72] Held[73] and others for having ignored 'the importance of the pregnant woman's experience as an element worthy of attention' that is a 'meaningful activity involving both choice and accommodation'.[74] Doucet analyses whether Ruddick's claim that fathers also 'mother' is correct, which she answers negatively.[75] Fathers engage in care in many ways which diverge from those of mothers but which must also be acknowledged as care, she argues – for example, in the activities of promoting children's independence and risk-taking[76] and through breadwinning.[77] Marvin expands Ruddick's philosophy 'in the context of trans and gender-creative youth'.[78] Particularly, Ruddick's idea of 'nurturance' and the way in which it is linked to 'nature' is challenged by the care that trans youth might need, as 'nature' might not be benign, might lead to negative outcomes for their wellbeing, and medical interventions might be required for beneficial growth.[79] Also Ruddick's centring of 'mothering' and 'kin work' fails to sufficiently account for the 'crucial form of care for trans youth through a larger gay, queer, and/or trans family-community', offering support particularly for the large numbers of trans youth rejected by their families.[80] Hill Collins contests the 'nearly universal' maternal activities described by Ruddick, and suggests that for mothers of colour 'survival, identity, and empowerment' are the primary goals. Survival for children of colour is not self-evident; their identity formation faces the challenges of a culture that devaluates Black or coloured identity; and empowerment is required for the mothers to be able to meet their children's and community's needs.[81] Finally, intersectional theorists[82] building on the work of Patricia Hill Collins, many from the Global South, have criticized Ruddick's work for not escaping white supremacy,[83] the rhetoric of the family that permeates 'intersecting inequalities of gender, race, class, sexuality and even constructions of national identity',[84] and 'a reductive and imaginary prism of white supremacy, heteronormativity, and sexism'.[85]

Rather than reject her work because of these limitations, we aim to acknowledge that, even though there remains much work to do, Ruddick's work was groundbreaking, not only for care theory. By challenging dominant ways of reasoning and pioneering a way out of dominant philosophical frameworks that excluded feminism and 'mothering' alike, she paved the way for other voices. By creating a new theoretical space for 'mothers' and 'carers' to be heard, Ruddick's work was the point of departure for many other groups to branch off and develop new theories on their ways of being, doing and thinking. Their common ground is their previous exclusion from dominant 'general' theories and their call to be heard as a call for epistemic justice.[86]

21.3 THE RISK OF 'FORCED IDENTITIES' FOR THE PREGNANT AND BIRTHING BODY

The fundamental care ethics' practice-based epistemology discussed in the previous section, remains one of its major pillars fitting its feminist goals. In this section we now turn to a profound analysis of practices which is relevant to Ruddick's (and following her lead: our) undertaking. For this we turn to another pathbreaking 'mother' of care ethics: Margaret Urban Walker. In her primary work Walker concurs with Ruddick in advocating a practice-based model for moral understandings, as opposed to the dominant theoretical-juridical model (see Table 21.1).[87] She argues that morality itself consists in practices, not in theories; that practices of responsibility are characteristic of morality; that morality is not socially modular; and that moral theorizing and moral epistemology need to be freed from impoverishing legacies of ideality and purity that makes most of most people's lives disappear, or render those lives unintelligible.[88]

With advocating the second, expressive-collaborative model of morality, Walker[89] suggests that practices (both action and speech) show what is important or valuable to people, by them assigning, accepting or deflecting responsibility,[90] in which they express their morality; and collaborative in the sense that practices are construed and established collectively around moral understandings that are fundamentally interpersonal.[91]

TABLE 21.1 Two models of morality, based on Walker[92]

Theoretical-juridical model	*Expressive-collaborative model*
Impersonally action guiding code within an agent	Morality consists in a family of practices
	that show what is valued by making people accountable to each other for it
Access by non-empirical reflection	Interpersonal: collaborative
Fuses tendencies: intellectualist, rationalist, individualist, impersonal, socially modular	What goes on morally between people is constrained and made intelligible by a background of understandings about what people are supposed to do, expect and understand
	Empirically saturated reflective analysis of what is going on in actual moral orders
	Intelligible, coherent, transparent
	Fully normative reflection = ideality

However, Walker also offers an alarming analysis of patterns and pitfalls inherent to practices that harm non-dominant groups.[93] We present her analysis of these groups and how they, as an effect of their subordinate positions, are facing an 'epistemic firewall' which makes their protests against their treatment as subservient ineffective. We follow her analysis closely, as Walker's rich view shows how power is all too often exercised over the bodies of subordinates (whose identity Walker terms 'necessary' in these power relations) to their detriment, while impeding their knowledge being noticed and their voices being heard. In what follows we draw upon research into obstetric care and midwifery-led birth, to exemplify each step of Walker's theory. By interweaving her theory and our research findings, we aim to show the pitfalls that are still there of connecting the pregnant, birthing and child-rearing body to 'care'.

Walker engages with a discussion on 'necessary identities' in which some identities are considered to have been 'necessary' in ancient Greece, whereas modernity is supposed to have rejected this idea.[94] She refers to Bernard Williams who contests this dichotomy as erroneous, since the Greeks did not see slavery as just or morally defendable, and they did see it as coerced, not natural.[95] In any case, a 'necessary identity' consists of 'a social role or status that is inevitably or comfortably well fitted to the people whose social position it is, because of some naturally occurring feature of those people'.[96] Walker elaborates the idea of 'necessary identities' as she considers it most relevant in her advocating the view that those involved in practices from various positions and perspectives also develop relevant moral understandings.

Necessary identities are socially constructed, hence not essential, meaning that certain persons consider themselves as well as others in a certain way, and are treated by others accordingly, while also expecting themselves to be treated that way, in a certain context. In Walker's words: 'A's are identified as B's by C's (themselves and/or others) in the context of certain institutions or practices, or to certain ends.'[97]

From our research, the comparison comes to mind of the 'natural occurring feature' of people in labour, who are often considered to be passive, irrational and ignorant. Labouring persons sometimes consider themselves irrational, are considered as irrational, and are treated as such. This perception contrasts distinctively with the features of the professional as active, rational, and 'knowing' and separates the labouring person from the midwife and other relations involved in birth.[98]

However, 'necessary identities' are not necessary because of something inalterable, as they are socially constructed and hence could also be changed socially. They are 'necessary identities' because of power relations: 'the necessity of certain identities is not, after all, for those who bear them, but for those who might otherwise have to account for the way they treat those people'.[99] These patterns show how practices and power are interrelated, in patterns of recognized power and epistemic authority:

> We should look for the apparent necessity of identities, then, in many facts about who has recognized power over whom [and] how the power is expected to be exercised. The power includes asymmetric or lopsided epistemic authority some have over others, and the muting or absence of the 'voice' of subordinates. ... These are facts about who gets to do what to whom, and who gets to talk about what gets done and is taken seriously by those with the power of authoritative judgment.[100]

These patterns, as this quote illustrates, create expectations of who gets to decide, who will be listened to and who will be silenced. But this is always dependent on particular circumstances, and would look awkward or downright wrong in other. This is the root cause for necessary identities: that some people are treated in ways that 'look "matter of course" where those treatments would be extraordinary for some other people, especially for those delivering the treatment'.[101]

Three processes and practices are involved in making these identities look 'matter of course': *naturalizing, privatizing* and *normalizing*.[102] *Naturalizing* identities is the process of making those identities 'no-entry/no-exit identities' – that is, identities that are 'conditions of birth, ceasing at death', in which one finds oneself 'from the point of self-consciousness, and others never know them otherwise'.[103] Examples are 'woman', 'coloured', 'black', which are identities that are conferred, but not seen as conferred but as 'natural' (see, for instance, de Beauvoir[104] and Butler[105] on the construction of 'woman'; and Davis[106] and Da Silva[107] on the social construction of race and racialized categories such as 'coloured' and 'black'). *Privatizing* happens when the treatment of certain identities is organized in such a way that their scrutiny is prevented, for instance literally, behind walls, doors, and fences, or virtually. The latter is described as '[e]ffected by customs, moral understandings, or laws that declare certain interactions outside legitimate or acceptable scrutiny, reaction, or public comment by others, even if those interactions take place in plain sight, or in places not private in the former sense'.[108] These processes can be recognized in obstetrics, for instance, where students in midwifery and obstetric medicine go through 'rites of passage' in which the naturalization and privatization of obstetric violence takes place.[109] Although they are trained to care for the labouring person, these rites introduce students to 'systemic tendencies that push students to cross ethical, social and political boundaries' and leads them to '[reproduce] the modern obstetric subject, the racialized (m)other, and institutionalized violence worldwide'.[110] In the Netherlands, research showed the prevalence of disrespect and abuse in obstetrics: 54 per cent of 12,239 participants experienced at least one form of disrespect and abuse. Of these, 21.1 per cent experienced 'harsh or rough treatment or physical violence'; 21.3 per cent 'lack of support'; 29.9 per cent 'lack of communication'; and 39.8 per cent 'lack of choices'. Those who were pregnant the first time (primiparity) and those with a migrant background were particularly at risk.[111] As a result of increased medicalization of birth, most obstetric practices take place in hospitals, therefore 'in plain sight' and 'not private' in the sense of the home, we can speak of naturalization and privatization of birth in the sense intended by Walker's quote above, as declaring these practices 'outside legitimate or acceptable scrutiny, reaction, or public comment by others' until recently.

And finally, the process of *normalizing* certain patterns of a practice makes certain identities 'matter of course'. This happens when 'practices that otherwise would look bad are rendered normal in these ways for certain contexts or certain people in them'.[112] When these 'otherwise bad' patterns of practice are normalized for 'certain contexts or certain people in them', three things happen: first, the presumptions underlying these patterns of behaviour are left unquestioned (e.g. when it is presumed that a person is irrational, the focus shifts from the coercion that they experience to actions that are permitted); second, normalizing then consists in the regulation of the patterns of practice, instead of prohibiting them (under conditions x and y, it is normal to overrule a person's right to consent); and third, the ones who demand to be heard or have self-control, are discredited. This last effect can be put in the words of Walker herself: normalizing practices make 'those who rebel against what "everybody" accepts appear as irrational freaks, malcontents, complainers, unstable deviants, or dangerous elements out of control'.[113] The effect of 'normalizing practices' is that people with claims against them 'prove' themselves that they are 'abnormal', 'even "prove" their unreliability as judges and informants, the incredibility of their testimonies'.[114] Walker puts it even more sharply:

> A reduced, circumscribed, or discredited status as knowers and claimers – being epistemically *marginalized* or *unauthorized* – is no small working part of the identities of those 'necessarily' subordinate. ... It is not just that their views don't count; given what those people are, their views can't count. ... No identity is so necessary as one that successfully precludes its bearer's confuting it. (emphasis in original)[115]

The result of these processes is the establishment of an 'epistemic firewall' that forms a wall between some who know and others who cannot know by 'sealing off recognizable injuries and credible complaints'.[116] This epistemic firewall is characteristic of many complex, uphill battles. Often those who protest, find themselves discredited. It is like in Heller's *Catch 22*: if you want to protest, your protest itself is proof that you are unfit; you are declared unfit, therefore your protest will not be listened to, as it is expressed by one who does not know what they say.

This is exactly what we can see happening in the battle against obstetric violence.[117] Here too we can see the distinction at work between people who are considered to be passive, irrational or unknowing labouring persons vs. the active, rational, 'knowing' professional, that we see so often depicted in movies and series. We noted the contrast between the labouring person as passive, suffering, unknowing and helpless, and the active, intervening, rescuing, knowing doctor or midwife. The normativity of the situation is often pervasive and internalized by all, as we noted, when labouring persons consider themselves to be irrational, others think so too and treat them as such. And this normativity is reproduced and reinscribed through the rites of passage of midwifery and obstetric medicine education. The general and sufficient goal that then becomes the focus of all attention is that of a good birthing outcome, meaning a healthy baby. Limiting the 'good birth outcome' to the baby's health and care's focus on this, perpetuates the mentioned processes on the labouring person. In this constellation, birthing people are treated in ways that look 'matter of course' – for instance, when obstetricians apply an episiotomy during birth without consent. Protesting against it effectuates the Catch 22 situation of making yourself unfit to assess anything concerning birth. Those charged with treating the labouring person then do so in manners that would be unacceptable for themselves.

21.4 REAPPRAISING RUDDICK'S EPISTEMOLOGY FOR MIDWIFERY PRACTICES

We have seen that acknowledgement of obstetric violence has been an uphill battle. We have shown how the processes as described by Walker can be detected here. But, like Walker and Ruddick, we do not believe that an ethics 'outside' these practices would suffice to correct the misconceptions that lead to harm. Instead, we maintain that care ethics with its relational ontology, practicalist epistemology and political ethics can correct and prevent the forms of abuse, disrespect and violence in obstetrics. We therefore follow in Ruddick's footsteps and develop a framework that is capable of alternative ideas of rationality to the dominant ones that divide and separate; to value practicalist ways of reasoning that arise out of needs and demands for care; and to fight against myths on mothers as 'naturally' loving and instead centring on social practices that present demands that require a response. Given the many limitations mentioned regarding Ruddick's work, and perhaps also assuming that professionals are not very keen to adapt a 'mothering framework' to their caring practice, we believe that relevant insights may come to the fore when we draw upon Ruddick's work for obstetric practices. We suggest that we follow this line of thought after which we discuss if the occurrence of obstetric violence can be countered by drawing upon a care ethics framework of mothering, underpinned by the expressive-collaborative model of morality offered by Walker.[118]

We have brought together the insights into Ruddick's idea of 'maternal thinking' and our suggestions for 'midwifery thinking'[119] in Table 21.2, 'Maternal thinking and midwifery thinking'.

In line with Ruddick's work, we return to practices as the touchstone for good maternity care. Ruddick's definition of practices is: 'practices are collective human activities distinguished by the aims that identify them and by the consequent demands made on practitioners committed to those aims'.[121] The aims of mothering practices are preservation, growth and social acceptability, which demand that mothers commit themselves to preservative love, nurturance and training.

Care for birth could, echoing Ruddick's view, be defined as practices committed to the aims of preservation of the birthing bodies, becoming (mother, baby, parent, sibling, grandparent, etc.), and supporting of relations and the environment. This demands that midwives and obstetricians give preservative care, nurturance and relational care. In these practices the critical touchstone, however, is to serve these aims for *both the labouring person and the foetus*, and additionally to the relational network. Similar to Ruddick's description of maternal practice, and instead of a singular focus upon the foetus, we argue that the obstetric practice is typically attuned to the particular demands made by each labouring person and the foetus/newborn. Whereas preservation during labour is a universal demand, now aimed at two involved, particularly the content and application of

TABLE 21.2 Maternal thinking and midwifery thinking

'Maternal thinking' (Ruddick)[120]	*'Midwifery thinking'*
Aims of mothering: – Preservation – Growth – Social acceptability	Aims of midwifery: – Preservation – Becoming – Supportive relations / environment
Demands of mothering: – Preservative love – Nurturance – Training	Demands of midwifery: – Preservative care – Nurturance – Relational care
Typical of 'maternal *practice*': – Attuned to the particular demands of each unique child – Historically and culturally different practices of 'nurturance' and 'training for social acceptability' – Goals may be simultaneously relevant and even conflicting from time to time	Typical of 'midwifery *practice*': – Attuned to the particular demands of each labouring person – Historically and culturally different practices of 'nurturing becoming' and 'care for relational environment' – Goals may be simultaneously relevant and conflicting
Typical of 'maternal *thinking*': – Strategic and conflict managing – Searching for meaning – Balancing the importance of goals – Mothering as a discipline emerges out of practices of thinking (identifying 'mothering' virtues) – Knowledge ≠ practising: struggle	Typical of 'midwifery *thinking*': – Strategic and conflict managing – Searching for meaning – Balancing the importance of goals – Midwifery as a discipline emerges out of practices of thinking (identifying 'midwifery' virtues) – Knowledge ≠ practising: struggle

the second and third demand may be historically and culturally varied. Views on the kind of nurturing demanded vary over time and between cultures, and also the kind of training for social acceptability. Further, all goals may be simultaneously relevant and conflicting and the ways these conflicts are solved depends upon many circumstances. We do not deny that obstetric practice often involves tensions – for example, between supporting and empowering the labouring person with the aim to preserve and nurture the labouring capacity (and thus the experience of bodily and personal power) while keeping an attentive eye on the bodily functions of the foetus. We have also seen that support for survival, identity, and empowerment take different shape for Black mothers and children, and for those of colour.[122] This already gives a clue of the typical characteristics of midwifery thinking, for which we can also make a comparison to Ruddick's description of maternal thinking: both maternal and midwifery thinking are strategic and conflict managing; searching for meaning; balancing the importance of goals; the discipline of 'midwifery' as emerging out of practices of thinking that for instance identifies 'midwifery virtues'; and the fact that having knowledge is not the same as practising, since it may be a struggle to put knowledge into practice.

In brief, like mothering practices, midwifery and obstetric practices require those caring for labouring persons to *think* and from this thinking a distinctive *discipline* emerges, that (like maternal thinking) *establishes criteria for determining failure and success*, *sets priorities* and *identifies virtues that the discipline requires*.[123] For midwifery and obstetric practices this also involves that the patterns and pitfalls of practices that Walker identified need to be avoided: the creating of 'necessary identities'; the processes of naturalizing, privatizing and normalizing subordination; and the creation of an 'epistemic firewall'.[124]

Midwifery thinking as a discipline might benefit from Ruddick's advice. Criteria for failure and success should be relational, i.e. not separating and individualizing the mother or (more probably) the foetus, but seeing them as intertwined, as both in need of ('demanding') care in its three forms: preservation, becoming, relational embeddedness. Failure then is everything that damages, obstructs personal processes and blocks relations. Failure consists in many forms (verbally, physically, through gestures, and symbolically) for which sensitivity needs to be trained. Priorities should be characterized by relationality as well: when one need is more urgent than the other, this can never be the cause to ignore, neglect, objectify or exploit the other. Rather the priority should always be the benefit of two persons who are valuable and dignified of humane treatment. And lastly, virtuous practice should be trained, in the essence of 'training to excel' in relational midwifery care. No blind eye should be turned to failures, mistakes, misconceptions or maltreatment. Open, honest, respectful communication in which all understandings from relevant perspectives are allowed to be expressed, listened to and acknowledged, is required for this. And lastly, storytelling helps. Only when the voices of people are heard, expressing their experiences and understandings, and their knowledge recognized as irreplaceable, practices can be improved.

ACKNOWLEDGEMENTS

We thank our colleagues and the editor of this volume for their helpful comments on this text.

NOTES

1. Nancy Chodorow, *The Reproduction of Mothering. Psychoanalysis and the Sociology of Gender* (Oakland: The Regents of the University of California, 1978).
2. Adrienne Rich, *Of Woman Born: Motherhood as Experience and Institution* (New York: Norton, 1976).
3. Many of the issues of the second feminist wave, including 'mothering', by the way, proved to be limited too, as they primarily pertained to middle- and upper-class women, ignoring those of Black women, women of colour and working-class women. This led to the third wave of feminism, to which we return below.
4. See: Sophie Bourgault, 'Attentive Listening and Care in a Neoliberal Era: Weilian Insights for Hurried Times', *Etica & Politica / Ethics & Politics* 18, no. 3 (2016): 311–37; Sophie Bourgault, 'Democratic Practice and "Caring to Deliberate": A Gadamerian Account of Conversation and Listening', in *Care Ethics, Democratic Citizenship and the State*, ed. Petr Urban and Lizzie Ward (London: Palgrave Macmillan, 2020), 31–51; Maurice Hamington, *Embodied Care: Jane Addams, Maurice Merleau-Ponty, and Feminist Ethics* (Champaign: University of Illinois Press, 2004).
5. Joan C. Tronto, *Moral Boundaries: A Political Argument for an Ethic of Care* (New York: Routledge, 1993).

6. Lisa Baraitser, *Maternal Encounters: The Ethics of Interruption* (Abingdon/New York: Routledge, 2009).
7. See: Andrea Doucet, 'Taking Off the Maternal Lens: Engaging with Sara Ruddick on Men and Mothering', in *21st Century Motherhood. Experience, Identity, Policy, Agency*, ed. Andrea O'Reilly (New York: Columbia University Press, 2010), 170–80; Amy Marvin, 'Groundwork for Transfeminist Care Ethics: Sara Ruddick, Trans Children, and Solidarity in Dependency', *Hypatia* 34, no. 1 (2018): 101–20; Amy Mullin, *Reconceiving Pregnancy and Childcare: Ethics, Experience, and Reproductive Labor* (Cambridge: Cambridge University Press, 2005).
8. Margaret Urban Walker, *Moral Understandings. A Feminist Study in Ethics* (Oxford: Oxford University Press, 2007).
9. Ibid.
10. Carol Gilligan, *In a Different Voice. Psychological Theory and Women's Development* (Cambridge, MA: Harvard University Press, 1982).
11. Inge van Nistelrooij and Carlo Leget, 'Against Dichotomies', *Nursing Ethics* 24, no. 6 (2016): 672, https://journals.sagepub.com/doi/10.1177/0969733015624475.
12. See: Eline Dalmijn, Merel Visse and Inge van Nistelrooij, 'Decision-Making in Case of an Unwanted Pregnancy: An Overview of What is Known About This Complex Process', *Journal of Psychosomatic Obstetrics & Gynecology* 45, no.1 (2024): 2321461; Clair Wills, 'Quickening, or How to Plot an Abortion: The Abortion Plot', *London Review of Books*, 16 March 2023, https://www.lrb.co.uk/the-paper/v45/n06/clair-wills/quickening-or-how-to-plot-an-abortion.
13. Nel Noddings, *Caring: A Feminine Approach to Ethics and Moral Education* (Oakland: University of California Press, 1984).
14. See also: Inge van Nistelrooij, 'The Fluidity of Becoming. The Maternal Body in Feminist Views of Care, Worship and Theology', in *Care Ethics, Religion and Spiritual Traditions*, ed. Inge van Nistelrooij, Maureen Sander-Staudt and Maurice Hamington (Leuven: Peeters, 2022).
15. Carol Gilligan, *In a Different Voice. Psychological Theory and Women's Development* (Cambridge, MA: Harvard University Press, 1993 [1982]), xiii, xix–xxiv.
16. Sara Ruddick, 'Maternal Thinking', *Feminist Studies* 6, no. 2 (1980): 346.
17. Noddings, *Caring*, 8.
18. Tronto, *Moral Boundaries*, 3.
19. Ibid., 1–3. See also: Van Nistelrooij, 'The Fluidity of Becoming'.
20. Van Nistelrooij, 'The Fluidity of Becoming'.
21. See also: Joan C. Tronto, *Caring Democracy: Markets, Equality, and Justice* (New York: New York University Press, 2013).
22. Andrea O'Reilly, 'Matricentric Feminism: A Feminism for Mothers', *Journal of the Motherhood Initiative* 10, no. 1–2 (2019): 13–26.
23. Dána-Ain Davis, *Reproductive Injustice. Racism, Pregnancy, and Premature Birth* (New York: New York University Press, 2019).
24. Michele Goodwin, *Policing the Womb: Invisible Women and the Criminalization of Motherhood* (Cambridge: Cambridge University Press, 2020).
25. See: Rachelle Chadwick, *Bodies that Birth: Vitalizing Birth Politics* (Abingdon and New York: Routledge, 2018); Rodante van der Waal and Inge van Nistelrooij, 'Reimagining Relationality for Reproductive Care: Understanding Obstetric Violence as "Separation"', *Nursing Ethics* 29, no. 5 (2022): 1186–97, https://doi.org/10.1177/09697330211051000; Rodante van der Waal et al., 'Obstetric Violence

Within Students' Rite of Passage: The Reproduction of the Obstetric Subject and its Racialised (M)other', *Agenda* 35, no. 3 (2021): 36–53, https://doi.org/10.1080/10130950.2021.1958553.
26. Davis, *Reproductive Injustice*.
27. Amrita Banerjee and Priya Sharma, 'Animating the Affect-Care-Labor Link in Wake of "The Surrogacy (Regulation) Bill": Care Ethics and Policy-Making on Indian Surrogacy', *Hypatia* 38, no. 3 (2023): 511–30.
28. Joke Struyf, 'Please Leave the Emergency Lane in an Orderly Fashion', *Tijdschrift voor Genderstudies* 26, no. 3/4 (2023): 217–34.
29. United Nations Population Fund, *The State of the World's Midwifery Report*, 2021, https://www.unfpa.org/sites/default/files/pub-pdf/21-038-UNFPA-SoWMy2021-Report-ENv4302.pdf.
30. For instance, for the narrative, proleptic care of a pregnant person and the care needed in pregnancy loss, see: Hilde Lindemann, 'Miscarriage and the Stories We Live By', *Journal of Social Philosophy* 46, no. 1 (2015): 80–90.
31. See: Bourgault, 'Attentive Listening and Care in a Neoliberal Era'; Virginia Held, 'Care and Justice, Still', in *Care Ethics & Political Theory*, ed. Maurice Hamington and Daniel Engster (Oxford: Oxford University Press, 2015), 19–36.
32. Fiona Robinson, 'Care Ethics, Political Theory, and the Future of Feminism', in *Care Ethics & Political Theory*, ed. Maurice Hamington and Daniel Engster (Oxford: Oxford University Press, 2015), 302.
33. Sara Ruddick, *Maternal Thinking. Towards a Politics of Peace* (Boston, MA: Beacon Press, 1989), 5.
34. She later acknowledges that this experience is primarily that of middle-class mothers. We return to this point below.
35. Ruddick, *Maternal Thinking*, 1989, 5.
36. Ibid., 4.
37. Ibid., 8–9.
38. See, for instance, references to her work in: Tronto, *Moral Boundaries*, 108–18.
39. Gilligan, *In a Different Voice*, 1993 [1982], ix.
40. Sara Ruddick, *Maternal Thinking. Towards a Politics of Peace* (Boston, MA: Beacon Press, 1995 [1989]), x.
41. Ibid., x–xi.
42. Gilligan, *In a Different Voice*, 1982.
43. Noddings, *Caring*.
44. Tronto, *Moral Boundaries*.
45. Walker, *Moral Understandings*.
46. Ruddick, 'Maternal Thinking', 347.
47. Robinson, 'Care Ethics, Political Theory, and the Future of Feminism', 304.
48. Ruddick, *Maternal Thinking*, xii.
49. Ruddick, 'Maternal Thinking', 347.
50. Ruddick, *Maternal Thinking*, 1989, 17.
51. Ibid., 18–23.
52. Ibid., 22–6.
53. Ruddick, 'Maternal Thinking', 349–57.
54. Ruddick, *Maternal Thinking*, 1989, 23–7.
55. Ibid., 24.
56. Ibid.

57. Ibid., 24–5.
58. Sarah LaChance Adams, *Mad Mothers, Bad Mothers, and What a 'Good' Mother Would Do: The Ethics of Ambivalence* (New York: Columbia University Press, 2014), 66.
59. Tronto, *Moral Boundaries*, 108.
60. Ibid., 109.
61. Ibid., 109–10.
62. Ibid., 105.
63. At this particular point, Tronto refers to Ruddick's work.
64. See: Bourgault, 'Attentive Listening and Care in a Neoliberal Era'; Bourgault, 'Democratic Practice and "Caring to Deliberate"'.
65. Hamington, *Embodied Care*, 35.
66. Baraitser, *Maternal Encounters*, 42–4.
67. Ruddick, 'Maternal Thinking', 347.
68. Ibid.
69. Ruddick, *Maternal Thinking*, xii–xxi.
70. Ibid., xvi.
71. Mullin, *Reconceiving Pregnancy and Childcare*, 107–8.
72. Ruddick, *Maternal Thinking*, 1989; and Sara Ruddick, 'Thinking Mothers/Conceiving Birth', in *Representations of Motherhood*, ed. Donna Bassin, Margaret Honey and Mahrer Kaplan (New Haven, CT: Yale University Press, 1994).
73. Virginia Held, 'Birth and Death', *Ethics* 99 (1989): 362–88.
74. Mullin, *Reconceiving Pregnancy and Childcare*, 108.
75. Doucet, 'Taking Off the Maternal Lens'.
76. Ibid., 177.
77. Andrea Doucet, 'Father Involvement, Care, and Breadwinning: Genealogies of Concepts and Revisioned Conceptual Narratives', *Genealogy* 4, no. 1 (2020): 1–17, https://doi.org/10.3390/genealogy4010014.
78. Marvin, 'Groundwork for Transfeminist Care Ethics', 105.
79. Ibid., 104–10.
80. Ibid., 110–11.
81. Patricia Hill Collins, 'Shifting the Center: Race, Class, and Feminist Theorizing about Motherhood', in *Mothering: Ideology, Experience, Agency*, ed. Evelyn Nakano Glenn, Grace Chang and Linda Rennie Forcey (Abingdon and New York: Routledge, 1994), 371–89.
82. Catherine Zufferey and Fiona Buchanan, 'Introduction', in *Intersections of Mothering. Feminist Accounts*, ed. Catherine Zufferey and Fiona Buchanan (Abingdon and New York: Routledge, 2020), 1–12.
83. Rebecca Aanerud, 'The Legacy of White Supremacy and the Challenge of White Antiracist Mothering', *Hypatia* 22, no. 2 (2007): 20–38.
84. Maxine Baca Zinn, 'Patricia Hill Collins Symposium. Patricia Hill Collins: Past and Future Innovations', *Gender & Society* 26, no. 1 (2012): 28–32.
85. Kaila Story, ed., *Patricia Hill Collins: Reconceiving Motherhood* (Bradford, ON: Demeter Press, 2014).
86. See: Bourgault, 'Attentive Listening and Care in a Neoliberal Era'; Bourgault, 'Democratic Practice and "Caring to Deliberate"'; Ann J. Cahill and Christine Hamel, *Sounding Bodies. Identity, Injustice, and the Voice* (London and New York: Bloomsbury Methuen Drama, 2023); Miranda Fricker, *Epistemic Injustice: Power and the Ethics of Knowing* (Oxford: Oxford University Press, 2007).
87. Walker, *Moral Understandings*, 7–14.

88. Ibid., 14–19.
89. Ibid.
90. Ibid., 10.
91. Ibid., 10–11.
92. Ibid., 7–14.
93. Ibid., 162–83.
94. Ibid., 161–2.
95. Ibid., 162.
96. Ibid.
97. Ibid., 177.
98. See: Van der Waal and Van Nistelrooij, 'Reimagining Relationality for Reproductive Care'; Rianne van Hassel, Rodante van der Waal and Inge van Nistelrooij, 'Mijn Belichaamde Kennis is van Waarde. Een Auto-etnografische, Zorgethische Analyse van Epistemisch Onrecht Binnen de Nederlandse Reproductieve Zorg [My Embodied Knowledge is Valuable. An Auto-ethnographic, Care-ethical Analysis of Epistemic Injustice in Dutch Reproductive Care]', *Tijdschrift voor Genderstudies* [*Journal of Gender Studies*] 25, no. 4 (2022): 339–62, https://doi.org/10.5117/TVGN.
99. Walker, *Moral Understandings*, 179.
100. Ibid., 178.
101. Ibid.
102. Ibid., 180–2.
103. Ibid., 180.
104. Simone de Beauvoir, *The Second Sex* (New York: Random House, 1997 [1949]).
105. Judith Butler, *Gender Trouble: Feminism and the Subversion of Identity* (New York: Routledge, 1990).
106. Angela Davis, *Women, Race, Class* (Harmondsworth: Penguin, 1981).
107. Denise Ferreira Da Silva, *Toward a Global Idea of Race* (Minneapolis: University of Minnesota Press, 2007).
108. Walker, *Moral Understandings*, 181.
109. Van der Waal et al., 'Obstetric Violence Within Students' Rite of Passage'.
110. Ibid.
111. Marit S. G. Van der Pijl et al., 'Disrespect and Abuse During Labour and Birth Amongst 12,239 Women in the Netherlands: A National Survey', *Reproductive Health* 19, no. 1 (2022): 1–16, https://doi.org/10.1186/s12978-022-01460-4.
112. Walker, *Moral Understandings*, 182.
113. Ibid.
114. Ibid., 183.
115. Ibid.
116. Ibid., 182.
117. Rodante van der Waal and Inge van Nistelrooij, 'Shroud Waving Self-Determination: A Qualitative Analysis of the Moral and Epistemic Dimensions of Obstetric Violence in the Netherlands', *PLOS One* 19, no. 4 (2024): e0297968.
118. Walker, *Moral Understandings*.
119. See also: Rodante van der Waal, Inge van Nistelrooij, Deborah Fox and Elizabeth Newnham, 'Somatophilic Reproductive Justice: On Technology, Feminist Biological Materialism, and Midwifery Thinking,' *Technophany: A Journal for Philosophy and Technology* 2, no. 1 (2023): 1–32. https://doi.org/10.54195/technophany.13801.
120. Ruddick, *Maternal Thinking*, 1989.

121. Ibid., 13–14.
122. Collins, 'Shifting the Center'.
123. See: Ruddick, *Maternal Thinking*, 1989, 24.
124. Walker, *Moral Understandings*.

BIBLIOGRAPHY

Aanerud, Rebecca. 'The Legacy of White Supremacy and the Challenge of White Antiracist Mothering', *Hypatia* 22, no. 2 (2007): 20–38.

Banerjee, Amrita, and Priya Sharma. 'Animating the Affect-Care-Labor Link in Wake of "The Surrogacy (Regulation) Bill": Care Ethics and Policy-Making on Indian Surrogacy', *Hypatia* 38, no. 3 (2023): 511–30.

Baraitser, Lisa. *Maternal Encounters. The Ethics of Interruption*. Abingdon/New York: Routledge, 2009.

de Beauvoir, Simone. *The Second Sex*. New York: Random House, 1997.

Bourgault, Sophie. 'Attentive Listening and Care in a Neoliberal Era: Weilian Insights for Hurried Times', *Etica & Politica / Ethics & Politics* 18, no. 3 (2016): 311–37.

Bourgault, Sophie. 'Democratic Practice and "Caring to Deliberate": a Gadamerian Account of Conversation and Listening', in *Care Ethics, Democratic Citizenship and the State*, edited by Petr Urban and Lizzie Ward, 31–51. London: Palgrave Macmillan, 2020.

Butler, Judith. *Gender Trouble: Feminism and the Subversion of Identity*. New York: Routledge, 1990.

Cahill, Ann J., and Christine Hamel. *Sounding Bodies: Identity, Injustice, and the Voice*. London and New York: Bloomsbury Methuen Drama, 2023.

Chadwick, Rachelle. *Bodies that Birth: Vitalizing Birth Politics*. Abingdon and New York: Routledge, 2018.

Chodorow, Nancy. *The Reproduction of Mothering: Psychoanalysis and the Sociology of Gender*. Oakland: The Regents of the University of California, 1978.

Collins, Patricia Hill. 'Shifting the Center: Race, Class, and Feminist Theorizing about Motherhood', in *Mothering: Ideology, Experience, Agency*, edited by Evelyn Nakano Glenn, Grace Chang and Linda Rennie Forcey, 371–89. Abingdon and New York: Routledge, 1994.

Dalmijn, Eline, Merel Visse and Inge van Nistelrooij. 'Decision-Making in Case of an Unwanted Pregnancy: An Overview of What is Known About This Complex Process', *Journal of Psychosomatic Obstetrics & Gynecology* 45, no. 1 (2024): 2321461.

Da Silva, Denise Ferreira. *Toward a Global Idea of Race*. Minneapolis: University of Minnesota Press, 2007.

Davis, Angela. *Women, Race, Class*. Harmondsworth: Penguin, 1981.

Davis, Dána-Ain. *Reproductive Injustice: Racism, Pregnancy, and Premature Birth*. New York: New York University Press, 2019.

Doucet, Andrea. 'Taking Off the Maternal Lens. Engaging with Sara Ruddick on Men and Mothering', in *21st Century Motherhood: Experience, Identity, Policy, Agency*, edited by Andrea O'Reilly, 170–80. New York: Columbia University Press, 2010.

Doucet, Andrea. 'Father Involvement, Care, and Breadwinning: Genealogies of Concepts and Revisioned Conceptual Narratives', *Genealogy* 4, no. 1 (2020): 1–17. https://doi.org/10.3390/genealogy4010014.

Fricker, Miranda. *Epistemic Injustice: Power and the Ethics of Knowing*. Oxford: Oxford University Press, 2007.

Gilligan, Carol. *In a Different Voice. Psychological Theory and Women's Development*. Cambridge, MA: Harvard University Press, 1982.

Gilligan, Carol. *In a Different Voice. Psychological Theory and Women's Development*. Cambridge, MA: Harvard University Press, 1993 [1982].

Goodwin, Michele. *Policing the Womb: Invisible Women and the Criminalization of Motherhood*. Cambridge: Cambridge University Press, 2020.

Hamington, Maurice. *Embodied Care: Jane Addams, Maurice Merleau-Ponty, and Feminist Ethics*. Champaign: University of Illinois Press, 2004.

Held, Virginia. 'Birth and Death', *Ethics* 99 (1989): 362–88.

Held, Virginia. 'Care and Justice, Still', in *Care Ethics & Political Theory*, edited by Maurice Hamington and Daniel Engster, 19–36. Oxford: Oxford University Press, 2015.

LaChance Adams, Sarah. *Mad Mothers, Bad Mothers, and What a 'Good' Mother Would Do. The Ethics of Ambivalence*. New York: Columbia University Press, 2014.

Lindemann, Hilde. 'Miscarriage and the Stories We Live By', *Journal of Social Philosophy* 46, no. 1 (2015): 80–90.

Marvin, Amy. 'Groundwork for Transfeminist Care Ethics: Sara Ruddick, Trans Children, and Solidarity in Dependency', *Hypatia* 34, no. 1 (2018): 101–20.

Mullin, Amy. *Reconceiving Pregnancy and Childcare: Ethics, Experience, and Reproductive Labor*. Cambridge: Cambridge University Press, 2005.

Noddings, Nel. *Caring: A Feminine Approach to Ethics and Moral Education*. Oakland: University of California Press, 1984.

O'Reilly, Andrea. 'Matricentric Feminism: A Feminism for Mothers', *Journal of the Motherhood Initiative* 10, no. 1–2 (2019): 13–26.

Rich, Adrienne. *Of Woman Born: Motherhood as Experience and Institution*. New York: Norton, 1976.

Robinson, Fiona. 'Care Ethics, Political Theory, and the Future of Feminism', in *Care Ethics & Political Theory*, edited by Maurice Hamington and Daniel Engster, 293–311. Oxford: Oxford University Press, 2015.

Ruddick, Sara. 'Maternal Thinking', *Feminist Studies* 6, no. 2 (1980): 342–67.

Ruddick, Sara. *Maternal Thinking: Towards a Politics of Peace*. Boston, MA: Beacon Press, 1989.

Ruddick, Sara. 'Thinking Mothers/Conceiving Birth', in *Representations of Motherhood*, edited by Donna Bassin, Margaret Honey and Mahrer Kaplan. New Haven, CT: Yale University Press, 1994.

Ruddick, Sara. *Maternal Thinking: Towards a Politics of Peace*. Boston, MA: Beacon Press, 1995 [1989].

Story, Kaila, ed. *Patricia Hill Collins: Reconceiving Motherhood*. Bradford, ON: Demeter Press, 2014.

Struyf, Joke. 'Please Leave the Emergency Lane in an Orderly Fashion', *Tijdschrift voor Genderstudies* 26, no. 3/4 (2023): 217–34.

Tronto, Joan C. *Moral Boundaries: A Political Argument for an Ethic of Care*. New York: Routledge, 1993.

Tronto, Joan C. *Caring Democracy: Markets, Equality, and Justice*. New York: New York University Press, 2013.

United Nations Population Fund. *The State of the World's Midwifery Report*, 2021. https://www.unfpa.org/sites/default/files/pub-pdf/21-038-UNFPA-SoWMy2021-Report-ENv4302.pdf.

Van der Pijl, Marit S. G., Corine J. Verhoeven, Rachel Verweij, Tineke van der Linden, Elselijn Kingma, Martine H. Hollander and Ank de Jonge. 'Disrespect and Abuse During Labour

and Birth Amongst 12,239 Women in the Netherlands: A National Survey', *Reproductive Health* 19, no. 1 (2022): 1–16. https://doi.org/10.1186/s12978-022-01460-4.
Van der Waal, Rodante, and Inge van Nistelrooij. 'Reimagining Relationality for Reproductive Care: Understanding Obstetric Violence as "Separation"', *Nursing Ethics* 29, no. 5 (2022): 1186–97. https://doi.org/10.1177/09697330211051000.
Van der Waal, Rodante, and Inge van Nistelrooij. 'Shroud Waving Self-Determination: A Qualitative Analysis of the Moral and Epistemic Dimensions of Obstetric Violence in the Netherlands', *PLOS One* 19, no. 4 (2024): e0297968.
Van der Waal, Rodante, Veronica Mitchell, Inge van Nistelrooij and Vivienne Bozalek. 'Obstetric Violence Within Students' Rite of Passage: The Reproduction of the Obstetric Subject and its Racialised (M)other', *Agenda* 35, no. 3 (2021): 36–53. https://doi.org/10.1080/10130950.2021.1958553.
Van der Waal, Rodante, Inge van Nistelrooij, Deborah Fox and Elizabeth Newnham. 'Somatophilic Reproductive Justice: On Technology, Feminist Biological Materialism, and Midwifery Thinking', *Technophany: A Journal for Philosophy and Technology* 2, no. 1 (2023): 1–32. https://doi.org/10.54195/technophany.13801.
Van Hassel, Rianne, Rodante Van der Waal and Inge Van Nistelrooij. 'Mijn Belichaamde Kennis is van Waarde. Een Auto-etnografische, Zorgethische Analyse van Epistemisch Onrecht Binnen de Nederlandse Reproductieve Zorg [My Embodied Knowledge is Valuable. An Auto-ethnographic, Care-ethical Analysis of Epistemic Injustice in Dutch Reproductive Care]', *Tijdschrift voor Genderstudies* [*Journal of Gender Studies*] 25, no. 4 (2022): 339–62. https://doi.org/10.5117/TVGN2022.4.004.HASS.
Van Nistelrooij, Inge. 'The Fluidity of Becoming: The Maternal Body in Feminist Views of Care, Worship and Theology', in *Care Ethics, Religion and Spiritual Traditions*, edited by Inge van Nistelrooij, Maureen Sander-Staudt and Maurice Hamington. Leuven: Peeters, 2022.
Van Nistelrooij, Inge, and Carlo Leget. 'Against Dichotomies', *Nursing Ethics* 24, no. 6 (2016): 694–703. https://doi.org/10.1177/0969733015624475.
Walker, Margaret Urban. *Moral Understandings. A Feminist Study in Ethics*. Oxford: Oxford University Press, 2007.
Wills, Clair. 'Quickening, or How to Plot an Abortion: The Abortion Plot', *London Review of Books*, 16 March 2023. https://www.lrb.co.uk/the-paper/v45/n06/clair-wills/quickening-or-how-to-plot-an-abortion.
Zinn, Maxine Baca. 'Patricia Hill Collins Symposium. Patricia Hill Collins: Past and Future Innovations', *Gender & Society* 26, no. 1 (2012): 28–32.
Zufferey, Catherine, and Fiona Buchanan. 'Introduction', in *Intersections of Mothering. Feminist Accounts*, edited by Catherine Zufferey and Fiona Buchanan, 1–12. Abingdon and New York: Routledge, 2020.

CHAPTER TWENTY-TWO

Care ethics and conflicts in needs

Balancing disabled and feminist perspectives and experiences in personalized social care services

KIRSTEIN RUMMERY

INTRODUCTION

In this chapter the development of 'personalization' – that is, care services that are commissioned by the state but are nominally under the control of service users (disabled and older people) rather than funders or providers – in social care in developed welfare states is discussed. Whilst these often result in greater independence, particularly for younger disabled people, they change the nature of social care, particularly for those providing it. This has overt and hidden gendered outcomes, but there are very few analyses that critically analyse these outcomes in a systematic comparative way. In this chapter an attempt is made to address this gap.

As has been well documented, there is a rising demand for social care services in developed welfare states, due to improved life expectancy and reduced mortality for both younger and older disabled people, and to demographic, cultural and political changes which have brought more women into the workforce and away from providing care. These are positive changes in social policy terms – indeed, they have been welcomed as one of the most significant successes of twentieth-century social policy.[1]

In this chapter, an approach to ethical care developed by Sevenhuijsen and others by using a framework of gender equity[2] is operationalized. This framework has been developed by Plantenga and Remery to produce the European Gender Equality Index (EGEI).[3] This framework is used to analyse the gendered outcomes of personalized versus state-run systems of delivering social care. Examples of different types of state-run and personalized schemes are used to draw out the ethical care-informed gender equity outcomes, and to compare different typologies of social care delivery with regard to balancing the needs of women and disabled people (as recipients of care). The analysis leads to the conclusion that formal personalized schemes offer better gender outcomes than more informal schemes, but whilst state-provided social care still offers the best gender outcomes overall, they do not necessarily provide ethical care for disabled people.

22.1 METHODS

To carry out comparative analysis meaningfully, it is important to be able to capture commonalities and differences across different policy contexts, and also to have some distance from the policies under review to be able to accurately judge outcomes.[4] For this reason, the author has chosen two sampling frames for social care policies. First, temporally, policies in operation between 2001 and 2016 have been selected. Rather than an exhaustive description of contemporary policies, which exists elsewhere, this enables sufficient temporal distance for the use of theoretical and empirical insights from scholars to be included in the analysis. Second, only countries with developed welfare states that would be judged to be mid-range or higher on the EGEI have been included. The purpose of this chapter is to compare gendered outcomes for personalized versus state-run social care services, which means the case studies had to be those where such services are in place, and where sufficient evidence has been provided to be able to judge gendered outcomes.

The data for this chapter are drawn from a systematic literature review, following the Campbell guidelines, of social care policies. An initial scoping review resulted in over 250 published articles and grey literature being grouped using qualitative comparative analysis methods.[5] Further inductive analysis of the themes in the empirical and published evidence from the chosen case studies was carried out. This resulted in the findings being synthesized into two models which internally shared dominant, relevant characteristics, and contrasted sharply on external factors. Further analysis revealed which characteristics were non-context-specific. This finally produced two models of state-run services (referred to herein as the universal and partnership models) and three models of personalized social care services (referred to herein as formal, semi-formal and informal) from which it was possible to describe simple, common elements, rather than a complex descriptive account of many case studies.

22.2 GENDER EQUITY AND SOCIAL CARE

Gender equality as a policy aim often takes the approach that gender-equal outcomes would involve men and women being treated the same even though nation-states have distinct histories and, for example, ways of framing the gendered division of labour between paid and unpaid work.[6] Gender equality in this approach means that men are the 'unit of assessment', and that gender equality is achieved when women are approaching equality with the male norm.

This approach is problematic in several ways. Using men as the norm ignores the social and economic advantages enjoyed by a society that overvalues their paid work in comparison to that of women and ignores the overrepresentation of women in those that undertake unpaid work (such as family care of older or disabled relatives) which means they are not able to participate full-time in the labour market. It also ignores the fact that whilst the market may not recompense women adequately for the unpaid care work they undertake, that does not mean that this work is unvalued by society. Indeed, one approach to equality advocates that there should be more equitable sharing of paid and unpaid work across the genders, rather than trying to recompense carers which has the result of reinforcing gendered divisions of labour.

Fraser and others have advocated using the idea of 'equity' (fairness) rather than 'equality', and recognizing that this is a complex idea. For Fraser, to achieve gender equity we should take neither the route of making women equal to men, nor compensating them for undertaking care, but find a way of achieving seven principles:

1. anti-poverty (addressing women's poverty specifically rather than poverty generally which can hide or even further women's poverty by not allowing for the gendered nature of the factors that lead to women's poverty);
2. anti-exploitation (not relying on the exploitation of women's unpaid or underpaid labour);
3. income equality (this includes access to income within the family);
4. leisure-time equality (addressing time inequality);
5. equality of respect (respecting the gendered roles equally);
6. anti-marginalization (addressing women's public oppression and marginalization due to the gendered nature of different roles); and
7. anti-androcentralization (addressing the inequality caused by women's biology and reproductive roles).

Fraser proposes that women's, instead of men's, current life patterns should become the 'norm' expected, so that people spend less time in the marketized labour force, and devote more time to other kinds of labour, such as care, activism and civic and political participation, a model she calls the 'universal caregiver model' of society.[7]

Social care is often neglected from a gender equity perspective (compared to, say, childcare) but it matters in several important ways. First, the ideology and theoretical approaches adopted by a country towards its social care provision have direct and indirectly gendered implications: if a country presumes that the family should have the primary responsibility for providing social care, then it is placing that burden disproportionately on women. Most intra-generational family care, particularly intimate personal care, is carried out by women. Mothers and daughters fall into gendered expectations, and this is at a great cost in terms of their labour market participation, risk of poverty and ill health, lack of independence and control over resources, and placing a serious strain on kinship ties. In contrast, if a country expects the state to be the main provider of social care, then it removes that burden from the family, and there is a reduced gendered impact or cost to providing care: women tend to be less disadvantaged in the labour market and to be at less risk of poverty and ill health. They also have greater control over their resources and play a much more prominent role in public life.

The second reason why social care matters to gender equity is that where care is provided by paid carers, these tend to be: (a) disproportionately (but not exclusively) jobs done by women; (b) considered to be relatively low skilled and therefore attract low rates of pay in the market. This reflects the low value given to care work precisely *because* it is gendered – it is a job that is done by women.

22.3 UNIVERSAL MODEL OF STATE-PROVIDED SOCIAL CARE

Countries that fell into this model had normative policy frameworks that were heavily focused on gender equality. Aspirations towards gender equality informed the constitutions of the countries, and also underpinned the development of welfare services. This means they provide public services on a universal basis, without stigma or loss of status. The twin commitment to gender equality and universality means that social care services have been part of state provision since the inception of the modern welfare state.

22.3.1 Denmark

Around one in six older people receive home care services in Denmark, which is provided free of charge. Recent changes include a reablement assessment and service before people are eligible for home care, and a very small direct payments scheme. Informal care is used but always considered to be supplemental to formal care.

Denmark scores relatively well on all gender equality indices. It works with a dual earner-carer model, whereby the assumption is that both paid work and unpaid care are equally shared between the genders, but this is more successful in long-term than in childcare policy: most parental leave is used by mothers, contributing in part to a gender pay gap of around 16 per cent.[8] Denmark and Iceland are commonly seen as the most ‘marketized’ or ‘neoliberal’ of the universal model countries, although the commitment to gender equality and universal social services remains strong.

22.3.2 Iceland

Until the early 1980s, most state care for older and disabled people was provided through institutional care (i.e. residential and nursing homes), but since 1982 policy changes have led to the development of home care services which are provided by municipalities (local government). User fees are charged for the non-health parts of the services – these vary but are modest (and income-related), so only 9.4 per cent of the total expenditure on home care services comes from these fees. Unpaid care by relatives plays a significant part in the provision of help and support for older people[9] with very small numbers receiving a working-age carer’s allowance. The main caregiver is usually a spouse (roughly gender-equal) but in 27 per cent of cases, this informal care is provided by daughters.[10]

22.3.3 Sweden

A longstanding commitment to publicly funded services to support gender equity through universal childcare has not necessarily extended to social care. Fourteen per cent of older people use home help services, and there has been a shift since the 1980s away from institutional towards home-based services. At the same time there has been a rise in daughters – particularly low-income daughters – providing unpaid care for their parents; higher-income families are in a better position to be able to pay for home-based and institutional social care.[11]

22.4 PARTNERSHIP MODEL OF STATE-PROVIDED SOCIAL CARE

Countries in the partnership model saw gender equity as important, but it was not the most important factor determining the development of social care policies. They had developed welfare states, but did not view the state as being necessarily the only or main provider of services. The state was seen more as a shaper of policy: it played a role in providing a legislative framework for funding and services, but in partnership with the market, with communities and families, and with individuals. There was a greater role played by municipal authorities than in the universal model, and thus sometimes a greater variation in the availability and quality of social care services. The state played a strong regulatory role, and individuals had important rights to access services.

22.4.1 Germany

The most significant recent change to social care policy occurred with the introduction of long-term care insurance. This is a national scheme that offers benefits based on three levels of need with fixed lump-sum benefits, along with cash payments for carers which can be supplemented by means-tested benefits. The purpose is to enable those who need care and support to purchase their own services from a mix of formal and family carers, using insurance-based state benefits topped up either through their own means or additional benefits.

Germany has opted to support women's care labour in social care by reimbursing them through cash payments, rather than encouraging women into the labour market and providing universal formal care services. Although cash benefits to recompense family carers were heralded as supporting and valuing care work undertaken by women, they have been criticized for leading to greater gender inequality, particularly among low-paid, low-skilled women for whom the cash benefits incentivize remaining away from the formal labour market for longer periods. This pattern (of higher-income women having more ability to use state benefits to avoid having to leave work to provide care themselves than lower-income women) is particularly noticeable in the results of the long-term care insurance policy.[12] Lower-income women are more likely to have a financial incentive to provide care to family members because they can receive payments through the long-term care insurance scheme and cash benefits directed at them.

22.4.2 The Netherlands

Social care in the Netherlands has recently undergone substantial change, separating out those with medically related chronic health problems (who are entitled to care within a health funded institution) from those with less severe needs (who are now eligible for support to help them stay in their own homes and participate in society). This is coupled with a reduction in eligibility for direct payments for disabled people, which enabled those living at home to employ their own carers (including family members). These changes are part of an ongoing policy drive to reduce costs by moving responsibility for the provision of social care from the public to the private purse.[13]

22.5 MEASURING GENDER EQUITY IN STATE-PROVIDED (I.E. NON-PERSONALIZED) SOCIAL CARE

TABLE 22.1 Universal provision: Denmark, Sweden and Iceland

Principle	*Progress (substantial; good; neutral; poor; very weak)*
Anti-poverty	**Substantial**, due to women's increased labour market participation and universal provision of services.
Anti-exploitation	**Good**, due to income protection and value placed on care work. More equitable sharing of unpaid care across genders needed.
Income equality	**Good**, due to women's increased labour market participation over life course. More progress needed on occupational segregation.
Leisure-time equality	**Good**, due to high levels of provision of social care. More progress needed on equitable sharing of unpaid care between genders.
Equality of respect	**Substantial**, due to high value placed on women's work, both paid and unpaid.
Anti-marginalization	**Substantial**, due to high levels of women's participation in public life.
Anti-androcentralization	**Neutral**, due to heteronormative models of family life and enduring gendered expectations around formal and informal social care.

TABLE 22.2 Partnership-based provision: Germany and the Netherlands

Principle	*Progress (substantial; good; neutral; poor; very weak)*
Anti-poverty	**Good**, because care which removes women from labour market is compensated for. However, it would be better if women were either encouraged to remain in labour market to increase their income or if compensation for care was at full market rates.
Anti-exploitation	**Good**, because care which removes women from labour market is compensated for.
Income equality	**Neutral**, because compensation for care work is set at level that does not encourage men into taking greater role in parenting or care of children. Also encourages low-paid women to withdraw from labour market to provide care, and increases inequality between low- and high-income women. However, greater encouragement (through shared and non-transferable parental leave) for men to share care work and for women to remain in labour market, as well as addressing occupational segregation, would further reduce income inequality.

Principle	*Progress (substantial; good; neutral; poor; very weak)*
Leisure-time equality	**Good**, due to support for flexible working for both genders (particularly in the Netherlands) and formal provision of social care.
Equality of respect	**Substantial**, due to recognition of and compensation for women's care labour. Formal care workers also supported as part of labour market.
Anti-marginalization	**Good**, due to value being given to women's care work. However, greater encouragement to remain in labour market and for men to take greater share of care work would reduce risk of marginalization for lower-income women.
Anti-androcentralization	**Poor**, due to reinforcement of gendered division of labour. However, more equal sharing of care work across genders would improve this.

22.6 DEVELOPING SERVICE USER-LED ('PERSONALIZED') MODELS OF SOCIAL CARE FOR DISABLED PEOPLE

There have been longstanding concerns within developed welfare states as to how to manage welfare and care policies in such a way as to cap the rising demand for resources, leading to a shifting of responsibilities across public sectors (for example, from health to social care, and from national to localized provision), and across sectors (for example, from state to private or third sector provision, or from state to family (or, indeed, family to state)). At the same time, a variety of international, national and local political, social and economic factors have led to changes in the governance of welfare, including increasing commodification of services and de-professionalization of practitioners.[14] Rising demand for support and services has also come not just from demographic changes but also from increasingly politicized 'user' movements (such as disability rights organizations in the UK and the Netherlands, and older people's organizations in the United States) who have rejected both family and informal care as exploitative (for both carers and cared-for) and state care as increasingly fragmented, unresponsive and dehumanizing – indeed, rejecting the rhetoric of 'care' altogether and demanding social rights, empowerment and control over the type and level of support received instead.[15] Increasing regulation of services in response to 'consumer' demand has only partially succeeded in responding effectively to these changes: new models of service delivery are being actively sought in response to these complex political, social and economic changes.[16]

These pressures have led to the development of personalization schemes across a range of developed welfare states. Although these vary considerably in their intentions, scope and the way they function, they are essentially mechanisms whereby a disabled or older person receives a cash benefit in order to purchase help or services themselves, in lieu of receiving services or support directly. They can be seen as a way of 'commodifying' care[17] and several different models have emerged: tightly controlled personal care budgets allowing direct employment of formal care workers; care allowances paid directly to disabled and older people but not directly governed; income maintenance approaches (whereby allowances are paid directly to carers to acknowledge or compensate for the loss of earned income, usually only available to low-income carers); and directly paying informal carers to replace publicly funded formal care. In some forms, particularly those paid directly to disabled and older people, their popularity among disabled and older people is well documented: they have been hailed as an important victory for social rights by campaigners in the UK, because of the way in which they have allowed disabled and older people to exert choice and control over the type of assistance and support they receive,[18] and the way they have enabled disabled people to combine different types of support (health and social care, formal and informal) in ways which have led to greater independence and social participation, without the 'burden of gratitude' experienced by people receiving informal care from family members or voluntary or paid workers not directly employed by the disabled or older person themselves.[19]

22.7 EXAMPLES OF PERSONALIZED SOCIAL CARE POLICIES

22.7.1 Formal

22.7.1.1 The Netherlands The Netherlands has seen the introduction in 1991 of a personal care allowance scheme that was extended in 1995 to become part of the national long-term care insurance scheme,[20] allowing recipients to choose to receive direct payments in lieu of directly provided services. This scheme is relatively strictly regulated, providing a degree of protection for directly employed care workers and making it impossible to directly pay workers on the 'black' or unregulated market. However, it can be used to purchase care from family members and thus enables recipients to combine formal and informal care arrangements flexibly. It is also relatively generously funded, leading to political concerns about rising demand, although, in common with other cash-for-care schemes, it is still cheaper than directly providing state-funded services.[21]

22.7.1.2 France France is usually viewed as a 'familialist' welfare state, with insurance-based health and social care payments coupled with a strong ethos of family-based care.[22] In 1997 the 'Prestation Spécifique Dépendance' (PSD) was introduced, which was replaced in 2002 by the 'Allocation Personnalisée à l'Autonomie' (APA). This is a payment made directly to older people (which can be supplemented by other means-tested benefits) which enables them to directly purchase their own care, either from a professional or a relative (but not from a spouse). It is most commonly used to purchase services from formal, not-for-profit social care organizations, rather than directly employing individuals. It has been argued that this formalized element to the payment is an important part of France's strategy of protecting the employment rights of care workers, as well as reinforcing gendered divisions of low-paid formal and informal labour.[23] The more formalized APA system has led to more employment protection for professional carers,[24] but it has not altered the gendered division of formal and informal care.[25]

22.7.2 Semi-formal

22.7.2.1 United Kingdom (UK) In the UK, a system of direct payments was introduced in 1996 which replaced previous ad hoc schemes. Disabled and older people are now able to apply for payments in lieu of directly provided services (the level of which is set according to a needs assessment) and these payments are usually used to directly employ formal care workers, or purchase care from not-for-profit care agencies. It is not possible to directly pay family members, as, unlike other schemes, it is intended to replace formal rather than informal care and support, and there is relatively low take-up among older people. A regulatory system is in place, although there is little formal employment protection for directly employed workers, and lack of formal assistance in recruitment of care workers is a problem for both users and employees. It is implemented locally, with the result that there is considerable regional variation in criteria, eligibility and access, although policy developments are in place to support more systematic take-up and to enable users to purchase a wider range of services (at present, the scheme is limited to 'social' care).[26]

22.7.2.2 United States A high degree of policy decentralization has led to considerable federal-level variation in American social care provision. Since 1981 Medicaid programmes in the United States have been allowed a greater discretion in providing services and support for older and disabled people, leading to a proliferation of 'consumer-choice' programmes allowing people to directly hire their own care workers, particularly through schemes such as the Cash and Counselling Demonstration pilots in Arkansas, Florida and New Jersey.[27] These schemes usually allow disabled and older people to directly employ workers with whom they have an ongoing relationship (through kinship or paid social care relationships) and have proved popular and successful, with the result that such 'private market solutions' are becoming part of mainstream social care policy.[28]

22.7.3 Informal

22.7.3.1 Italy Italy has historically seen very little development of formal residential or community-based care services, explained in part by very decentralized state provision of services generally (leading to substantial regional variations) and a reliance on family and informal care,[29] accompanied by a reluctance to develop formal, central-state-driven responses to the rising demand for social care.[30] The 'Indennita di accompagnamento' is a non-means-tested benefit available to disabled and older people who are certified as 'dependent'. It is not tempered according to need, and no restrictions are placed upon its use. This comparative lack of regulation means that it is most often used to employ care workers, often on the black (unregulated) labour market.[31] Local means-tested care allowances, which are subject to local variations in terms of eligibility and access, are also available and are also used primarily to purchase care from individual workers and family members, reinforcing gendered divisions of labour – or sometimes as a supplement to the family income and not paid out directly for care.[32]

22.7.3.2 Austria Austria has traditionally been viewed as a strong social-democratic state with an emphasis on a gendered division of labour and the 'male breadwinner' model of welfare provision, resulting in low levels of provision of formal care services.[33] In 1993 the long-term care allowance ('Pflegegeld') system was introduced, a tax-financed non-means-tested benefit paid directly to the disabled or older person.[34] It is generally used to purchase care from either organizations or individuals, or to reimburse family members.[35] They have tended to be used to fund informal care or migrant/'grey' labour market workers (often from neighbouring accession states), reinforcing traditions of low-paid workers (often women) with very little employment protection whilst also reinforcing gendered divisions of labour within the familial sphere.[36]

22.7.4 Ethically balancing the needs of users and carers: governance issues

Two issues pertinent to the governance of personalized schemes emerge from an analysis of the six schemes under discussion. First, there is the issue of national versus regional/local governance. Where schemes have been developed which allow for a degree of localized discretion in their implementation (e.g. the UK, the United States and, to a certain degree, Italy) there is considerable scope for inequalities and inequities inherent in the system to have a gendered impact (for example, in the different types of employment protection available to workers, and the differential impact commodifying care can have on family relationships). Second, there is the issue of the governance of the schemes themselves: how they are operated, how users are made to account for how they spend money, and the level of policing and surveillance that gives the state over individuals' lives. Some schemes (e.g. the UK, the Netherlands, France) are highly regulated, which, on the one hand, offers a degree of protection both to potentially vulnerable users and workers (and, particularly in the case of France, offers valuable employment protection to potentially exploited groups of care workers who are overwhelmingly women), but which, on the other hand also gives the state a great deal of power to police the lives of women.

22.7.5 Life course and social divisions

In some respects, the introduction of a marketized, consumerist mechanism such as cash-for-care schemes into an area that was previously the domain of either the private, familial sphere or the public, statutory sphere is likely to create and exacerbate social divisions already apparent between different social groups. For example, the evidence on take-up of such schemes in the UK suggests that it is generally articulate, younger, well-educated disabled people who are disproportionately represented among those who choose to use them.[37] Take-up among older people, ethnic minorities and learning-disabled adults remains comparatively low. These findings echo concerns across other areas of welfare provision that consumerist-driven reforms will tend to favour those best placed to benefit from the market by exercising choice, voice and exit.[38] In other words, the gulf between middle-class and poorer disabled and older people is likely to be made greater by the introduction of cash-for-care schemes, as is the gulf between middle-class and poorer carers, with the former being more able to exercise choice about the level and type of care work they undertake than the latter. As discussed above, cash-for-care schemes are also likely to lead to a widening gulf between carers working in regulated, professionalized and protected formal care employment and those working in private, unregulated employment, whether this be for a family member, direct employer or through the grey/black labour market. They are likely to further disenfranchise low-skilled, poorly paid women in comparison to their wealthier, better-educated sisters and to widen social division within and across genders.

Furthermore, the impact of personalized schemes on power relationships within the family sphere across the life course and across generations remains unexplored, but there are reasons to voice concern about several aspects. First, in low-income families where the use of the cash payment is fairly unregulated (for example, in Italy) it is likely, based on what we already know about the distribution and use of money in low-income households, that gender differentials will emerge, with women more likely to use the payments to purchase care and men being more likely to use the payments as part of the general household income,[39] leading to a reinforcement of gendered power differences within families. Second, where personalized schemes are used to route money to informal family carers, this can have the effect of creating or reinforcing dependency relationships both intergenerationally (for example, between learning-disabled adult children and parent/carers; or between daughters/daughters-in-law and parents) and intragenerationally (for example, between spouses). Finally, the use of unregulated and unsupervised cash-for-care payments, both to pay family carers and directly employ unskilled care workers, has the result of commodifying intimate and sometimes unarticulated relationships and expectations, with the possibility of exploitation and abuse of vulnerable parties on both sides.[40] Money, after all, in a highly consumer-oriented capitalist society, is power, and the person controlling the money in a care relationship is in a position to be able to exert power and influence over the person who does not; and any relationship involving the exertion of power and control over another person is open to the possibility of the abuse of that power and control. Again, better-educated, better-skilled and better-paid women are likely to be in a better position to avoid the potential abuse and exploitation suffered by lower-education, lower-skilled and lower-paid women in these situations, leading to greater inequalities between different groups of women (and sometimes men).

22.7.6 Wellbeing and citizenship for users and carers

Notwithstanding the issues and concerns raised above, the evidence across all the schemes, particularly in comparative and qualitative studies[41] suggests that such schemes do appeal to both users and formal and informal carers, and it is worth exploring some of the gendered dimensions of why this is the case. First, cash-for-care schemes are a way of recognizing the complexity and reciprocity that characterize many caring relationships. One thing that both feminist and disability rights researchers and campaigners have pointed out is that people's identities within the social world are not easily divided into binary distinctions: public versus private, user versus carer, worker versus non-worker. It is possible – indeed, usual – for disabled and older people to simultaneously be employers (for example, of personal care workers), carers (for example, of spouses, children or grandchildren), workers (whether full- or part-time, paid or unpaid, voluntary or involuntary, or a combination of all of these) and to be exercising citizenship rights and duties in other complex ways.[42] The advantage of cash-for-care schemes over the alternatives (i.e. formal state provision or informal family provision of care and support) is that giving choice and control to disabled and older people enables them to purchase care and support that fits in with both statutory and informal networks, and enables them to carry out their own caring and other duties.[43]

Second, personalized schemes are a very effective way of filling in gaps between service provision that are not easily addressed by formal provision – for example, by enabling users to employ workers who cross the 'health/social' care divide, or by allowing users to purchase support for themselves in a caring role (e.g. as a parent) – which can have the result of ameliorating the effects of power dependencies within families. The effects of freeing people up (to be parents, spouses and children, rather than carers and/or cared-for) can have a significantly positive effect on the wellbeing and relationships of all concerned. Exercising choice and control is empowering not only for users but also for carers: being able to choose when and how to care and being able to choose not to care can reduce the disempowering effects of having to provide care because no other options are available. As women are still the primary carers in families their concerns are with the wellbeing of all their families, and a policy development that has the effect of increasing the wellbeing of all members of the family is one to be welcomed.

Finally, if we move away from a neoliberal economic analysis of cash-for-care schemes as being a way of trapping women into low-paid, unskilled care work towards a more nuanced understanding of the value of care work and an 'ethic of care',[44] both for carers and cared-for, we can conceivably argue that giving women the opportunity to engage in that work for payment, even if that payment is low, is possibly opening up citizenship opportunities in a way that is preferable to some of the alternatives available. For example, engaging in care work, particularly if freely chosen, is arguably less dangerous and exploitative to low-paid migrant workers than other black-market alternatives; any gendered analysis would have difficulty asserting that contributing to the wellbeing of disabled and older people is of less importance than contributing to the wellbeing of the purchasers of sexual services, for example.

22.7.7 Personalized social care and gender equity

TABLE 22.3 France and the Netherlands: formal schemes

Principle	*Progress (substantial; good; neutral; poor; very weak)*
Anti-poverty	• **Good** because of reasonable rates of pay for formal carers and lack of incentives for unpaid carers.
Anti-exploitation	• **Substantial** because family carers are not forced to provide care in absence of suitable alternatives.
Income equality	• **Good**, due to rates of pay for formal carers, and ability of potential family carers to engage in labour market rather than provide unpaid care.
Leisure-time equality	• **Good** because lack of pressure to provide informal care. • Could be improved by more gender equality among those who 'fill in gap' between formal paid care.
Equality of respect	• **Substantial**, due to rates of pay for formal carers – seen as citizenship right for users.
Anti-marginalization	• **Good** because lack of pressure to provide informal care. • Could be improved by more gender equality among those who 'fill in gap' between formal paid care.
Anti-androcentralization	• **Good** because lack of pressure to provide informal care. • Could be improved by more gender equality among those who 'fill in gap' between formal paid care, and by more men providing paid care.

TABLE 22.4 The UK and the United States: semi-formal schemes

Principle	*Progress (substantial; good; neutral; poor; very weak)*
Anti-poverty	• **Poor,** due to lack of comprehensive cover of scheme and low rates of pay for formal carers.
Anti-exploitation	• **Poor,** due to low rates of pay and lack of substantive legal protection for carers.
Income equality	• **Very weak,** due to low rates of pay for carers, pressure for women to fill in gaps left by formal care and removal of informal carers from labour market.
Leisure-time equality	• **Poor,** due to pressure on women to fill in gaps left by formal care.
Equality of respect	• **Poor** due to low rates of pay for care and negligible benefit rates for those providing unpaid care.
Anti-marginalization	• **Poor,** due to low rates of pay and respect for paid carers and low rates of income for family carers.
Anti-androcentralization	• **Very weak,** with both paid and unpaid care done mainly by women, very little incentive to share care work more equitably across genders.

TABLE 22.5 Austria and Italy: informal schemes

Principle	*Progress (substantial; good; neutral; poor; very weak)*
Anti-poverty	• **Very weak,** due to low rates of pay for formal carers, and gendered expectations leading to women removing themselves from labour market to provide unpaid care to fill in gaps.
Anti-exploitation	• **Very weak,** due to low rates of pay and no substantive legal protection for paid carers.
Income equality	• **Very weak,** due to low rates of pay for formal care and high risk of poverty for women expected to leave labour market to provide unpaid care.
Leisure-time equality	• **Very weak,** due to demands on women's time to provide unpaid care.
Equality of respect	• **Poor,** due to low rates of pay, although unpaid care valued as citizenship contribution.
Anti-marginalization	• **Poor,** due to low rates of pay for formal carers and incentives to remove themselves from labour market to provide care for low-income women.
Anti-androcentralization	• **Very poor,** due to gendered nature of paid and unpaid care and lack of incentives for more gender equity in caring responsibilities.

CONCLUSIONS: WHAT KIND OF SOCIAL CARE LEADS TO BETTER GENDER EQUITY AND PROVIDES ETHICAL CARE FOR WOMEN AND DISABLED PEOPLE?

If our only consideration is to look at social care policies that score highly on Fraser's gender equity index, then clearly the provision of universal state social care provides the best gender outcomes. Denmark, Sweden and Iceland clearly score well on all seven of Fraser's domains, by recompensing care work fairly and not making the family (and thus women) the default providers of social care.

However, if we want to balance the needs of users AND carers then formal personalized schemes, such as those in France and the Netherlands, score as highly as universal state provision. These schemes have the added bonus that they provide more choice, control and independence for disabled and older people who need social rather than direct state provision. On balance, if we want gender equity AND independence for disabled people, then we should be developing formal personalized social care policies.

If we want state involvement, but also more flexibility to meet family needs, then state-sponsored social care, like that in Germany and the Netherlands, provides a balanced approach to gender equity and users' needs. It allows the use of both formal and informal care and flexible options to reflect family circumstances and different cultural and ideological expectations of social care.

The worst options in terms of gender equity outcomes are semi-formal and informal personalized social care schemes, such as those found in the UK, the United States, Austria and Italy. These rely heavily on the undervaluing of paid care and the willingness of unpaid family members, usually women, to provide unpaid care to fill in the gaps left by paid provision.

NOTES

1. Alan Walker and Ariela Lowenstein, 'European Perspectives on Quality of Life in Old Age', *European Journal of Ageing* 6, no. 2 (2009): 61–6.
2. Nancy Fraser, *Justice Interruptus: Critical Reflections on the Post-Socialist Condition* (New York: Routledge, 1997).
3. Janneke Plantenga and Chantal Remery, *Flexible Working Time Arrangements and Gender Equality, European Commission: A Comparative Review of 30 European Countries* (European Commission Directorate-General for Employment, Social Affairs and Equal Opportunities. Luxembourg: Publications Office of the European Union, 2009).
4. Linda Hantrais, *International Comparative Research: Theory, Methods and Practice* (London: Palgrave, 2009).
5. Jaquelina Hewitt-Taylor, 'Use of Constant Comparative Analysis in Qualitative Research', *Nursing Standard* 15, no. 42 (2001): 39–42.
6. Janine Goetschy, 'The European Employment Strategy: Genesis and Development', *European Journal of Industrial Relations* 5, no. 2 (1999): 117–37.
7. Fraser, *Justice Interruptus*, 48.
8. NOSOSCO, *Social Protection in the Nordic Countries 2007–2008: Scope, Expenditure and Financing* (Copenhagen: Nordic Social-Statistical Committee, 2009).
9. Sigurveig H. Sigurðardóttir and Ingemar Kåreholt, 'Informal and Formal Care of Older People in Iceland', *Scandinavian Journal of Caring Sciences* 28, no. 4 (2014): 802–11.

10. Sigurveig H. Sigurðardóttir, Gerdt Sundström, Bo Malmberg and Marie Ernsth Bravell, 'Needs and Care of Older People Living at Home in Iceland', *Scandinavian Journal of Public Health* 40 (2012): 1–9.
11. NOSOSCO, *Social Protection in the Nordic Countries 2007–2008*.
12. Hildegard Theobald and Kristine Kern, 'The Introduction of Long-Term Care Policy Schemes: Policy Development, Policy Transfer and Policy Change', *Policy and Politics* 39, no. 3 (2011): 325–42.
13. Ellen Grootegoed and Diana van Dijk, 'The Return of the Family? Welfare State Retrenchment and Client Autonomy in Long-Term Care', *Journal of Social Policy* 41, no. 4 (2012): 677–94.
14. Janet Newman, 'Constructing Accountability: Network Governance and Managerial Agency', *Public Policy and Administration* 19, no. 4 (2005): 17–33.
15. Jenny Morris, 'Independent Living and Community Care: A Disempowering Framework', *Disability & Society* 19, no. 5 (2004): 427–42.
16. Clare Ungerson and Sue Yeandle, eds. *Cash for Care in Developed Welfare States* (Basingstoke: Palgrave Macmillan, 2007).
17. Clare Ungerson, 'Social Politics and the Commodification of Care', *Social Politics* 4, no. 3 (1997): 362–81.
18. Kirstein Rummery, 'Disabled Citizens and Social Exclusion: The Role of Direct Payments', *Policy and Politics* 34, no. 4 (2006): 633–50.
19. Rose Galvin, 'Challenging the Need for Gratitude: Comparisons Between Paid and Unpaid Care for Disabled People', *Journal of Sociology* 40, no. 2 (2004): 137–55.
20. Marja Pijl and Claire Ramakers, 'Contracting One's Family Members: The Dutch Care Allowance', in *Cash for Care in Developed Welfare States*, ed. Clare Ungerson and Sue Yeandle (Basingstoke: Palgrave Macmillan, 2007), 81–103.
21. Sylvia Weekers and Marja Pijl, *Home Care and Care Allowances in the European Union* (Utrecht: NIZW, 1998).
22. Claude Martin and Blanche Le Bihan, 'Cash for Care in the French Welfare State: A Skilful Compromise?' in *Cash for Care in Developed Welfare States*, ed. Clare Ungerson and Sue Yeandle (Basingstoke: Palgrave Macmillan, 2007), 32–59.
23. Claude Martin, 'Atouts et limites de l'expérimentation: l'exemple de la prestation dépendance', *Revue Française des Affaires Sociales* 1, no. 1 (2000): 47–58.
24. Sophie Bresse, 'Le personnel des services d'aide à domicile en 1999', *Études et résultats* 297 (Paris: DREES, 2004).
25. Blanche Le Bihan and Claude Martin, 'A Comparative Case Study of Care Systems for Frail Elderly People: Germany, Spain, France, Italy, United Kingdom and Sweden', *Social Policy & Administration* 40, no. 1 (2006): 26–46.
26. Rummery, 'Disabled Citizens and Social Exclusion'.
27. Kevin J. Mahoney, Kristin Simone and Lori Simon-Rusinowitz, 'Early Lessons for the Cash and Counselling Demonstration and Evaluation', *Generations* 24, no. 3 (2000): 41–6.
28. Sharon Keigher, 'Consumer Direction in an Ownership Society: An Emerging Paradigm for Home and Community Care in the United States', in *Cash for Care in Developed Welfare States*, ed. Clare Ungerson and Sue Yeandle (Basingstoke: Palgrave Macmillan, 2007), 166–87.
29. Cristiano Gori, 'Applicare i Livelli Essenziali nel Sociale', *Prospettive Sociali e Sanitarie* 15, no. 7 (2003): 1–8.

30. Emmanuele Pavolino and Costanzo Ranci, 'New Trends of Elderly Care Policy in Western Europe: Towards a Social Market of Care Services?' (presented at XVI ISA World Congress of Sociology, Durban, 2006).
31. See: Cristiano Gori and Barbara Da Roit, 'The Commodification of Care – The Italian Way', in *Cash for Care in Developed Welfare States*, ed. Clare Ungerson and Sue Yeandle (Basingstoke: Palgrave Macmillan, 2007), 60–80; Costanzo Ranci, 'Crisis and Transformation of the Italian Care Model: Beyond Familism, the Role of the Market and Public Policies' (presented at ESPA-Net Annual Conference, Vienna, 2007).
32. Gori and Da Roit, 'The Commodification of Care – The Italian Way'.
33. Francesca Bettio and Janneke Plantenga, 'Comparing Care Regimes in Europe', *Feminist Economics* 10, no. 1 (2004): 85–113.
34. August Oesterle, *Equity Choices and Long-Term Care Policies in Europe: Allocating Resources and Burdens in Austria, Italy, the Netherlands and the United Kingdom* (Aldershot: Ashgate, 2001).
35. Elisabeth Hammer and August Oesterle, 'Welfare State Policy and Informal Long-Term Care Giving in Austria: Old Gender Divisions and New Stratification Processes Among Women', *Journal of Social Policy* 32, no. 1 (2003): 37–53.
36. See: Margareta Kreimer and Helene Schiffbaenker, 'The Austrian Care Arrangement and the Role of Informal Care for Social Integration', in *Care and Social Integration in European Societies*, ed. Birgit Pfau-Effinger and Birgit Geissler (Bristol: Policy Press, 2005), 173–95; Oesterle, *Equity Choices and Long-Term Care Policies in Europe*.
37. Helen Spandler, 'Friend or Foe? Towards a Critical Assessment of Direct Payments', *Critical Social Policy* 24, no. 2 (2004): 187–209.
38. Perri 6, 'Giving Consumers of British Public Services More Choice: What Can Be Learned from Recent History?', *Journal of Social Policy* 32, no. 2 (2003): 239–70.
39. Carlyn Vogler and Jan Pahl, 'Social and Economic Change and the Organisation of Money Within Marriage', *Work, Employment and Society* 7, no. 1 (1993): 71–95.
40. Clare Ungerson, 'Whose Empowerment and Independence? A Cross-National Perspective on "Cash-for-Care" Schemes', *Ageing & Society* 24, no. 2 (2004): 189–212.
41. For example, see: Caroline Glendinning and Peter A. Kemp, *Cash and Care: Policy Challenges in the Welfare State* (Bristol: Policy Press, 2006); Kirstein Rummery, 'Caring, Citizenship and New Labour: Dilemmas and Contradictions for Disabled and Older Women', in *Women and New Labour: Engendering Politics and Policy?*, ed. Claire Annesley, Francesca Gains and Kirstein Rummery (Bristol: Policy Press, 2007), 175–91; Ungerson and Yeandle, eds, *Cash for Care in Developed Welfare States*.
42. See: Liz Lloyd, 'Caring About Carers – Only Half the Picture?', *Critical Social Policy* 20, no. 1 (2000): 136–50.
43. Rummery, 'Disabled Citizens and Social Exclusion'.
44. Selma Sevenhuijsen, *Citizenship and the Ethics of Care: Feminist Considerations on Justice, Morality, and Politics* (London: Routledge, 1998).

BIBLIOGRAPHY

6, Perri. 'Giving Consumers of British Public Services More Choice: What Can Be Learned from Recent History?' *Journal of Social Policy* 32, no. 2 (2003): 239–70.

Bettio, Francesca, and Janneke Plantenga. 'Comparing Care Regimes in Europe', *Feminist Economics* 10, no. 1 (2004): 85–113.

Bresse, Sophie. 'Le personnel des services d'aide à domicile en 1999', *Études et résultats* 297. Paris: DREES, 2004.

Fraser, Nancy. *Justice Interruptus: Critical Reflections on the Post-Socialist Condition.* New York: Routledge, 1997.

Galvin, Rose. 'Challenging the Need for Gratitude: Comparisons Between Paid and Unpaid Care for Disabled People', *Journal of Sociology* 40, no. 2 (2004): 137–55.

Glendinning, Caroline, and Peter A. Kemp. *Cash and Care: Policy Challenges in the Welfare State.* Bristol: Policy Press, 2006.

Goetschy, Janine. 'The European Employment Strategy: Genesis and Development', *European Journal of Industrial Relations* 5, no. 2 (1999): 117–37.

Gori, Cristiano. 'Applicare i Livelli Essenziali nel Sociale', *Prospettive Sociali e Sanitarie* 15, no. 7 (2003): 1–8.

Gori, Cristiano, and Barbara Da Roit. 'The Commodification of Care – The Italian Way', in *Cash for Care in Developed Welfare States*, edited by Clare Ungerson and Sue Yeandle, 60–80. Basingstoke: Palgrave Macmillan, 2007.

Grootegoed, Ellen, and Diana van Dijk. 'The Return of the Family? Welfare State Retrenchment and Client Autonomy in Long-Term Care', *Journal of Social Policy* 41, no. 4 (2012): 677–94.

Hammer, Elisabeth, and August Oesterle. 'Welfare State Policy and Informal Long-Term Care Giving in Austria: Old Gender Divisions and New Stratification Processes Among Women', *Journal of Social Policy* 32, no. 1 (2003): 37–53.

Hantrais, Linda. *International Comparative Research: Theory, Methods and Practice.* London: Palgrave, 2009.

Hewitt-Taylor, Jaquelina. 'Use of Constant Comparative Analysis in Qualitative Research', *Nursing Standard* 15, no. 42 (2001): 39–42.

Keigher, Sharon. 'Consumer Direction in an Ownership Society: An Emerging Paradigm for Home and Community Care in the United States', in *Cash for Care in Developed Welfare States*, edited by Clare Ungerson and Sue Yeandle, 166–87. Basingstoke: Palgrave Macmillan, 2007.

Kreimer, Margareta, and Helene Schiffbaenker. 'The Austrian Care Arrangement and the Role of Informal Care for Social Integration', in *Care and Social Integration in European Societies*, edited by Birgit Pfau-Effinger and Birgit Geissler, 173–95. Bristol: Policy Press, 2005.

Le Bihan, Blanche, and Claude Martin. 'A Comparative Case Study of Care Systems for Frail Elderly People: Germany, Spain, France, Italy, United Kingdom and Sweden', *Social Policy & Administration* 40, no. 1 (2006): 26–46.

Lloyd, Liz. 'Caring About Carers – Only Half the Picture?', *Critical Social Policy* 20, no. 1 (2000): 136–50.

Mahoney, Kevin J., Kristin Simone and Lori Simon-Rusinowitz. 'Early Lessons for the Cash and Counselling Demonstration and Evaluation', *Generations* 24, no. 3 (2000): 41–6.

Martin, Claude. 'Atouts et Limites de L'experimentation: L'exemple de la Prestation Dépendance', *Revue Française des Affaires Sociales* 1, no. 1 (2000), 47–58.

Martin, Claude, and Blanche Le Bihan. 'Cash for Care in the French Welfare State: A Skilful Compromise?', in *Cash for Care in Developed Welfare States*, edited by Clare Ungerson and Sue Yeandle, 32–59. Basingstoke: Palgrave Macmillan, 2007.

Morris, Jenny. 'Independent Living and Community Care: A Disempowering Framework', *Disability & Society* 19, no. 5 (2004): 427–42.

Newman, Janet. 'Constructing Accountability: Network Governance and Managerial Agency', *Public Policy and Administration* 19, no. 4 (2005): 17–33.

NOSOSCO. *Social Protection in the Nordic Countries 2007–2008: Scope, Expenditure and Financing.* Copenhagen: Nordic Social-Statistical Committee, 2009.

Oesterle, August. *Equity Choices and Long-Term Care Policies in Europe: Allocating Resources and Burdens in Austria, Italy, the Netherlands and the United Kingdom*. Aldershot: Ashgate, 2001.

Pavolino, Emmanuele, and Costanzo Ranci. 'New Trends of Elderly Care Policy in Western Europe: Towards a Social Market of Care Services?', presented at XVI ISA World Congress of Sociology, Durban, 2006.

Pijl, Marja, and Claire Ramakers. 'Contracting One's Family Members: The Dutch Care Allowance', in *Cash for Care in Developed Welfare States*, edited by Clare Ungerson and Sue Yeandle, 81–103. Basingstoke: Palgrave Macmillan, 2007.

Plantenga, Janneke, and Chantal Remery. *Flexible Working Time Arrangements and Gender Equality, European Commission: A Comparative Review of 30 European Countries*. European Commission Directorate-General for Employment, Social Affairs and Equal Opportunities. Luxembourg: Publications Office of the European Union, 2009.

Ranci, Costanzo. 'Crisis and Transformation of the Italian Care Model: Beyond Familism, the Role of the Market and Public Policies', presented at ESPA-Net Annual Conference, Vienna, 2007.

Rummery, Kirstein. 'Disabled Citizens and Social Exclusion: The Role of Direct Payments', *Policy and Politics* 34, no. 4 (2006): 633–50.

Rummery, Kirstein. 'Caring, Citizenship and New Labour: Dilemmas and Contradictions for Disabled and Older Women', in *Women and New Labour: Engendering Politics and Policy?*, edited by Claire Annesley, Francesca Gains and Kirstein Rummery, 175–91. Bristol: Policy Press, 2007.

Sevenhuijsen, Selma. *Citizenship and the Ethics of Care: Feminist Considerations on Justice, Morality, and Politics*. London: Routledge, 1998.

Sigurðardóttir, Sigurveig H., Gerdt Sundström, Bo Malmberg and Marie Ernsth Bravell. 'Needs and Care of Older People Living at Home in Iceland', *Scandinavian Journal of Public Health* 40 (2012): 1–9.

Sigurðardóttir, Sigurveig H., and Ingemar Kåreholt. 'Informal and Formal Care of Older People in Iceland', *Scandinavian Journal of Caring Sciences* 28, no. 4 (2014): 802–11.

Spandler, Helen. 'Friend or Foe? Towards a Critical Assessment of Direct Payments', *Critical Social Policy* 24, no. 2 (2004): 187–209.

Theobald, Hildegard, and Kristine Kern. 'The Introduction of Long-Term Care Policy Schemes: Policy Development, Policy Transfer and Policy Change', *Policy and Politics* 39, no. 3 (2011): 325–42.

Ungerson, Clare. 'Social Politics and the Commodification of Care', *Social Politics* 4, no. 3 (1997): 362–81.

Ungerson, Clare. 'Whose Empowerment and Independence? A Cross-National Perspective on "Cash-for-Care" Schemes', *Ageing & Society* 24, no. 2 (2004): 189–212.

Ungerson, Clare, and Sue Yeandle, eds. *Cash for Care in Developed Welfare States*. Basingstoke: Palgrave Macmillan, 2007.

Vogler, Carlyn, and Jan Pahl. 'Social and Economic Change and the Organisation of Money Within Marriage', *Work, Employment and Society* 7, no. 1 (1993): 71–95.

Walker, Alan, and Ariela Lowenstein. 'European Perspectives on Quality of Life in Old Age', *European Journal of Ageing* 6, no. 2 (2009): 61–6.

Weekers, Sylvia, and Marja Pijl. *Home Care and Care Allowances in the European Union*. Utrecht: NIZW, 1998.

CHAPTER TWENTY-THREE

Cultivating moral epiphanies through care

MAURICE HAMINGTON

INTRODUCTION

Imagine sitting down to enjoy viewing a comedy television programme. You watch it because it is funny, the characters are engaging, and the situations are absurd but relatable. Even though the protagonists are significantly different from you, their humanity contributes to a connection and affinity whereby you want to know how they evolve and root for them. You like them. This description is common for many successful comedies. Absorbing stories can have powerful effects. When taken on a narrative flight, our imagination can allow us to inhabit previously unfamiliar realities and a glimpse into the lives of others. Imaginative connection can be true even in the case of fictional characters.[1] Empathy and understanding can emerge as interest is sparked and maintained. Although we are physically passive as television spectators, our imaginations actively form relationships with the characters. Our involvement with stories has moral implications. As psychiatrist Robert Coles describes, 'all in all, not a bad start for someone trying to find a good way to live this life: a person's moral conduct responding to the moral imagination of writers and the moral imperative of fellow human beings in need'.[2]

Will & Grace was one such absorbing television show. Airing in the United States on the NBC network from 1998 to 2006 (with a revival from 2017 to 2020), the comedy was popular and acclaimed, winning eighteen Emmy Awards. The show follows the lives of two people who share an apartment: Eric McCormack as Will Truman, a corporate lawyer, and Debra Messing as Grace Adler, an interior decorator. It also features Megan Mullally as Karen Walker, who works for Adler, and Sean Hayes as Jack McFarland, Truman's childhood friend. The 'situation' in this situation comedy is that McCormack and McFarland are gay; thus, Adler and McFarland are close friends who live together but are not intimate. All four characters are quirky and played by skilled comic actors, engaging in hilarious hi-jinks every episode. Many outstanding comedy television shows exist; what makes this one unique is its impact on viewers' LGBTQ sensitivities and familiarity. It was the first and most successful prime-time television show in the United States to feature gay men (although Ellen DeGeneres had broken ground for lesbians with *Ellen* a few years earlier).

When *Will & Grace* first aired, only about 30 per cent of Americans supported same-sex marriage, and state bans on same-sex marriage were on the rise. In the 2010s, a massive shift in cultural mores took place. Today, 70 per cent of Americans support same-sex marriage, and since a 2015 Supreme Court ruling, it has been legal in every state. As political scientist Don Haider-Markel states, 'you can't find another issue where attitudes have shifted so rapidly'.[3] Of course, it must be noted that acceptance of same-sex marriage neither entails sexual orientation parity nor does it signal the end of homophobia. Furthermore, for some feminist and gay rights advocates, marriage carries too much heterosexual patriarchal baggage to be a marker of a breakthrough.[4] For them, gay marriage represents a mainstreaming of same-sex relationships that may diminish their socially provocative edge. Conversely, it can be argued that the prevalence of same-sex marriage could alter the norms of traditional heterosexual marriage towards different familial power relations as well as a normalization of sexual diversity that represents inclusive moral progress.[5]

Despite the debates over its merits, the shift in attitudes regarding same-sex marriage can be employed as a crude yet measurable proxy for a moral transformation that was relatively quick and substantial. What did *Will & Grace* have to do with the country's attitude change? The answer is contested. In 2012, then Vice President Joe Biden stated on national television, 'I think "Will & Grace" probably did more to educate the American public than almost anything anybody has ever done so far'[6] and then proceeded to declare his comfort with same-sex marriage before the Obama administration had officially taken that position. Biden's enthusiasm aside, like most social transformations, the causal link between changes in attitudes on same-sex marriage and a commercial television programme is not so straightforward. Although *Will & Grace* may have contributed to the public's familiarity and comfort with gay characters, many factors led to the progress in acceptance.[7]

Furthermore, *Will & Grace* is not without its critics who cite the show's failure to deal with many LGBTQ issues directly and its leveraging of common gay social stereotypes for comic effect.[8] Nevertheless, there is no denying that it was a groundbreaking and widely watched television comedy that significantly altered attitudes about the LGBTQ community. For this chapter, the role of *Will & Grace* in modifying moral views is a catalyst for thinking about morality, moral progress and epiphanies from the perspective of care ethics. Because viewers cared about the characters, Will and Jack, their empathetic imaginations allowed them to begin to think about the morality of same-sex relationships differently.

Care ethics is a relational approach to morality developed through the work of many international feminist scholars as a paradigm shift in thinking about the nature of the ethical. Rather than a system for adjudicating moral dilemmas (i.e. following rules or choosing the most good for the most number of people) or a plan for individual moral development (i.e. virtue ethics), care theory poses a way of being in the world that is responsive to the needs of others and the self that fosters connected growth. In recent years, outstanding new and differently situated voices have enriched the understanding of care theory, making it a highly dynamic and rich field of study.[9] In this chapter, I argue that care is an ethical process that cultivates moral epiphanies – moments of enlightenment and understanding. Ultimately, such moral epiphanies have the capacity to foment change of hearts and minds that can lead to greater appreciation and compassion for others.

Moral epiphanies are vital for ethical growth. They can shake us out of the dogmatic slumber of our ethical habits and traditions to visualize new and different possibilities and recognize alternative standpoints. Moral epiphanies are the stuff of moral progress if they are socially enacted.

This chapter first discusses the nature of moral epiphanies and then the elements of care theory to argue why care is a vital incubator for such epiphanies.

23.1 EPIPHANIES

Epiphanies are the subject of considerable recent studies. The idea is expressed variously as insight, eureka moments, 'a-ha' experiences, revelations, 'eye-openers' and the like. As with most concepts, a critical analysis of epiphanies reveals their complexity. Philosopher Sophie Grace Chappell describes an epiphany as a '(1) overwhelming (2) existentially significant manifestation of (3) value, (4) often sudden and surprising, (5) which feels like it "comes from outside" – it is something given, relative to which I am a passive perceiver – which (6) teaches us something new, which (7) "takes us out of ourselves," and which (8) demands a response'.[10] Chappell's definition connotes a potentially moral element in all epiphanies as the new knowledge is not just an encounter with a surprising fact but rather a transformative experience.

For this project, the focus is explicitly on *moral* epiphanies – ethical insight that challenges our established ethical frameworks or values. Such an experience can cause dissonance – it is not always easy to admit being wrong or misguided about essential ideas. Part of the struggle can be reconciling the new information against biases of confirmation and conformity. Thus, a moral epiphany is a subversion of the accepted ethical structure. Yet, grappling with new ideas can result in growth and development. For example, resistance and denial might occur when one initially discovers the privileges associated with one's identity. Still, as the knowledge becomes actuated and incorporated, the potential for change can result. As a white male, I do not routinely fear my encounters with law enforcement officers. However, if through personal experience, watching the news or through fictional accounts, I learn most Black men in the United States do not share this privilege, my moral understanding is challenged, and I am compelled to determine how this epiphany alters my attitudes and/or actions.

Although the suddenness of epiphanies is experientially correct, their manifestation may be subject to internal and external variables. Internally, a person can fall on a continuum from openness to resistance when encountering new moral insight. An open person might welcome being touched emotionally and cognitively by a new understanding. At the same time, a resistant individual may avoid such knowledge, as described by epistemic ignorance[11] – the study of why we do not know things, including motivations for ignorance. Furthermore, external circumstances can promote or hinder epiphanies. Exposure to new and different ideas creates more opportunities for an a-ha moment. This exposure can take the form of education, novels, plays, poetry, art or even commercial television shows.

Epiphanies have a substantial epistemological character. Epiphanies are discoveries of something unexpected – realizations of significance. They are commonly thought of as sudden illuminations but do not have to be.[12] Epiphanies are experiences that stand out as unique from ordinary knowledge acquisition.

Moral epiphanies stand at the crossroads between individual and collective social progress. It is unlikely that one person's epiphany has never been considered previously by others. Since moral progress is uneven across individuals, one person's realization may be regarded as common knowledge to someone else. As mentioned in the introduction, when *Will & Grace* first aired in 1998, 30 per cent of Americans supported same-sex marriage – meaning over 80 million people in the United States had reached that particular milestone in inclusive moral progress. For those people, the events that catalysed the shift in social thinking to accept gay rights over the next two decades did not constitute an epiphany, or at least not to the same degree as it did for the other 70 per cent of the public. For many, the hours of television watching two likeable gay men may have resulted in a moral epiphany – a realization that the negative stereotypes used to marginalize gay men might be inaccurate.

Many epiphanies occur haphazardly; something along the course of natural experiential events triggers insight. However, epiphanies can also be *cultivated*. I know that I have often said to students that if, during their college careers, they don't come across some challenge to their beliefs, then we are not doing our jobs as teachers. There is nothing nefarious about this expectation. The presentation of information, something universities do a great deal of, can lead to rational and logical conclusions that might prompt an epiphany. However, there can also be an emotional dimension to epiphany beyond a cognitive realization. Specifically, empathy can lead to epiphany. When one feels with someone else, it can spark realizations that challenge one's beliefs. A television comedy like *Will & Grace* is thin on rational arguments or data about queer life. Still, it is an opportunity to make empathetic connections to characters like Will McCormack and Jack McFarland and discover that they and their desires are not so much different than our own. The heart can bring us to an epiphany, perhaps even more so than the mind. Of course, the language I have used here is an unnecessary dualism. The heart and mind work together when we learn and grow.

23.2 THE MORAL GOOD OF EMBODIED CARE

We cannot interrogate the relationship of care to moral epiphanies without addressing the nature of morality. Narratives of moral progress employ spatial and directional metaphors. Accordingly, if morality is to progress, what is it progressing to? What is the state of ethics that would indicate progress has been made? Although the nature of morality is the constant companion of philosophers, there are no settled answers to these questions. From a care perspective, I would argue that accepting others' identities and promoting their relationships, as in same-sex marriage, qualifies as moral progress. However, some would say that *Will & Grace* did not contribute to moral progress because they contend that a world welcoming different forms of gender and sexual expression is not moral. For example, religious dogmatism based on selective readings of biblical passages and natural law arguments often finds diversion from heterosexual gender normativity a violation – a sin. However, the Jewish and Christian sacred texts are complex ancient documents, and drawing interpretations regarding modern concepts such as sexual identity or abortion is fraught with complications.[13] Furthermore, care ethics is anti-dogmatic; it responds to human needs rather than rules or principles. Acceptance from others as one is rather than what traditions indicate one should be is a significant human need.[14]

So why does care theory have a valid and compelling argument for what constitutes morality? To answer this question, I begin by recognizing that all ethical systems are human constructs. Then, I examine the ontological assumptions of care and conclude that care is the central moral good of society.

Feminist theorists have long argued that morality is a social construction of reality. Norms of valuation and conduct are collective decisions. Such norms may appear natural because widely held beliefs are taken for granted and reinforced by conventions in religion, politics, economics, education, etc. Collectively, we have chosen specific rules, consequences and/or virtues as moral ones; therefore, they are not sacred or immutable. Thus, the door is open for other arguments regarding what constitutes morality. If they think about ethics at all (often moral norms are passed on from generation to generation with limited reflection on their efficacy), communities decide that a particular deontological, teleological, or virtue moral system (or some combination) is more persuasive than others in guiding decisions and behaviours. The relational approach that care theory represents is a relatively new and less familiar way of thinking about morality. Rather than considering morality primarily about judgement, as in 'right versus wrong', a more expansive view considers what is good. Each moral system has a theory of the good, which has implications for what is right. Ethical approaches all provide ethical insight, but reducing the totality of morality to any specific set of variables is fraught with reductionist challenges, given the complexity of the human (and non-human) condition. So, for this discussion, moral progress emphasizes the moral good over the right.

Philosopher Charles Larmore describes a moral good as 'worth having or doing and enhances the life of those who possess it'.[15] Larmore's description suggests that the moral good is both an end, 'worth having', and a means, 'worth doing'. This distinction is consistent with care as it is a practice; there are positive implications of the caring activities – for example, the epistemic agency that comes when being listened to – and there are positive results of caring where someone has needs met, such as the physical benefits of being given food or medical attention. In discussing care as a good, care theorist Luigina Mortari favours the idea that care is a core moral good but problematizes the notion of 'good', as it has been sometimes invoked in the Western philosophical tradition. She wishes to avoid any dogmatic understanding of the good and, thus, any universalization or reification.[16] A process approach to care theory avoids ossified accounts of the good.

Caring is essential to humanity and, thus, should be the centrepiece of morality. Without care, humans do not survive. Fairness and justice, classic and significant measures of morality, coexist with care. Concepts like fairness and justice depend on other understandings; their definition is not settled and universally applied. Indeed, care impacts how we come to understand fairness and justice. This complementary view ostensibly opposes the understanding of care and justice as divergent; the latter conception represented in Carol Gilligan's original framing of care theory was in contrast to that of a justice approach as 'different ideologies'.[17] However, Gilligan was naming the previously unnamed, so the distinction helped articulate the new ground that care thinking was occupying. Even in laying out this bifurcated territory in 1982, Gilligan wrote that as people mature, they find a convergence between the two in judgement.[18] Similarly, Nel Noddings recognized that pitting justice against care is a false dichotomy: 'care theorists usually seek ends compatible with justice, but we try to achieve them by establishing conditions in which caring itself can flourish'.[19] Rules and rights are essential moral considerations. Still, they are not substitutes for the hard work of parsing out the particulars of a situation, including the web of relationships of the humans involved. Justice may be a moral good, but as Virginia Held argues, 'there can be care without justice ... There can be no justice without care.'[20] For Held and others, the problem with maintaining historical justice approaches is that they fail to answer today's questions by ignoring the fundamental role of relationships. She suggests that care ethics should be the overarching moral approach while retaining traditional justice thinking in particular social domains: 'I have come to think that the ethics of care is potentially a comprehensive moral theory constructed from an understanding of care *and* the justice already so theorized and thought about for centuries.'[21] The justice and care relationship has different formulations, but the trajectory is one of decreasing separation.

One persuasive advantage that care theorists have regarding care as central to ethics is their recognition that humans are fundamentally embodied and relational beings. Therefore, the ontological assumptions make care the starting point for understanding the nature of morality. Our bodies all need care. As much as we value independence, humans are interdependent at their core. We are born vulnerable and face vulnerability throughout our lives despite the illusions of sovereignty that affluence and social privilege can bring us. Furthermore, many uncaring social, political and economic forces foist additional precarity on people.[22] Humans need one another, and there is no avoiding this condition. Furthermore, we are embodied beings, and those bodies are the starting point for need. Our primary and richest experiences of care come through the body and are delivered through the body.[23]

23.3 CARE AS A PROCESS MORALITY

Caring is a process. A process approach to care theory assists in understanding morality as more than a decision science. Making difficult decisions is indeed an essential part of ethics; it is not the only part. Moral decision making can sometimes reduce morality to a snapshot of deciding the 'right' course of action. However, morality also deals with the nature of the good and how to promote that good. In this case, that good is care. Developing the skills of care at the personal level or the ethos of care at the community level is a process. To interrogate care as a process, I examine what Alfred North Whitehead and those he influenced had to say about process philosophy.

Whitehead lived from 1861 to 1947 in the United Kingdom and the United States. A polymath, he made scholarly contributions to mathematics, logic, physics and philosophy. He came to philosophy late in his career and focused primarily on metaphysics.[24] Whitehead argued that reality consists of processes rather than material objects and that these processes were all in dynamic relationships with one another. His philosophy became known as process philosophy and would be applied to many humanities and social sciences fields, notably theology. Theologian, environmentalist and philosopher John B. Cobb is the most prominent contemporary process theorist. Cobb created the think tank Center for Process Studies at the Claremont School of Theology, which spawned twenty-three such process-oriented academic centres worldwide. Process philosophy represents a niche field within philosophy, yet it remains the source of study.

Whitehead was a prolific writer who is eminently quotable.[25] He famously stated, 'the safest general characterization of the European philosophical tradition is that it consists of a series of footnotes to Plato'.[26] Nevertheless, his philosophical writings are quite dense and demanding. Whitehead's commentators admit this challenge and have offered numerous books and webpages explaining Whiteheadean terminology and offering summary elucidations.

Drawing from these commentaries, in perhaps too reductionist a fashion, one can say that Whitehead's process philosophy describes the universe as in continual process with those processes being relationally engaged with one another. Philosopher and theologian C. Robert Mesle claims, 'process thinkers insist that our failure to recognize that reality is a relational process is a source of great harm'.[27] Furthermore, emphasis is placed on particularity and experience over abstraction. Given its relational metaphysics, process ethics values harmonious living between humans, non-humans and the earth. Philosopher and theologian Jay McDaniel characterizes process thinking as a worldview:

> Process thinking is an attitude toward life emphasizing respect and care for the community of life. It is concerned with the well-being of individuals and also with the common good of the world, understood as a community of communities of communities. It sees the world as a process of becoming and the universe as a vast network of inter-becomings. It sees each living being on our planet as worthy of respect and care.[28]

Note the phrase 'respect and care' appears twice in the quotation. There are apparent resonances between care theory and process philosophy.

Despite the similarities in approach, most contemporary feminist engagement with process thinking has come through feminist theologians. These scholars are attracted to the dynamic sense of being, including a process understanding of God that challenges fixed masculine theological approaches.[29] However, the emphasis on theology in Whitehead, Cobb and other process thinkers' writing may be why so few feminist philosophers or care theorists have engaged in it. Care theory is not antithetical to religious belief; however, it foregrounds an experiential and relational approach that is agnostic regarding the existence of a deity or one's religious spirituality.

Framing care theory as a process morality has advantages. In particular, process thinking supports the idea of care ethics as a non-ideal theory capable of negotiating an intersectional existence. A process approach also 'thickens' the temporal dimension of care as contrasted with an adjudicative method of moral assessment. Rich relational care – good care – takes time because it is a process. Accordingly, Tronto claims, 'among the most important considerations in rethinking society from a caring perspective, then, is creating time and space for care'.[30] Feminist philosophers have often described care as a practice. Care is commonly thought of as a disposition, which it can be. Still, as Tronto contends, 'unless we also understand care in its richer sense of a practice, we run the risk of sentimentalizing and in other ways containing the scope of care in our thinking'.[31] This quote comes from Tronto's groundbreaking book, *Moral Boundaries,* and expresses her concern for how care has been marginalized and how to bring it to the centre. A practice is a process that can be combined with other practices to form more extensive caring processes. For example, active listening is a set of learned skills – paying attention, signalling focus on the one speaking, deferring judgement, asking questions for clarification, etc. Listening can be a significant practice of caring. When combined with empathetic imagination and the practice of taking responsive action, a rich moral process of good care can be achieved.

If care is a practice, then by implication, one can improve upon it. We improve at many processes by attending to them with greater reflection and through mindful practice. If we want to deliver better speeches, we might practise, ask for feedback on our speeches, study great speakers or read about the elements of good speaking. However, we do not commonly think about morality or caring that way. If good care is marked by humble inquiry, inclusive connection and responsive action, we want to engage in activities that assist in being better inquirers, open to greater inclusivity, and more responsive in our actions. In other words, better carers.

Allowing ourselves to discover and understand the plights of others is perhaps one of those activities.

23.4 CARING AS GENERATIVE OF MORAL EPIPHANIES

Caring can incubate moral epiphanies through at least three processual characteristics: *time and space*, *imagination* and *security*.

Because we are embodied beings, care has a significant temporal and spatial dimension, particularly as we consider deep, relational care. Indeed, there can be moments of care between strangers – picking up a dropped wallet, a welcoming smile, the fast action of a capable healthcare provider in a crisis. However, serious or profound care comes through a proximal relationship over time. Familiarity breeds understanding that increases the opportunity for connection. There is a common sense understanding of such bonds as it is generally assumed that one cares for the friends and family members that one spends time with. Students and teachers who experience a term together can better understand one another and build connections. Time and spatial closeness build familiarity. The person with whom I spend time becomes less of a mystery. No one completely knows someone else, even when they have lived with them for half a century. However, time together fosters trust and a sense of commonality despite differences in culture, religion or political stances. In getting to know someone else, I discover aspects of myself. Epiphanies, large and small, are possible, such as I can enjoy the company of someone different than myself. This person values something so strongly, perhaps veganism; I wonder why they feel that way. We can still care for someone at great distances, but it has its foundational reality in our iterative embodied interactions.[32] The realizations we can have through close encounters have the potential to engender moral epiphanies.

A second relatively unheralded aspect of care that can foment moral epiphanies is the imagination. Good care engages imaginative explorations. The humble inquiry that can spark care provides our minds with information that allows us to imagine the other's experience, feelings and needs – empathy. Although empathy can be characterized as an intellectual or an emotional understanding, in either case, one takes the empirical evidence presented and extends it beyond the caregiver's immediate experience. If someone tells me of being imprisoned and deprived of contact and food for an extended time, I could never say that I fully 'know' what that experience is like. Still, I can use my imagination in combination with their description and my own limited experiences to have an intellectual and visceral inkling or glimpse of what that might be like. The imagination can be initiated through direct experience as well as through the arts.[33] These imaginative connections can catalyse moral epiphanies: taking someone else's plight seriously. Stepping into someone else's shoes can spark a previously absent idea into reality that challenges our ethical presuppositions.

The care relationship's temporal, spatial and imaginative aspects emphasize fostering moral epiphanies in the one providing care. However, those who receive good care may also be afforded opportunities for moral epiphanies. The realization that comes with an epiphany assumes some opportunity for reflection. One could watch *Will & Grace* and only laugh at the comedy and never take a moment to pause and realize that the gay characters desire lives of fulfilment and joy like I, a viewer, do. It is challenging (although not impossible) to have the opportunity for epiphanies if one lives an insecure existence, whether food, housing or physical insecurity. When one is cared for, the mind is freer to make the appropriate epiphanic connections. As care political theorist Fiona Robinson describes, 'The word "security" is derived from the Latin root *secures*, which means "without care." Care in this sense refers to concern, worry, fear, or anxiety: thus, to be secure is to be "carefree," or without anxiety.'[34] This relationship of care to security is analogous to understanding what is necessary to seek higher-order needs according to Abraham Maslow's hierarchy of needs. Accordingly, one is motivated to seek higher-order needs such as relational, esteem and self-actualization only once basic safety and physiological needs are met. The latter becomes all-consuming when present.[35] Thus, care can be a crucible for greater opportunities for moral epiphany.

Most systems of ethics are focused on determining right action. Care theory is a broader understanding of morality that includes a way of being in the world with generative opportunities for moral discovery.

CONCLUSION: CULTIVATING MORAL EPIPHANIES THROUGH A CARE ETHOS

This chapter argues that care can be a resource for moral epiphanies. It began with an imperfect example of moral progress regarding evolving dispositions towards same-sex marriage in the United States. It foreshadowed cultivating epiphanies by describing the tenuous relationship between the television show *Will & Grace* and that transformation. The chapter argued that care is a worthy centrepiece of moral progress, given that it is necessary for human sustainability and flourishing. An essential clarification is offered with the claim that not any form of care will do for moral improvement but that care needs to be good or effective, given that it has historically been invoked in numerous distinctly non-caring ways. The nature of moral progress was discussed with an emphasis on inclusive and egalitarian forms. Then, it was argued that care is a process morality and, as such, lends itself well to the process of progress. Such progress includes moral epiphanies that reveal our connection to others.

In conclusion, I address a care ethos as a method for cultivating caring moral progress. Laws, principles and practices that underwrite greater inclusive moral progress through care, such as supporting social infrastructure, the rights of marginalized people, and better economic assistance for those in need, are vital steps towards a more caring society. Moreover, such progress is bolstered and reified through a widespread spirit or ethos of care. Thus, state-sponsored structures need the presence of community members to enact their purpose of achieving social changes in moral norms. For example, if trans rights were suddenly enshrined in law, that does not mean that social oppression would disappear. Similarly, suppose the federal government initiated programmes to move more people out of poverty. The result would not be that individuals and communities no longer have to engage in mutual aid to help those in need. Furthermore, without an expanded care ethos, any legal or programmatic victories are vulnerable to dismantling if the people's will does not support them, as witnessed with civil rights and abortion rights in the United States.

What do I mean by a care ethos? Although care is a practice – the enactment of healing and meeting needs – it can originate in a disposition. The definition of reasonable care offered above includes humble inquiry, inclusive connection and responsive action. Note that humble inquiry has a bit of an oxymoronic character to it. 'Humility' generally connotes modesty and a diminishment of ego in exchanges with others. However, 'inquiry' signals an assertive approach to knowledge production: seeking answers. 'Humble inquiry' suggests an active openness to others and their plights, the readiness of someone to listen and ask questions without pretence other than they want to help. Mesle describes Whitehead's process philosophy as exhibiting a 'bold humility' whereby, according to Whitehead, 'speculative boldness must be balanced by complete humility before logic and fact'.[36] Neither Whitehead nor Mesle addresses care ethics, yet we can see that the contrasting elements can be applied to a care ethos: one can actively seek information from others to be cared for while remaining humble before their needs and concerns.

Such a care ethos can be framed as looking for epiphanies. If we are humble and open to the plight of others, their stories may change us. I might have a preconceived notion about someone wearing the trappings of a political ideology I abhor. Still, given the opportunity to listen and spend time with them, I might better understand their motivations and experiences. I might have a moral epiphany regarding an unfamiliar other. This claim is not to suggest that someone with a care ethos is a moral reed blowing in the wind, that someone will change their ethical convictions because they are sympathetic to someone's backstory. However, better knowledge of others and their needs and fears is a significant hope for the future of making common cause in the world. The point is that a care ethos can increase the opportunities for moral epiphanies.

We care through our bodies and minds; like other practices, caring involves skills that can be exercised and improved through progress. Care theory is a non-ideal theory of improvement rather than moral perfection. Humble inquiry, inclusive connection and responsive action are skills that can develop with practice or, conversely, atrophy through disuse. However, we can cultivate our caring skills to serve an ethos of good care. Exposure to art and literature, social exchanges and even talking to strangers are opportunities to enhance care skills. By extension, these experiences make moral epiphanies possible. Education theorist Kevin Gary argues that moral epiphanies can be cultivated in school settings: 'given that egotism is often our natural default setting, we are in need of constant epiphanic awakening to rouse us from our moral apathy and slumber. We need to be on the lookout for moral epiphanies, not from on high, but in the daily run of things.'[37]

Teachers can cultivate epiphanies in schools, but people can as well. We can cultivate our epiphanies through quality experiences of broad exposure to others different from ourselves, whether in person or through the arts. Any exchange with someone else is an opportunity for a moral epiphany if we are open to it.

One final note: *Will & Grace* also had the advantage of being a comedy. The misdirection of humour can often allow provocations and social commentary to be heard when serious narratives might not have been listened to. There can sometimes be a message behind the absurd. Here is a snippet of dialogue from the second season of *Will & Grace*:

> Jack: Heterosexual marriage is just wrong! If God had intended a man and a woman to be together, he would have given them both penises!
> Will: I believe I heard Pope RuPaul II say that.[38]

NOTES

1. Howard Sklar, *Art of Sympathy in Fiction: Forms of Ethical and Emotional Persuasion* (Amsterdam: John Benjamins Publishing Company, 2013).
2. Robert Coles, *The Call of Stories: Teaching and the Moral Imagination* (Boston, MA: Houghton Mifflin Company, 1989), 205.
3. Don Haider-Markel quoted in Samantha Schmidt, 'Americans' Views Flipped on Gay Rights. How Did Minds Change So Quickly?' *The Washington Post*, 7 June 2019.

4. Claudia Card, 'Against Marriage and Motherhood', *Hypatia* 11, no. 3 (1996): 1–23.
5. Dorothy C. Miller, 'The Potential of Same-Sex Marriage for Restructuring Care and Citizenship', in *Socializing Care: Feminist Ethics and Public Issues*, ed. Maurice Hamington and Dorothy C. Miller (Lanham, MD: Rowan & Littlefield, 2006), 89–103.
6. David Eldridge, 'Biden "Comfortable" with Gay Marriage, Cites "Will & Grace"', *The Washington Times*, 6 May 2012, https://www.washingtontimes.com/news/2012/may/6/biden-will-grace-educated-public-about-gays/.
7. Stacey L. Sobel, 'Culture Shifting At Warp Speed: How the Law, Public Engagement, and *Will & Grace* Led to Social Change for LGBT People', *St John's Law Review* 89 (2015): 143–94.
8. Jack Myers, '"Will & Grace" – The TV Series that Changed Gay Rights in America', *mediavillage.org*, 28 September 2017, https://www.mediavillage.com/article/will-grace-the-tv-series-that-changed-gay-rights-in-america/print/.
9. For example, a special issue of *Essays in Philosophy* 24, no. 1–2 (2023), titled 'Care Ethics Otherwise', edited by Hil Malatino, Amy McKiernan and Sarah Clark Miller, sought to 'push the boundaries of contemporary care ethics in subversive and inclusive new directions including essays engaging with critical race theory, queer theory, disability justice, environmental ethics, and animal ethics', 1.
10. Sophie Grace Chappell, 'Introducing Epiphanies', *Zemo* 2 (2019): 95.
11. Gaile Pohlhaus, 'Epistemic Oppression, Ignorance, and Resistance', in *The Oxford Handbook of Feminist Philosophy*, ed. Kim Q. Hall and Ásta (Oxford: Oxford University Press, 2021), 418–28.
12. Chappell, 'Introducing Epiphanies', 101.
13. Ken Stone, 'Homosexuality and the Bible or Queer Reading? A Response to Martti Nissinen', *Theology and Sexuality* 14 (2001): 107–18.
14. Ra Keum Huh, 'Revisiting Feminist Care Ethics for the Age of the "Pluralistic Family"', *Asian Journal of Women's Studies* 26 (2020): 22–35.
15. Charles Larmore, 'Right and Good', *Routledge Encyclopedia of Philosophy* (London: Taylor and Francis, 1998), https://www.rep.routledge.com/articles/thematic/right-and-good/v-1.
16. Luigina Mortari, *The Philosophy of Care* (Wiesbaden: Springer VS, 2022).
17. Carol Gilligan, *In a Different Voice: Psychological Theory and Women's Development* (Cambridge, MA: Harvard University Press, 1982), 167.
18. Ibid., 174.
19. Nel Noddings, 'Care, Justice, and Equity', in *Justice and Caring: The Search for Common Ground in Education*, ed. Michael S. Katz, Nel Noddings and Kenneth A. Strike (New York: Teachers College Press, 1999), 19.
20. Virginia Held, *The Ethics of Care: Personal, Political, and Global* (New York: Oxford, 2006), 17.
21. Virginia Held, 'Care and Justice, Still', in *Care Ethics and Political Theory*, ed. Daniel Engster and Maurice Hamington (New York: Oxford, 2015), 34.
22. Maurice Hamington and Michael Flower, eds, *Care Ethics in the Age of Precarity* (Minneapolis: University of Minnesota Press), 2021.
23. Maurice Hamington, *Embodied Care: Jane Addams, Maurice Merleau-Ponty, and Feminist Ethics* (Urbana-Champaign: University of Illinois Press, 2004).
24. C. Robert Mesle, *Process-Relational Philosophy: An Introduction to Alfred North Whitehead* (West Conshohocken, PA: Templeton Press, 2008), 8.

25. A. H. Johnson, 'The Wit and Wisdom of Whitehead', *Philosophy of Science* 13, no. 3 (1946): 223–51.
26. Alfred North Whitehead, *Process and Reality*, corrected edition, ed. David Ray Griffin and Donald W. Sherburne (New York: Free Press, 1978), 39.
27. Mesle, *Process-Relational Philosophy*, 8.
28. Jay McDaniel, 'Twenty Key Ideas', *Open Horizons*, https://www.openhorizons.org/process-worldview.html.
29. Monica Coleman, *Making a Way Out of No Way: A Womanist Theology* (New York: Fortress Press, 2008); Marjorie Hewitt Suchocki, *God Christ Church: A Practical Guide to Process Theology* (New York: Crossroad, 1989); Monica A. Coleman, Nancy R. Howell and Helene Tallon Russell, *Creating Women's Theology: A Movement Engaging Process Thought* (Eugene, OR: Wipf and Stock, Pickwick Publications, 2011); Marilyn Thie, 'Feminist Concerns and Whitehead's Theory of Perception' *Process Studies* 8, no. 3 (Fall, 1978): 186–91.
30. Joan C. Tronto, *Caring Democracy: Markets, Equality, and Justice* (New York: New York University Press, 2013), 167.
31. Joan C. Tronto, *Moral Boundaries: A Political Argument for an Ethic of* Care (New York: Routledge, 1993), 119.
32. Maurice Hamington, *Embodied Care.*
33. Ce Rosenow and Maurice Hamington, 'A Careful Poetics: Caring Imagination, Caring Habits, and Haiku', *Juxta* 3 no. 1 (2017), https://thehaikufoundation.org/juxta/juxta-3-1/a-careful-poetics-caring-imagination-caring-habits-and-haiku/.
34. Fiona Robinson, *The Ethics of Care: A Feminist Approach to Human Security* (Philadelphia, PA: Temple University Press, 2011), 7.
35. Abraham H. Maslow. 'A Theory of Human Motivation', *Psychological Review* 50, no. 4 (1943): 370–96.
36. Whitehead, *Process and Reality*, 17.
37. Kevin Gary, 'Cultivating Moral Epiphanies', *Educational Theory* 71, no. 3 (2021): 387.
38. James Burrows, director, 'An Affair to Forget', *Will & Grace*, season 2, episode 19, aired 18 April 2000.

BIBLIOGRAPHY

Card, Claudia. 'Against Marriage and Motherhood', *Hypatia* 11, no. 3 (1996): 1–23.

Chappell, Sophie Grace. 'Introducing Epiphanies', *Zemo* 2 (2019): 95–121.

Coleman, Monica. *Making A Way Out of No Way: A Womanist Theology*. New York: Fortress Press, 2008.

Coleman, Monica A., Nancy R. Howell and Helene Tallon Russell. *Creating Women's Theology: A Movement Engaging Process Thought*. Wipf and Stock: Pickwick Publications, 2011.

Coles, Robert. *The Call of Stories: Teaching and the Moral Imagination*. Boston, MA: Houghton Mifflin Company, 1989.

Eldridge, David. 'Biden "Comfortable" with Gay Marriage, Cites "Will & Grace"', *The Washington Times*, 6 May 2012. https://www.washingtontimes.com/news/2012/may/6/biden-will-grace-educated-public-about-gays/.

Gary, Kevin. 'Cultivating Moral Epiphanies', *Educational Theory* 71, no. 3 (2021): 371–88.

Gilligan, Carol. *In A Different Voice: Psychological Theory and Women's Development*. Cambridge, MA: Harvard University Press, 1982.
Hamington, Maurice. *Embodied Care: Jane Addams, Maurice Merleau-Ponty, and Feminist Ethics*. Urbana-Champaign: University of Illinois Press, 2004.
Hamington, Maurice, and Michael Flower, eds. *Care Ethics in the Age of Precarity*. Minneapolis: University of Minnesota Press, 2021.
Held, Virginia. *The Ethics of Care: Personal, Political, and Global*. New York: Oxford University Press, 2006.
Held, Virginia. 'Care and Justice, Still', in *Care Ethics and Political Theory*, edited by Daniel Engster and Maurice Hamington, 18–36. New York: Oxford University Press, 2015.
Huh, Ra Keum. 'Revisiting Feminist Care Ethics for the Age of the "Pluralistic Family"', *Asian Journal of Women's Studies* 26 (2020): 22–35.
Johnson, A. H. 'The Wit and Wisdom of Whitehead', *Philosophy of Science* 13, no. 3 (1946): 223–51.
Larmore, Charles. 'Right and Good', in *Routledge Encyclopedia of Philosophy*. London: Taylor and Francis, 1998. https://www.rep.routledge.com/articles/thematic/right-and-good/v-1.
McDaniel, Jay. 'Twenty Key Ideas', *Open Horizons*. https://www.openhorizons.org/process-worldview.html.
Miller, Dorothy C. 'The Potential of Same-Sex Marriage for Restructuring Care and Citizenship', in *Socializing Care: Feminist Ethics and Public Issues*, edited by Maurice Hamington and Dorothy C. Miller, 89–103. Lanham, MD: Rowan & Littlefield, 2006.
Mortari, Luigina. *The Philosophy of Care*. Wiesbaden: Springer VS, 2022.
Myers, Jack. '"Will & Grace" – The TV Series that Changed Gay Rights in America', *mediavillage.org*, 28 September 2017. https://mediavillage.com/article/will-grace-the-tv-series-that-changed-gay-rights-in-america/print/.
Noddings, Nel. 'Care, Justice, and Equity', in *Justice and Caring: The Search for Common Ground in Education*, edited by Michael S. Katz, Nel Noddings and Kenneth A. Strike, 7–20. New York: Teachers College Press, 1999.
Pohlhaus, Gaile. 'Epistemic Oppression, Ignorance, and Resistance', in *The Oxford Handbook of Feminist Philosophy*, edited by Kim Q. Hall and Ásta, 418–28. Oxford: Oxford University Press, 2021.
Robinson, Fiona. *The Ethics of Care: A Feminist Approach to Human Security*. Philadelphia, PA: Temple University Press, 2011.
Rosenow, Ce, and Maurice Hamington. 'A Careful Poetics: Caring Imagination, Caring Habits, and Haiku', *Juxta* 3, no. 1 (2017). https://thehaikufoundation.org/juxta/juxta-3-1/a-careful-poetics-caring-imagination-caring-habits-and-haiku/ (accessed 31 January 2024).
Schmidt, Samantha. 'Americans' Views Flipped on Gay Rights. How Did Minds Change So Quickly?', *The Washington Post*, 7 June 2019.
Sklar, Howard. *Art of Sympathy in Fiction: Forms of Ethical and Emotional Persuasion*. Amsterdam: John Benjamins Publishing Company, 2013.
Sobel, Stacey L. 'Culture Shifting at Warp Speed: How the Law, Public Engagement, and Will & Grace Led to Social Change for LGBT People', *St John's Law Review* 89 (2015): 143–94.
Stone, Ken. 'Homosexuality and the Bible or Queer Reading? A Response to Martti Nissinen', *Theology and Sexuality* 14 (2001): 107–18.
Thie, Marilyn. 'Feminist Concerns and Whitehead's Theory of Perception', *Process Studies* 8, no. 3 (1978): 186–91.

Tronto, Joan C. *Moral Boundaries: A Political Argument for an Ethic of Care*. New York: Routledge, 1993.

Tronto, Joan C. *Caring Democracy: Markets, Equality, and Justice*. New York: New York University Press, 2013.

Whitehead, Alfred North. *Process and Reality*. Corrected edition, edited by David Ray Griffin and Donald W. Sherburne. New York: Free Press, 1978.

CHAPTER TWENTY-FOUR

Feminist care ethics and temporality

SOPHIE BOURGAULT

INTRODUCTION

Across the world, women are more often time poor than men. Indeed, in every single country on earth, women are more likely than men to have insufficient discretionary time (i.e. time for rest and leisure) and more likely to experience time pressures and health problems due to an unequal distribution of unpaid care work. According to recent surveys, when unpaid and paid labour are combined, women across the globe work, on average, one hour more than men each day.[1] This is, no doubt, old news. Scholars have known for a long time now that, within heterosexual couples, women tend to do the bulk of household care work[2] – work that is unremunerated, undervalued, invisibilized. While the gender gap in unpaid care work has decreased over the years in many places, researchers estimate that the pace of change is so slow that it might take another 210 years to close it.[3] And this 'optimistic' temporal estimate might even be thrown off completely by climate change, which complicates access to water and is thus likely to increase women's time poverty in the Global South.[4]

Now, if some scholars are slightly hopeful for women in the Global North,[5] other researchers have argued that feminist advances in 'temporal justice'[6] made since the 1990s have been compromised by the legacies of neoliberal policies and by social acceleration – a structural and cultural phenomenon that exacerbates time pressures and mental distress in workers.[7] Sociologist Hartmut Rosa is one of many who argues that the acceleration of technological and social change, mixed with the acceleration of life's daily rhythm, is responsible for high rates of burnout and a growing inability to enter into meaningful (or, to use his term, '*resonant*') relationships.[8] If Rosa himself was quite silent on the gendered dimensions of social acceleration and of time poverty, some feminist scholars have shown how gender (as well as race and class) deeply affects the character of our experience of time: for instance, women are less likely to have access to unfragmented leisure time. If access to sufficient and uninterrupted free time is an important component of gender equality and wellbeing, as some have argued,[9] it is evident that this issue still needs scholarly attention – something that Covid-19 pandemic lockdowns (periods in which women took on increased unpaid labour and whose career progression and health suffered) made painfully clear.[10]

This chapter discusses how feminist care ethics has contributed to this research on time, care work and gender; it also makes an argument for care ethics' *critical* potential and considers a series of remedies for creating a more *caring temporality*. While few readers might intuitively associate care ethics with a very deep concern for temporality, I want to argue that time is, on the contrary, absolutely central for care ethics' normative and political aims. Indeed, the crafting of more decent ethico-political and work lives calls for significant change in both our *distribution* of free time and in our dominant *perspective on* time. The goals of this chapter are thus twofold: first, I provide readers with an overview of what care scholarship has said about time and care, focusing on some specific places and occupations where gender inequities have been considered. My second objective is to indicate what care ethics, as a distinct analytical lens, adds to the existing research. What I propose is that feminist care ethics offers critical insights about the importance of analysing the *temporality* of care work. One of such insights is that time must always be analysed relationally, and with an eye to context and to particularity. Care ethics also places great emphasis on the ethico-political significance of maintenance and repair – a view that offers, as I argue below, an interesting avenue for theorizing a feminist caring chronopolitics.

The chapter will proceed as follows. Section 24.1 will examine various time pathologies tied to the care work that takes place in the private sphere, and then Section 24.2 will turn to the gendered temporalities found in institutional settings – with a particular focus placed here on the labour that takes place in healthcare and university settings. Finally, in my third and last section, I draw the contours of a feminist caring temporality, offering readers a brief overview of a few measures to be considered in our efforts to increase temporal justice.

24.1 TIME AND CARE IN INTIMATE SETTINGS

While there have been numerous accounts of care ethics proposed since the 1980s (grounded in diverse methodological, disciplinary and political sensibilities), one can suggest that the bulk of them understand care as referring at once to ethical/moral dispositions and to practices/work. Most care ethicists are also fairly comfortable with Joan Tronto and Berenice Fischer's widely cited definition of care as 'a species activity that includes *everything that we do to maintain, continue and repair our "world"* so that we can live in it as well as possible. That world includes our bodies, our selves, and our environment' (emphasis added).[11] As underscored here, care is thus understood as a kind of repair and daily *maintenance* labour – one that is geared towards enabling the mere perpetuation of human existence, its basic functioning.

24.1.1 Caring for needy bodies and dirty floors

Certainly the caring for 'mere life', for the survival of human bodies by feeding, washing them and attending to various other needs, is one of the most studied areas of gender temporal inequalities. Indeed, since the 1970s (hence, before care ethics), numerous social scientists and governments have conducted time-use studies that track – to varying degrees of sophistication – gendered inequalities in unpaid work. Many of these studies show that in heterosexual[12] couples, women (including those who work full-time) tend to perform a disproportionate amount of household work (e.g. care for children, elderly relatives, cooking). Again, while some of this disproportion has diminished in many industrialized countries since the 1990s, it has not disappeared yet and is particularly striking among women in the 30–44 age group who have children.[13] In their large scale cross-national survey of people's discretionary time, Robert Goodin and colleagues[14] have shown that women in all countries studied enjoy less discretionary time than men, and have half-jokingly concluded that women interested in having more quality free time would do best to move to Sweden and to avoid having children (and, if they do, to never get a divorce). But let us note here that even in Sweden – a beacon of gender equality for many – women still do 50 minutes more of unpaid care work than men each day.[15]

Researchers have also devoted considerable effort to showing the *effects* of these inequities in unpaid care work and discretionary time: for instance, diminished physiological wellbeing, consequences for career progression, financial security/pensions.[16] Nedelsky and Malleson have also recently noted that time poverty fuels a widespread and undesirable resentment in us all against care activities, and compromises the degree to which we are capable of truly paying attention to others.[17] Other consequences flowing from excessive unpaid labour are those tied to mental health – to the impact of what has been labelled the 'mental charge' (or mental load). A recent systematic review of research published in *The Lancet*[18] indicates that the *doing itself* of unpaid labour tends to have adverse effects on women's mental health, whereas this is not the case for men. The author of the survey suggests that the added health strain on women might partially be the result of the *particular type* of household tasks done by men, which tend, on average, to be less time-sensitive, more likely to be done outside (which can boost mental health), and less likely to be interrupted or done while multitasking.[19]

24.1.2 Care ethics' insights

Several care ethics scholars have built on this research, but they have also contributed to it in a distinctive manner. The first thing that feminist care ethics has added, as an analytical lens, is a heightened focus on particularities and contextual considerations when analysing ethical dilemmas or social policies. 'An ethic of care eschews universalizable moral principles that can be applied across time and space', correctly notes Fiona Robinson. '[It] demands attention to context – to the particularities of social location, historical background, structural conditions and relationships between relevant moral actors.'[20] Readers may recall that Gilligan's *In a Different Voice* clearly sought to rehabilitate the nuanced perspective of Amy – one of the girls she interviewed for her study. For Gilligan, Amy's discomfort with universal, impartial rules and her cautious answer to the question 'how should one choose when faced with conflicting ethical responsibilities?' (her reply was 'well, it really *depends on the situation*' (emphasis added)[21]) was not a sign of moral immaturity or weakness, but of maturity.

Ever since Gilligan, this focus on particulars has been crucial for care scholarship, and I argue that this serves as a healthy corrective to the dominant narratives about acceleration proposed in social science and philosophy,[22] which have neglected gender. As care ethicists Tronto[23] and Julie White have rightly emphasized in their work, not all individuals are equally 'time poor'; some people have *too much* time and suffer from this excess (e.g. the forcibly unemployed or isolated elderly).[24] As Tronto also correctly observes, not everyone has the same resources to deal or cope with time poverty: 'as time and money become more unequal, care resources and care itself become more and more unequal, too'.[25] Indeed, societal groups experience temporalities in different manners, and these experiences vary greatly depending on the level of infrastructural and relational support individuals have access to.[26] It is also crucial, from a care ethics perspective, to acknowledge that some groups are not subject to the effects of a generalized 'speeding up' but, rather, that they are subjected to the *slow-paced* and unspectacular unfolding of a discreet kind of structural violence and economic marginalization (a type of violence described by Lauren Berlant under the label 'slow death'. In her well-known piece on the subject, Berlant describes 'slow death' as a gradual and 'ordinary' wearing down of the bodies (and minds) of marginalized populations, who tend to be more hardly impacted by late capitalism's failures.)[27] For these individuals, the fast-paced work, technological and living conditions decried by more privileged labourers take on quite a different meaning.

Care ethics' attunement to particulars and context is also helpful for underscoring the limitations of time-use studies – several of which have not sufficiently considered the *qualitative* dimensions of time use and temporalities' intricate connections to class, gender and race. From a care ethics perspective, simply looking at an aggregate number of minutes of time spent on unpaid care or at minutes available per day for a particular task, or merely adding minutes of 'discretionary time' possessed by individuals, is inadequate. A care ethics perspective compels researchers to attend to the qualitative dimensions of discretionary time – to consider, for instance, whether the forty-six total daily minutes of leisure time is fragmented in small chunks of ten minutes or enjoyed in one block, or whether it is spent in the company of young children (are there, indeed, opportunities for leisure in solitude?). Mattingly and Blanchi's work speaks to this – having shown the varying *quality* of free time experienced by distinctive groups (with employed women's free time more frequently broken up by children's needs and non-leisure tasks).[28] In France, Bessin and Gaudart[29] and Damamme and Paperman[30] have also made a case for care ethics' ability to foreground that our relationship to time is definitely not gender neutral.

In a recent piece on time use and unpaid work, Canadian care ethicist Andrea Doucet has underscored the insufficiency of looking chiefly at quantitative markers of time poverty and of methodologies that solely invoke an account of 'clock time' to analyse unpaid work and gender inequities (Nancy Folbre similarly argues for the need to 'look beyond the clock').[31] While Doucet does not call for completely setting aside 'standard' time-use studies or time diaries, she insists on looking at care responsibilities through the lens of a conception of time that is more relational, messier and non-linear (for one thing, many care-related tasks accomplished daily in homes overlap). She argues that care responsibilities and activities tend to be experienced as '*process time*' rather than clock time, and for this reason, invites researchers to never assume that 'an hour is an hour is an hour' – for methodological, political and feminist reasons all at once.[32]

The second element foregrounded by care ethics when it approaches unpaid care work is a focus on relationality. Care ethics has been relational through and through, from its first articulations in Gilligan and Ruddick to its most recent expressions in the likes of Hamington, Robinson or Puig della Bellacasa. In *Caring Democracy,* Tronto sums things up quite simply: 'the world consists not of individuals who are the starting point for intellectual reflection, but of humans who are always in relations with others. To make sense of human life requires a relational perspective.'[33] For care ethicists, we simply cannot approach ethico-political questions without working with the ontological premise that humans are, *always,* interdependent beings. One of the several things that flows from this in my view is that relationships, in and of themselves, constitute a *good* worth protecting, nurturing and ameliorating. If some care ethicists might recoil from the invocation of a thick language of 'the Good', most might agree with the thesis that a decent human life is one where individuals experience frequent moments of meaningful and non-violent relationality.[34] Most care ethicists seem to embrace Gilligan's rehabilitation of the young

Amy's position and reasoning – and more specifically, the importance Amy attached to figuring out what is a proper *response* to others and what can be done to ensure that relationships survive.

If a great deal of feminist researchers have insisted on the inequalities between men and women in the provision of care work, this has sometimes slipped into an outlook where caring work is chiefly perceived as a *burden* unequally shared. Care ethics, I argue, insists on the centrality of such caring activities *to the good life* – thus the core of the care theorists' charge is not simply that there is an unfair distribution of burdensome duties (though that is a crucial part of the charge), but that the duties themselves should be placed front and centre in our political projects. If, for instance, the unequal distribution of care work in a household were remedied by the hiring of a nanny, this might solve the problem of the unjust distribution of personal leisure time, but it would not satisfy the egalitarian feminist care ethicist, who wishes rather to see the care tasks both *valued* and *shared equally* (two things which go together).

24.1.3 Relationality's significance

For the specific subject matter that concerns us here, I now wish to highlight two crucial implications issuing from care ethics' emphasis on relationality. The first is that addressing inequalities in the distribution of unpaid care work needs to be done in a relational manner: we need to redistribute responsibilities or shift some labour from some to others (or institutions), which requires serious reflection on care work as a shared, relational good and responsibility. Second, care ethics' account of *relationships* calls on us to admit the significant amount of work, energy and time relationships require – time that cannot readily be accounted for in quantitative research (for one, there is no category labelled 'relationship maintenance'). Indeed, to state what might seem obvious, but which is understated in social sciences, relationships do not maintain themselves without significant effort, care and time. Relationship creation and relationship maintenance is *work* (one that is not always pleasant or easy). Several care ethics have foregrounded this simple thesis in their research. Tronto, for instance, writes in unequivocal terms: 'care is about relationships. And relationships require, *more than anything else*, two things: sufficient time and proximity. Among the most important considerations in rethinking society from a caring perspective, then, is creating time and space for care'[35] (emphasis added).

Anchored in care ethics, Stéphanie Mayer's research also highlights the amount of time and emotional labour relationships necessitate, and she proposes that gender justice requires much more awareness for the way *relationship-building work* tends to be poorly distributed within heterosexual couples (with many shirking this labour because of gendered socialization/norms).[36] In a similar manner, Ellie Anderson has recently brought our attention to gender inequities in 'hermeneutic labour' (i.e. the work done to understand people's emotions and reactions in order to address conflict or avoid relationship breakdown).[37] Anderson shows the extent to which women tend to perform more of this labour than men and what the consequences of this unequal sharing are. One thing to flag here is that Gilligan, Mayer and Anderson are certainly *not* saying that *all* relationships are worth nurturing/protection or are worthy of our time; some ought to be severed or refused. One could suggest that it is in fact a crucial task for feminist theory to be able to distinguish (and to insist on the distinction) between various types of relationships – as scholars like Held,[38] Gilligan and Snider,[39] and FitzGerald[40] have also noted.

24.2 CARE AND TEMPORALITY IN INSTITUTIONAL, PUBLIC SETTINGS

While considerable attention has been paid by care scholars to the intimate sphere and to the temporal inequalities tied to unpaid care work in the private sphere (including, as just noted, the work tied to relationships themselves), paid labour and care in the public sphere has also been an important object of research.[41] Over the years care ethicists have analysed work dynamics within a wide variety of settings – including front-line welfare service counters, janitorial care, morgues – with the two most frequently discussed occupational spheres being healthcare and education.

24.2.1 Healthcare and time

With regard to healthcare workers and time, one central issue discussed by care scholars has been the impact of the 'time squeeze' (associated with neoliberal austerity policies and with technological change) on the provision of care. For Tronto, the experience of time in which care is anchored jars with our productivist outlook on time – one that seeks efficiencies, good 'outputs' or 'good returns'.[42] Indeed, from a care perspective, it is often the case that spending time (or, rephrased in the language of management, 'wasting' time) is '*itself* a part of the activity ... *simply spending time with another*, listening to stories' (emphasis added).[43] Indeed, Tronto has often insisted that many (albeit not all) care tasks cannot be accelerated (or commodified) without significantly altering their nature.

One reason why care cannot be sped up is that one of its core elements – attentiveness – is radically at odds with speed. Readers mildly familiar with care ethics will recall that in Tronto's widely embraced account of care, attentiveness is one of the foremost ethical qualities required. Ruddick had also noted, in her early piece 'Maternal Thinking', the significance of attentiveness, describing it (in a manner largely upheld by care ethicists to this day) as a state of hyper-receptivity to others' needs, and an ability to listen.[44] For care ethicists Sandra Laugier[45] and Marie Garrau,[46] attention/attentiveness could even be regarded as the *core* of ethics itself.

Now, for care scholars, attentive and genuine listening to others (both in institutional and intimate settings) require sufficient time and a moderate pace.[47] Care ethicist Helen Kohlen has also maintained, in an unequivocally titled text 'Time Matters a Lot in Care Practices', that time pressures in clinical settings compromise the ability of healthcare professionals, family members and patients to have meaningful relationships or, as she puts it (here drawing on Hartmut Rosa), into 'resonance relations'.[48] Hamington has also underscored the fact that more time spent with a patient tends to decrease the likelihood of 'empathetic errors' – mistaken interpretations of patients' needs or wishes offered by well-meaning healthcare professionals.[49]

Care ethicists are concerned about increased time pressures in clinical/institutional settings not only because these pressures can compromise the 'warmth' or 'resonance' of care giving/receiving, but also because they increase the likelihood of abuse and epistemic injustice. Indeed, some care ethicists[50] have drawn on the research in bioethics and feminist epistemology that shows that time pressures have a significant impact on healthcare workers' ability to listen to patients in a non-prejudicial manner – and here we put aside any hope for 'warmth' in care delivery, we are just concerned with basic competent care and *absence of harm*.[51] These risks of prejudicial treatment are obviously not unique to medical settings: for most large institutions, one can find data indicating that, when pressed for time, front-line bureaucrats are more likely to have their judgement compromised by negative group-based prejudices.[52]

Several care ethicists have argued that there is 'mis-fit' or (dys)synchronization between the pace of decent care, our dominant cultural ethos and the pace of many contemporary workplaces. As Julie White puts it: 'care work is slow work and its marginalization is in part about being subject to deceleration in an economy and politics that are oriented to acceleration as the aesthetic of efficient production. Care is dyssynchronous with the dominant temporal regimes.'[53] None of this is to suggest that for care ethicists, time is a panacea or a sufficient condition for decent care; they all insist quite clearly on the significance of other structural and ethical conditions.

24.2.2 Time and higher education

Universities are another setting where care ethicists have studied the impact of temporal pressure and of our accelerated ethos. Based on a series of interviews, a recent study by Stéphanie Gaudet et al. concluded that female professors tend, on average, to do more hours of 'academic housework' (administrative/community service) and mentoring than male professors, and that this has negative impacts on their health and career advancement.[54] While the women interviewed admit cherishing the relational goods they spend so much time on, they feel that these goods are not acknowledged or appreciated by their employers. The professors interviewed report experiencing a deep inner conflict between their employers' quantified performance-based expectations, and the relational (and non-quantifiable) pull of caring practices.[55] This is not exclusively a North American reality: a Colombian study informed by care ethics offers similar observations about gender expectations, care work and time. A survey conducted by Isaura Castelao-Huerta with professors led her to conclude that 'care work is considered "domestic" work of the organization … women usually are disproportionately encouraged and pressured to do it, and [yet] this work is under-recognized and underappreciated'.[56] Gaudet et al.[57] insist that several universities are increasingly characterized by an ethos of *carelessness*, which feeds gender inequality.[58] Once again, quantified performance assessment is ill suited to account for relational and unquantifiable caring *processes* and for the 'care' labour that decent workplaces require. As Canadian scholars calling on universities to adopt an ethics of care put it: 'counting culture leads to intense, insidious forms of institutional shaming … and self-surveillance. It compels us to enumerate and self-audit, rather than listen and converse.'[59]

While there were obviously pressures on academics before the advent of neoliberal metrics or the university's corporatization, research suggests that time pressures have increased in the last decade.[60] One reason to worry, for some, is that these pressures have become insidious or discreet, more ordinary – partially because of the ubiquitousness of information and communication technology (ICT).[61] The growing presence of ICT in our lives twenty-four hours a day is clearly one that affects all teaching and administrative staff (not simply female professors); but since time experiences often tend to be more fragmented among women in academia (or at least those with children or sick parents)[62] and given that ICT tends to increase time fragmentation, the impact of technology may have had more serious effects on them.[63]

24.2.3 What care ethics foregrounds

Here, as above, what care ethics adds to the research on time and gender is an emphasis on particulars. As White notes in her research, much of the social acceleration literature 'homogenizes the impact of acceleration. But the organization of time is a critical way in which privilege is organized and this is particularly and differently true in the context of care work.'[64] To state the obvious: untenured, racialized or female professors tend to be affected in particular ways by acceleration, and – quite importantly – their distinctive 'timespaces' are all entangled, as a relational perspective on this problem suggests. What this means, in part, is that when some exhausted or more strategically minded workers refuse to take on unrewarded or underappreciated care work in institutions, someone *else* often (though not always) may pick up the slack. As such, we need to find ways of responding to 'neoliberal' and fast-paced work tempo in a manner that takes these different and interlocked 'temporalities' seriously, and that tries to foster open debates (uncomfortable ones, no doubt) about the urgency of considering care work as a shared responsibility.

Moreover, what several care ethics scholars have foregrounded in their research on time and institutions is the need to 'blur boundaries'. Indeed, several insist on the need to look at 'time pathologies' (and at measures that might mitigate them) in a holistic manner – one that troubles binaries between ethics and politics, and private and public (a core principle of care ethics, as Robinson has shown).[65] Among many others, Tronto has made the case that we need to attend to these time pathologies not only because these can damage our health or turn us into inadequate or harried parents/spouses, but also because they turn us into inadequate *citizens* (by depriving us of the time needed to participate in civic life).[66] In her work, Jorma Heier highlights some of the intricate connections between time, decent deliberation and epistemology: 'if "democratic caring with" is to disrupt epistemic misconceptions about the needs and situations and contributions of our fellow citizens and to arrive at more just distributions of caring responsibilities, *learning about* all people's lives through our democratic practices and incorporating that knowledge into our *democratic caring* is indispensable'.[67]

For care ethics, then, a democratic life worthy of the name must include decent dialogical exchange and sufficient knowledge about other groups for citizens to be able to make sense of their claims, desires and frustrations (a sobering and timely insight in our highly polarized political times). And many emphasize that sufficient time is needed to cultivate the skills needed for dialogue. Robinson writes: 'an ethics of care suggests that this kind of [dialogical] process requires patience, and takes time. ... dialogue should be understood as something that happens *over the very long term* ... Dialogue of this nature involves learning how to listen effectively. Care ethics reminds us that listening to others is ... developed *in and through relations*' (emphasis added).[68]

Before turning to our last section, I would like to emphasize another insight a care ethics lens offers on time and gender within institutional settings: namely, that what is needed is not only or chiefly 'more time', but rather, a *different temporal regime* altogether – one that could act as a counterweight to our productivist ethos. What this might partially entail is an interrogation of what we mean by 'productive', and what is considered unproductive or wasteful. As White puts it:

> hours spent keeping the lonely company or holding hands with the dying are not hours 'wasted'. Similarly, hours spent deliberating are not 'wasted' when we fail to accomplish agreement. *Democracy as a process of relating*, educating and caring for one another is slow. But it is this kind of pace and space that generates both citizen-subjects and citizen *relationships* critical to robust democracy[69] (emphasis added).

24.3 TOWARDS A FEMINIST CARING TEMPORALITY

What I have sought to accomplish above is to give readers a taste for some of care ethics' critical and distinctive insights about the intersection between time, gender and care. In lieu of a conclusion, I would like to shift gears in a more prescriptive mode and briefly consider five[70] 'remedies' informed by care ethics that might help mitigate, in my view, the effects of acceleration or of the uneven distribution of care responsibilities.

24.3.1 Shorten the work week; and consider the ethical and the political simultaneously

One recent scholarly proposal regarding how to deal with the high level of stress and depletion among women (especially single mothers) is that made by Jennifer Nedelsky and Tom Malleson in *Part-Time for All*. Building partially on care scholarship (most notably Ruddick and Tronto), Nedelsky and Malleson argue that the distress that accompanies the irreconcilable demands of full-time work and unpaid care labour might be diminished by moving towards a 'society of PTfA' (part-time work for all). The authors are unequivocal: 'we will *never* obtain gender equality until we rearrange the distribution of [unpaid] care, which itself requires the transformation of paid work'.[71] Their proposed framework for greater gender equality and a healthier temporality requires, *for all* individuals (regardless of gender): quality *part-time* jobs; time sovereignty; economic security (e.g. via public services or universal income schemes); and care-friendly policies (e.g. 'forced' paternity leave). There is no space to discuss the PTfA proposal at length, but allow me to underscore one of the book's crucial claims, since it resonates with care ethics: namely, the view that transformative measures must be proposed at both the workplace/policy level and cultural/normative level, and be adopted *simultaneously*. Like most care ethicists, Nedelsky and Malleson believe that we cannot sever these, and that in fact, it is precisely our failure to deal with both policies/institutions and norms/ethics *simultaneously* that explains our slow progress in gender equality. The view that working fewer hours is desirable for feminist reasons is also espoused by Tronto, who emphasizes at once the simplicity and radical nature of such measures: 'a "caring-with" alternative would require everyone to work less ... to really effect this change would require us to revolutionize how we think about our time, the place of work in our lives, and how we are compensated for our labour'.[72] Surely many more scholars could be cited here, so common is the view that working less might lead to greater wellbeing for women, ameliorate civic participation and diminish our environmental footprint.[73]

While I am very sympathetic to these proposals for shorter hours (especially in the North American work context), I nevertheless think that they ought not be accompanied by the (sometimes implicit, sometimes explicit) view that a decent life *must necessarily* accord greater importance to the tasks, pleasures or relationships located in homes than in workplaces. That is, these proposals sometimes give the impression that there is a moral hierarchy among human activities and that paid work is at the very bottom of it. In efforts to address the conflicting pressures of work and family life, we ought to avoid drawing *necessary* associations between work, pain and alienation. And here the research by Pascale Molinier might offer a helpful, quite nuanced perspective.[74] Molinier's research vividly shows the *joys* and sense of belonging paid work provide, while also acknowledging the inevitable moments of frustration, alienation or suffering (which vary significantly along class, racial and gender lines). Hers is an analysis that is instructive for its ability to thread with nuance the blurry line between care as painful, 'dirty work' and as joyful, meaningful 'labour of love'.

24.3.2 'Count What Others Don't'[75] and insist that all employers do so

Now, to stress the joys of work is not to ignore the many things that must be done to *improve workplaces*. One of those might be to campaign for a shift in the dominant ways of recognizing, approaching or 'counting' work – and more specifically, to find ways to give more explicit public recognition of the time spent on informal care, on relations and mentoring. We noted above the frustration expressed by depleted professors of having what they viewed as significant be invisibilized by 'performance assessments' or of facing an unequal distribution of service work. Partial solutions to this might obviously entail redistributing this care more equally, but might also entail changing *the way* employers view, 'count' and reward work.

One might object that the entire ethos of 'counting' is precisely the problem, and that 'counting' (or framing things in terms of distributive justice) is radically at odds with care ethics. While there are tensions here, I still wish to briefly entertain the question posed by the feminist geographers care collective: 'what if we counted *differently*?'[76] Is there a way to better acknowledge, reward and 'count' the more discreet work done in institutions that sustain workplace solidarity, health or relationships? This proposal of 'counting differently' partially resonates with the United Nations' outlook on ways to address gender inequalities in unpaid care – the UN having moved from a '3R' policy/research approach (recognize, reduce and redistribute unpaid care work) to a '5R' approach, which also includes represent and *reward*. Now, some readers might (rightly) recoil at the idea of professors doing more mentoring or more extensive listening out of a desire to get a pay bonus or their dean's praise. But could the resort to a 'carrot' – especially with individuals who do little care work in institutions – help uncaring employees discern the pleasures, importance or difficulty of 'caring'? Besides, to 'reward' the care work done in large bureaucratic institutions need not be thought of in monetary terms; we can think of alternative ways to acknowledge or recompense the time spent by some on this discreet labour.

24.3.3 Redistribute unpaid care within households: contest privileged irresponsibility

Redistributing care work within *private* settings is also part of the solution to gender inequalities in time use, as Malleson and Nedelsky argue (with the authors insisting, once again, on the inseparability between workplace and parental leave policies and this measure).[77] We ought to heed Tronto's invitation to take away the 'free passes' possessed by some – this may include some men in heterosexual couples, but also, more generally, privileged individuals (of all genders) who unreflexively purchase (and poorly remunerate) large amounts of housework services without much concern for the time poverty or precarity experienced by those hired. 'Taking away free passes' is a measure that may lead to some resentment or open conflict within couples, as Mayer has underscored in her work.[78] Mayer invites her feminist readers to reconsider their dismissal of the value of a (certain type) of conflict, discomfort or disagreement with the intimate sphere (here she draws on feminist agonists).[79] Mayer also insists that the goal is not to have a perfectly equal number of minutes spent on tasks daily – something Tronto also described as patently 'absurd'.[80] But for both Tronto and Mayer, what is crucial and long overdue is to orchestrate sustained and open discussions about the defective ways we currently allocate care responsibilities.

24.3.4 Refuse individualizing responses to depletion: insist on structural transformation

Another way to make workplaces more 'caring' is to object to the individualist/ individualizing remedies proposed by many (neoliberal) employers and governments. This is an outlook in which much of the responsibility (and blame when there is substandard performance or sickness tied to excessive temporal pressures) is placed on the *individual* employees themselves. Examples of 'individualizing' remedies to stress and temporal pressures I have in mind are things like yoga and meditation retreats; hiring the services of a nutritionist or sleep expert; health/mood self-tracking apps; online 'time-management and resilience' workshops.

We ought to be wary of individualized efforts to resist acceleration or time poverty not only because these individual resistance efforts might be less potent for social transformation (and besides, our temporalities are all entangled), but also because these individual 'solutions' to depletion are clearly not accessible to all. And here I mean not only in terms of financial resources, but also in terms of things like job security. A fully tenured professor might 'resist' her workplace's norms by no longer stressing about publishing outputs, and a nurse with job security might be able to ignore menacing (or guilt-inducing) pressures for her to take on overtime shifts. But not all workers have this luxury. As Mountz et al. rightly acknowledge, 'slowness might be possible for some and leave others behind'; indeed, they insist, 'slow, self-determined work [has to be] possible for everyone'.[81]

24.3.5 Embrace a careful chronopolitics that celebrates the unhurried pace of maintenance work

Last but not least, I wish to come back to the idea briefly evoked above that what we need is not simply more time, but a different outlook on temporality and 'what matters'. For this, we might want to look anew at Tronto and Fisher's definition of care, and to unpack further what the 'maintaining and repairing' of bodies/things/worlds might signify for our outlook on time, and for feminist resistance.[82]

We noted above that care for human beings has been a crucial object of study in much feminist scholarship. But what has been a less frequent object of discussion (and of celebration) has been the care given to *things* – whether those inside our homes (floors, toilets, dishes) or outside (roads, public spaces, buildings, infrastructure). (Notable exceptions to my observation here, in care ethics, include Molinier,[83] della Bellacasa[84] and Prattes.)[85] As Fanny Ambjörnsson notes, this relatively low interest on the part of feminist scholars is unsurprising: in the 1970s and 1980s, most feminists regarded domestic labour as a major source of women's exploitation.[86] But Ambjörnsson suggests that something else might explain the feminist scholarly neglect for household cleaning: namely, the fact that it is commonly associated with a monotonous, slow and repetitive tempo. Material housework is seen, in a way, as 'stuck in time'; and acts of cleaning do not seem to *produce* anything *new*. At best, cleaning is regarded as serving the (uninteresting) function of maintaining the status quo, or of *slowing down* decay and the passage of time.[87] Hence, to neglect the subjects of cleaning or maintenance work is not surprising given our dominant cultural and economic ethos, which is driven by a forward-looking ethos of progress, performance and productivity. But for Ambjörnsson,[88] it is precisely because it is at odds with this forward-looking, productivist and fast-paced ethos that maintenance/cleaning work and its sluggish tempo might offer the basis for a feminist chronopolitics of resistance.[89] With Ambjörnsson, I think that critics of acceleration might wish to turn to the slower temporality of maintenance work, as one way to orchestrate a reappraisal of the value of the care we give objects but also the care of bodies, public infrastructure and relationships.

The ethico-political and temporal significance of maintaining or of 'mending' things, bodies and relationships was there already in Tronto and Fischer's 1987 definition of care – and it was also in Gilligan's *In a Different Voice.* The central moral problem for Amy, and for Gilligan herself in my view, was for (non-violent) relationships to be nurtured and for fractures of (decent) relationships to 'be mended'. As Gilligan explains: '[Amy's] central tenet of nonviolent conflict resolution, and her belief in the restorative activity of care, lead her to see the actors in the dilemma arrayed not as opponents in a contest of rights but as members of a network of relationships on whose continuation they *all* depend.'[90] To take care of relationships – and to mend those that are fragile or appear broken – is time-consuming work, but it is work on which we *all* depend. And we suffer (collectively and individually) when such work is neglected.

To insist on a better acknowledgement of the *time* needed for nurturing relationships might strike some as a little simplistic, or as hardly an urgent matter for policy or politics. But perhaps the World Health Organization's (WHO's) recent report on the severe consequences of the growing 'epidemic of loneliness' (and its announcement of a two-year *Commission on Social Connection*) might succeed in lending more credence to that view. The WHO's urgent call to pay much more attention to how to strengthen connection *as a matter of public health* and justice might convince some sceptical readers. Feminist care ethics, I argue, gives us some of the tools needed to make a strong case for *why* relationships matter, and give us the tools to analyse the infrastructural, technological, political and *temporal* conditions decent relationships require.

NOTES

1. See: M. Moyser and A. Burlock, *Time Use: Total Work Burden, Unpaid Work, and Leisure*, Report for Women in Canada: A Gender-based Statistical, Report no. 89–503–X (Statistics Canada, 2018); UN Women, 'World Survey on the Role of Women in Development: Why Addressing Women's Income and Time Poverty Matters for Sustainable Development', Secretary General, 2019, https://www.unwomen.org/sites/default/files/Headquarters/Attachments/Sections/Library/Publications/2019/World-survey-on-the-role-of-women-in-development-2019.pdf.
2. According to a 2020 UN report, 'women continue to do the lion's share [of unpaid care work]. On an average day, women globally spend about three times as many hours on unpaid domestic and care work as men (4.2 hours compared to 1.7). In Northern Africa and Western Asia that gender gap is even higher, with women spending more than seven times as much as men on these activities.'
3. Jacques Charmes, *The Unpaid Care Work and the Labour Market: An Analysis of Time Use Data Based on the Latest World Compilation of Time-use Surveys* (Geneva: ILO, 2019), https://www.bollettinoadapt.it/wp-content/uploads/2020/01/wcms_732791.pdf.

4. See: Jessica S. Marter-Kenyon et al., 'Who Has the Time? A Qualitative Assessment of Gendered Intrahousehold Labor Allocation, Time Use and Time Poverty in Rural Senegal', *Frontiers in Sustainable Food Systems* 7 (2023); UN Women, 'The Climate-Care Nexus: Addressing the Linkages between Climate Change and Women's and Girls' Unpaid Care, Domestic and Communal Work', Working paper, 2023, https://www.unwomen.org/sites/default/files/2023-11/working-paper-the-climate-care-nexus-en.pdf.
5. See: Joan García Román and Pablo Gracia, 'Gender Differences in Time Use across Age Groups: A Study of Ten Industrialized Countries, 2005–2015', *PloS One* 17, no. 3 (2022): e0264411.
6. Robert E. Goodin, 'Temporal Justice', *Journal of Social Policy* 39, no. 1 (2010): 1–16.
7. Jennifer Ervin et al., 'Gender Differences in the Association Between Unpaid Labour and Mental Health in Employed Adults: A Systematic Review', *The Lancet Public Health* 7, no. 9 (2022): e775–e786; Heather Menzies and Janice Newson, 'Time, Stress and Intellectual Engagement in Academic Work: Exploring Gender Difference', *Gender, Work, and Organization* 15, no. 5 (2008): 504–22.
8. Hartmut Rosa, *Resonance: A Sociology of Our Relationship to the World* (Cambridge: Polity, 2019).
9. See: Michael Bittman and Judy Wajcman, 'The Rush Hour: The Character of Leisure Time and Gender Equity', *Social Forces* 79, no. 1 (2000): 165–89; Goodin, 'Temporal Justice'.
10. OECD, 'Caregiving in Crisis: Gender Inequality in Paid and Unpaid Work during COVID-19', report by Valerie Frey and Lyydia Alajääskö, 2022, https://www.oecd-ilibrary.org/view/?ref=1122_1122019-pxf57r6v6k&title=Caregiving-in-crisis-Gender-inequality-in-paid-and-unpaid-work-during-COVID-19.
11. Berenice Fisher and Joan C. Tronto, 'Toward a Feminist Theory of Care', in *Circles of Care: Work and Identity in Women's Lives*, ed. Emily Abel and Margaret Nelson (Albany: SUNY Press, 1991).
12. This chapter focuses on heterosexual couples largely because of the sparse data we have on time use in queer couples. It also deals exclusively with high-income countries – partially in light of care ethics' own focus until quite recently, and because doing justice to the variations between high/medium/low-income countries would require much more space than available here.
13. For example, see: Charmes, *The Unpaid Care Work and the Labour Market*; Moyser and Burlock, *Time Use.*
14. Robert E. Goodin, *Discretionary Time: A New Measure of Freedom* (Cambridge: Cambridge University Press, 2008).
15. Ervin et al., 'Gender Differences in the Association Between Unpaid Labour and Mental Health in Employed Adults'.
16. For examples, see: Bittman and Wajcman, 'The Rush Hour'; Charmes, *The Unpaid Care Work and the Labour Market*; Shira Offer and Barbara Schneider, 'Revisiting the Gender Gap in Time-use Patterns', *American Sociological Review* 76, no. 6 (2011): 809–33.
17. Jennifer Nedelsky and Tom Malleson, *Part-Time for All* (New York: Oxford University Press, 2023): 11–12.
18. Ervin et al., 'Gender Differences in the Association Between Unpaid Labour and Mental Health in Employed Adults'.
19. Offer and Schneider show that women are more likely to multitask and to suffer deleterious effects from it. (See: Offer and Schneider, 'Revisiting the Gender Gap in Time-use Patterns'.)
20. Fiona Robinson, 'Feminist Foreign Policy as Ethical Foreign Policy? A Care Ethics Perspective', *Journal of International Political Theory* 17, no. 1 (2021): 31.

21. Carol Gilligan, *In a Different Voice* (Cambridge, MA: Harvard University Press, 1993), 35.
22. See: Robert Hassan, *The Age of Distraction* (New York: Routledge, 2012); Rosa, *Resonance*.
23. Joan C. Tronto, 'Time's Place', *Feminist Theory* 4, no. 2 (2003): 123.
24. Julie White, 'Time for Caring Democracy: Resisting the Temporal Regimes of Neoliberalism', in *Care Ethics, Democratic Citizenship and the State*, ed. Petr Urban and Lizzie Ward (New York: Palgrave Macmillan, 2020).
25. Joan C. Tronto, *Who Cares? How to Reshape a Democratic Politics* (Ithaca, NY: Cornell University Press, 2015), 25–6.
26. Andrea Doucet, 'Care is Not a Tally Sheet: Rethinking the Field of Gender Divisions of Domestic Labour with Care-centric Conceptual Narratives', *Families, Relationships and Societies* 12, no. 1 (2023): 10–30.
27. Lauren Berlant, 'Slow Death (Sovereignty, Obesity, Lateral Agency)', *Critical Inquiry* 33, no. 4 (2007): 754–80.
28. Marybeth Mattingly and Suzanne M. Blanchi, 'Gender Differences in the Quantity and Quality of Free Time: The US Experience', *Social Forces* 81, no. 3 (2003): 999–1030.
29. Marc Bessin and Corinne Gaudart, 'Les temps sexués de l'activité: La temporalité au principe du genre?' *Temporalités* 9 (2009): 979.
30. Aurélie Damamme and Patricia Paperman, 'Temps du Care et Organisation Sociale du Travail en Famille', *Temporalités* 9 (2009): 1036.
31. Nancy Folbre, 'Beyond the Clock: Rethinking the Meaning of Unpaid Childcare in the US', *Time & Society* 32, no. 4 (2023): 367–84.
32. Andrea Doucet, ''Time is Not Time is Not Time': A Feminist Ecological Approach to Clock Time, Process Time, and Care Responsibilities', *Time & Society* 32, no. 4 (2023): 451.
33. Joan C. Tronto, *Caring Democracy: Markets, Equality, and Justice* (New York: New York University Press, 2013), 36.
34. I specify meaningful/non-violent because the question here is *not* whether one can live relationally or not (relationality is inevitable).
35. Tronto, *Caring Democracy*, 166.
36. Stéphanie Mayer, 'Irresponsabilités relationnelles, asymétries de pouvoir et injustices ordinaires du quotidien,' *Canadian Journal of Political Science* 54, no. 4 (2021): 791–808.
37. Ellie Anderson, 'Hermeneutic Labor: The Gendered Burden of Interpretation in Intimate Relationships between Women and Men,' *Hypatia* 38, no. 1 (2023): 1–21.
38. Virginia Held, 'Can the Ethics of Care Handle Violence?' *Ethics and Social Welfare* 4, no. 2 (2010): 115–29.
39. Carol Gilligan and Naomi Snider, *Why Does Patriarchy Persist?* (Cambridge: Polity Press, 2021).
40. Maggie FitzGerald, 'Violence and Care: Fanon and the Ethics of Care on Harm, Trauma, and Repair', *Philosophies* 7, no. 3 (2022): 64.
41. The private/public distinction around which my chapter is structured is for presentation purposes only. With care ethics, I will insist below on the desirability of blurring boundaries and on tackling the problem of temporal inequalities with private and public measures *simultaneously*.
42. 'Time caring is not about mastery and control but about maintenance and nurturance. [… thus] little in caring can be enhanced by being "forced" in a time/space compression: not learning, healing … dying.' (See: Tronto, 'Time's Place', 123.)
43. Tronto, *Caring Democracy*, 121.
44. Sara Ruddick, 'Maternal Thinking', *Feminist Studies* 6, no. 2 (1980): 342–67.

45. Sandra Laugier, 'L'éthique comme politique de l'ordinaire', *Multitudes* 37–38, no. 2 (2009): 80–8.
46. Marie Garrau, *Care et attention* (Paris: PUF, 2014).
47. See: Maurice Hamington, 'Care Ethics and Corporeal Inquiry in Patient Relations', *International Journal of Feminist Approaches to Bioethics* 5, no. 1 (2012): 52–69; Fiona Robinson, 'Stop Talking and Listen: Discourse Ethics and Feminist Care Ethics in International Political Theory', *Millennium* 39, no. 3 (2011): 845–60.
48. Helen Kohlen, '"Time Matters a Lot in Care Practices". Palliative Care Meets Care Ethics', in *The Ethics of Care: The State of the Art*, ed. Andries J. Baart, Frans Vosman and Jaco Hoffman (Leuven: Peeters Publishers, 2020), 234.
49. Hamington, 'Care Ethics and Corporeal Inquiry in Patient Relations', 64–5.
50. See: Sophie Bourgault, 'Attention, injustices épistémiques et humilité', *Politique et Sociétés* 42, no. 3 (2023): 135–61; Hamington, 'Care Ethics and Corporeal Inquiry in Patient Relations'.
51. See: Ian James Kidd and Havi Carel, 'Epistemic Injustice and Illness', *Journal of Applied Philosophy* 34, no. 2 (2017): 172–90; Irena Stepanikova, 'Racial-Ethnic Biases, Time Pressure and Medical Decisions', *Journal of Health and Social Behavior* 53, no. 3 (2012): 329–43.
52. See: Sophie Bourgault, 'Epistemic Injustice, Face-to-Face Encounters and Caring Institutions', *International Journal of Care and Caring* 4, no. 1 (2020): 91–107; Laura Hand, 'A Virtuous Hearer: An Exploration of Epistemic Injustice and an Ethic of Care in Public Encounters', *Administrative Theory & Praxis* 43, no. 1 (2021): 117–33.
53. White, 'Time for Caring Democracy', 162.
54. Stéphanie Gaudet et al., 'Women and Gender Equity in Academia through the Conceptual Lens of Care', *Journal of Gender Studies* 31, no. 1 (2022): 74–86.
55. Gaudet et al., 'Women and Gender Equity in Academia through the Conceptual Lens of Care', 81–2.
56. Isaura Castelao-Huerta, 'Beyond the Neoliberalized Academy: Caring and Careful Practices of Women Full Professors', *Gender and Education* 35, no. 3 (2023): 236.
57. Gaudet et al., 'Women and Gender Equity in Academia through the Conceptual Lens of Care'.
58. See also: Vivienne Bozalek, Michalinos Zembylas and Joan Tronto, *Posthuman and Political Care Ethics for Reconfiguring Higher Education Pedagogies* (New York: Routledge, 2020); Emilie Dionne, 'Slowing Down with Non-human Matter: The Contribution of Feminist New Materialism to Slow Scholarship', in *Posthuman and Political Care Ethics for Reconfiguring Higher Education Pedagogies*, ed. Vivienne Bozalek et al. (New York: Routledge, 2020), 91–106; Nedelsky and Malleson, *Part-Time for All.*
59. Alison Mountz et al., 'For Slow Scholarship: A Feminist Politics of Resistance through Collective Action in the Neoliberal University', *ACME* 14, no. 4 (2015): 1243.
60. Dionne, 'Slowing Down with Non-human Matter'.
61. Heather Menzies and Janice Newson, 'No Time to Think: Academics' Life in the Globally Wired University', *Time & Society* 16, no. 1 (2007): 83–98.
62. 'Nearly 20% women in Canada performed housework and/or caregiving *at the same time as leisure activities* in 2015, compared with 6.0% of men.' (See: Moyser and Burlock, *Time Use.*)
63. See: Menzies and Newson, 'No Time to Think', 92; Menzies and Newson, 'Time, Stress and Intellectual Engagement in Academic Work'.
64. White, 'Time for Caring Democracy', 164.

65. Fiona Robinson, 'Resisting Hierarchies through Relationality in the Ethics of Care', *International Journal of Care and Caring* 4, no. 1 (2020): 11–23.
66. Tronto, *Caring Democracy*.
67. Jorma Heier, 'Democratic Inclusion Through Caring Together with Others', in *Care Ethics, Democratic Citizenship and the State*, ed. Petr Urban and Lizzie Ward (New York: Springer, 2020), 64.
68. Robinson, 'Stop Talking and Listen', 856. See also: Sophie Bourgault, 'Democratic Practice and "Caring to Deliberate": A Gadamerian Account of Conversation and Listening', in *Care Ethics, Democratic Citizenship and the State*, ed. Petr Urban and Lizzie Ward (London: Palgrave Macmillan, 2020); Cliona Loughnane, Carol Kelleher and Claire Edwards, 'Care Full Deliberation? Care Work and Ireland's Citizens' Assembly on Gender Equality', *Critical Social Policy* 43, no. 4 (2023): 697–717.
69. White, 'Time for Caring Democracy', 175.
70. This is obviously not an exhaustive list; due to space constraints, I am only considering a few here.
71. Nedelsky and Malleson, *Part-Time for All*, 6.
72. Tronto, *Caring Democracy*, 176; and Tronto, *Who Cares?*, 31.
73. Juliet B. Schor, 'Sustainable Consumption and Worktime Reduction', *Journal of Industrial Ecology* 9, no. 1–2 (2005): 37–50.
74. Pascale Molinier, 'The Work of Care: Beyond Femininity and the Maternal', in *Care Ethics in yet a Different Voice*, ed. S. Bourgault and F. Vosman (Leuven: Peeters Publishers, 2020).
75. Mountz et al., 'For Slow Scholarship', 1249.
76. Ibid., 1243.
77. Nedelsky and Malleson, *Part-Time for All*.
78. Mayer, 'Irresponsabilités relationnelles, asymétries de pouvoir et injustices ordinaires du quotidien', 805.
79. See also: Stéphanie Mayer, 'Les irresponsabilités relationnelles en matière de care dans le couple et la famille: le conflit comme levier de transformation', in *La Justice, La Vulnérabilité et Le Politique Autrement* (Quebec: Presses de l'Université Laval, 2022), 285–308.
80. Tronto, *Who Cares?*, 141.
81. Mountz et al., 'For Slow Scholarship', 1249. See also: Dionne, 'Slowing Down with Non-human Matter'; and Tronto, *Who Cares?*
82. Fisher and Tronto, 'Toward a Feminist Theory of Care', 35–62.
83. Pascale Molinier, *Le travail du care* (Paris: La Dispute, 2013).
84. Maria Puig de la Bellacasa, *Matters of Care: Speculative Ethics in More than Human Worlds* (Minneapolis: University of Minnesota Press, 2017), 90–132.
85. Riikka Prattes, '"I Don't Clean up after Myself": Epistemic Ignorance, Responsibility and the Politics of the Outsourcing of Domestic Cleaning', *Feminist Theory* 21, no. 1 (2020): 25–45.
86. Fanny Ambjörnsson, 'Time to Clean', *Sociologisk Forskning* 56, no. 3/4 (2019): 275–88.
87. Ibid., 279–81.
88. Ambjörnsson, 'Time to Clean'.
89. Here I am particularly inspired by the work of Ambjörnsson and that of Sarah Sharma (*In the Meantime*) and of Lisa Baraitser (*Enduring Time*), which I am currently analysing in another research project. I am convinced that feminist care ethics might find in their writings some insights that largely resonate with their own.
90. Gilligan, *In a Different Voice*, 31.

BIBLIOGRAPHY

Ambjörnsson, Fanny. 'Time to Clean', *Sociologisk Forskning* 56, no. 3/4 (2019): 275–88.

Anderson, Ellie. 'Hermeneutic Labor: The Gendered Burden of Interpretation in Intimate Relationships between Women and Men', *Hypatia* (2023): 1–21.

Berlant, Lauren. 'Slow Death (Sovereignty, Obesity, Lateral Agency)', *Critical Inquiry* 33, no. 4 (2007): 754–80.

Bessin, Marc, and Corinne Gaudart. 'Les temps sexués de l'activité: La temporalité au principe du genre ?', *Temporalités* 9, no. 9 (2009): 979.

Bittman, Michael, and Judy Wajcman. 'The Rush Hour: The Character of Leisure Time and Gender Equity.' *Social Forces* 79, no. 1 (2000): 165–89.

Bourgault, Sophie. 'Democratic Practice and "Caring to Deliberate": A Gadamerian Account of Conversation and Listening', in *Care Ethics, Democratic Citizenship and the State*, edited by Petr Urban and Lizzie Ward, 31–51. London: Palgrave Macmillan, 2020.

Bourgault, Sophie. 'Epistemic Injustice, Face-to-Face Encounters and Caring Institutions', *International Journal of Care and Caring* 4, no. 1 (2020): 91–107.

Bourgault, Sophie. 'Attention, injustices épistémiques et humilité', *Politique et Sociétés* 42, no. 3 (2023): 135–61.

Bozalek, Vivienne, Michalinos Zembylas and Joan Tronto. *Posthuman and Political Care Ethics for Reconfiguring Higher Education Pedagogies*. New York: Routledge, 2020.

Castelao-Huerta, Isaura. 'Beyond the Neoliberalized Academy: Caring and Careful Practices of Women Full Professors', *Gender and Education* 35, no. 3 (2023): 234–49.

Charmes, Jacques. *The Unpaid Care Work and the Labour Market: An Analysis of Time Use Data Based on the Latest World Compilation of Time-use Surveys*. Geneva: ILO, 2019. https://www.bollettinoadapt.it/wp-content/uploads/2020/01/wcms_732791.pdf.

Damamme, Aurélie, and Patricia Paperman. 'Temps Du Care et Organisation Sociale Du Travail En Famille', *Temporalités* 9, no. 9 (2009): 1036.

Dionne, Emilie. 'Slowing Down with Non-Human Matter: The Contribution of Feminist New Materialism to Slow Scholarship', in *Posthuman and Political Care Ethics for Reconfiguring Higher Education Pedagogies*, edited by Vivienne Bozalek et al., 91–106. New York: Routledge, 2020.

Doucet, Andrea. 'Care is Not a Tally Sheet: Rethinking the Field of Gender Divisions of Domestic Labour with Care-centric Conceptual Narratives', *Families, Relationships and Societies* 12, no. 1 (2023): 10–30.

Doucet, Andrea. '"Time is Not Time is Not Time": A Feminist Ecological Approach to Clock Time, Process Time, and Care Responsibilities', *Time & Society* 32, no. 4 (2023): 434–60.

Ervin, Jennifer, Yamna Taouk, Ludmila F. Alfonzo, Belinda Hewitt and Tania King. 'Gender Differences in the Association Between Unpaid Labour and Mental Health in Employed Adults: A Systematic Review', *The Lancet Public Health* 7, no. 9 (2022): e775–e786.

Fisher, Berenice, and Joan C. Tronto. 'Toward a Feminist Theory of Care', in *Circles of Care: Work and Identity in Women's Lives*, edited by Emily Abel and Margaret Nelson, 35–62. Albany: SUNY Press, 1991.

FitzGerald, Maggie. 'Violence and Care: Fanon and the Ethics of Care on Harm, Trauma, and Repair', *Philosophies* 7, no. 3 (2022).

Folbre, Nancy. 'Beyond the Clock: Rethinking the Meaning of Unpaid Childcare in the US', *Time & Society* 32, no. 4 (2023): 367–84.

Garrau, Marie. *Care et attention*. Paris: PUF, 2014.

García Román, Joan, and Pablo Gracia. 'Gender Differences in Time Use across Age Groups: A Study of Ten Industrialized Countries, 2005–2015', *PloS One* 17, no. 3 (2022): e0264411.

Gaudet, Stéphanie, Isabelle Marchand, Merridee Bujaki and Ivy Lynn Bourgeault. 'Women and Gender Equity in Academia through the Conceptual Lens of Care', *Journal of Gender Studies* 31, no. 1 (2022): 74–86.

Gilligan, Carol. *In a Different Voice*. Cambridge, MA: Harvard University Press, 1993.

Gilligan, Carol, and Naomi Snider. *Why Does Patriarchy Persist?* Cambridge: Polity Press, 2021.

Goodin, Robert E. *Discretionary Time: A New Measure of Freedom*. Cambridge: Cambridge University Press, 2008.

Goodin, Robert E. 'Temporal Justice', *Journal of Social Policy* 39, no. 1 (2010): 1–16.

Hamington, Maurice. 'Care Ethics and Corporeal Inquiry in Patient Relations', *International Journal of Feminist Approaches to Bioethics* 5, no. 1 (2012): 52–69.

Hassan, Robert. *The Age of Distraction*. New York: Routledge, 2012.

Heier, Jorma. 'Democratic Inclusion Through Caring Together with Others', in *Care Ethics, Democratic Citizenship and the State*, edited by Petr Urban and Lizzie Ward, 53–76. New York: Springer, 2020.

Held, Virginia. 'Can the Ethics of Care Handle Violence?', *Ethics and Social Welfare* 4, no. 2 (2010): 115–29.

Kidd, Ian James, and Havi Carel. 'Epistemic Injustice and Illness', *Journal of Applied Philosophy* 34, no. 2 (2017): 172–90.

Hand, Laura. 'A Virtuous Hearer: An Exploration of Epistemic Injustice and an Ethic of Care in Public Encounters', *Administrative Theory & Praxis* 43, no. 1 (2021): 117–33.

Kohlen, Helen. '"Time Matters a Lot in Care Practices": Palliative Care Meets Care Ethics', in *The Ethics of Care: The State of the Art*, edited by Andries J. Baart, Frans Vosman and Jaco Hoffman, 233–60. Leuven: Peeters Publishers, 2020.

Laugier, Sandra. 'L'éthique comme politique de l'ordinaire', *Multitudes* 37–38, no. 2 (2009): 80–8.

Loughnane, Cliona, Carol Kelleher and Claire Edwards. 'Care Full Deliberation? Care Work and Ireland's Citizens' Assembly on Gender Equality', *Critical Social Policy* 43, no. 4 (2023): 697–717.

Marter-Kenyon, Jessica S., S. Lucille Blakeley, Jacqueline Lea Banks, Codou Ndiaye and Maimouna Diop. 'Who Has the Time? A Qualitative Assessment of Gendered Intrahousehold Labor Allocation, Time Use and Time Poverty in Rural Senegal', *Frontiers in Sustainable Food Systems* 7 (2023).

Mattingly, Marybeth, and Suzanne M. Blanchi. 'Gender Differences in the Quantity and Quality of Free Time: The US Experience', *Social Forces* 81, no. 3 (2003): 999–1030.

Mayer, Stéphanie. 'Irresponsabilités relationnelles, asymétries de pouvoir et injustices ordinaires du quotidien', *Canadian Journal of Political Science* 54, no. 4 (2021): 791–808.

Mayer, Stéphanie. 'Les irresponsabilités relationnelles en matière de care dans le couple et la famille: le conflit comme levier de transformation', in *La Justice, La Vulnérabilité et Le Politique Autrement*, 285–308. Quebec: Presses de l'Université Laval, 2022.

Menzies, Heather, and Janice Newson. 'No Time to Think: Academics' Life in the Globally Wired University', *Time & Society* 16, no. 1 (2007): 83–98.

Menzies, Heather, and Janice Newson. 'Time, Stress and Intellectual Engagement in Academic Work: Exploring Gender Difference', *Gender, Work, and Organization* 15, no. 5 (2008): 504–22.

Molinier, Pascale. *Le travail du care*. Paris: La Dispute, 2013.

Molinier, Pascale. 'The Work of Care: Beyond Femininity and the Maternal', in *Care Ethics in yet a Different Voice*, edited by S. Bourgault and F. Vosman. Leuven: Peeters Publishers, 2020.

Mountz, Alison, Anne Bonds, Becky Mansfield, Jenna Loyd, Jennifer Hyndman, Margaret Walton-Roberts, Ranu Basu et al. 'For Slow Scholarship: A Feminist Politics of Resistance through Collective Action in the Neoliberal University', *ACME* 14, no. 4 (2015): 1235–59.

Moyser, M., and A. Burlock. *Time Use: Total Work Burden, Unpaid Work, and Leisure*. Report for Women in Canada: A Gender-based Statistical. Report no. 89–503–X. Statistics Canada, 2018.

Nedelsky, Jennifer, and Tom Malleson. *Part-Time for All*. New York: Oxford University Press, 2023.

OECD. 'Caregiving in Crisis: Gender Inequality in Paid and Unpaid Work during COVID-19', Report by Valerie Frey and Lyydia Alajääskö, 2021. https://read.oecdilibrary.org/view/?ref=1122_1122019-pxf57r6v6k&title=Caregiving-in-crisis-Gender-inequalityin-paid-and-unpaid-work-during-COVID-19.

Offer, S., and B. Schneider. 'Revisiting the Gender Gap in Time-use Patterns', *American Sociological Review* 76, no. 6 (2011): 809–33.

Prattes, Riikka. '"I Don't Clean up after Myself": Epistemic Ignorance, Responsibility and the Politics of the Outsourcing of Domestic Cleaning', *Feminist Theory* 21, no. 1 (2020): 25–45.

Puig de la Bellacasa, Maria. *Matters of Care: Speculative Ethics in More than Human Worlds*. Minneapolis: University of Minnesota Press, 2017.

Robinson, Fiona. 'Stop Talking and Listen: Discourse Ethics and Feminist Care Ethics in International Political Theory', *Millennium* 39, no. 3 (2011): 845–60.

Robinson, Fiona. 'Resisting Hierarchies through Relationality in the Ethics of Care', *International Journal of Care and Caring* 4, no. 1 (2020): 11–23.

Robinson, Fiona. 'Feminist Foreign Policy as Ethical Foreign Policy? A Care Ethics Perspective', *Journal of International Political Theory* 17, no. 1 (2021): 20–37.

Rosa, Hartmut. *Resonance: A Sociology of Our Relationship to the World*. Cambridge: Polity, 2019.

Ruddick, Sara. 'Maternal Thinking', *Feminist Studies* 6, no. 2 (1980): 342–67.

Schor, Juliet B. 'Sustainable Consumption and Worktime Reduction', *Journal of Industrial Ecology* 9, no. 1–2 (2005): 37–50.

Stepanikova, Irena. 'Racial-Ethnic Biases, Time Pressure and Medical Decisions', *Journal of Health and Social Behavior* 53, no. 3 (2012): 329–43.

Tronto, Joan C. 'Time's Place', *Feminist Theory* 4, no. 2 (2003): 119–38.

Tronto, Joan C. *Caring Democracy: Markets, Equality, and Justice*. New York: New York University Press, 2013.

Tronto, Joan C. *Who Cares? How to Reshape a Democratic Politics*. Ithaca, NY: Cornell University Press, 2015.

UN Women. 'World Survey on the Role of Women in Development: Why Addressing Women's Income and Time Poverty Matters for Sustainable Development', Secretary General, 2019. https://www.unwomen.org/sites/default/files/Headquarters/Attachments/Sections/Library/Publications/2019/World-survey-on-the-role-of-women-in-development-2019.pdf.

UN Women. 'The Climate-Care Nexus: Addressing the Linkages between Climate Change and Women's and Girls' Unpaid Care, Domestic and Communal Work'. Working paper, 2023. https://www.unwomen.org/sites/default/files/2023-11/working-paper-the-climate-care-nexus-en.pdf.

White, Julie. 'Time for Caring Democracy: Resisting the Temporal Regimes of Neoliberalism', in *Care Ethics, Democratic Citizenship and the State*, edited by Petr Urban and Lizzie Ward, 161–77. New York: Palgrave Macmillan, 2020.

INDEX

Addams, Jane 1
ageing
and care needs 17, 146, 321, 410–11
and Covid-19 267–70
and the concept of a completed life 83–6
and frailty 43
and public policy 252–60, 377–90
and technology 231
as a focus of care ethics research 18
altruism 12–13, 18–26, 31–3, 67, 357
Arendt, Hannah 82
Aristotle 25, 340
assisted Dying 83–4
autism 299–310
autonomy
and assisted dying 83
and care practice 276
and dependency 26–7, 30–3, 48–50, 151, 169, 207, 271
and disability 46–7
and human nature 98, 102
and interdependence 308–10
and liberalism 114, 119–22, 124, 143, 149, 207
as a focus of the ethics of justice 10, 144, 146, 204, 206–7, 301
as a 'masculine' value 44, 196
relational autonomy 52, 208, 301

benevolence 11, 22, 206–7
Buber, Martin 9, 18

Chinese philosophy 1–2, 4, 11–16, 239
Christianity 1, 18–20, 398
climate change 158–70, 187, 342–3, 409
colonialism 18, 21, 23, 183, 255
Confucianism 2, 11
Covid-19 43, 187, 267–79, 342–3, 409

dementia 29, 31, 165, 253
democracy
and caregiving 66, 185, 205, 207–8, 260, 268–9, 336, 416
and empathy 143
and liberalism 67
and public administration 339
and public space 136
and structural injustice 168
in South Korea 251, 260
dependency
and altruism 20
and asymmetric relationships 23, 26–33, 42
and autonomy 207
and disability 45–6
and domination 47
and equality 149–53
and feminism 44–5, 142
and intimacy 224–5
and illness 270
and liberalism 4, 67, 100, 114, 122–3, 125, 142, 148–9, 318
and power 23
and responsibility– 164–70, 207
and stigma –309
and the ageing society 254–5
and the welfare state 385, 387
and utilitarianism 101
as a fact of human nature 1–2, 43, 67, 97–8, 102, 251, 259, 286–7, 301, 318
as foundational to care ethics 4, 41–53, 97–102, 146–9, 157–8
fear of 84
disability
activism 68, 285
and asymmetric relationships 17, 19–20, 23, 26, 31
and dependency 41–9, 318
and equality 152
and intimacy 215–27
and liberalism 148–9
and mothering 299–310
and race 123–4
and the welfare state 377–90
domination
and activism 284, 287
and colonialism 22, 183, 185
and critical theory 134–9
and dependency 2, 26, 47, 152

and equality 151–2
and feminism 71–3
and norms 63, 65
and public administration 336–7, 340
and structural injustice 158–9
In care relationships 26, 47, 147, 152, 207

education
and caregiving 89
and criminal justice 320, 323
and morality 397–8
and public administration 338–9, 344–5
and time 415
as a care need 29, 208
emotional labour 258, 337–8, 413
empathy
and care 9–12, 16, 104, 143–5, 267–8
and emotional maturity 106–7
and moral deliberation 162–70
and moral development 395–402
and social media 267, 275
epistemology
and morality 72, 89–90, 181–6, 397
and rationality 15
and the care relationship 23–4, 33–4, 206, 358–62
Definition of 13
epistemic injustice 362–8, 414, 416
equality
and colonialism 183
and dependency 42–52
and the system of caregiving 114–22, 357–8, 377–89
gender equality 99, 135–58, 357, 377–89, 409–11, 415, 417
income inequality 187
interactions with care ethics 2, 4, 19, 141–55, 275
moral equality 70
power inequality 251
racial equality 72, 357
exploitation
and colonialism 183
and critical theory 135–8
and dependency 23, 30, 32–4
and gender 99, 419
and human survival 105
and the welfare state 379–89
as a core concern of care ethics 20–1, 44, 46
in research 220
in the system of caregiving 113–114, 123–6, 149, 318

feminism
and dependency 43–9
and liberalism 113–19, 142
and maternity 355–62
and morality 398–9
and normativity 61–73
and theology 401
and time 409–20
and social scientific research 301–5
care ethics as a branch of feminist philosophy 1–4, 18–26, 32, 99, 144, 180–9, 195–6, 204–7
feminist crisis management 343–4
the feminist philosophy of Nancy Fraser 133–5
film and television 199–204, 365, 395–403
Foucalt, Michel 133
freedom
activism 284–5
and dependency 26–7
and recognition 138
interactions with care ethics 2, 22, 24, 305
of speech 144, 339
of the will 13
to care 113–26

gender
and altruism 18–21
and capitalism 135–6
and moral psychology 1–2, 204, 356–7
and public space 136–7
and norms 62–3
and socialization 24–5
and the distribution of care 47–9, 98–9, 113–19, 123–4, 142, 144, 149, 258–9
and the welfare state 377–90
and time 409–20
and values 44, 180
essentialism 3, 206, 360
gendered conceptions of care 32–4, 47–9, 272, 335
gender identity and expression 290, 398
Gilligan, Carol 1–2, 9–10, 18, 20, 23–4, 62, 89, 141, 162, 184–5, 195–7, 204–8, 336, 350, 355–9, 399, 411–13, 420
globalization 115, 124, 138

healthcare 88, 216–19, 231–45, 414
Heidegger, Martin 18–19, 87–8
Held, Virginia 2, 24, 33, 36–7, 42, 68, 98–102, 126, 144–5, 148–52, 165, 173, 184, 217, 282–92, 301, 361, 399, 413

housing 254, 292, 300, 321, 402
Hume, David 1, 9, 67, 89, 114, 181

interdependence
and covid-19 267, 271
and equality 150
and structural injustice 158–63
as a fact of human nature 1, 67, 99, 251, 259, 286, 291, 308, 310, 317–19, 400, 412
as an alternative to dependency 41, 48–9, 52–3
In caring relationships 300–1
international relations 179–89
intimacy 106, 119–20, 215–27, 282, 410–14

justice
and care 98–102, 141–53, 284–7, 305, 310, 339–41, 399–400
and gender 44, 134–9
and liberalism 51, 114–15, 118–25
criminal justice 299–302, 319–27
ethics of 2, 9–10, 62, 196, 198, 204–8
global justice 179–90
reproductive justice 355–67
structural injustice 157–71
temporal justice 409–20

Kant, Immanuel 10, 67, 70, 89, 98–9, 104, 142, 179, 181–3, 205, 233
Kittay, Eva F. 2, 24, 30, 37, 42–3, 45, 47–9, 52, 65–6, 74–5, 98, 100–2, 104, 133, 141, 148–53, 163–5, 170, 320
Kohlberg, Lawrence 1, 89, 356–7

Levinas, Emmanuel 18, 85, 89, 361
liberalism
and dependency 43, 51, 53, 318
and equality 141–53
in international relations 182
liberal dependency care 113–26
of John Rawls 66–67, 69, 207
Locke, John 9, 99–100
Lorde, Audre 20, 283–4, 286, 292

Marx, Karl 114, 134–5
metaethics 18–19, 62–73, 201
migration 117, 119, 125, 134, 146, 170, 269, 292, 326, 365, 385, 388
moral development 1, 89, 97, 145, 356, 398

Noddings, Nel 1, 10, 18, 24, 26, 30–1, 42–3, 46–8, 63, 68, 89, 184–5, 196, 310, 346, 357, 359, 399
nursing 3, 18–22, 27–8, 43, 88, 185, 216, 231, 237–8, 241–4, 253, 258, 299, 318–19, 419

ontology
and dependency 44–9, 53
and interdependence 412
and phenomenology 87
developmentalist 183
of care 398–400
of the particular 198–9
relational 18–19, 23–7, 32–4, 89, 115, 139, 184, 305, 366
social 118–19
oppression
and activism 282–8
and dependency 45–6, 49
of trans people 403
of women 2–3, 19–21, 113–14, 184–7, 358, 379
race-based 114, 187

parenting and childcare 17, 37, 45, 106–7, 252–60, 318, 358–60, 379–82
patriarchy 23, 116–17, 123, 134, 180–3, 283, 355–61
phenomenology 18–23, 43, 69, 81–90, 162, 216–18, 225, 232–6, 241
poetry 88, 233–4, 243–4, 291, 397
power
and equality 105–52, 251, 355–7, 362–364
and human survival 105
and international relations 180–9
and norms 62–71
and politics 133
and public administration 335–7
and research 217–18, 222, 226
and social media 273
and structural injustice 159–67
and the erotic 284
and the welfare state 269, 386–8
in caring relationships 18–30, 42–5, 307, 318–19, 396
narrative power 301
precariousness 41–42, 48, 51–3, 227, 257, 260, 286
pregnancy and childbirth 256, 355–68
psychology
and dependency 48, 164

and emotional development 103, 106–7
descriptive psychology 82, 87
evolutionary psychology 104
moral psychology 2, 62–3, 70, 89
psychological functioning and philosophy 11–15, 68
psychological harm 21

queer theory and the LGBTQ+ community 62, 64–5, 281–92, 362, 405, 421

race 18–32, 62–72, 113–29, 134–9, 146–9, 188, 207, 283, 356–64, 409–18
rationality
and care ethics 10, 196, 202, 359, 366
and communication 368
and equality 151
and justice 151
and morality 13, 104, 113, 181, 345
and the social contract 100
and yin-yang 15–16
epistemic 15
practical 12–13, 15
Rawls, John 2, 10, 66–7, 69, 99–102, 114, 122, 133, 145, 148–9, 151, 153, 171, 182, 205–7
respect
and anthropology 222
and care ethics 143, 163, 165, 288, 318–26, 336, 359, 401
and equality 138, 379, 382–3, 388–9
and obstetrics 364–6
and utilitarianism 101
for autonomy 121, 124, 151
for difference 106
for others 144
Ruddick, Sara 18, 24, 42–3, 46, 48, 89, 271, 293, 355–62, 366–69, 412, 414, 417

self-respect 29, 101, 149, 323
Smith, Adam 1
social contract 52, 99–100, 142, 148, 207, 251
social status 21, 115–23, 138, 151–2, 251–9, 363–5, 380

Tronto, Joan 1, 3, 24–5, 42, 47–8, 62, 65–6, 98, 102, 133, 147, 165, 168, 170, 172, 180, 185, 196, 204–7, 231, 244, 268, 270–4, 318–21, 335–6, 350, 355, 357, 360–1, 401, 410–14, 416–20

violence 64–5, 105, 117–23, 183–8, 281–2, 285, 300–10, 356–66
virtue
and altruism 20
and benevolence 11
and care ethics 17, 81, 98, 145, 147, 185, 207
and oppression 2
and politics 133, 145
and rationality 11
and yin-yang 13, 15
interpersonal reciprocity as a virtue 124, 126
kindness as a virtue 201
love as a virtue 360
midwifery virtues 367
mothering virtues 360, 367–8
sensitiveness as a virtue 202
virtue ethics 10, 25, 98, 396–9
vulnerability
and care practices 301–310, 339–47
and covid-19 267–75
and inequality 115–18
and pleasure activism 285–90
and the welfare state 386–7
as a fact of human nature 26–34, 67–71, 83–5, 139, 142–52, 318–25, 400–3
as a source of moral obligation 162–9, 199–208
as an alternative to dependency 41–53
in research 216–26

wellbeing
and covid-19 269
and global justice 180
and interests 101
and race 20, 123
and research 220, 222
and status inequality 116, 123, 362
and structural injustice 167–8
and time 401–17
and the welfare state 387–8
and the workplace 338
in asymmetric relationships 28, 32, 195
of carers 150
of strangers 44
mental wellbeing 324
welfare state 135, 138, 335, 377–90
Wittgenstein, Ludwig 195–200, 206

yin-yang 11–16

www.ingramcontent.com/pod-product-compliance
Ingram Content Group UK Ltd.
Pitfield, Milton Keynes, MK11 3LW, UK
UKHW050418051026
15470UKWH00022B/1599

9 781350 428379